Medical Management of Liver Disease

Clinical Guides to Medical Management

Consulting Editor

BURTON E. SOBEL, M.D.
Medical Center Hospital of Vermont
University of Vermont
Burlington, Vermont

Medical Management of Heart Disease, edited by Burton E. Sobel

Medical Management of Rheumatic Musculoskeletal and Connective Tissue Diseases, edited by Jan Dequeker, Gabriel Panayi, Theodore Pincus and Rodney Grahame

Medical Management of Atherosclerosis, edited by John LaRosa

Medical Management of Liver Disease, edited by Edward L. Krawitt

Medical Management of Pulmonary Diseases, edited by Gerald S. Davis, Theodore W. Marcy, and Elizabeth A. Seward

ADDITIONAL TITLES IN PREPARATION

Medical Management of Kidney and Electrolyte Disorders, edited by F. John Gennari

Medical Management of Liver Disease

edited by

Edward L. Krawitt
University of Vermont College of Medicine
Burlington, Vermont
Dartmouth College
Hanover, New Hampshire

MARCEL DEKKER, INC. NEW YORK • BASEL

ISBN: 0-8247-1968-9

This book is printed on acid-free paper.

Headquarters
Marcel Dekker, Inc.
270 Madison Avenue, New York, NY 10016
tel: 212-696-9000; fax: 212-685-4540

Eastern Hemisphere Distribution
Marcel Dekker AG
Hutgasse 4, Postfach 812, CH-4001 Basel, Switzerland
tel: 41-61-261-8482; fax: 41-61-261-8896

World Wide Web
http://www.dekker.com

The publisher offers discounts on this book when ordered in bulk quantities. For more information, write to Special Sales/Professional Marketing at the headquarters address above.

Current printing (last digit):
10 9 8 7 6 5 4 3 2 1

PRINTED IN THE UNITED STATES OF AMERICA

This book is dedicated to
Laura Prange Krawitt

Preface

Interest has been rekindled in the treatment of liver diseases and their complications, fueled in part by the enormous recent progress in the area of liver transplantation. During the same time period, changes in health-care delivery systems have mandated that, in some cases, patients with a variety of serious liver diseases will be treated by primary care and intensive care physicians rather than by gastroenterologists and hepatologists.

We concluded, therefore, that a practical, moderate-sized book devoted to the treatment of liver disease would be an important addition to the libraries of practicing primary care physicians, intensive care physicians, gastroenterologists, and hepatologists, and would also be helpful to students and physicians-in-training.

Part I, Approach to the Patient with Hepatobiliary Disease, will be most helpful to physicians less experienced in caring for patients with liver disease, particularly considering the array of diagnostic studies available at this time. Parts II through VIII are designed to help physicians develop a treatment plan for specific liver diseases. It is divided into chapters that cover viral hepatitis, autoimmune liver diseases, alcoholic liver disease, gallstones, liver infections, and hepatobiliary neoplasms, as well as a variety of other less common liver diseases. Part IX outlines the management of both common and rare complications of liver disease and Part X details important measures in the management of patients before and after liver transplantation.

We hope that this book will serve as a practical, concise, and up-to-date reference for physicians managing patients with a variety of liver diseases of varying complexity.

Edward L. Krawitt

Contents

Part X. Management of Patients Before and After Liver Transplantation

Contributors

Victoria Alagiozian-Angelova, M.D. University of California, Irvine Medical Center, Orange, California

W. Kemper Alston, M.D. University of Vermont College of Medicine, Burlington, Vermont

Paul Angulo, M.D. Mayo Clinic and Mayo Foundation, Rochester, Minnesota

Andrew Bedford, M.D. Harvard Medical School and Beth Israel Hospital, Boston, Massachusetts

Martin Black, M.D. Temple University Hospital, Philadelphia, Pennsylvania

Victorino Spinelli Barreto University Hospital of Pernambuco, Recife, Brazil

Herbert L. Bonkovsky, M.D., F.A.C.G., F.A.C.P. University of Massachusetts Medical Center, Worcester, Massachusetts

Richard F. Branda, M.D. University of Vermont College of Medicine, Burlington, Vermont

Azade Çakir-Yedidag University of Iowa, Iowa City, Iowa

Robert L. Carithers, Jr., M.D. University of Washington, Seattle, Washington

Kelly L. Carson, M.D. Duke University Medical Center, Durham, North Carolina

Michael Charlton, M.D. Mayo Clinic and Foundation, Rochester, Minnesota

Sanjiv Chopra, M.D. Harvard Medical School and Beth Israel Hospital, Boston, Massachusetts

Philippe Chossegros, M.D. Hôtel-Dieu Hospital and INSERM U271, Lyon, France

Ram Chuttani, M.D. Harvard Medical School and Beth Israel Hospital, Boston, Massachusetts

Luiz Guilherme Costa Lyra University Hospital of Bahia, Salvador, Brazil

Scott J. Cotler, M.D. RUSH-Presbyterian-St. Luke's Medical Center, Chicago, Illinois

Helma P. Cotrim, M.D. Universidade Federal da Bahia, Salvador, Brazil

Ana Lúcia Coutinho Domingos University Hospital of Pernambuco, Recife, Brazil

Douglas T. Dieterich New York University School of Medicine, New York, New York

Gregory T. Everson, M.D. University of Colorado School of Medicine, Denver, Colorado

Lawrence S. Friedman, M.D. Harvard Medical School and Massachusetts General Hospital, Boston, Massachusetts

Hans Fromm, M.D. The George Washington University Medical Center, Washington, D.C.

Gabriel Garcia, M.D. Stanford University School of Medicine, Palo Alto, California

Fredric D. Gordon, M.D. Beth Israel Deaconess Medical Center and Harvard Medical School, Boston, Massachusetts

Christopher J. Grace, M.D. University of Vermont College of Medicine, Burlington, Vermont

Stephen Crane Hauser, M.D. Harvard Medical School and Brigham and Women's Hospital, Boston, Massachusetts

Robert D.J. Henihan, M.D. Harvard Medical School and Massachusetts General Hospital, Boston, Massachusetts

John C. Hoefs, M.D. University of California, Irvine Medical Center, Orange, California

Christine M. Hunt, M.D. Duke University Medical Center, Durham, North Carolina

Ira M. Jacobson, M.D. New York-Presbyterian Hospital (Cornell Campus), New York, New York

Lennox Jeffers University of Miami and Veterans Affairs Medical Center, Miami, Florida

Roger L. Jenkins, M.D., F.A.C.S. Beth Israel Deaconess Medical Center and Harvard Medical School, Boston, Massachusetts

Donald M. Jensen, M.D. RUSH-Presbyterian-St. Luke's Medical Center, Chicago, Illinois

Frederick C. Johlin, Jr., M.D. University of Iowa, Iowa City, Iowa

Marshall M. Kaplan, M.D. New England Medical Center, Boston, Massachusetts

Emmet B. Keeffe, M.D. Stanford University Medical Center, Stanford, California

Jason Kelley, M.D. University of Vermont College of Medicine, Burlington, Vermont

Afshin Khatibi, M.D. University of California, Irvine Medical Center, Orange, California

Jonathan M. Koff, M.D. Boston University School of Medicine, Boston, Massachusetts

Raymond S. Koff, M.D. Professor, University of Massachusetts Medical School, Worcester, Massachusetts

Kris V. Kowdley, M.D., F.A.C.P. University of Washington, Seattle, Washington

Edward L. Krawitt, M.D. University of Vermont College of Medicine, Burlington, Vermont

Annette Kyprianou, M.D. MetroHealth Medical Center, Cleveland, Ohio

Douglas R. LaBrecque University of Iowa, Iowa City, Iowa

John R. Lake, M.D. University of Minnesota Medical School, Minneapolis, Minnesota

Anne M. Larson, M.D. University of Washington, Seattle, Washington

Jose A. Lavergne, M.D. University of Miami School of Medicine, Miami, Florida

Samuel S. Lee, M.D., F.R.C.P.C. University of Calgary, Calgary, Alberta, Canada

William M. Lee, M.D. University of Texas Southwestern Medical Center, Dallas, Texas

Young-Mee Lee, M.D. New England Medical Center, Boston, Massachusetts

W. David Lewis, M.D. Beth Isreal Deaconess Medical Center and Harvard Medical School, Boston, Massachusetts

Keith D. Lindor, M.D. Mayo Clinic and Mayo Foundation, Rochester, Minnesota

Zenghua Ma, M.D., Ph.D. University of Calgary, Calgary, Alberta, Canada

Enrique J. Martinez LifeLink Transplant Institute, Tampa General Hospital, Tampa, Florida

Ian G. McFarlane, Ph.D., D.Sc.(Med.) King's College Hospital, London, England

Savant Mehta Harvard Medical School and Beth Israel Hospital, Boston, Massachusetts

Philippe Merle, M.D. Hôtel-Dieu Hospital and INSERM U271, Lyon, France

Dilip K. Moonka, M.D. Henry Ford Health Systems, Detroit, Michigan

Eneya Mulagha, M.D The George Washington University Medical Center, Washington, D.C.

Kevin D. Mullen, M.B., F.R.C.P MetroHealth Medical Center, Cleveland, Ohio

Christopher B. O'Brien University of Miami, Miami, Florida

Gerd R. Pape, M.D. University of Munich, Munich, Germany

Raymundo Paraná, M.D., Ph.D. University Hospital of Bahia, Salvador, Brazil

Edward L. Parrish Hospital for Special Surgery–Cornell University Medical College, New York, New York

David H. Perlmutter, M.D. Washington University School of Medicine and St. Louis Children's Hospital, St. Louis, Missouri

Michael A. Poles, M.D. University of California School of Medicine, Los Angeles, California

Gottumukkala Raju Harvard Medical School and Beth Israel Hospital, Boston, Massachusetts

Mary Beth Ramundo, M.D. University of Vermont College of Medicine, Burlington, Vermont

K. Rajender Reddy, M.D. University of Miami School of Medicine, Miami, Florida

Vinod K. Rustgi, M.D. Georgetown University School of Medicine, Washington, D.C.

Arun J. Sanyal, M.D. Medical College of Virginia–Virginia Commonwealth University, Richmond, Virginia

Steedman A. Sarbah, M.D. MetroHealth Medical Center, Cleveland, Ohio

Gerd H. Sauter, M.D. University of Munich, Munich, Germany

Thomas D. Schiano, M.D. University of Chicago Hospitals, Chicago, Illinois

Michael L. Schilsky, M.D. Marion Bessin Liver Research Center, Albert Einstein College of Medicine, Bronx, New York

Frank V. Schiødt University of Copenhagen, Copenhagen, Denmark

Mitchell L. Shiffman, M.D. Medical College of Virginia–Virginia Commonwealth University, Richmond, Virginia

Roshan Shrestha, M.D. University of Colorado School of Medicine, Denver, Colorado

Irmin Sternlieb National Center for the Study of Wilson's Disease, St Luke's/Roosevelt Hospital Center, New York, New York

Norman L. Sussman, M.D. Amphioxus Cell Technologies, Inc., Houston, Texas

Christian Trepo, M.D. Claude Bernard University, INSERM U271, Lyon, France

Bruce Y. Tung, M.D. University of Washington, Seattle, Washington

Russell H. Wiesner, M.D. Mayo Clinic, Rochester, Minnesota

Medical Management of Liver Disease

1

Approach to the Patient with Elevated Serum Enzyme Levels

Edward L. Krawitt
University of Vermont College of Medicine, Burlington, Vermont

Although elevated circulating enzyme levels are frequently seen in patients who are symptomatic or jaundiced, they are also seen in asymptomatic patients. The latter situation is becoming more common in the present era of screening, blood donation, data bank configuration, and examinations required for schooling, employment, and insurance. Thus, it is inevitable that serum enzyme levels above the established upper limits of normal will be found in otherwise apparently healthy patients. More specifically, these enzyme elevations are of alanine aminotransferase (ALT), aspartate aminotransferase (AST), alkaline phosphatase (AP) and/or gamma glutamyl transpeptidase (GGT). Although these measurements do not test liver function in a physiological or biochemical sense, they are often referred to as liver function tests (LFTs). Their elevation generally represents evidence of liver damage; since these enzymes may be released into the circulation from other organs, however, on occasion, they may reflect muscle or bone disease.

THE SEVEN-PLUS APPROACH

An approach to the problem of elevated serum enzyme levels, often phrased as abnormal LFTs (coded 794.8), that I have found helpful is one that I have named the "seven-plus approach." This method considers the laboratory abnormalities from an etiological perspective, focusing on the most common causes of abnormalities seen in practice. In brief, when analyzing subjective and objective information on such patients, one must consider seven broad etiological categories clustered, for ease in recall, into the "big four" and the "little three" (Table 1). Needless to say, these seven categories do not encompass all abnormalities of liver disease; thus others must be considered in the broadest of categories, that of "plus."

The "big four" includes medication-induced liver disease, alcohol-induced liver disease, viral hepatitis, and biliary disease, while the "little three" encompasses genetic hemochromatosis, nonalcoholic fatty liver, and autoimmune liver disease. The entities included in the "big four" and "little three" can be subdivided as indicated in Table 1.

Table 1 The Seven-Plus Approach

"Big four"	Drug-induced disease
	Alcohol-induced disease
	a. Alcoholic steatosis
	b. Alcoholic hepatitis
	c. Cirrhosis
	Viral hepatitis
	a. Acute: hepatitis A, B, C, D, E
	b. Chronic: hepatitis B, C, D
	Biliary disease
	a. Gallstone-associated
	b. Non-gallstone-associated
"Little three"	Nonalcoholic fatty liver
	a. Nonalcoholic steatosis
	b. Nonalcoholic steatohepatitis (NASH)
	c. Cirrhosis
	Genetic hemochromatosis
	Autoimmune liver disease
	a. Autoimmune hepatitis
	b. Primary biliary cirrhosis
	c. Primary sclerosing cholangitis
	d. Overlap syndromes
"Plus"	Neoplasms
	a. Benign
	b. Malignant
	Infectious diseases
	Granulomatosis hepatitis
	Genetic diseases
	Cystic diseases
	Collagen-vascular diseases
	Pregnancy-associated
	Etc.

If initially the diagnosis is not clear cut or likely, one must also consider the "plus" group, which comprises everything else—namely, any and all other liver diseases that might apply. Consideration of some of these diseases will be obvious, such as metastatic disease in the patient known to have cancer, diseases specifically associated with pregnancy, liver involvement in the patient known to have polycystic kidney disease, and so on. Others will be less apparent.

Aminotransferase Elevations

With moderate elevations of transaminases, both ALT and AST are generally abnormal; but with mild elevations, particularly in nonalcoholic liver disease, an ALT elevation may be an isolated abnormality. Indeed, many patients with low-level elevations of ALT secondary to chronic hepatitis C present with an ALT that may be only minimally elevated ($\leq$ 1.5 times the upper limit of normal) and accompanied by a normal AST. Elevated transaminases are, however, seen in a variety of liver diseases. For the most part, when ALT and AST are both elevated and the liver disease is in the precirrhotic phase, the ALT exceeds the AST. The reverse may occur when cirrhosis has appeared. This should not be confused with the situation in which acute alcohol-induced liver damage is present and the ratios of AST:ALT can achieve levels of 4–5. When AST elevations exceed those of AST in cirrhosis, the AST:ALT ratio is generally $\leqslant 2$.

Transaminase elevations are common in drug-induced and alcohol-induced disease as well as in viral hepatitis. Elevation of an aminotransferase in the absence of a concomitant elevation of AP would be very unlikely in the presence of extrahepatic biliary obstruction from either a malignant or a benign cause. Abnormal values are also seen in nonalcoholic fatty liver and may be the only abnormality seen in early hemochromatosis. Transaminases are characteristically elevated in autoimmune hepatitis. In primary biliary cirrhosis and primary sclerosing cholangitis, the elevation of AP is more impressive than in autoimmune hepatitis. On occasion, a transaminase elevation may be due to muscle disease (skeletal or cardiac), and in that sense it may not represent a liver test. Transaminase elevations have also been reported in patients with thyroid disease.

Alkaline Phosphatase Elevations

AP, when elevated in the presence of frank jaundice or conjugated hyperbilirubinemia, is almost always a reflection of intrahepatic or extrahepatic obstruction and forms part of the picture of cholestasis (see Chap. 3). In this situation, the cause of the extrahepatic obstruction (benign or malignant) or of intrahepatic obstruction (medication-induced, alcohol-induced, etc.) must be sought. When AP and aminotransferase elevations occur concomitantly, they generally reflect an etiology from the same disease process, but elevated bone AP may confound the workup.

An isolated AP abnormality may present a difficult diagnostic problem on occasion. In the patient with obvious systemic disease, it sometimes is merely a nonspecific reflection of disease, especially if elevations are $\leqslant 2$ times normal. Such a mild elevation of circulating liver AP reflects systemic disease, as does an elevated erythrocyte sedimentation rate or an elevated serum ferritin. On the other hand, an isolated AP may reflect the presence of a variety of liver diseases—namely, those of the "big four" and "little three" and those in the "plus" category: granulomatous disease, malignancy, fatty liver, primary biliary cirrhosis, and so on. A not unusual presentation of primary biliary cirrhosis, the most common of the autoimmune diseases (see Chap. 12) is that of an elevated AP with a normal bilirubin in a middle-aged woman who often complains of pruritus. Although extrahepatic obstruction is almost unheard of without an elevated serum AP, it must be emphasized that the presence of an elevated level of AP, or of conjugated bilirubin for that matter, does not differentiate between intrahepatic or extrahepatic disease. This distinction may be made on the basis of an imaging or cholangiographic study.

If the AP is abnormal in the presence of unconjugated hyperbilirubinemia, however, one needs to sort out the cause of the unconjugated hyperbilirubinemia—which, in general, is secondary to Gilbert's syndrome or erythrocyte hemolysis—independent of evaluating the AP elevation.

Gamma Glutamyl Transpeptidase Elevation

The presence of an elevated GGT is frequently a sensitive indicator of liver disease but may also merely reflect enzyme induction. Elevations of GGT after alcohol ingestion may last as long as 8 weeks and a variety of drugs induce GGT; this may confound the picture when one is searching for evidence of liver disease. An elevated circulating AP sometimes represents enzyme of bone origin. The growing adolescent has higher circulating levels of AP than do adult patients. Benign or malignant bone disease can result in AP elevation. In those cases, fractionation of the enzyme into bone and liver components is often helpful. Alternatively, measuring GGT may be helpful, as GGT should reflect liver involvement. Similarly, a GGT should be normal when elevated circulating intestinal AP is secondary to renal failure.

AN ALGORITHM

The "seven-plus approach" can be facilitated by plugging it into a diagnostic algorithm (see Fig. 1). Most of the pertinent information for drug and alcohol-induced diseases will be obtained from a detailed history. Important subjective information regarding viral hepatitis should include history of exposure, including contact with individuals with hepatitis; multiple sexual partners; exposure to blood-product transfusions; and also evidence of potential parenteral exposure via intravenous drug use, cocaine snorting, body piercing, tattoos, acupuncture, and so on. Often, biliary disease is marked by a history that includes abdominal pain and/or jaundice, but "silent" gallstone disease also occurs. Obstruction from stricturing or pancreatic disease may also be painless.

Genetic hemochromatosis may be uncovered through a family history, although frequently when patients give a family history of liver disease or liver cancer it has been assumed that the etiology was alcoholism. The prototypical patient with nonalcoholic fatty liver is an obese diabetic woman; this entity, however, can be found in the absence of any of those three features. It is often seen in patients with hyperlipidemia. Rheumatological systems may be apparent in patients who eventually turn out to have autoimmune liver disease. Concurrent or family disease of other autoimmune disorders such as autoimmune thyroiditis, diabetes mellitus, Raynaud's phenomenon, Sjögren's disease, autoimmune hemolytic anemia, or autoimmune thrombocytopenia may suggest concurrent autoimmune liver diseases. The presence of ulcerative colitis should alert the physician to the possibility of autoimmune hepatitis or primary sclerosing cholangitis; approximately 70% of patients with primary sclerosing cholangitis have concomitant nonspecific ulcerative colitis.

History for the "plus" category may present obvious possibilities, as noted, with previously diagnosed malignancies, sarcoidosis, systemic lupus erythematosus, polycystic kidney disease, cystic fibrosis, Wilson's disease, alpha$_1$-antitrypsin deficiency, endocrinopathy, etc.

The physical examination can be helpful in providing evidence of a systemic disease or stigmata of chronic liver disease such as spider angiomas, palmar erythema, and finger clubbing or of parental exposure (tattoos, piercing, needle scars). A careful examination of the abdomen can reveal hepatomegaly or splenomegaly. If advanced liver disease is present, jaundice, shifting dullness, peripheral edema, asterixis, or gynecomastia may be present.

As indicated in Figure 1, depending on the subjective and objective data obtained during the history and physical examination and contingent on the laboratory data at hand, one has the choice of obtaining additional objective data using laboratory determinations or of pursuing imaging and/or cholangiographic studies (see Table 2). Alternatively, it may be clear that a liver biopsy is the next logical diagnostic step.

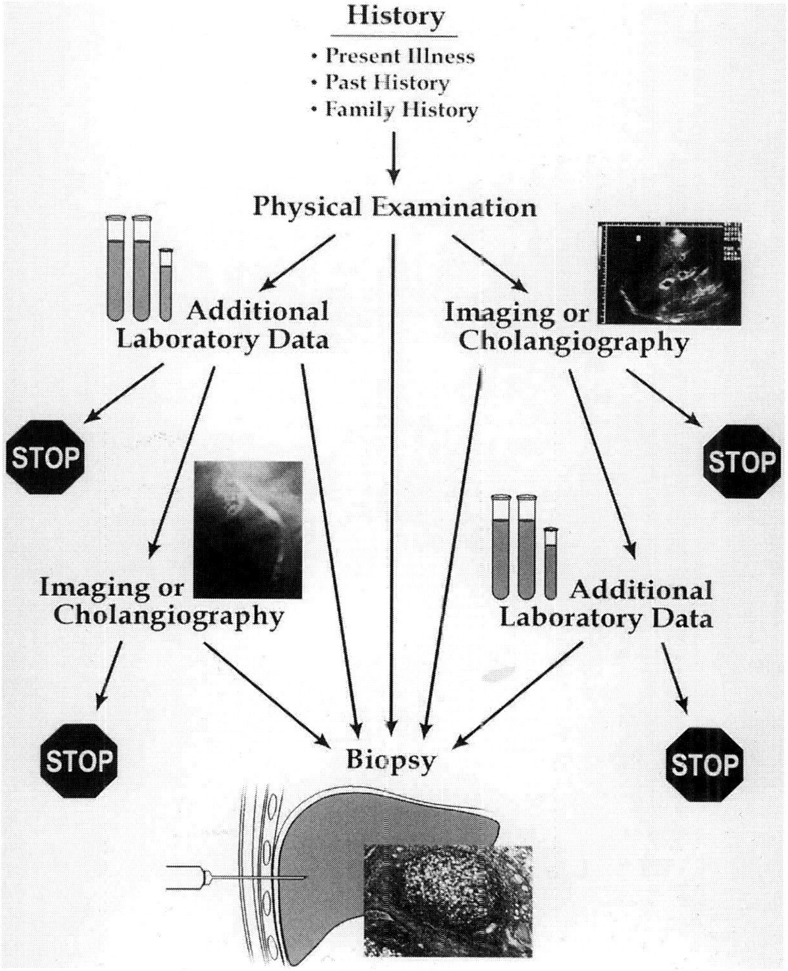

Figure 1 An algorithm for the diagnosis of conditions causing abnormal LFTs.

Additional Laboratory Data

A serological hepatitis profile should be obtained to uncover the presence of acute or chronic hepatitis. Measurements of HBV DNA and HCV RNA may also be necessary (see Chap. 4).

In general, serum ferritin, iron, and iron-binding capacity (or transferrin) are used to screen for this common disease, which has a prevalence of 3–4/1000 in North America. The percent transferrin saturation (iron/transferrin ×100) is the most sensitive measure for hemochromatosis. Although elevated serum ferritin is frequently seen in this disease, abnormalities also occur in a variety of liver diseases, notably chronic viral hepatitis, alcoholic liver disease, and nonalcoholic steatosis. In families with a history of hemochromatosis, screening may evolve to searching directly for the specific allele of HLA HFE (originally named HLA H) (see Chap. 27).

Table 2 Commonly Performed Diagnostic Studies

Serum determinations
Hepatitis screening
Hepatitis A antibody, hepatitis Bs antigen, hepatitis Bc antibody, hepatitis Bs antibody
Hepatitis C antibody
Hepatitis D antibody
Hepatitis B virus DNA, hepatitis C virus RNA
Iron studies
Iron, iron-binding capacity (transferrin), ferritin
Protein studies
Total protein/albumin (total protein − albumin = total globulin)
Protein electrophoresis
Quantitative immunoglobulin
Autoantibodies
Antinuclear antibody
Smooth muscle antibody
Antimitochondrial antibody
Antineutrophil cytoplasmic antibody
Radiological studies
Ultrasonography
Computed tomography
Magnetic resonance imaging
Hepatic scintigraphy
Cholangiography
Percutaneous
Endoscopic retrograde
Magnetic resonance
Liver biopsy
Percutaneous
Transjugular
Laparoscopic

Hyperglobulinemia and circulating autoantibodies are hallmarks of autoimmune liver disease. Serum protein electrophoresis and/or quantitative immunoglobulin measurement may be helpful. The first line of autoantibodies to consider when there is a suspicion of autoimmune liver disease includes antinuclear antibody (ANA), smooth muscle antibody (SMA), antimitochondrial antibody (AMA), and antineutrophil cytoplasmic antibody (ANCA). ANA and SMA are characteristic of autoimmune hepatitis, AMA of primary biliary cirrhosis, and ANCA of primary sclerosing cholangitis, but overlapping and concurrent autoantibodies occur. AMA in primary biliary cirrhosis, however, is the most sensitive and specific of these autoantibodies. In children, in whom autoimmune hepatitis is suspected, an antiliver kidney microsome type 1 (ALKM-1) antibody should be ordered (see Chap. 11).

Radiological Studies

In lieu of or in addition to the above laboratory studies—depending upon the clinical situation—imaging studies such as ultrasonography and computed tomography may be required (see Fig. 1). Imaging studies are crucial to differentiate intrahepatic from extrahepatic cholestasis and are often helpful in establishing the presence of certain conditions such as steatosis, cysts, tumors, and so on. In some cases, hepatic scintigraphy or magnetic resonance imaging may be more appropriate. In other situations, physicians elect to obtain cholangiography, either percutaneous transhepatic (PTC), endoscopic retrograde (ERC) or, if available and appropriate, magnetic resonance cholangiography (MRC). The latter serves as a noninvasive cholangiographic technique but is not readily available and depends on sophisticated software programming (see Chap. 2).

Liver Biopsy

Once the data from additional laboratory measurements and/or radiological studies are available, a liver biopsy may be the next appropriate diagnostic step. Alternatively, it may have been clear that additional studies were not required prior to a percutaneous, transjugular, or laparoscopic liver biopsy or that a biopsy need not be performed.

BIBLIOGRAPHY

Craxi A, Almasio P. Diagnostic approach to liver enzyme elevation. J Hepatol 1996; 25:1:47–51.

Kamath PS. Clinical approach to the patient with abnormal liver test results. Mayo Clin Proc 1996; 71:1089–1095.

Sherman KE. Alanine aminotransferase in clinical practice. Arch Intern Med 1991; 151:260–265.

2
Approach to the Patient with Abnormal Imaging Studies

Jose A. Lavergne and K. Rajender Reddy
University of Miami School of Medicine, Miami, Florida

INTRODUCTION

The frequent use of imaging studies has led to the identification of mass lesions in the liver that may or may not be symptomatic. Improvement in imaging technology has also been helpful in identifying small lesions and heterogeneous processes such as iron deposition and fatty infiltration. The assessment of an abnormal imaging study of the liver involves a fundamental knowledge of the imaging characteristics of these abnormalities and their associated clinical features.

A stepwise workup is possible in most cases, but there are exceptions where different approaches may be considered. Local expertise and availability of the various imaging studies dictate variations in evaluation.

In this chapter, we attempt to give a comprehensive review of the relevance of various imaging studies in the evaluation of hepatobiliary abnormalities and then discuss cases to illustrate their usefulness in approaching patients with abnormalities.

HEPATIC SCINTIGRAPHY

In the evaluation of hepatobiliary diseases, a wide variety of scintigraphic studies are employed. These include the technetium 99m (^{99m}Tc) sulfur colloid scan, ^{99m}Tc red blood cell (RBC) blood-pool scintigraphy, iminodiacetate (IDA) scintigraphy, and single-photon-emission computed tomography (SPECT); each of these has inherent advantages and indications. More recently, newer imaging modalities like computed tomography (CT) and magnetic resonance imaging (MRI) have led to a decrease in the use of nuclear imaging studies.

The ^{99m}Tc-labeled sulfur colloid scan involves the principle of phagocytosis of the radionucleotide material by the reticuloendothelial (RE) cells of the liver, thereby allowing for the visualization of different areas of the liver according to the degree of RE activity. The degree of radiation exposure of other organs is low because of the use of low doses and the short half-life of ^{99m}Tc. Hepatic inflammation and fibrosis cause abnormal hepatic

RE cell function, which, in turn, produces a shift of the radionucleotide material to the spleen and bone marrow. It seems to have a greater role in the diagnosis of chronic liver disease. Increased uptake in the spleen and bone marrow is observed in both acute hepatitis and cirrhosis.

Hepatic hemangiomas are large, blood-filled, endothelium-lined spaces separated by fibrous septa; although blood-filled, these hemangiomas have a sluggish flow. The ^{99m}Tc RBC blood-pool scan is the scintigraphic procedure of choice for the evaluation of lesions suspicious for hepatic hemangiomas. It is obtained after the intravenous administration of ^{99m}Tc-labeled autologous erythrocytes. Hemangiomas classically show decreased blood flow on the dynamic flow images and slow, delayed, uniform tracer accumulation in the lesion that peaks 30 to 50 min postinjection. This appearance has been termed a *perfusion/blood pool mismatch.* Rare cases of angiosarcoma and hepatoma have demonstrated a similar scintigraphic appearance. Also, atypical images of actual hemangiomas can be seen when these lesions have undergone significant fibrosis or are full of blood clots. Planar imaging has adequate sensitivity for detecting hemangiomas larger than 3 cm, but it has poor sensitivity for lesions smaller than 2 cm. Routine SPECT imaging has improved this sensitivity, especially for lesions 1 to 2 cm in size, for which SPECT has a sensitivity of as high as 90%.

Focal nodular hyperplasia (FNH) is another lesion that can have characteristic scintigraphic features. Histologically, FNH is a well-circumscribed region of hyperplastic liver parenchyma containing a central stellate fibrous scar, from which fibrous septa containing vascular structures and proliferating bile ducts radiate. Although RE cells are contained in this type of lesion, the sulfur colloid uptake varies.

FNH can show a normal uptake (30%), increased uptake (30%), or even decreased uptake compared with normal parenchyma (30%). However in 10% of cases, the uptake is intense, a finding considered specific for FNH. Scintigraphy appears to be more specific than ultrasound (US), CT, or angiography for the diagnosis of FNH when the characteristic image is seen.

Hepatocellular carcinoma (HCC) appears in sulfur colloid liver imaging as a nonspecific focal defect due to the lack of RE cells. Gallium-67 scanning has been used to diagnose HCC, as 90–95% of these lesions accumulate this radiotracer, with 50% having greater uptake than the surrounding parenchyma. Gallium scans can also be used to differentiate HCC from regenerating nodules in patients with cirrhosis, as only about 10% of the latter pick up gallium. Therefore, gallium scans should be used in conjunction with sulfur colloid images to assess the differential uptake of hepatic lesions in suspected cases of HCC. Gallium scintigraphy is interpreted as abnormal when a lesion that shows decreased activity on a sulfur colloid liver scan demonstrates increased or normal gallium uptake compared with the surrounding liver. However, the clinical presentation remains important, as lymphomas, hepatic abscesses, and occasional metastases can demonstrate a similar scintigraphic appearance.

Routine nuclear scanning has good sensitivity for detecting liver metastases (80–85%); sensitivity is, however, related to the size of the lesions. SPECT imaging has only marginally improved sensitivity for hepatic metastases as compared with the planar imaging technique. Its specificity is limited by the difficulty in differentiating small lesions from normal vessels, the biliary tree, and variations in the normal contour.

The main pitfalls of scintigraphic studies are false-positive scans caused by extrahepatic tumors, the right kidney, inferior vena cava, porta hepatis, and gallbladder and by anatomic variations in the size, shape, and position of the liver. Cirrhosis, diffuse fatty infiltration of the liver, alcoholic hepatitis, biliary obstruction, and passive congestion of the liver due to heart failure may be mistaken for multiple space-occupying intrahepatic lesions. Furthermore, superficial lesions smaller than 2 cm and deep lesions (especially those within the right lobe) of even 3 to 4 cm in diameter are poorly detected.

Scintigraphy has also been used in the evaluation of patients suspected to have biliary pathology. IDA cholescintigraphy is used to evaluate the patency of the cystic duct. The failure to visualize the gallblader after 4 h of scanning has greater than 90% sensitivity and specificity for acute cholecystitis. Morphine can be used to shorten the imaging period from 4 h to 90 min by inducing spasm of the sphincter of Oddi and increased bile flow into the gallbladder through a patent cystic duct. IDA scintigraphy has a high sensitivity but a low specificity for acalculous cholecystitis.

ULTRASONOGRAPHY

US is the least invasive and simplest radiological test for the evaluation of liver lesions. The basis of this imaging study is the transmission of sound pulses through tissues and detection of the amplitude and depth of the reflected sound. The degree of reflection of the sound waves depends upon the interface between tissues with different acoustic properties. The degree of echogenicity depends on the ability of the media being evaluated to reflect and absorb the ultrasound waves. Echogenicity is compared with the normal surrounding parenchyma. The larger the difference between tissues, the stronger the reflection. Nowadays, US utilizes computerization to process the different signals, which has allowed better definition of even smaller lesions (not less than 1 cm). Its major advantages are its availability, low cost, and portability. One of the major advantages of an inexpensive and easy-to-perform modality such as US is its ability to facilitate monitoring of lesions, such as hepatic abscesses or hematomas, that are likely to change with time. Further it has a high resolution in differentiating cystic lesions from solid lesions, including delineating septation in a cystic lesion. Although US can define a solid lesion, it is not specific, as it cannot assess the vascularity of the lesions. The other main disadvantages are that it is operator-dependent, and both adipose tissue and overlying bowel gas interfere with proper interpretation.

Computed Tomography (CT Scan)

This technique is based on passing fine x-ray beams through the patient, with detectors located on the opposite site of the body to record the amount of radiation not attenuated by the tissues. The information is then processed by a computer, which calculates the attenuation values in reference to the water value of zero (Hounsfield units). Intravenous iodine contrast can be used to determine the vascularity of lesions compared with that of normal liver. However, intravenous iodine contrast must be administered with accurate timing, taking into consideration the suspected clinical condition and nonenhanced image, so as not to mask lesions that can become isodense with the parenchyma once contrast has been administered.

Successful CT of the liver can be obtained despite significant obesity, overlying bowel gas, or ascites and can provide considerable information about extrahepatic anatomy, which may offer additional clues to the etiology of hepatic lesion being scanned. Conventional CT scan is considered less sensitive than ultrasound at detecting lesions smaller than 1–2 cm; it is also more expensive and involves the risk of radiation and exposure to intravenous iodine contrast.

Helical or spiral CT scan is a technique aimed at optimizing the detection rate and lesion characterization of hypervascular lesions that are missed by the conventional incremental contrast-enhanced CT. Conventional contrast-enhanced CT predominantly enhances the liver parenchyma and is a good technique to detect hypovascular lesions such as metastases from nonhypervascular tumors (colon, pancreas, and lung) and infrequently hepatocellular carcinoma. In contrast, helical CT obtains images during the hepatic artery phase by scanning during the first 20–30 s of a high rate contrast infusion. Thus, helical CT provides the advantage of scanning through the entire liver twice: once during the hepatic artery–dominant phase and another during the conventional portal venous–dominant phase. This technique is superior to conventional CT in detecting hepatocellular carcinoma.

Helical or spiral CT should be utilized in patients with known or suspected hypervascular neoplasms, such as hepatocellular carcinoma, metastases from renal cell carcinoma, neuroendocrine (islet cell) tumors, breast cancer, thyroid carcinoma, and sarcomas.

Magnetic Resonance Imaging (MRI)

MRI is based on the utilization of a strong magnetic field to align the axes of rotating hydrogen protons within the body. As the protons realign to the main magnetic field, measurements of energy released are sampled at various time intervals. The signal intensity is calculated for small boxes of tissue (voxels) from the degree of realignment within a given time period. Cross-sectional images are obtained based on a gray scale, with tissues being presented from a low to a high signal intensity. The degree of signal intensity is dependent on the water and fat content of tissues as well as to the presence of certain substances such as hemosiderin. The T1 relaxation time refers to the time required for protons to realign themselves with an external magnetic field after a radiowave pulse. The T2 relaxation time describes the rate at which protons get out of phase with one another because of the effect of adjacent protons. This measurement will affect the signal intensities and thus the appearance of the image; for instance water has a low signal intensity (dark) on T1-weighted images but a high signal intensity (light) on T2-weighted images. The reverse is true for fat. MRI can therefore demonstrate abnormal signal intensity of hepatic masses as compared with normal parenchyma and can identify blood flow without intravenous contrast. Gadolinium-diethylenetriaminepentacetic acid (DTPA) can be used as a contrast agent to enhance the liver image in order to obtain further information about the vascular supply of a lesion.

The advantages of MRI include excellent contrast resolution, multiplanar imaging, reproducibility, and lack of need for iodinated contrast in patients with renal failure. MRI and CT enhance lever lesions to a similar degree. The major disadvantages are motion artifacts, high cost, lack of ready availability, and the claustrophobia experienced by some patients. Additionally, CT is considered superior to MRI for the evaluation of extrahepatic organs and spaces and for identifying calcifications.

The consensus among clinicians and radiologists is that MRI and CT are comparable, with MRI being preferred for the evaluation of HCC, cavernous hemangioma, and focal fatty infiltration. Hemangiomas characteristically appear as well-circumscribed homogeneous masses with high signal intensity on T2-weighted images. A giant hemangioma can be more irregular and inhomogeneous. After gadolinium injection, a hemangioma demonstrates enhancement similar to that seen on bolus-contrast CT. Because hepatic scintigraphy is less expensive, MRI should be used for those patients whose lesions are smaller than 2 cm, or are located adjacent to the heart or to major intrahepatic vessels, as they can be difficult to define by RBC blood-pool studies. MRI has also been exceptionally helpful in the evaluation of hypervascular metastatic liver lesions, such as islet cell carcinoma, carcinoid tumors, thyroid tumors, and melanoma, which can be difficult to evaluate with CT.

MRI has also been very helpful in the evaluation of masses in patients with well-established cirrhosis, where the possibility of HCC should be differentiated from regenerative nodules. Malignant degeneration within a cirrhotic liver should be suspected when a nodule or a mass is hyperintense (or heterogeneous with zones of hyperintense signal) on T2-weighted images. Regenerative nodules usually remain low in signal intensity on T2-weighted images and mimic the signal intensity of normal hepatic parenchyma. Almost half of these malignant tumors have homogeneously increased signal intensity on T1-weighted images. The cause of this increased signal is thought to be steatosis, hemorrhage, or possibly deposition of copper in the tumor. MRI may also show evidence of vascular invasion by large hepatic tumors.

MRI is also very reliable in discriminating between focal fatty infiltration and other hepatic masses. Using the difference in processional frequency between fat and water protons, fat can be distinguished from other types of hepatic tissues. Similarly, iron overload can be defined by using MRI. Patients with primary hemochromatosis can have decreased signals in the liver and pancreas, whereas those with secondary iron overloading (reticuloendothelial deposition) may have decreased signals in the liver, spleen, and bone marrow. The spleen is not commonly affected in primary hemochromatosis. There can be overlap of these features.

FNH is another lesion that can be evaluated by MRI. It characteristically shows a well-circumscribed mass that is isointense on both T1- and T2-weighted images. Unfortunately, the characteristic hyperintense central scar on the T2-weighted images is seen in only half of cases.

Ferumoxides are tissue-specific iron particles used as MRI contrast agents for the detection of hepatic tumors. They are taken up by the reticuloendothelial system (Kupffer cells), and cause them to have a decreased signal on T2-weighted images. Hepatic lesions, which lack Kupffer cells, will not take up ferumoxide and will appear bright against a black background. The use of this contrast agent increases the sensitivity for hepatic lesions compared to unenhanced MRI and contrast-enhanced dynamic CT. An advantage of ferumoxide over gadolinium MRI is that the patients need not hold their breath while images are obtained.

MR cholangiography (MRC) and MR cholangiopancreatography (MRCP) are noninvasive techniques to evaluate the biliary and pancreatic systems based on heavily T2-weighted pulses. As a result, stationary fluids, including bile and pancreatic secretions, have a high signal intensity, while solid organs have a low signal intensity. Flowing blood also has little or no measurable signal. An advantage of this technique is that it does not require preparation of the patient or injection of contrast medium, and it takes between 20 and 30 min. MRCP has a high sensitivity and specificity for choledocholithiasis and malignant strictures of the biliary tree. This modality is, however, not widely available and is in the process of being perfected. At present, it is being considered more frequently in patients with suspected primary sclerosing cholangitis and those who have had unsuccessful endoscopic retrograde cholangiopancreatography (ERCP) surgical bypass procedures (BII anastomosis, hepatico-jejunostomy), or acute pancreatitis, and in those with low clinical suspicion for choledocholithiasis.

DIAGNOSTIC LAPAROSCOPY

Diagnostic laparoscopy is an underutilized technique for the evaluation of the patient who has had abnormal imaging studies. In the hands of an experienced operator, diagnostic laparoscopy can evaluate patients with abnormal liver chemistries, abnormal imaging studies, unexplained ascites, hepatomegaly, suspected metastatic liver disease, or jaundice; it is also useful in the preoperative staging of malignant tumors.

Laparoscopy is most helpful in the diagnosis of small focal hepatic lesions, cirrhosis, and peritoneal disease. In case of suspected malignancy, a laparoscopic evaluation of the liver is particularly helpful for detecting very small lesions (< 1 cm) not seen on routine ultrasonography or CT scanning of the abdomen. Laparoscopy may be useful in the staging of hepatocellular carcinoma; pancreatic, esophageal, and gastric cancers; and lymphomas.

TUMOR MARKERS

Tumor markers can be a useful adjunct to the clinical picture in determining the nature of a hepatic lesion discovered by imaging. The most common markers used in clinical practice for this purpose are carcinogenic embryonic antigen (CEA), alpha-fetoprotein (AFP), and CA 19-9.

CEA is the most widely used. It is present in most carcinomas but has been mainly evaluated in colorectal, breast, and lung cancer. Its highest levels are found in colon cancer, where is used as a marker of recurrent disease and as a test of effectiveness of treatment.

AFP is a glycoprotein produced in the yolk sac, liver, and intestines. After birth, levels remain low. HCC presents with elevations of this marker in approximately 70% of cases. Levels above 400 ng/mL in the right clinical setting are considered specific for HCC. Marked elevations of AFP have also been seen, however, after massive or submassive hepatic necrosis; these cannot be explained only by regeneration, as these elevations are not seen after partial hepatic resections. Fibrolamellar carcinoma, a variety of HCC, characteristically is not associated with an elevated AFP level.

CA 19-9 is an asialylated Lewis blood group antigen that is detected by a monoclonal antibody. It is elevated in colorectal cancer (20%), gastric cancer (42%), and HCC (22–51%) but is more frequently elevated in patients with pancreatic cancer (70–100%). A combination of CA 19-9 and CEA has been used for the detection of pancreatic cancer. Its specificity is lowered by elevations in patients with pancreatitis and liver diseases; however, these elevations typically will not exceed 120 U/mL with benign pancreatitis. Unfortunately, early pancreatic cancer tends to have a low CA 19-9 level, and very high levels predict unresectable disease, as shown by the fact that less than 5% of patients with a CA 19-9 level of 1000 U/mL have resectable disease.

CASE ILLUSTRATIONS

Case 1: Evaluation of a Cystic Mass

A 48-year-old professional woman who set up national corporate meetings was evaluated for a cystic mass discovered by an abdominal CT scan. She presented with upper abdominal discomfort associated with early satiety and had also noticed a prominent fullness in her epigastric region. There was no history of fever, weight loss, jaundice, or pruritus. She related no history of alcohol abuse or travel outside the United States and had spent all her life in a metropolitan area of Florida. She was a nonsmoker and had no risk factors for viral hepatitis, such as transfusion, intravenous drug abuse, or sexual promiscuity. She was not taking contraceptive steroids or other medications.

On examination, her blood pressure was 140/70; heart rate, 70 beats per minute;

respiratory rate, 18 per minute; and temperature, of 98.4 °F. There were no stigmata of chronic liver disease; her lungs were clear and the heart had a normal rhythm. There was prominence in the epigastric area, with a firm, smooth surface fullness without well-defined borders.

Pertinent laboratory data revealed normal hemoglobin, white blood cell count, and platelet count. The patient's prothrombin time and biochemical panel were normal except for an elevated alkaline phosphatase of 191 U/L (normal ranges up to 155 U/L). Tumor markers were negative. CT scan demonstrated a cystic lesion in the liver (Fig. 1).

Discussion

The CT scan of the abdomen demonstrates a predominantly cystic abnormality in the left lobe of the liver. The differential diagnosis of cystic lesions should include simple cyst, echinococcal cyst disease, biliary cystadenoma or cystadenocarcinoma, and, infrequently, congenital intrahepatic biliary dilatation (Caroli's disease) and congenital biliary dilatation that may be intrahepatic or extrahepatic (choledochal cyst). The infrequently encountered cystic disease of the biliary tree is characteristically associated with dilated bile ducts, which are not evident on the CT scan. An important observation on this imaging study is that septations are identified, which would make a simple cyst highly unlikely unless there has been hemorrhage into a simple cyst, resulting in a heterogeneous cystic appearance. A partially necrotic but solid malignancy may have a hypodense appearance, but in this case it is highly unlikely, since the wall of this cystic lesion is quite regular and thin. An

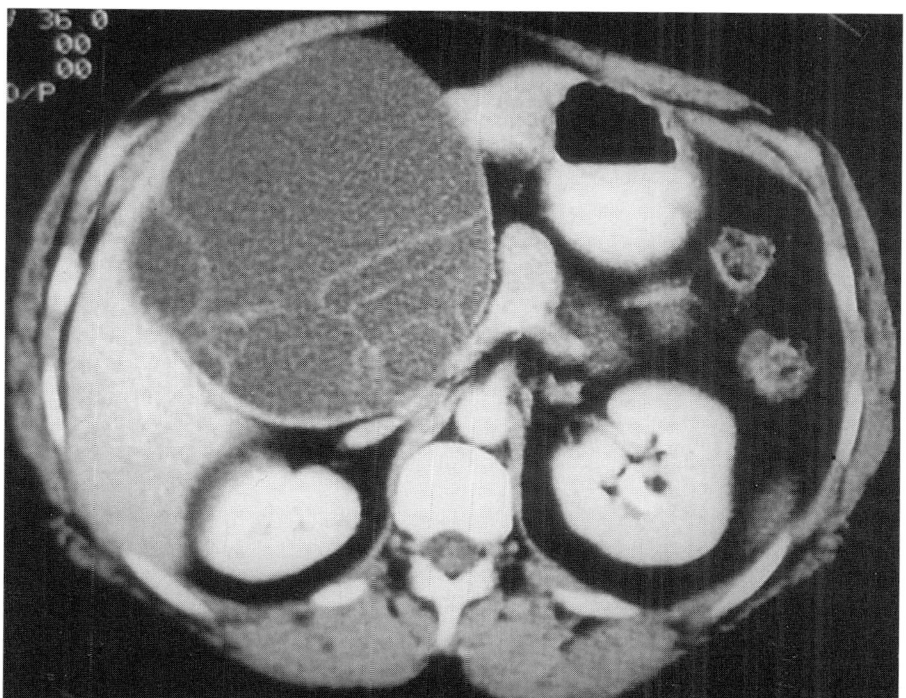

Figure 1 A cystic abnormality with septations and a thin wall in the left lobe of the liver. The lesion is hypodense and homogeneous.

echinococcal cyst is not a serious consideration given the lack of travel to an endemic area and the absence of calcification. Further, an echinococcal cyst is likely to have a wall of varying thickness, with heterogeneous density due to daughter cysts. A serious consideration in this patient is of a biliary cystadenoma or a cystadenocarcinoma. This lesion occurs almost exclusively in middle-aged women, and the cyst has a lining of mucin-secreting columnar or cuboidal epithelium. Abdominal discomfort is the most common presenting system and CT scan, as noted here, demonstrates a septated cystic lesion. Percutaneous aspiration of these abnormalities reveals mucinous and/or gelatinous nonserous fluid. The prognosis is excellent, although in up to 25% of cases malignant change over several years has been described. The recognition of such an abnormality leads to appropriate care in that surgical resection is indicated.

Case 2: Evaluation of Multiple Cystic and Solid Lesions in the Liver

A 62-year-old male physician was referred for further evaluation of liver abnormalities that had been detected on a CT scan. Metastatic carcinoma of the liver was suspected. He related a 9-month history of pain in his feet and calves, particularly in the morning. Over the next 2 to 3 months, the pain progressed to the thighs and hips and then developed in the upper arms. These symptoms were associated with a slight loss of appetite and weight but not with fever or chills. The physical evaluation failed to demonstrate hepatomegaly or lymphadenopathy. The complete blood count was normal, with hemoglobin of 14 g/dL and a hematocrit of 42%. The erythrocyte sedimentation rate was 40 but later dropped to 20. Serum CEA was normal on three occasions; serum aldolase was normal and the biochemical panel was normal on repeated testing except for a slightly elevated alkaline phosphatase of 90 U/L (normal, 30–80 U/L) on one occasion. AFP and CA-19-9 were normal. In view of the slightly elevated alkaline phosphatase, a CT scan of the abdomen was performed, which revealed multiple small lesions throughout the hepatic parenchyma; these mostly had low attenuation consistent with cysts, although some had an increased density suggestive of solid elements (Fig. 2). MRI showed that the lesions had both cystic and solid components and revealed additional multiple minute lesions throughout the entire liver parenchyma.

A diagnostic laparoscopy was performed. It demonstrated multiple small lesions and cysts over the entire liver (Fig. 3) as well as a large 3-cm cyst on the lateral segment of the left lobe. The lesions were well circumscribed, whitish-gray, and 2 to 3 mm in diameter; some of them were indented. A clear, acellular yellowish fluid was obtained by needle aspiration of the large cyst. Biopsy specimens taken from lesions in the right and left lobes showed bile duct hamartomas (Fig. 4). There was no evidence of tumor within the liver or peritoneum.

Discussion

In this case a malignant disease was suspected because of the multiple lesions on a background of anorexia, weight loss, and an elevated alkaline phosphatase. The CT scan demonstrated cystic and solid lesions. One approach would have been to do an imaging–guided biopsy, which would have ruled out a malignancy but would have not been helpful in establishing a precise diagnosis because of the small nature of the lesions. At laparoscopy, several small cystic lesions were observed and aspiration of one of these revealed clear fluid with acellularity consistent with simple cysts. Additionally, tiny, well-circumscribed,

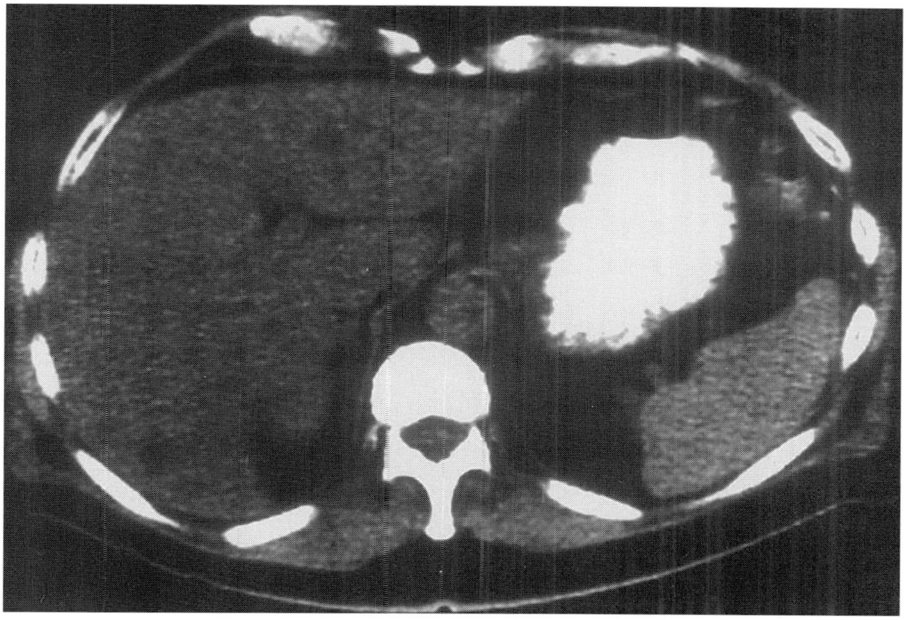

Figure 2 A CT scan showing several small abnormalities in the liver that are partly cystic and solid.

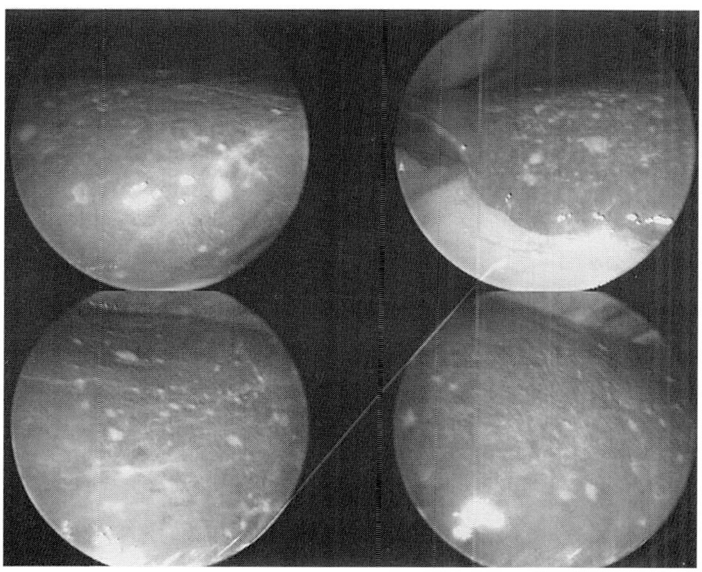

Figure 3 A laparoscopic photograph of the left lobe of the liver. Note the small grayish-black abnormalities, which represent cysts. The several small, white indented areas represent bile duct hamartomas.

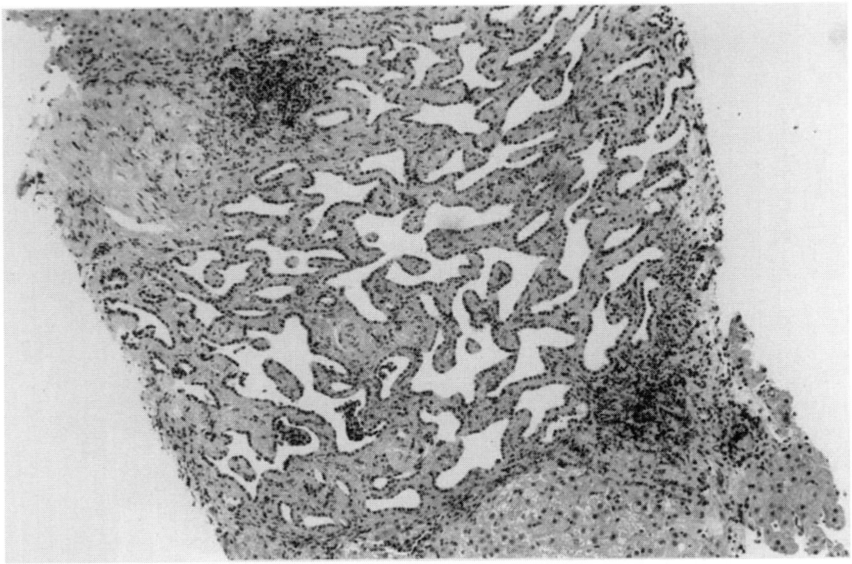

Figure 4 Liver biopsy demonstrating several redundant bile ducts in a portal area with normal biliary epithelium characteristic of a Von Myenberg complex.

mostly indented areas were observed which, on biopsy, proved to be bile duct hamartomas (Von-Meyenburg complexes). These are usually asymptomatic and are either diagnosed incidentally or found at autopsy. They contain a group of dilated and redundant bile ducts that may contain inspissated bile. These hamartomas fall in the spectrum of fibropolycystic diseases and may be associated with polycystic liver disease, as was the case here (see Chap. 32).

Case 3: Evaluation of a Diffusely Hypodense Liver on a CT Scan

A 52-year-old woman complained of vague right-upper-quadrant abdominal pain, which was constant and not related to meals. There was no history of fever, nausea, vomiting, or weight loss. She had a history of diabetes mellitus and hyperlipidemia treated with oral medications for several years. On physical exam, she was slightly overweight and had normal vital signs. There was no goiter, palpable lymph nodes, evidence of heart failure, or stigmata of liver disease. Her abdomen was soft, with an easily palpable, round-edged nonpulsatile liver; it was slightly tender. Complete blood count, prothrombin time, and biochemical panel were normal except for an AST of 60 U/L, ALT 120 U/L, and a slightly elevated alkaline phosphatase of 90 U/L (normal, 30–80 U/L). A CT scan of the abdomen revealed a hypodense liver (Fig. 5). A percutaneous liver biopsy was subsequently done, which revealed steatohepatitis (Fig. 6).

Discussion

The CT scan obtained demonstrated a markedly hypodense liver. This can be appreciated when the density is compared with that of other structures, particularly the spleen. A

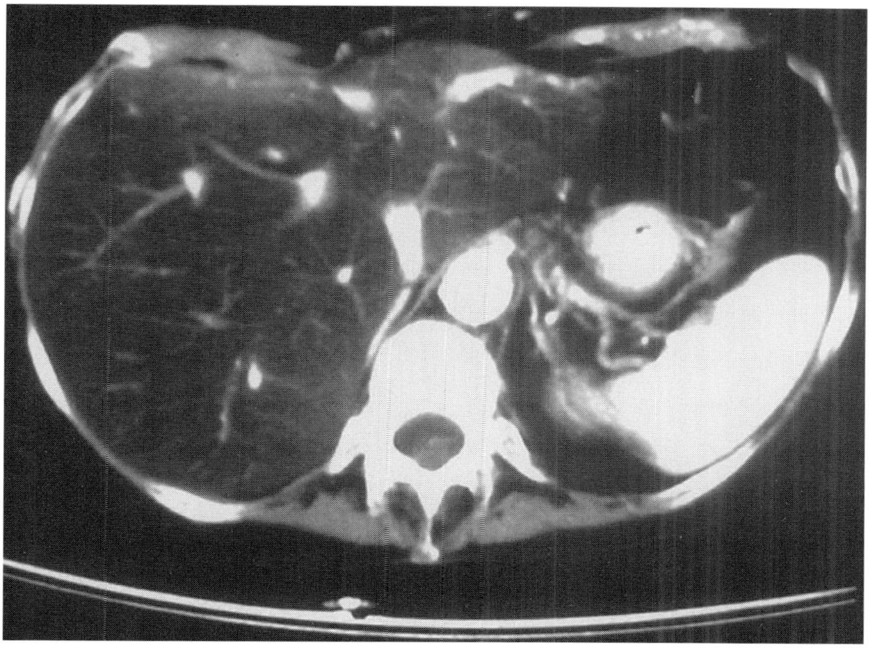

Figure 5 A CT scan of the liver demonstrating a diffusely hypodense liver, characteristic of fatty infiltration.

contrasting clinical condition is of hemochromatosis, where the density of the liver is significantly increased relative to that of other organs. With such a dramatic appearance of the liver, there is nothing else that would need to be considered in a differential diagnosis, and identification of etiological conditions would be appropriate. Typically, fatty liver is associated with diabetes mellitus, obesity, and alcohol abuse; it may be related to medications such as corticosteroids. Fat can be focal, presenting as multiple low-density abnormalities on a CT scan. Focal fat may mimic infiltrative disease; therefore, a biopsy in such cases is necessary to eliminate the possibility of malignant disease.

A liver biopsy was done in this case to establish the severity of the fatty liver for prognostic purposes. The patient was found to have nonalcoholic steatohepatitis. This typically demonstrates polymorphonuclear leukocyte infiltration and occasional Mallory's hyaline. A pericentral fibrosis can also be observed. This stage is infrequent as opposed to the more commonly observed clinical picture of bland steatosis. Fatty liver is generally benign and can improve with treatment of the underlying factors (see Chap. 26).

Case 4: Evaluation of a Heterogeneous Abnormality in the Liver of a Young Woman Who Presents with Severe Abdominal Pain

A 26-year-old woman was admitted with acute right-upper-quadrant abdominal pain. She had similar episodes over the previous several weeks; some associated with a temperature of 101 °F. An ultrasound of her right upper quadrant obtained during a previous episode of abdominal pain failed to show evidence of cholelithiasis or cholecystitis. Her medications included oral contraceptives for the past 3 years. On physical exam, her blood

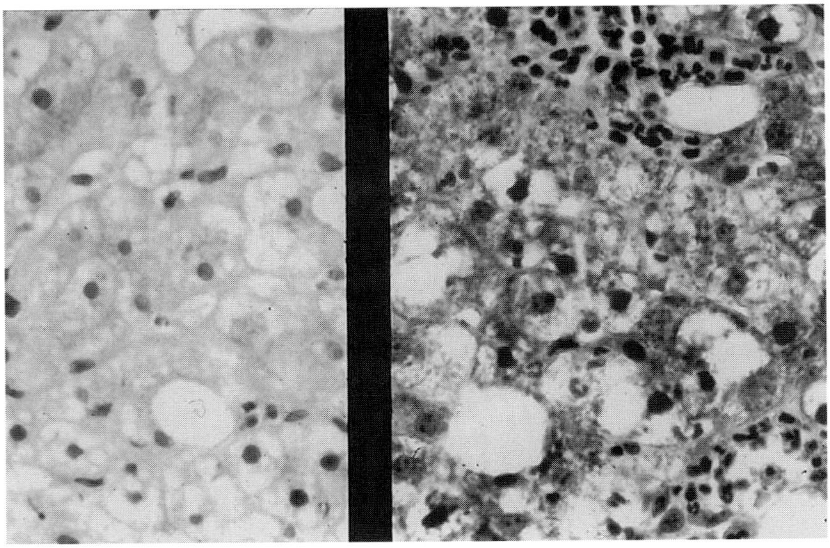

Figure 6 Low- and high-power photographs of a liver biopsy demonstrating fatty change with polymorphonuclear leukocyte infiltration.

pressure was 84/60, pulse 134 beats per minute, and a temperature of 101.2 °F. She was anicteric, without stigma of liver disease; tenderness was present in her epigastrium and abdominal right upper quadrant area, precluding an adequate evaluation of her liver. Her white blood cell count was 13,000 with a left shift; hemoglobin, 9.4 g/dL; platelet count, 685,000; and mean corpuscular volume (MCV) of 94. Prothrombin time was 13.6 s. Her AST and ALT levels were normal; alkaline phosphatase was elevated at 185 U/L (normal, 30–80 U/L). A pregnancy test was negative. A scan with dimethyl iminodiacetic acid showed a good and rapid visualization of the gallbladder. Given the absence of evidence of acute cholecystitis, a CT scan of the abdomen was obtained, showing significant hepatomegaly, a low-density space-occupying lesion of the lateral margin of the right lobe, and a normal-appearing left lobe (Fig. 7).

Discussion

In this case, CT scan demonstrated a heterogeneous abnormality in the right lobe of the liver, predominantly under the capsule of the liver. The CT scan had to be interpreted with a proper knowledge of several aspects of the clinical history. This was a young woman who had been on oral contraceptives and presented with a dramatic onset of severe right-upper-quadrant abdominal pain associated with hemodynamic instability and anemia. Serious consideration here would be bleeding from a hepatic adenoma related to the long-time use of oral contraceptives. The heterogeneous nature of the abnormality by CT scanning suggests bleeding due to a mass lesion that perhaps is obscured by blood. Also, the abnormality seems to be confined to the liver; if bleeding had occurred, it would be confined to the liver. Free bleeding into the peritoneum can have the catastrophic consequence of exsanguinating hemorrhage. It is also possible that the abnormality had nothing to do with previous contraceptive steroid use. A variety of tumors that include hepatocellular carcinoma can bleed into the liver, and a differential diagnosis should also include bleeding into a cyst.

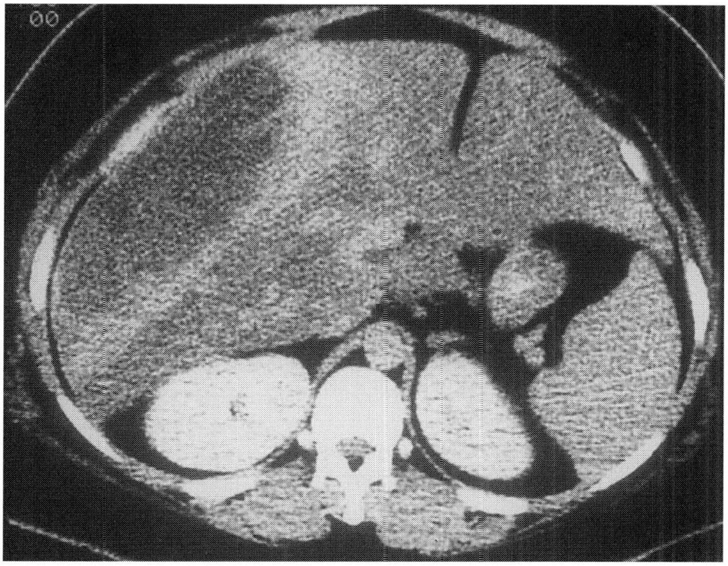

Figure 7 A heterogeneous abnormality under the capsule of the right lobe of the liver as seen on a CT scan.

Other causes for spontaneous intrahepatic bleeding include the use of oral anticoagulants, particularly associated with an overdose of anticoagulants and rupture of the liver due to toxemia of pregnancy. In this patient, a subcapsular hematoma in the liver was evacuated and a small hepatocellular adenoma was resected.

Case 5: Evaluation of an Incidentally Noted Mass in the Liver

A 38-year-old woman was referred for evaluation of a liver mass found incidentally during a renal ultrasound for nephrolithiasis. She denied abdominal pain, fever, or weight loss and had no medical history other than kidney stones. She denied current or previous use of oral contraceptives, history of smoking, and use of alcohol or intravenous drugs. She was born in the United States and had no history of travel to other countries. Her physical exam showed a well-developed and well-nourished woman in no apparent distress, without the stigmata of liver disease or lymphadenopathy. The liver and spleen were not palpable. The complete blood count and biochemical panel were normal, including AST 32 U/L, ALT 30 U/L, and an alkaline phosphatase of 60 U/L (normal, 30–80 U/L). An MRI revealed a hemangioma (Fig. 8).

Discussion

This patient was found to have an "incidentaloma" of the liver during ultrasound evaluation of her kidneys. It demonstrated an irregular but hyperdense abnormality. Because of the incidental nature of this finding in an asymptomatic patient with normal hepatic biochemical tests, it was suspected to be a hemangioma. This was confirmed by MRI, which demonstrated a hyperintense lesion on a T2-weighted image, typical of hemangiomas. Note

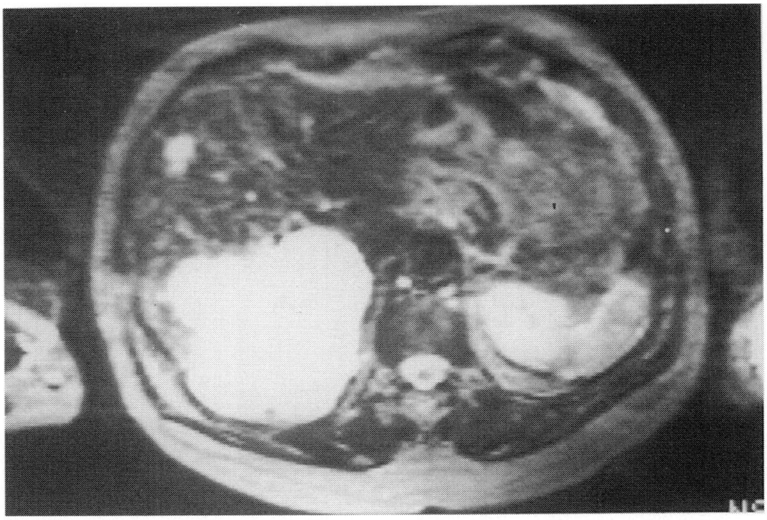

Figure 8 An MRI showing a hyperintense T2-weighted image of a lesion in the right node of the liver. Note the irregular borders, which should help differentiate a hemangioma from a simple cyst.

that the borders of the abnormality are irregular, indicating that this is not likely to be a simple cyst, which can also be hyperintense on a T2-weighted image. This lesion was not removed because this was an asymptomatic hemangioma, and these abnormalities are not known to rupture. Therefore, they pose no risk of exsanguinating hemorrhage. They may grow in size over time, however, particularly during pregnancy or with use of oral contraceptives or steroids. Also, thrombosis may occur, leading to severe abdominal pain.

BIBLIOGRAPHY

Bennett, WF, Bona JG. Review of hepatic imaging and a problem-oriented approach to liver masses. Hepatology 1990; 12:4:761–775.

Bluenke DA, Soyer, P, Fishman EK. Helical (spiral) CT of the liver. Radiol Clin North Am 1995; 33:863–885.

Davis LP, McCarroll K. Correlative imaging of the liver and hepatobiliary system. Semin Nucl Med 1994; 24(3):20–218.

Johnson CD. Magnetic resonance imaging of the liver: current clinical applications. Mayo Clin Proc 1993; 68:147–156.

Oliver JH III, Baron RL. Helical biphasic contrast enhanced CT of the liver: technique, indications, interpretations, and pitfalls. Radiology 1996; 201(1):1–14.

Reddy KR, Schiff ER. Approach to a liver mass. Semin Liver Dis 1993; 13:4:423–435.

Rubin RA, Lichtenstein GR. Hepatic scintigraphy in the evaluation of solitary solid liver masses. J Nucl Med 1993; 34:697–705.

Rubin RA, Mitchel DG. Evaluation of the solid hepatic mass. Med Clin North Am 1996; 80:907–928.

Salvatori, M. Imaging of hepatic focal lesion by nuclear medicine. J Surg Oncol Suppl 1993; 3: 189–191.

3
Approach to the Patient with Jaundice

Stephen Crane Hauser
Harvard Medical School and Brigham and Women's Hospital, Boston, Massachusetts

Jaundice, due to an abnormal increase in the serum bilirubin concentration, is evident upon physical examination. Patients with jaundice have a yellow discoloration of the skin, mucous membranes, and sclera (scleral icterus) when the serum bilirubin concentration exceeds 2.5–3.0 mg/dL (50 μmol/L). Lesser degrees of hyperbilirubinemia (1.0–2.5 mg/dL) do not produce jaundice. Patients with jaundice may be entirely well (e.g., Gilbert's syndrome), or they may be desperately ill (e g., jaundice associated with bacterial sepsis). Some patients with jaundice also suffer from cholestasis or diminished bile flow (e.g., extrahepatic biliary obstruction due to a gallstone impacted in the distal common bile duct), while other patients have jaundice without cholestasis (e.g., the Dubin-Johnson syndrome). A thorough understanding of bilirubin metabolism facilitates the clinical approach to the jaundiced patient.

BILIRUBIN CHEMISTRY

Bilirubin IXα (Z,Z) is by far the most abundant naturally occurring bilirubin isomer found in humans. The conventionally written structure [Fig. 1(a)] shows the methene bridge double bonds adjacent to the outer pyrrole rings (A and D) in the Z,Z position. However, bilirubin IXα (Z,Z) is not a linear tetrapyrrole but an involuted structure [Fig. 1(b)], which is stabilized by six intramolecular hydrogen bonds linking the propionic acid groups to the nitrogens and oxygen of the opposite pyrrole rings. This hydrogen bonding accounts for the water-insolubility of bilirubin. Hepatic conjugation of the propionic acid groups with glucuronic acid prevents the formation of hydrogen bonds and results in water-soluble derivatives (bilirubin glucuronides), which, unlike bilirubin itself, are readily excreted in bile. During phototherapy with blue or green light, the outer pyrrole rings of bilirubin IXα (Z,Z) flip over, resulting in the formation of unstable geometric (configurational) isomers, or photobilirubin [bilirubin IXα (Z,E), bilirubin IXα (E,Z), and bilirubin IXα (E,E) photoisomers]. These photoisomers are unable to form intramolecular hydrogen bonds and

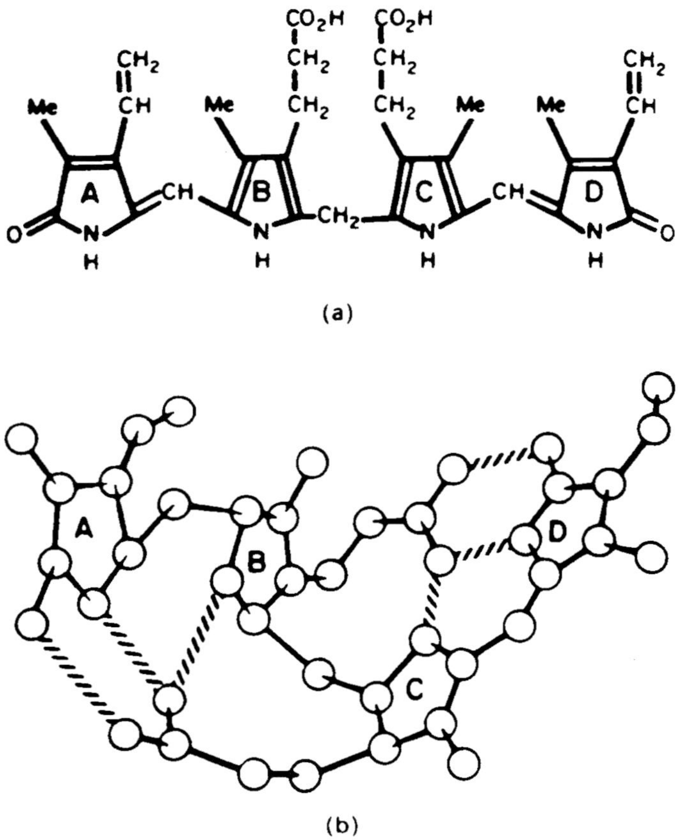

Figure 1 Structure of bilirubin IXα (Z,Z). (a) Conventionally written structure. (b) Involuted hydrogen-bonded structure in which the propionic acid groups of pyrrole rings B and C are linked to the nitrogens of the opposite pyrrole rings (interrupted lines).

hence are more polar and are excreted into bile without the need of conjugation. Once in bile, these unstable photoisomers may rapidly revert to the more stable bilirubin IXα (Z,Z). Structural isomerization or cyclization of bilirubin IXα (E,Z) in the presence of further light absorption results in a much more stable, water-soluble photoisomer known as lumirubin (cyclobilirubin, photobilirubin II), which is the predominant bilirubin species found in the bile of jaundiced neonates undergoing phototherapy.

FORMATION OF BILIRUBIN

Bilirubin is a degradation product of heme catabolism. Heme is dissociated from its apoprotein (e.g., globin) and transferred to the microsomal enzyme heme oxygenase, which is present in reticuloendothelial cells, Kupffer cells, hepatocytes, and renal tubular cells. The iron-containing protoporphyrin (heme) ring is cleaved selectively at the α-methene carbon bridge; iron is released; and the green, water-soluble pigment biliverdin IXα is formed. This reaction requires molecular oxygen (O_2) and NADPH-cytochrome *c* reductase and yields carbon monoxide. Heme oxygenase is the rate-limiting step in the transformation of heme to bilirubin. Unlike iron-protoporphyrin, tin-protoporphyrin binds to and inhibits heme oxygenase. Biliverdin IXα is rapidly converted to bilirubin IXα by the plentiful and ubiquitous cytosolic NADPH-dependent enzyme biliverdin reductase, which is found in reticuloendothelial cells, Kupffer cells, and hepatocytes.

SOURCES OF BILIRUBIN

Total daily bilirubin production averages 250–350 mg in adults. Destruction of the heme moiety of hemoglobin derived from senescent red blood cells in the reticuloendothelial system (bone marrow, spleen, liver) accounts for 70–80% of total daily bilirubin production. The remaining 20–30% is due to turnover of other hemoprotein in the liver (e.g., cytochrome P-450, catalase), and heme derived from the destruction of erythrocyte precursors in the bone marrow prior to their maturation or release.

PLASMA TRANSPORT OF BILIRUBIN

Nearly all of the bilirubin in the plasma of healthy adults is unconjugated bilirubin. This bilirubin is mostly bound to albumin by one high-affinity [1:1 binding would require a serum bilirubin of 35 mg/dL (600 μmol/L) at a serum albumin concentration of 4 g/dL] and at least two low-affinity sites. Hence, there is only an extremely small amount of free or unbound bilirubin in plasma. Only very small amounts of conjugated bilirubin (bilirubin glucuronides) are found in the plasma of healthy adults (e.g., 0.1 mg/dL). Although plasma-conjugated bilirubin is less tightly bound to albumin than unconjugated bilirubin, less than 1% of conjugated bilirubin is unbound or free. When jaundice includes increased plasma-conjugated bilirubin, this free, nonbound fraction is filtered by the glomeruli, and a fraction of it is not reabsorbed by the proximal convoluted tubules, resulting in bilirubinuria. Furthermore, when jaundice includes increased plasma-conjugated bilirubin, a fraction of the conjugated bilirubin becomes covalently bound to albumin (delta bilirubin, delta fraction, biliprotein, Bil-alb) and hence is not excreted in urine. Delta bilirubin, once formed, is very slowly cleared from plasma, because albumin has a long half-life (12–14 days). Delta bilirubin is not present in normal persons or patients with unconjugated hyperbilirubinemia.

HEPATIC TRANSPORT AND CONJUGATION

Uptake of bilirubin (unconjugated bilirubin in health and, in disease states, conjugated bilirubin) across the hepatocyte sinusoidal membrane occurs by carrier-mediated mechanisms, which are shared by other organic anions (e.g., sulfobromophthalein, indocyanine green) but not in most instances by bile acids. The uptake process is rapid, has a great capacity, and is not rate-limiting for hepatic bilirubin transport. Thus, the plasma bilirubin concentration in health is less than 1 mg/dL (17 μmol/L). Several carrier proteins that mediate bilirubin uptake into the hepatocyte have been identified. Once inside the hepatocyte, bilirubin appears to interact with membrane lipids such that it may transfer from membrane to membrane (e.g., plasma membrane to endoplasmic reticulum). Bilirubin within the hepatocyte can also bind to cytoplasmic proteins (e.g., glutathione-S-transferase or ligandin). Once bilirubin IXα reaches the endoplasmic reticulum, the COOH groups of one or both of its propionic acid side chains are esterified (conjugated) with glucuronic acid by the enzyme bilirubin UDP-glucuronosyltransferase (one of a family of isoforms of UDP-glucuronosyltransferases), to form bilirubin monoglucuronides and bilirubin diglucuronide. Under normal conditions, the majority of bilirubin conjugates in bile are bilirubin diglucuronide (80%). When UDP-glucuronosyltransferase is deficient (e.g., Gilbert's syndrome) or when the amount of the cofactor UDP-glucuronic acid is decreased (e.g., decreased availability due to fasting, or enhanced utilization with acetaminophen overdose), relatively less bilirubin diglucuronide is formed relative to bilirubin monoglucuronides.

The process involved in the transport of bilirubin glucuronides to and across the canalicular membrane and into the bile are poorly understood. The hepatocyte microtubular system, hepatic bile salt excretion, and membrane carrier proteins all appear to facilitate the excretion of bilirubin glucuronides into bile. The process of biliary excretion, the rate-limiting step in bilirubin transport, is susceptible to damage from a variety of acquired liver diseases, which leads to an increased concentration of serum-conjugated bilirubin. Bilirubin conjugates reflux from bile or from the hepatocyte itself into plasma via poorly defined mechanisms. In addition, a small fraction of these bilirubin conjugates are deconjugated, resulting in increased plasma unconjugated as well as conjugated bilirubin levels in these disorders (e.g., jaundice due to drugs such as chlorpromazine, viral hepatitis, extrahepatic obstruction). Finally, most of these disorders are characterized by concomitant diminished bile salt excretion (cholestasis), hence elevated serum bile salt levels.

SERUM BILIRUBIN DETERMINATION

Serum bilirubin levels are measured in most clinical laboratories by the Van den Bergh method. Bilirubin in the presence of sulfanilic acid is split into two dipyrroles to form stable red-violet azopigments, which can be quantified by spectroscopy. Conjugated bilirubin gives an immediate, direct reaction, whereas unconjugated bilirubin, due to its hydrophobic, internally hydrogen-bonded structure, requires the addition of an accelerator (e.g., methanol, caffeine benzoate) to disrupt the hydrogen bonding and thus allow the diazotization reaction to take place. Up to 30% (0.3 mg/dL, or 5.1 μmol/L) of the total bilirubin in health is direct-reacting, even though only extremely small amounts of plasma-conjugated bilirubin exist in normal persons. This is because the direct fraction is overestimated, due to other compounds in plasma that react with sulfanilic acid and because a small portion of unconjugated bilirubin reacts in the absence of an accelerator. More accurate methods using high-performance liquid chromatography (HPLC) have been developed for measurement of bilirubin and its conjugates. In general, however, these methods are not available or necessary for the clinical evaluation of jaundiced patients.

APPROACH TO THE JAUNDICED PATIENT

Jaundice or hyperbilirubinemia can be due to predominantly unconjugated hyperbilirubinemia or to conjugated hyperbilirubinemia (see Table 1). Unconjugated hyperbilirubinemia

Table 1 Causes of Jaundice

Unconjugated hyperbilirubinemias
Hemolysis
Ineffective erythropoiesis
Impaired hepatic uptake of bilirubin
Crigler-Najar syndromes (types I and II)
Gilbert's syndrome
Physiological jaundice of the newborn
Conjugated hyperbilirubinemias
Dubin-Johnson syndrome
Rotor's syndrome
Hepatic storage disease
Hepatocellular diseases
Intrahepatic cholestasis
Extrahepatic cholestasis

(i.e., when the total serum bilirubin concentration exceeds 1.0–1.2 mg/dL and the direct fraction is less than 20–30% of the total) occurs when there is an increase in bilirubin production, impaired hepatic uptake of bilirubin, or diminished conjugation. Conjugated hyperbilirubinemia (i.e., an elevated total serum bilirubin concentration, with more than 30% of the total due to the direct fraction) is due to decreased biliary excretion of bilirubin with or without impaired bile flow. Conjugated hyperbilirubinemia with cholestasis is usually divided into intrahepatic and extrahepatic disorders. An algorithmic approach similar to that suggested in Chapter 1 may be helpful in determining etiology.

UNCONJUGATED HYPERBILIRUBINEMIA

Increased Bilirubin Production

Increased bilirubin production may occur with hemolysis or ineffective erythropoiesis. In both instances, the total serum bilirubin level (principally unconjugated bilirubin) rarely exceeds 4–5 mg/dL, and there is no bilirubinuria or serum delta bilirubin. Concomitant liver dysfunction in the presence of increased bilirubin production can result in increased serum levels of conjugated bilirubin as well. Common causes of hemolysis include sickle cell hemolytic crises, hereditary spherocytosis, paroxysmal nocturnal hemoglobinuria, and hemolytic anemias due to cold and warm autoantibodies. Ineffective erythropoiesis due to premature red blood cell destruction may cause an unconjugated hyperbilirubinemia, such as that seen with thalassemia and pernicious anemia. Bleeding into extravascular spaces with subsequent hemolysis (i.e., hematomas, hemothorax) also can result in unconjugated hyperbilirubinemia.

Impaired Hepatic Uptake of Bilirubin

Defects in hepatic bilirubin uptake are rare. Drugs such as rifampicin, rifamycin, and probenecid may interfere with bilirubin uptake and cause a reversible mild unconjugated hyperbilirubinemia.

Diminished Conjugation of Bilirubin

Crigler-Najjar type I syndrome is an autosomal recessive disorder in which there is no bilirubin UDP-glucuronosyltransferase activity. Essentially no bilirubin glucuronides are found in the bile. Mutations within exons common to all isoforms of UDP-glucuronosyltransferases as well as mutations affecting only exons of the bilirubin-conjugating isoform have been identified in these patients. Newborns with this disorder have serum bilirubin levels that usually exceed 20 mg/dL, virtually all of it unconjugated. Other liver function tests are normal. Nearly all of these children will develop severe neurological damage (i.e., kernicterus) despite treatment with phototherapy or plasmapheresis. Hepatic histology is normal. Phenobarbital therapy is ineffective because there is no enzyme present that can be induced. Thus, liver transplantation is the treatment of choice.

Crigler-Najjar type II syndrome is an inherited disorder, either autosomal dominant with incomplete penetrance or autosomal recessive, in which there is greatly reduced bilirubin UDP-glucuronosyltransferase activity due to mutations affecting exons of the bilirubin-conjugating isoform. Patients rarely if ever develop neurological disorders and usually live normal lives. Periodically, these patients may develop jaundice, with plasma bilirubin levels up to 6 to 25 mg/dL, largely unconjugated. Other liver function tests and hepatic histology are normal. The bile of these patients contains bilirubin conjugates, predominantly bilirubin monoglucuronides. This is most likely to occur during prolonged fasting or other illnesses. Phenobarbital therapy by enhancing enzyme activity results in a fall in plasma unconjugated bilirubin concentration and can be used for cosmetic reasons.

Gilbert's syndrome, in contrast to the two Crigler-Najjar syndromes, is much more common. Up to 7% of the population have Gilbert's syndrome, with a male-to-female ratio of about 4:1. Autosomal recessive inheritance seems likely. As in the Crigler-Najjar syndromes, liver histology and liver function tests are normal except for unconjugated hyperbilirubinemia. In Gilbert's syndrome, the plasma bilirubin level is less than 6 mg/dL, often less than 3 mg/dL. Patients with Gilbert's syndrome are well; their fluctuating hyperbilirubinemia may be exacerbated by stress, other illnesses, or fasting and ameliorated by phenobarbital or corticosteroid administration. Hyperbilirubinemia in some Gilbert's syndrome patients may be more pronounced by the concomitant presence of mild hemolytic disorders. Some Gilbert's patients have also been found to have mild defects in the hepatic uptake and intracellular transport of organic anions. However, the principal defect in Gilbert's syndrome is a mild decrease in bilirubin UDP–glucuronosyltransferase activity. An abnormality in the promoter region of bilirubin UDP–glucuronosyltransferase (TATA box sequence variation) has been identified in Gilbert's patients but may not be the only defect. Thus, an asymptomatic adult with periodic mild elevations of the plasma unconjugated bilirubin level with normal plasma aminotransferase and alkaline phosphatase levels and no signs of hemolysis can be assumed to have Gilbert's syndrome, a benign disorder.

Unconjugated hyperbilirubinemia is a common occurrence in the newborn—so-called physiological jaundice. Plasma-unconjugated bilirubin is normal at birth but rises in some neonates to 3–5 mg/dL in the first week, returning to normal in the second week. In some cases, the plasma bilirubin level can become much higher, putting the infant at risk for neurological disorders. The cause of physiological jaundice of the newborn is multifactorial, due primarily to the immaturity of the enzyme bilirubin UDP–glucuronosyltransferase but also to increased red cell destruction, diminished intracellular binding by ligandin, decreased biliary excretion of bilirubin conjugates, and increased intestinal deconjugation and reabsorption of bilirubin. Other conditions, such as hypothyroidism, must be excluded. Treatment of more severe cases of physiological jaundice of the newborn includes phototherapy, exchange transfusion, and avoidance of drugs (e.g., aspirin, sulfa drugs) and conditions (e.g., acidosis) that displace bilirubin from albumin. Tin protoporphyrin may be of use in the future.

CONJUGATED HYPERBILIRUBINEMIA

Decreased Biliary Excretion of Bilirubin Without Cholestasis

The Dubin-Johnson syndrome is a benign hereditary disorder characterized by recurrent episodes of jaundice. The inheritance of this disorder is autosomal recessive, and the defect involves the transport of conjugated bilirubin and other organic anions across the canalicular membrane. Periodically, patients develop a conjugated hyperbilirubinemia without cholestasis. Serum bile salt levels are normal, and besides jaundice, patients with Dubin-Johnson syndrome are asymptomatic. Because of the conjugated hyperbilirubinemia, delta bilirubin may be found in the plasma. Macroscopically the liver is darkly pigmented, due to retention of nontoxic epinephrine-like compounds. This pigment may disappear after a bout of viral hepatitis. The plasma bilirubin level usually is 2–5 mg/dL but may be much higher with pregnancy or estrogen administration. Pregnancy in patients with Dubin-Johnson syndrome may be complicated by fetal loss more often than in normal persons. Because of the defect in canalicular excretion of organic anions, these patients may have nonvisualization of the gallbladder on oral cholecystography, and with dimethyliminodiacetic acid usually shows prompt, intense homogenous and prolonged visualization of the liver with no visualization of the biliary tree and gallbladder. Urinary coproporphyrin analysis demonstrates normal total coproporphyrins with coproporphyrin I accounting for over 80% of the total (coproporphyrin III is normally 75% of the total).

Two other extremely rare and poorly defined disorders, Rotor's syndrome and Hepatic storage disease, are also characterized by intermittent conjugated hyperbilirubinemia without other symptoms and without cholestasis. These disorders appear to involve defective uptake and storage of bilirubin conjugates and other organic anions and are inherited in an autosomal recessive manner.

Decreased Biliary Excretion of Bilirubin with Cholestasis

Most adult patients with jaundice are cholestatic, with elevated serum bile salt levels. Usually, the hepatic alkaline phosphatase level (see Chap. 1) is also increased, along with that of delta bilirubin. Jaundice with cholestasis can be characterized as intrahepatic (i.e., hepatocellular, bile canalicular, or bile ductular or involving the intrahepatic bile ducts) or extrahepatic (i.e., obstruction of the extrahepatic bile ducts). The differential diagnosis for intrahepatic cholestasis with jaundice (e.g., drugs, hormones, hepatitic viruses, toxins, immunological disease, infections, total parenteral nutrition, inherited metabolic disorders, fatty liver disorders, primary biliary cirrhosis, sarcoidosis, cholestatic jaundice of pregnancy, postoperative jaundice, tumors, cysts, abscesses, and granulomas) and for extrahepatic cholestasis with jaundice (e.g., gallstones, tumors and strictures of the extrahepatic bile ducts, ampullary carcinoma, cancer of the head of the pancreas, choledochal cyst, biliary atresias, and primary and secondary sclerosing cholangitis) is large. Imaging studies (see

Chaps. 1 and 2), such as ultrasound and computed tomography, are useful in differentiating large-duct, extrahepatic from intrahepatic causes of cholestatic jaundice. More invasive diagnostic tests (i.e., liver biopsy, cholangiopancreatography) may then be indicated.

BIBLIOGRAPHY

Berk PD, Noyer C, eds. Bilirubin metabolism and the hereditary hyperbilirubinemias. Semin Liver Dis 1994; 14:321–394.

Bosma PJ, Chowdhury JR, Bakker C, Gantla S, de Boer A, Oostra BA, Lindhout D, Tytgat GN, Jansen PL, Oude Elferink RP, Chowdhury NR. The genetic basis of the reduced expression of bilirubin UDP-glucuronosyltransferase 1 in Gilbert's syndrome. N Engl J Med 1995; 333:1171–1175.

Bosma PJ, Seppen J, Goldhoorn B, Bakker C, Oude Elferink RP, Chowdhury JR, Chowdhury NR, Jansen PL. Bilirubin UDP-glucuronosyltransferase 1 is the only relevant bilirubin glucuronidating isoform in man. J Biol Chem 1994; 269:17960–17964.

Crawford JM, Gollan JL. Bilirubin metabolism and the pathophysiology of jaundice. In: Schiff L, Schiff ER, eds. Diseases of the Liver. Philadelphia: Lippincott, 1993:42–84.

Hauser SC, Gollan J. Bilirubin metabolism and hyperbilirubinemic disorders. In: Millward-Sadler GH, Wright R, Arthur MJP, eds. Wright's Liver and Biliary Disease. London: Saunders, 1992:317–370.

Seppen J, Bosma PJ, Goldhoorn BG, Bakker CT, Chowdhury JR, Chowdhury NR, Jansen PL, Oude Elferink RP. Discrimination between Crigler-Najjar type I and II by expression of mutant bilirubin uridine diphosphate-glucuronosyltransferase. J Clin Invest 1994; 94:2385–2391.

4

Interpretation of Serological and Virological Tests for Hepatitis

Dilip K. Moonka
Henry Ford Health Systems, Detroit, Michigan

Christopher B. O'Brien
University of Miami, Miami, Florida

INTRODUCTION

Viral hepatitis represents a worldwide health problem of enormous magnitude. Fortunately, the understanding of viral hepatitis has grown dramatically and has benefited from advances in modern molecular biology. These advances in the biology of viral hepatitis have led to a growing array of antiviral therapies. It is important to understand the complex group of diagnostic assays when determining appropriate antiviral therapy. This chapter provides a practical discussion of diagnostic modalities available to practicing physicians. The discussion includes the principles and uses of classic serological assays, as well as newer assays based on molecular methodologies. Emphasis is placed on the advantages and limitations of each in the diagnosis of viral hepatitis.

The physician should always have a systematic approach to the evaluation of a patient with suspected liver disease. A positive test result does not always mean that the physician can end the evaluation of the patient, as it is not uncommon for a patient to have more than one etiology for liver disease. The clinical diagnosis of viral hepatitis is made by establishing the presence of hepatic inflammation, identifying laboratory evidence of one or more of the hepatitis viruses, and excluding noninfectious causes of liver disease. There are five classic hepatitis viruses: hepatitis A (HAV), hepatitis B (HBV), hepatitis C (HCV), hepatitis D (HDV), and hepatitis E (HEV). Although there was a tentative description of a hepatitis F, subsequent investigators have been unable to confirm the identification. There is also much current interest in the hepatitis G virus (HGV); while it is discussed briefly, it is not clear at this time that HGV is a true hepatic pathogen.

Principles of Serological Diagnostic Assays

Serological assays remain the primary means to detect viral hepatitis at the present time. These assays provide indirect but generally accurate evidence of viral infection by identifying antibody produced by a patient in response to the presence of a virus.

Serological assays have the advantages that they are widely available through commercial labs, easy to perform, and highly reproducible. For HAV, HBV, and HEV, serological assays have the additional potential to distinguish between acute and chronic infection. Antibody of the IgM class is the first class of antibody to appear in response to a foreign antigen and usually becomes undetectable within several (5 to 7) months after the initial infection. This IgM response precedes the IgG antibody response, which can last for many years. Unfortunately, serological assays for the IgM antibody in HCV and HDV have not been able to distinguish acute versus chronic disease. Serological assays also have another disadvantage in that they lack the sensitivity to detect the cause of hepatitis early in its clinical presentation.

Enzyme Immunoassay (EIA)

The primary serological assay currently in use is an enzyme immunoassay (EIA). Radioimmunoassays (RIA) are still commercially available for some serological assays. But, RIAs are used less and less because EIAs are now as accurate as RIA, easier to use, and avoid problems that arise from the use of radioactive material. Enzyme-linked immunosorbent assays (ELISAs) are a form of EIA.

The general concepts behind an EIA or ELISA are relatively straightforward (see Fig. 1). Serum or plasma from a patient is added to a well coated with viral proteins (antigens). If the patient has antibody specific to the virus, it will bind the viral proteins, forming an antigen-antibody complex. If antiviral antibody is not present, the complex will not form. Unbound material is then washed off and a detector antibody is added. The detector antibody is typically an antibody generated in mice or goats directed against the constant region of the human antibody. This detector antibody is conjugated with an enzyme, usually horseradish peroxidase (HRPO), that produces a chemiluminescent product when provided with the appropriate substrates, usually *o*-phenylenediamine (OPD) and hydrogen peroxide. After the detector antibody is allowed to bind to the antiviral antibody and unbound reagents are washed off, an enzyme substrate is added and the presence of virus-specific antibody confirmed by the generation of the chemiluminescent product.

There are many variations on the basic EIA. If the detector antibody is generated specifically against the human IgM heavy-chain constant region, the EIA can assay directly for an IgM antibody against a particular virus (indicator of acute infection). In addition, combinations of viral proteins can be used to coat the wells, instead of a single protein, to improve sensitivity and specificity, as has been done with second- and third-generation assays for anti-HCV antibody. Finally, EIA assays can be constructed to provide quantitative assessments of antibody against a specific virus.

Recombinant Immunoblot Assay (RIBA)

The RIBA-2 (Chiron; Emeryville, CA) is an immunoassay with four recombinant HCV antigens placed as individual bands bound to a nitrocellulose strip. If the patient's serum contains HCV antibody, it will bind to the complementary HCV antigen on the RIBA test strip. Goat antihuman IgG labeled with horseradish peroxidase (HRPO) will bind to the HCV antibody that is immobilized on the RIBA strip. This HRPO produces a brown band

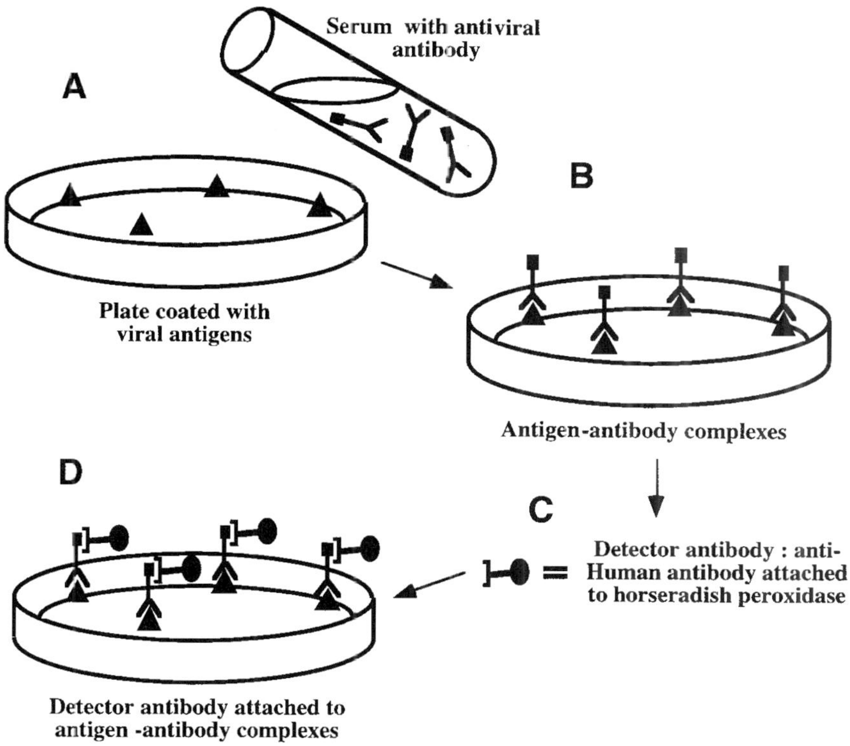

Figure 1 Enzyme immunoassay (EIA) technique. Panel A: serum containing the antiviral antibody is added to a plate (or more often a well) coated with the viral antigens. Panel B: antibody and antigen bind to form complexes. Panel C: detector antibody is added. This antibody is directed against human immunoglobulin and conjugated to the enzyme horseradish peroxidase. Panel D: The detector antibody binds to the antibody-antigen complexes and produces a chemiluminescent product when the appropriate enzyme substrate is added.

when developed with OPD and hydrogen peroxide. The advantage of the RIBA format is that it allows the detection of antibody to individual antigens or bands.

Principles of Molecular Diagnostic Techniques

The array of tools that molecular biologists can bring to the study of biological systems is now extensive. These molecular techniques, which include the cloning of all hepatitis viruses, have allowed major advances in the understanding of the natural history of these viral infections. However, the methods that are of most immediate relevance to clinicians are those that allow the detection and quantitation of viral nucleic acids in patient serum. These assays are used primarily in the evaluation of patients with hepatitis B and C infections.

The most frequently used molecular assays of viral nucleic acids are molecular hybridization, branched-chain DNA assays, and the polymerase chain reaction (PCR).

There are both advantages and disadvantages to the application of these assays in the evaluation of patients with viral hepatitis. They offer more direct evidence of viral replication that does not rely on a functioning immune system. The sensitivity and specificity of these assays often compare favorably with those of serological assays. They can also identify infection very early, at a time when serological and biochemical tests may not yet be abnormal. Furthermore, the assays can usually distinguish between persistent and resolved infections, measure levels of virus, and monitor response to antiviral therapy. These methods, however, are technically demanding. PCR, in particular, is so sensitive that there is significant potential for false-positive tests from laboratory contamination. Finally, because many of these tests are just now entering into widespread practice, their reliability, precise interpretation, and roles are still being defined.

Molecular Hybridization

One of the first and simplest approaches to the detection of viral RNA or DNA is molecular hybridization. In this method, RNA or DNA is extracted from patient serum and then fixed to nitrocellulose or nylon membranes (see Fig. 2). The transfer of viral RNA or DNA is often accomplished with a slot or dot device. The resulting assay is, therefore, termed either a slot- or dot-blot hybridization. The membranes are then exposed to probes. These probes are short pieces of DNA called oligonucleotides which contain a nucleotide sequence that is complementary to viral nucleic acid sequences. The probes are labeled with radioactive isotopes, chemiluminescent markers, or an enzyme (similar to those used for EIA, described above) that produces a signal if the probe binds to the viral nucleic acids. Hybridization assays can be standardized to provide quantitative data about the amount of viral nucleic acid present in serum because the amount of probe that binds to the membrane is in proportion to the quantity of viral nucleic acid present. The major drawback to hybridization techniques is that they lack the sensitivity of PCR techniques. Slot- and dot-blot techniques are still used commercially for the detection of HBV DNA but not HCV RNA, because titers of circulating HBV DNA are typically many logs higher than those of HCV RNA.

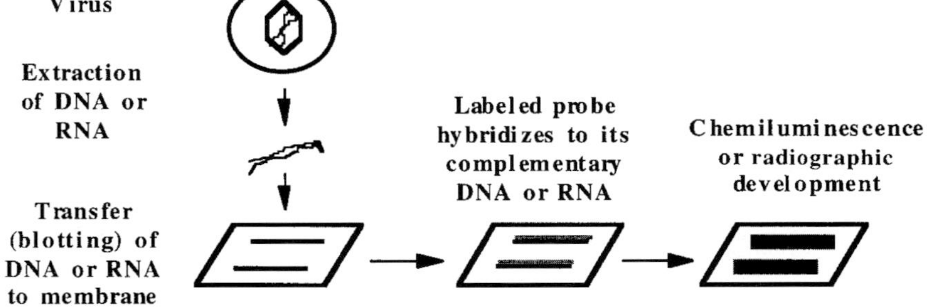

Figure 2 Technique of molecular hybridization. Viral RNA or DNA is extracted and then fixed ("blotted") onto a nitrocellulose membrane. The membrane is then exposed to probes specific for the viral nucleic acid and unbound probe is washed off. Bound probe is detected through either radioactive or chemiluminescent markers attached to the probe.

Branched DNA (bDNA) Amplification

The branched DNA (bDNA) signal-amplification assay is a widely used test. The advantage of the assay is that it is relatively easy to use and provides a highly standardized, reproducible quantitation of viral nucleic acids. In this assay, serum RNA or DNA is added to microwells coated with oligonucleotide probes specific for viral nucleic acids. The "capture" probes hybridize to the viral nucleic acids and immobilize them in the wells. Additional "target" probes are then added that bind to exposed sequences of the immobilized viral nucleic acids. The "target probes," in turn, bind to "reporter" probes consisting of branched chains of DNA complexed to alkaline phosphatase. A substrate is added for the alkaline phosphatase, resulting in a chemiluminescent product that is measured to provide a quantitation of the viral nucleic acid present. The branched DNA amplifies the signal approximately 10,000:1. The bDNA amplification assays have proven to be reproducible and easier to perform than PCR assays. As with hybridization assays, they lack the sensitivity of PCR to detect very low levels of virus, and this has again been a problem specifically in the detection and quantitation of HCV RNA in serum or plasma.

Polymerase Chain Reaction (PCR)

The most sensitive of the molecular assays for the detection of virus is PCR, which allows even minute quantities of DNA to be amplified to easily detectable levels. In theory, PCR conditions can be adjusted so that even a single copy of viral DNA can be successfully amplified. PCR, in the simplest terms, can be thought of as a reaction consisting of repeated cycles in which the target DNA in a tissue sample is doubled in number with each cycle. Hence, if there is 1 copy of viral DNA present at the start of a PCR, there will be 2 copies after one cycle, 4 after two cycles, and 2^{10} or approximately 1000 copies after 10 cycles. Because PCR amplifications typically consist of 30–40 cycles, millions of copies of DNA can be amplified from small numbers of original target DNA, and this amount of DNA is readily detectable.

A brief description of PCR is provided in Figure 3. Each cycle of PCR consists of three steps called *denaturation*, *annealing*, and *extension*. Total DNA extracted from a tissue sample, a pair of primers, free nucleotides, and a thermostable DNA polymerase are combined in a reaction tube. The primers are small pieces of DNA or oligonucleotides that are synthesized to be complementary and specific to the target DNA at its ends or flanking regions. The reaction is first heated so that the double-stranded DNA separates or "denatures" into two single strands. The reaction is then cooled so that primers can bind or "anneal" to the target DNA. The reaction is then heated to an intermediate temperature that is optimal for the activity of the DNA polymerase. The DNA polymerase attaches to the primer and uses the free nucleotides to synthesize a new strand in a step called "extension." At the end of the cycle two new double-stranded copies of the target DNA exist for each original copy. The cycle is then repeated. Critical to the reaction are the programmable PCR thermocyclers or heating blocks that can move precisely between the three temperatures necessary for each of the three steps and the thermostable DNA polymerases that are not destroyed by the high temperatures required by the denaturation step.

PCR will amplify only DNA and not RNA. To amplify viral RNA—as is necessary for RNA viruses such as HAV, HCV, HDV, HEV, and HGV—an additional step is necessary. The RNA is extracted from tissue or serum and then reverse transcriptase, an enzyme, is used to make a copy of DNA (cDNA) from each RNA molecule. The cDNA can then be amplified as described. Reverse transcriptase is abbreviated RT, and the term

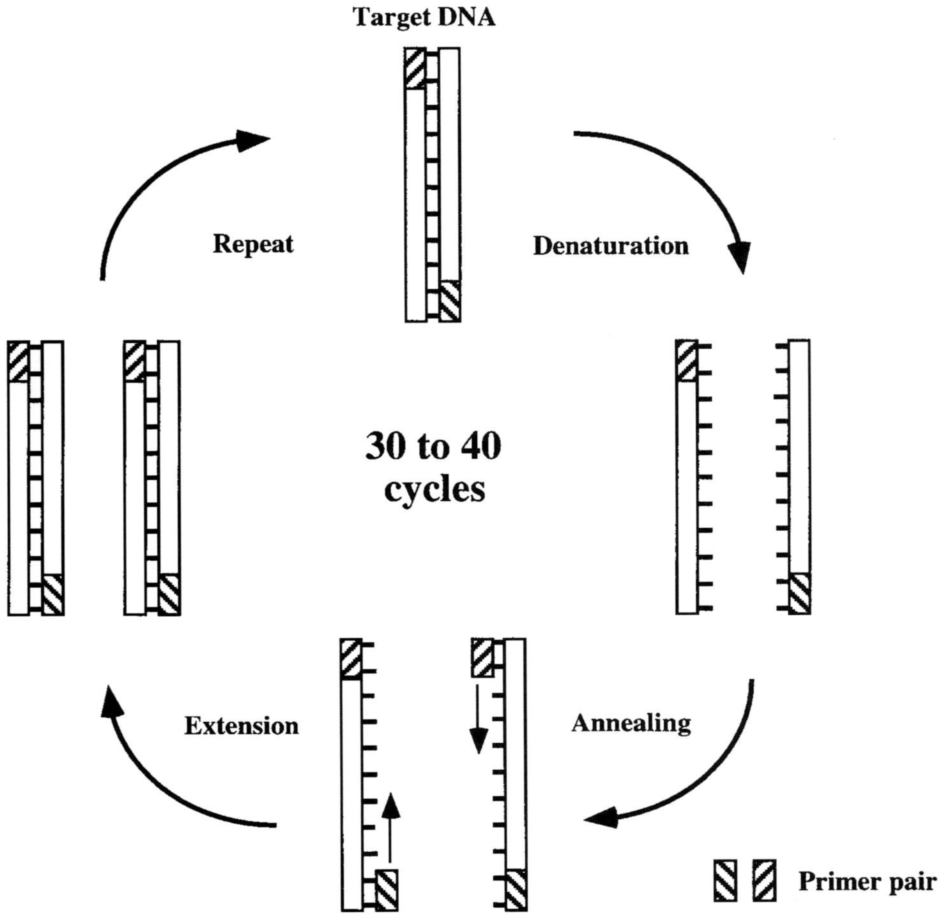

Figure 3 Polymerase chain reaction (PCR). PCR consists of repeated cycles. In each cycle the target DNA is "denatured" by heating it to separate the double-stranded DNA into single strands. The reaction is then cooled to allow primers specific to the target DNA to bind or "anneal" to their complementary sites. The reaction is then heated to an intermediate temperature ideal for the thermostable DNA polymerase to "extend" or complete the new strand. The cycle is then repeated.

RT-PCR is commonly used to describe the PCR reaction used to amplify and identify an RNA target.

Quantitative PCR

PCR amplifications are used not only to determine whether viral DNA or RNA is present in a patient's serum (qualitative PCR) but also to quantitate the amount of virus present (quantitative PCR). The primary concern with quantitative PCR is that the amplification of the target DNA is so powerful that it may not accurately reflect the amount of target initially present. A variety of approaches are used to address this concern. Control PCR reactions are typically run with a variety of known concentrations of viral DNA, which provide a curve to quantitate the amount of viral DNA in serum or tissue samples. In addition, the original tissue sample can be "spiked" with known amounts of a synthetic RNA or DNA. The synthetic nucleic acid is designed to be identical to the target nucleic acid at the ends where the primers bind, so that both the target and synthetic nucleic acids are amplified simultaneously. The efficiency of nucleic acid extraction and PCR or RT-PCR of the synthetic RNA or DNA can be determined and used to correct the quantitation of the amount of viral RNA or DNA originally present in the sample.

With both quantitative and qualitative PCR, contamination is a critical concern. Because PCR is so sensitive, even minute amounts of PCR produced from previous amplifications can easily contaminate subsequent PCR reactions, giving false-positive results. This potential can be reduced significantly by use of negative controls, methods to destroy products of previous PCR methods, and through the careful physical separation of prior PCR products from fresh serum samples. A variety of both quantitative and qualitative PCR assays are commercially available to clinicians. Unfortunately, contamination and varying reproducibility have been problems. The use of assays with published validation of the assay has simplified the management of our patients with chronic viral hepatitis.

HEPATITIS A

The hepatitis A virus (HAV) is an RNA virus of the Picornaviridae family. It is spread by the fecal-oral route, usually from ingestion of food or water contaminated with human fecal material. This virus is endemic in the developing world and approximately 80% of adults in areas of Africa and Asia have serological evidence of exposure. In the United States, approximately 40% of adults will be exposed to HAV in their lifetimes. There is no chronic form of HAV infection. Approximately 1% of infected patients can develop a fulminant viral hepatitis resulting in death or need for liver transplantation. The remainder recover without chronic sequelae, though a small percentage of patients can experience relapsing disease for up to 6 months. There is no specific therapy for HAV infection and the role of diagnosis is to exclude other forms of liver disease, prevent exposure of other individuals, and provide prophylactic therapy to individuals who were exposed.

Serological Assays for HAV

Diagnosis of acute HAV infection is made by a serological EIA for IgM anti-HAV. This assay is directed against parts of the VP1 capsid protein that do not vary significantly among different HAV strains. Symptoms typically occur within 20–45 days of exposure; the IgM anti-HAV is almost always detectable at that time and remains detectable for up to 6 months (see Fig. 4).

Conversely, HAV RNA levels in stool and blood decline at this time, which explains why patients are usually not infectious at the time of presentation. The IgM anti-HAV assay has both a sensitivity and a specificity of over 99%. There are only rare reported cases in which the IgM anti-HAV was not elevated at the time of presentation but was detectable on repeat testing several weeks later. While total anti-HAV (IgM, IgG) tests are available, they are not useful in the diagnosis of acute infection because the IgG may be elevated from a distant prior infection, especially in populations with high HAV prevalence rates. RT-PCR assays for HAV RNA in both serum and stool are used in research settings but have not found a role in clinical practice.

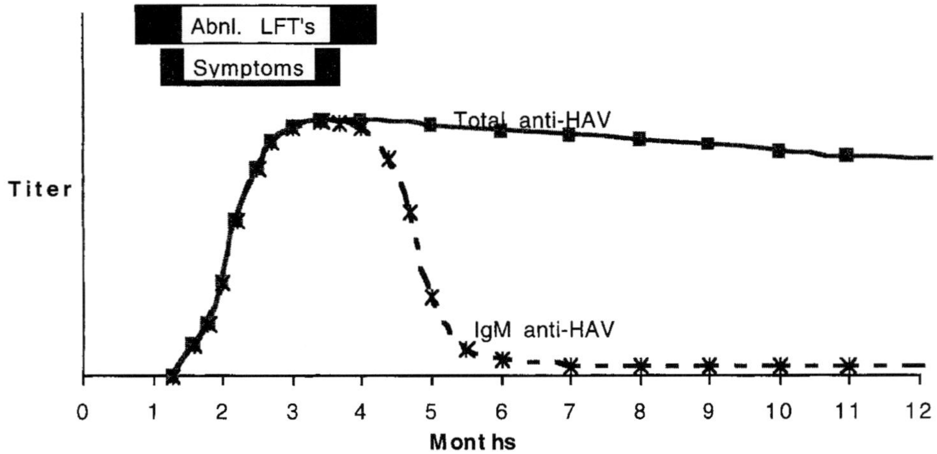

Figure 4 Hepatitis A serologies. Time courses of clinical events and antiviral serological response to a hepatitis A infection. The total anti-HAV consists of both the IgM anti-HAV and the IgG anti-HAV. The IgM component declines over time and only the IgG fraction remains detectable after 6 months.

Serological Assays After Use of Immune Serum Globulin or HAV Vaccines

Issues arise in the interpretation of anti-HAV serologies in patients who have received either immune serum globulin (ISG) or hepatitis A vaccines. While ISG can contain a significant amount of IgG anti-HAV and result in a positive test for total anti-HAV antibody, ISG does not contain a detectable amount of IgM anti-HAV. A positive IgM test even in a patient who has received ISG signifies an acute HAV infection. Vaccination with both the HAVRIX (SmithKline Beecham Biologicals, Inc.) and VAQTA (Merck & Company, Inc.) results in levels of IgG anti-HAV that are typically 10- to 100-fold less than those produced by natural infection. Nevertheless, vaccination can result in detectable levels of IgG anti-HAV using standard assays but rarely results in detectable levels of the IgM anti-HAV. In some instances, the clinician may wish to confirm the presence of protective levels of anti-HAV antibody after vaccination. Modification of assays from both Abbott Laboratories (Abbott Park, IL) and SmithKline Biologicals can detect anti-HAV antibody as low as the minimal protective level of 20 MIU/mL. The clinician should contact his reference laboratory about the availability of these assays. In any case, administration of either ISG or vaccination should not interfere with the diagnosis of acute HAV infection with the IgM anti-HAV assay.

HEPATITIS B

Chronic hepatitis B viral infection remains one of the world's major medical problems and is a leading cause of morbidity and mortality. The hepatitis B virus (HBV) is a small, double-stranded, circular, DNA virus of the Hepadnaviridae family. The diagnosis of hepatitis B is dependent upon detection of the presence of the hepatitis B surface antigen

(HBsAg). A typical patient will acquire hepatitis B and successfully clear the virus within several months. Resolution of hepatitis B occurs when the patient mounts a successful immune response. This immune response consists of a high titer, neutralizing antibody to the hepatitis B surface antigen (hepatitis B surface antibody: anti-HBs), with subsequent loss of the HBsAg. Unfortunately, approximately 5–10% of adults do not lose detectable HBsAg within a 6-month period of time and develop chronic infection.

In addition to testing for hepatitis B, all patients should be tested for coinfection with the hepatitis C virus (HCV) and the hepatitis D virus (HDV).

Diagnosis of Acute Hepatitis B

The hepatitis B surface antigen appears very early (within 3–4 weeks) in the blood of patients with acute hepatitis B. The serum aminotransferases soon rise, and shortly thereafter the patient typically develops symptoms of acute viral hepatitis. Both the IgM and the IgG antibodies to the hepatitis B core (anti-HBc) become detectable and peak within 10–14 weeks after their initial appearance in serum (see Fig. 5).

The diagnosis of an acute hepatitis B infection is dependent upon the detection of the IgM antibody to the core protein of the hepatitis B virus (IgM anti-HBc). This IgM antibody occurs early, within 4–6 weeks of exposure. The IgM anti-HBc typically peaks after 12–16 weeks; with resolution of the infection, it becomes nondetectable within 6 months. The IgG anti-HBc is slower to resolve and remains detectable for years. It is important to test for the IgM anti-HBc because not all patients who present with symptoms and a positive HBsAg have acute hepatitis B. A patient who presents for the first time with a positive HbsAg may have either recently acquired acute hepatitis B or a superimposed hepatitis due to hepatitis A, hepatitis C, hepatitis D, or a hepatotoxic medication.

The hepatitis B "e" antigen (HBeAg) has been the most commonly used marker of active viral replication. This protein is produced at the same time that the HBV DNA is produced and is detected shortly after the HBsAg (see Fig. 6). It is during this time period

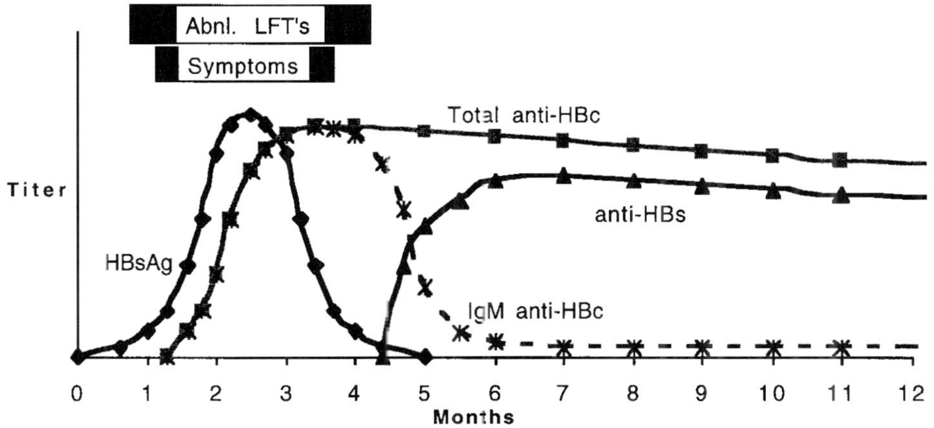

Figure 5 Generalized time course of clinical events and hepatitis B serologies for an acute, self-limited hepatitis B infection. The HBsAg peaks and becomes undetectable within 6 months. The total anti-HBV consists of both the IgM anti-HBV and the IgG anti-HBV. The IgM component declines over time and only the IgG fraction remains detectable after 6 months.

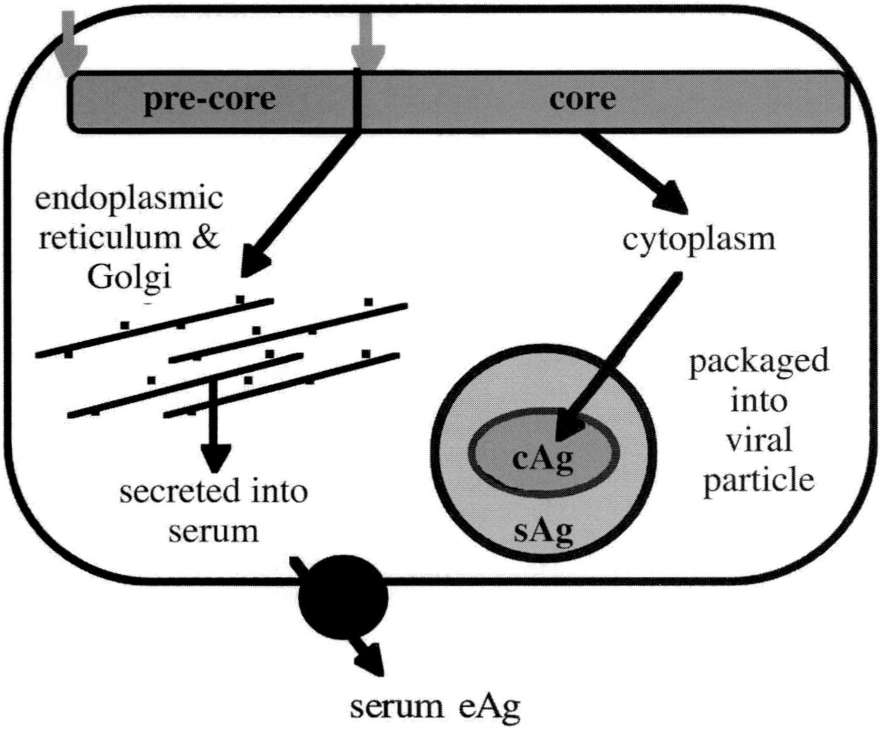

Figure 6 Hepatitis B "e" Antigen. The top arrows designate the two possible starts of transcription of the HBV nucleocapsid protein (the core of the virus). The HBV's DNA polymerase can transcribe both the precore and core segments. The mRNA is processed through the rough endoplasmic reticulum and then the Golgi apparatus. The protein is secreted into the serum as the "e" antigen. Alternatively, only the shorter core segment is transcribed, processed in the cytoplasm, and packaged into the viral particle as its nucleocapsid.

that the patient is the most infectious. The hepatitis B virus is thought to generate the HBeAg in an attempt to induce a state of tolerance from the patient's immune system, thereby enabling the virus to set up a chronic infection. The loss of the HBeAg with the development of anti-HBe implies that the patient is on the way to clearance of the hepatitis B.

Direct testing for hepatitis B viral DNA (HBV DNA) has now replaced serological detection of "e" antigen as the preferred marker for viral replication. Originally, circulating HBV DNA was felt to be present in serum only during the early period of an acute infection. This was based on observations using slot- or dot-blot hybridization assays to detect HBV DNA. Recently, many diagnostic testing laboratories have adopted the branched-chain DNA (bDNA) assay as a more accurate quantitative assay with an improvement in sensitivity (approximately 10^5 genome equivalents per milliliter) over the slot-blot technique (approximately 10^6 genome equivalents per milliliter). Even more recently, PCR techniques have become available for the detection of HBV DNA (sensitivity of 10^2 genome equivalents per milliliter). With the advent of the bDNA (Chiron Corporation, Emeryville, CA) and PCR assays (National Genetics Institute, Culver City, CA), it is now clear that HBV DNA usually persists despite the conversion of the HBeAG to anti-HBe. Neither assay is FDA-approved for this indication at the present time. At present, both the bDNA and PCR determinations of HBV DNA titers are performed for research purposes only.

Diagnosis of Chronic Hepatitis B

Evolution to chronic hepatitis B infection occurs if hepatitis B surface antigen (HBsAg) persists in serum for over 6 months (see Fig. 7). This is due to the inability of the patient's immune system to produce sufficient quantities of the hepatitis B surface antibody (anti-HBs), an antibody directed against HBsAg, which is neutralizing and protective and usually heralds resolution of infection. Approximately 10–15% of patients can have both detectable HBsAg and anti-HBs.

Patients who are persistently HBsAg-positive should undergo evaluation to determine the activity of the HBV replication. The evaluation should include serum HBV DNA, HBeAg, and anti-HBe. Those patients with active hepatitis B viral replication will usually have both detectable HBV DNA and HBeAg. The presence of circulating HBV DNA and HBeAg identifies patients who may benefit from antiviral therapy and provides the means to follow their response to therapy (see Chap. 7).

Viral replication also may slowly decrease over time, or the viral activity can fluctuate from periods of apparent quiescence to dynamic viral reproduction. The periods of viral inactivity (or low replication) are characterized by HBsAg positivity, nondetectable serum HBV DNA, nondetectable HBeAg, and normal serum aminotransferases. Patients with this latent viral state are termed *healthy carriers*. It is debatable whether this is an accurate description of the true state of affairs.

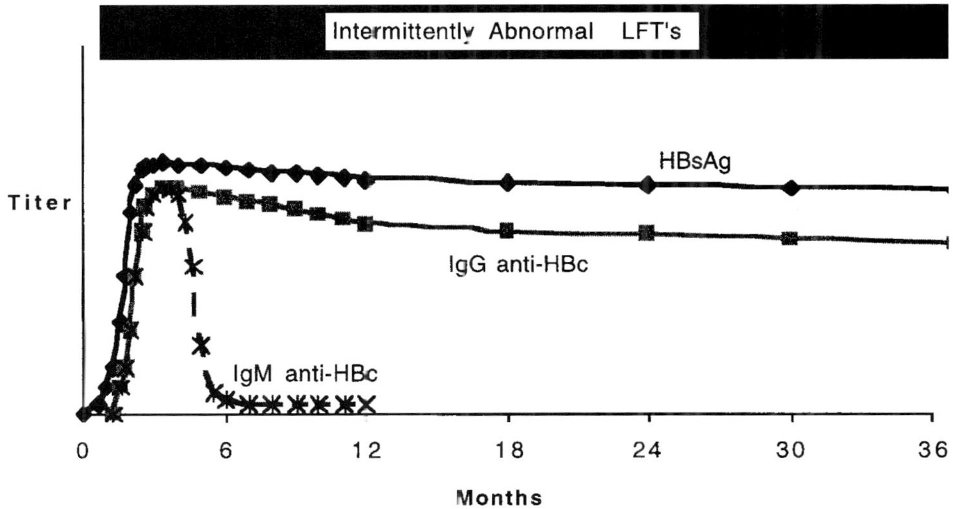

Figure 7 Time course of clinical events and hepatitis B serologies for chronic hepatitis B infection. Those patients that are unable to successfully clear HBsAg within 6 months develop chronic infection with the virus. The hepatitis B surface antibody (anti-HBs) usually does not become detectable by conventional serologies.

Table 1 Hepatitis B: Classical Serological Patterns

Presentation	HBsAg	HBcAb IgM	HBcAb IgG	HBsAb
Acute	+++	+++	+++	
Chronic	+++	+++	+++	
Recovered			+++	+++
Vaccinated				+++

The above description is classic for the serological patterns found with chronic hepatitis B (see Table 1). It now appears that this description is, to some degree, an oversimplification that reflects the limited sensitivity of current testing methods. Typical cutoff sensitivities of the present serological tests are greater than 1 million copies per milliliter of serum. Because the hepatitis B virus is typically found at levels much higher than this (10^9 to 10^{12}), currently available serological tests will allow an accurate diagnosis most of the time. But more sensitive molecular testing methods (available on a research basis only) demonstrate that virtually all patients with chronic hepatitis B harbor both HBsAg and anti-HBs, both HBeAg and anti-HBe, and low levels of HBV DNA at all times. The viral antigen forms complexes with its complementary antibody. Whatever remains in excess is detected by the current serological assays. The substance in lower titer is completely bound in antigen-antibody complexes and is not available to be measured. It is the relative shifts in the balance between viral replication and the magnitude of the patient's immune response to the virus that determine the final serological results. With some newer, more sensitive serological assays, almost 10–40% of patients will have simultaneous detection of anti-HBs and HBsAg.

Serological Pattern After Vaccination

A patient who has received the hepatitis B vaccination will develop detectable anti-HBs. Since the vaccine contains only the surface antigen of the virus, there can be no immunity to the core region of the virus. Therefore, a patient who has developed immunity after vaccination should have no detectable anti-HBc. Any patient that has both anti-HBs and anti-HBc has gained immunity by exposure to the actual virus and not through vaccination. Overall, the titer of anti-HBs tends to be higher in those patients who acquire immunity after exposure to the hepatitis B virus and declines more slowly than the anti-HBs that develops after vaccination.

Patients with Atypical Serological Patterns

Isolated Positive Antibody to the Hepatitis B Core Antigen (HBcAb)

This may occur in two different ways. The first situation occurs when a patient has had hepatitis B for a very long time. This patient is a chronic carrier and has an anti-HBs that actually is positive but has declined over time to a low titer, just below the limits of detectability of the standard assays. In this situation, if the patient is given the hepatitis B vaccine, there will be a prompt, amnestic response in the titer of the antibody so that it can be detected by the conventional anti-HBs assay.

The second possibility is that the patient could have a very low level viral infection with an HBsAg that is positive, but below the limits of detection for the HBsAg assay. To resolve this issue, the patient could be vaccinated with the hepatitis B vaccine, and the lack of an anti-HBs in 2 months would suggest inability to mount an immune response because of the continued (very low level) presence of the virus. Alternatively, PCR could be used to detect low-level HBV DNA in serum, demonstrating continued presence of the virus.

Precore Mutation Pattern

Some patients present with a positive HBsAg and a positive HBV DNA but no detectable HBeAg (see Table 2). Many of these patients have a particular "precore" mutation that introduces a "stop" codon into the HBV nucleotide sequence and prevents production of the HBeAg (see Fig. 8). This particular form of HBV infection, while described first in the Mediterranean countries, also occurs throughout Europe and the United States. When compared to the "wild-type" HBeAg-positive patients, patients infected with the precore mutant HBV have a decreased response to interferon-alpha and higher rates of relapse posttherapy.

Active Hepatitis B and (−) HBV DNA

Some patients will present with a positive HBsAg and elevated aminotransferases but undetectable HBV DNA and HBeAg. In these patients it is critical to rule out other causes of liver disease. It is likely that some of these patients do have HBV DNA present in their serum, but at a level that is too low to detect with current commercial HBV DNA assays. Newer quantitative PCR assays are currently under development. Their increased sensitivity may identify HBV DNA in some of these patients.

Coinfection with Hepatitis B and Hepatitis C

Approximately 10% of patients with HBV are also coinfected with HCV, although this number varies depending upon the patient population. The treatment of this group of patients is complicated by the observation that these patients tend to have more severe disease than seen with either virus alone. The viruses appear to "interfere" with or "suppress" the replication of each other. Most of the patients will have "low replication" HBV with positive anti-HBe and no detectable HBeAg or HBV DNA by commercial laboratory assay.

Serologies for Monitoring Therapy

Multiple studies have demonstrated that those patients most likely to respond to therapy with interferon-alpha have evidence of a strong, preexisting immune response to HBV, as suggested by low serum HBV DNA (less than 100 pg/mL) and high serum aminotransferases (ALT > 100 IU/L). Patients with high serum HBV DNA (greater than 100 pg/mL) and little evidence of hepatic inflammation (ALT < 100 IU/L) are least likely to respond.

Table 2 Chronic Hepatitis B: Markers of Viral Replication and Activity

Presentation	ALT	HBV DNA	HBeAg	HBeAb
Wild-type hepatitis	+++	−++	+++	
Precore mutant variant	+++	−++		+++
Healthy carrier				+++

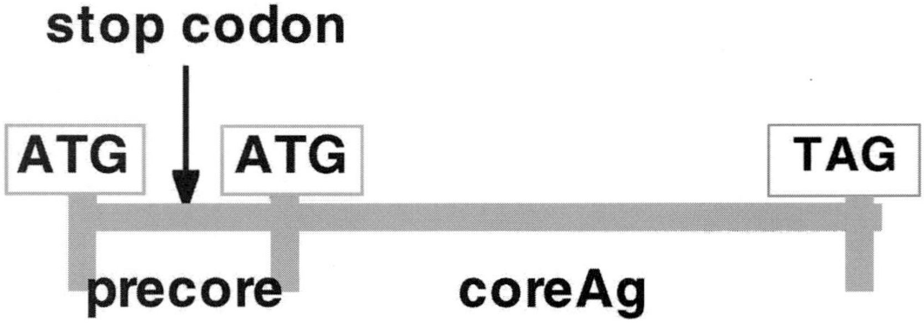

Figure 8 Hepatitis B precore mutants. The ATG codons are signals for the HBV's polymerase to initiate transcription of the downstream region (gene). A mutation in the precore region can produce a signal (stop codon) to stop the DNA polymerase from reading the encoded HBV DNA for the entire "e" antigen. These patients have no detectable "e" antigen. Since the second initiation site (for the core protein) is unaffected, the core (nucleocapsid) can be manufactured and incorporated into the viral particle.

As discussed, the endpoints used to determine "response" to therapy are the loss of serum HBV DNA and HBeAg and normalization of elevated serum aminotransferases. These are the most commonly used markers of active viral replication.

Despite the successes seen with interferon-alpha therapy for chronic hepatitis B, most patients do not respond. The most promising new drugs currently being used for hepatitis B are the nucleoside analogue compounds. The serological responses after therapy with this group of medications are not entirely clear at the present time.

HEPATITIS C

The hepatitis C virus (HCV) is an RNA virus of the Flaviviridae family which was first cloned in 1988. It was soon determined to be the cause of over 90% of non-A, non-B hepatitis infections in the world. While HCV infection can cause acute hepatitis, its most dramatic impact on world health is as a cause of chronic liver disease affecting hundreds of millions of individuals (see Chap. 9). After initial exposure, HCV RNA can be detected in blood within 1–3 weeks and anti-HCV antibodies subsequently appear. Over 90% of patients demonstrate detectable antibody within 3 months (see Fig. 9). In approximately 15% of patients, infection will resolve. The remainder develop chronic hepatitis with persistent viremia.

The development of serological tests for HCV has been critical in the diagnosis of HCV and in the prevention of transfusion-related HCV infection. However, serological assays have the disadvantages that they often do not detect anti-HCV antibody until months after infection, do not distinguish between persistent and resolved infection, and cannot monitor response to antiviral therapy. These limitations have resulted in the development of newer molecular assays that directly detect viral RNA in serum.

Serological Assays for HCV

Cloning of hepatitis C led directly to an enzyme immunoassay directed against a recombinant antigen, c100-3, from an HCV nonstructural protein (NS4). This first-generation anti-

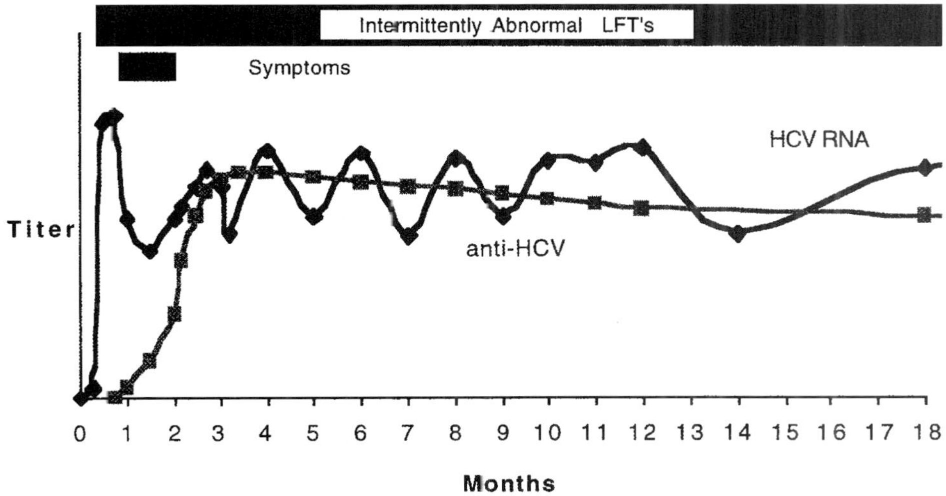

Figure 9 (Chronic) hepatitis C: time course of serologies. The HCV RNA rises very rapidly and becomes detectable at high titer within 1 to 2 weeks of the initial exposure. This titer then declines and tends to stabilize at a "characteristic level" for an individual patient. The HCV antibody (anti-HCV) usually takes 4 to 8 weeks to become positive. This antibody remains positive whether the patient resolves the infection or develops chronic hepatitis.

HCV test had suboptimal sensitivity and specificity. It was often not positive for 6 months or longer from the time of exposure. As a result, second- and third-generation tests and supplemental assays were developed that use multiple recombinant HCV antigens to detect anti-HCV antibodies. The second-generation Abbott (Abbott Park, IL) HCV EIA (v2.0) uses antigens from the core (C), NS3, and NS4 proteins. Using tests for HCV RNA as a "gold standard," this assay has a sensitivity of over 99% in low-prevalence populations and 92–95% in high-prevalence populations. Over 90% of infected patients have a positive result at 3 months after exposure. A third-generation EIA assay is now available that uses an additional antigen from the NS5 region. While this assay provides some incremental improvement in sensitivity, it does not provide the marked improvement seen with the second-generation tests.

Supplemental Serological Assays for HCV

A major concern with serological assays for hepatitis C is the high rate of false-positive tests (low specificity) seen when the test is used in low-prevalence populations. In groups such as blood donors, over half of all positive results can be false-positive. Supplemental tests, most notably the second-generation recombinant immunoblot assay (RIBA-2; Chiron, Emeryville, CA), are used to eliminate these false-positive results. The RIBA-2 is essentially an immunoassay with four recombinant HCV antigens arranged as individual bands on a nitrocellulose membrane. The RIBA format allows the detection of antibody to individual antigens or bands. If two or more bands are positive, the result is positive; if one band is positive, the result is indeterminate; and if no bands are positive, the result is negative. In low-prevalence populations with positive HCV EIA v2.0, 40–65% of RIBA-2 assays will be negative. But in high-prevalence populations—patients with risk factors for HCV transmission and elevated serum transaminases—over 90% of RIBA-2 tests will be positive.

Indeterminate RIBA-2 results can be evaluated for HCV RNA by RT-PCR. The number of indeterminate RIBA-2 assays that are positive for HCV RNA also varies with the prevalence rate of HCV in the particular population. In high-prevalence groups, approximately 20–50% of RIBA-2 indeterminate specimens are positive for HCV RNA, with much lower numbers for low-prevalence groups. For comparison, approximately 85% of RIBA-2 positive patients are positive for HCV RNA and almost no RIBA-2 negative patients have HCV RNA in their serum. It now appears that most positive and some indeterminate RIBA-2 assays with negative HCV RNA probably indicate patients with resolved HCV infection. A RIBA-3 test has been developed and is being evaluated in Europe. The test was designed to lower the number of indeterminate results and it remains to be seen whether it will achieve that goal.

Role of HCV RNA Assays

The precise role of assays for HCV RNA is still being defined, but there are clearly circumstances in which these assays provide important information to clinicians. In several clinical settings, results from serological tests may not provide an accurate assessment of the presence of HCV infection in an individual. These settings include those involving patients recently infected with HCV in whom serological tests have not yet become positive, immunocompromised patients (including organ transplant recipients) who may not be able to mount a detectable antibody response to HCV, patients who have an indeterminate RIBA assay result, and neonates who may not be infected with HCV (but who may have passively received anti-HCV antibody from their mothers). In the past, hepatitis C serologies could be misleading in patients who had received either immune serum globulin or intravenous immunoglobulin. However, this should no longer be a concern, because HCV positive donors are now excluded in the preparation of these products.

Molecular assays of HCV RNA also have an emerging role in determining therapy of chronic HCV infection (see Chap. 9). All patients with positive anti-HCV serological assays who are being considered for interferon-alpha therapy should be tested for serum HCV RNA. In up to 15% of these patients, HCV RNA will not be detected presumably because the positive serological assay reflects a resolved infection for which interferon-alpha is not indicated. HCV RNA assays can also be used to monitor response to therapy. Biochemical tests do not always reflect the presence or level of viremia. Interferon-alpha is generally given for 12 months for chronic HCV infection. However, patients who have received 3 months of interferon-alpha and have persistent elevation of serum ALT levels or presence of HCV RNA in serum have an extremely low likelihood of response, and their therapy can be discontinued. The definition of sustained response to therapy now includes the absence of detectable HCV RNA in serum 6 months after therapy has been completed.

Molecular Assays for HCV RNA

bDNA and RT-PCR

The branched DNA signal-amplification assay (bDNA) and RT-PCR are two approaches available to determine the presence and level of HCV RNA in serum. RT-PCR assays have traditionally varied enormously in accuracy and reliability from one reference laboratory to another. Standardization of results has proven difficult. For this reason, the bDNA assay (Chiron, Emeryville, CA) was originally an attractive alternative. This assay has been extensively evaluated and is highly standardized. Because the assay signal is amplified and not the HCV RNA target, there is less chance of product from one assay contaminating the results of another. The primary drawback to the bDNA assay is that it is less sensitive than RT-PCR. The lower limit of detectability is less than 400,000 copies per milliliter. This is of concern because patients with low viral titers are favorable candidates for interferon therapy. These patients may not be identified by the bDNA assay. Some hepatologists have advocated routine use of the bDNA assay to assess HCV RNA followed by RT-PCR for all negative bDNA results.

RT-PCR Assays

Recently two RT-PCR assays have emerged with better-documented standardization and reliability. The two assays are the Amplicor HCV Monitor (Roche Molecular Diagnostics, Branchburg, NJ) and the SuperQuant (National Genetics Institute, Culver City, CA) assays. Both provide quantitative and qualitative HCV RNA results. The Amplicor assay is a test kit with built-in controls for sensitivity and specificity. The quantitative Amplicor assay uses a known quantity of an internal standard RNA that is coamplified with the HCV RNA to control for the efficiency of the RT-PCR reaction. The Amplicor assays use novel technology to help prevent PCR contamination. The qualitative assay has been studied extensively and compared with optimized RT-PCR assays in research laboratories. It has excellent sensitivity and detects levels of serum HCV RNA with lower limits of detectability at 100 copies per milliliter with a specificity of 97–99%. The qualitative assay has a report linear range from 500 to 5×10^5 copies per milliliter. The SuperQuant assay also has a sensitivity of 100 copies of HCV RNA per milliliter and a reported quantitation range of 100 to 5×10^6 copies per milliliter. For both Amplicor and assays, titers greater than 5×10^6 copies per milliliter can be determined by serial dilutions. The SuperQuant assay is performed by National Genetics Institute at its central licensed clinical laboratory under fully automated, highly controlled conditions. Serum must be frozen immediately and shipped on dry ice by overnight delivery. The Amplicor assay is currently under evaluation for FDA approval.

HCV Genotyping

The clinician should be aware of the significance of the term *genotype* as it pertains to hepatitis C. HCV is classified on the basis of characteristic nucleotide sequences in certain regions of the hepatitis C genome. There are at least six major genotypes and numerous additional subtypes. Different genotypes of HCV vary in terms of geographic distribution and response to interferon. For instance, the most common genotypes in the United States by far are genotypes 1a and 1b; these are particularly resistant to interferon therapy. Genotyping is offered by National Genetics Institute (Culver City, CA) using the Inno-LiPA (Innogenetic, Belgium) assay. This assay is a reverse molecular hybridization assay in which probes specific for each of the six major genotypes are fixed to a membrane as individual bands. The membrane is immersed in a solution containing HCV RNA PCR product, and the product is allowed to hybridize to the appropriate band.

Approach to the Evaluation of HCV Infection

Current serological assays for HCV have excellent sensitivity. Specific situations are discussed above in which serological studies can be misleading, and the clinician should be alert to these situations. In practice, it is unusual to see a chronic hepatitis patient with negative serologies and a positive HCV RNA result. Patients with positive serologies, on the other hand, must have confirmation of detectable HCV RNA prior to therapy. A significant percentage of patients with positive serologies will not have detectable HCV RNA.

This is because false-positive results are still possible, even with a supplemental RIBA II/III test, and because up to 15% of patients infected with HCV spontaneously resolve their infection. Therapy is not indicated in these patients. A positive HCV RNA result indicates a patient is infected with the virus and may be an appropriate candidate for therapy.

The choice of which method to use to measure HCV RNA is not straightforward. At this time, no one test has emerged as being clearly superior to another. The practitioner should be aware of the actual test(s) being performed by his or her clinical laboratory and should understand that a negative result from a bDNA assay should be followed with a RT-PCR assay to confirm that HCV RNA is truly undetectable. It is hoped that as individual RT-PCR assays are further validated in on-going clinical trials, they will provide a single accurate test to detect and quantitate HCV RNA. While genotyping provides prognostic information and is available, its use is not recommended in standard patient care because it does not typically affect therapeutic decisions.

HEPATITIS D

In North America, HDV is most commonly found in intravenous drug users and in individuals who have received multiple transfusions, such as hemophiliacs. It is a small, defective RNA virus that is unable to manufacture its own surface coat. HDV requires the presence of the hepatitis B surface antigen to encapsulate its genome. As a result, individuals can become infected with HDV only if they are currently infected with HBV.

The simultaneous acquisition of both HDV and HBV is called a *coinfection*. Those patients who are chronic carriers of the HBV who acquire HDV later in time are said to have developed a *superinfection*. While patients with simultaneous acute HBV and HDV (coinfection) can develop a fulminant hepatitis more often than patients infected only with HBV, simultaneous infection usually follows the course of acute HBV. As with HBV, the vast majority of patients will resolve their infection and only approximately 5–10% of coinfected patients will develop chronic liver disease. Patients with chronic HBV infection who become superinfected with HDV, however, almost always develop a concomitant aggressive liver disease with chronic HDV (see Chap. 8).

Coinfection

The typical serological profile of a patient who acquires simultaneous hepatitis B and hepatitis D resembles that of a patient with acute hepatitis B alone.

Figure 10 shows the sequence of events of hepatitis D overlaid on those of hepatitis B. The hepatitis D antigen (HDAg) becomes detectable simultaneously with HBsAg and later disappears when the HBsAg is lost. IgM anti-HD rises after IgM anti-HBc and usually more slowly. This IgM anti-HD falls rapidly and is therefore useful for the diagnosis of acute coinfection with HBV and HDV. The IgG anti-HD appears later than its IgM component; it tends to decline more rapidly and persist for a shorter period of time than the IgG anti-HBc.

The only test commonly available for the diagnosis of hepatitis D is anti-HDV antibody. Similar to hepatitis B, the viral nucleic acids (in this case a RNA genome) can be identified by the use of slot-blot hybridization or the RT-PCR assay. The direct detection of HDAg is not commercially available and can only be obtained from a university or government research laboratory.

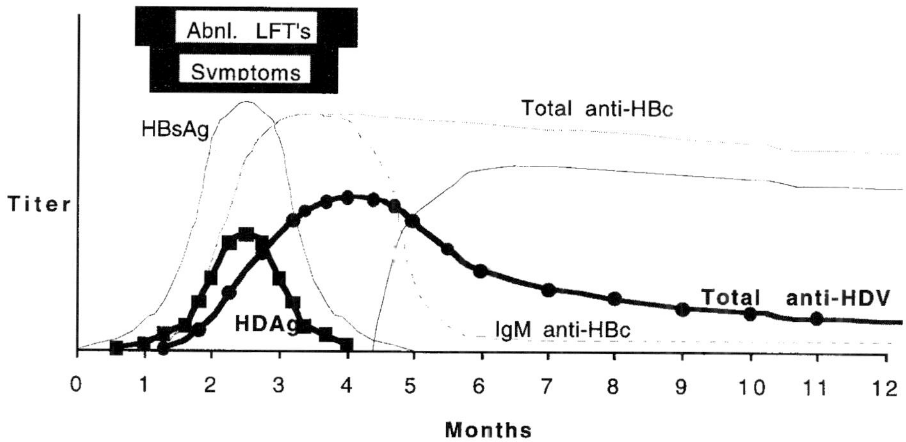

Figure 10 Hepatitis D coinfection serologies (acute HBV and acute HDV). The hepatitis D viral antigen and the HBsAg are both detectable in the blood around the same time. The HDAg and the HBsAg decline in titer in parallel and disappear as their respective antibodies appear. The IgG component of anti-HDV falls much more rapidly than total anti-HBc and becomes negative usually within 1 to 2 years postresolution of acute hepatitis D.

Superinfection

When a patient who has chronic hepatitis B acquires hepatitis D, there is the concurrent development of the HDAg in the serum and a transient decline in the level of the hepatitis B viral surface antigen. Hepatitis D virtually always progresses to chronicity, as demonstrated by the persistence of the HDAg in the serum. Despite the persistence of the HDAg, patients also develop large amounts of the IgM as well as the IgG forms of anti-HD. All components are measurable in the serum (see Fig. 11).

HEPATITIS E

Hepatitis E (HEV) is an RNA virus similar to viruses in the Caliciviridae family. It is typically transmitted by fecal contamination of water supplies. Although a major cause of hepatitis in Asia, Africa, and Mexico, HEV is vanishingly rare in the United States and is found only in patients who have recently traveled to endemic areas. The disease is almost always self-limiting except in pregnant women, where mortality can be as high as 15–25%. There is no chronic form of HEV infection. The incubation period is approximately 40 days, with a range of 15–60 days. Serological tests for IgM anti-HEV are typically positive at the time of presentation.

Serological Assays for HEV

As with HAV, the diagnosis of acute HEV infection is made by a serological EIA for IgM anti-HEV. EIAs are now available using multiple recombinant proteins for both structural and nonstructural antigens, and these assays have improved sensitivity over earlier versions. Product information provided by GeneLabs Diagnostic (Redwood City, CA) notes

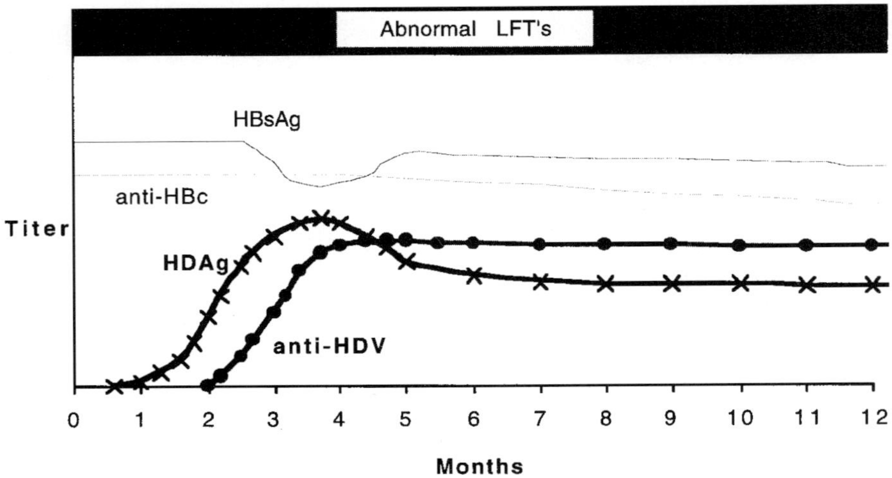

Figure 11 Hepatitis D superinfection serologies (chronic HBV and acute HDV). The hepatitis D superinfection of a chronic HBV carrier results in transient suppression of the HBV viral replication. This suppression of HBV viral replication causes a decrease in the HBV DNA level in the blood. Since the patient's immune system was unable to clear the original HBV infection, the HDV also invariably becomes chronic as well. persistent HDV infection is characterized by continuous high levels of both the IgM anti-HDV and IgG anti-HDV.

that their IgM anti-HEV has a sensitivity of 95% and a specificity of 97%. These numbers may vary depending upon the isolate and the prevalence of disease in the population. As noted, IgM anti-HEV is usually detectable at the time patients present with symptoms and remains positive for several months. Some 50% of patients are still positive at 4 months, and 6% are positive at 7 months (see Fig. 12). The IgG response declines more slowly,

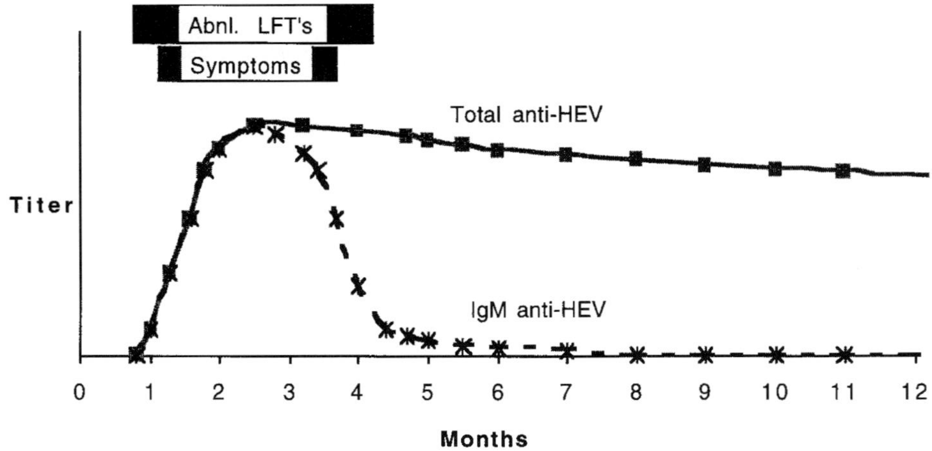

Figure 12 Generalized time course of clinical events and antiviral serological response to a hepatitis E infection. The total anti-HEV consists of both the IgM anti-HEV and the IgG anti-HEV. The IgM component declines over time and only the IgG fraction remains detectable after 6 months.

and up to 50% of patients remain positive at 14 years. HEV RNA is detectable by RT-PCR in both serum and stool, though these tests are performed only in research laboratories and are not commercially available.

HEPATITIS G

Abbott Laboratories (Abbott Park, IL) identified three novel hepatotrophic viruses of the Flaviviridae family using molecular techniques. The first two of these viruses, GBV-A and GBV-B, were identified in the blood of a primate by a subtractive PCR technique. Indications now are that the GBV-A is a virus found only in primates. It also appears that GBV-B probably is confined to monkey species as well. However, sequence analysis of the GBV-C isolate has shown that it is closely related to another member of the Flaviviridae named hepatitis G virus (HGV), which was simultaneously cloned by Genelabs (Redwood City, CA).

While it was certain, early in its identification and cloning, that the HCV was a definite hepatotrophic virus, the same cannot be said for GBV-C/HGV. Even the name of this virus has yet to be resolved. Despite the fact that it is an RNA virus in the same family as HCV, it is not yet clear whether HGV causes significant if any liver disease. Virtually all patients infected with GBV-C/HGV have normal LFTs despite the continued presence of the virus in their blood, this virus may not actually be a cause of liver disease in humans. The only way to identify GBV-C/HGV is through the RT-PCR detection of the viral RNA in serum. Although not FDA-approved, serum may be sent to either Abbott Laboratories or Genelabs on a research basis only.

BIBLIOGRAPHY

Brunetto MR, Giarin M, Oliveri F, Saracco G, Barbera C. "e" antigen defective hepatitis B virus and course of chronic infection. J Hepatol 1991; 13:S82–S86.

Centers for Disease Control. Prevention of hepatitis A through active or passive immunization: recommendations of the Advisory Committee on Immunization Practices (ACIP). MMWR 1996; 45(RR-15):1–30.

De Medina M, Schiff E. Hepatitis C: diagnostic assay. Semin Liver Dis 1995; 15:33–40.

Eisenstein BI. The polymerase chain reaction: a new method of using molecular genetics for medical diagnosis. N Engl J Med 1990; 322:178–183.

Hoofnagle JH, Shafritz DA, Popper H. Chronic type B hepatitis and the "healthy" HBsAg carrier state (review). Hepatology 1987; 7:758–763.

Hu K-Q, Vierling JM. Molecular diagnostic techniques for viral hepatitis. Gastroenterol Clin North Am 1994; 23:479–498.

Liaw YF. Role of hepatitis C virus in dual and triple hepatitis virus infection (review). Hepatology 1995; 22:1101–1108.

Linnen J, Wages J, Jr., Zhang Keck ZY, Fry KE, Krawczynski KZ, Alter H, Koonin E, Gallagher M, Alter M, Hadziyannis S, Karayiannis P, Fung K, Nakatsuji Y, Shih JWK, Young L, Piatak M, Jr., Hoover C, Fernandez J, Chen S, Zou JC, Morris T, Hyams KC, Ismays S, Lifson JD, Hess G, Foung KH, Thomas H, Gradley D, Margolis H, Kim JP. Molecular cloning and disease association of hepatitis G virus: A transfusion-transmissible agent. Science 1996; 271: 505–508.

Mast EE, Krawczynski K. Hepatitis E: an overview. Annu Rev Med 1996; 47:257–266.

Monjardino J. Replication of hepatitis delta virus. J Viral Hepatitis 1996; 3:163–166.

Polish LB, Gallagher M, Fields HA, Hadler SC. Delta hepatitis: molecular biology and clinical and epidemiological features (review). Clin Microbiol Rev 1993; 6:211–229.

Schlauder GG, Dawson GJ, Simons JN, Pilot-Matias TJ, Gutierrez RA, Heynen CA, Knigge MF, Kurpiewski GS, Buijk SL, Leary TP, Muerhoff AS, Desai SM, Mushahwar IK. Molecular and serologic analysis in the transmission of the GB hepatitis agents. J Med Virol 1995; 46:81–90.

Simons JN, Leary TP, Dawson GJ, Pilot-Matias TJ, Muerhoff AS, Schlauder GG, Desai SM, Mushahwar IK. Isolation of novel virus-like sequences associated with human hepatitis. Nature Med 1995; 1:564–569.

Sjögren MH. Serologic diagnosis of viral hepatitis. Med Clin North Am 1996; 80:929–957.

Tong MJ, Hwang SJ. Hepatitis B virus infection in Asian Americans (review). Gastroenterol Clin North Am 1994; 23:523–536.

Urdea MS. Branched DNA signal amplification: does bDNA represent post-PCR amplification technology? Biotechnology 1994; 12:926–927.

Weltman MD, Brotodihardjo A, Crewe EB, Farrell GC, Bilous M, Grierson JM, Liddle C. Coinfection with hepatitis B and C or B, C and delta viruses results in severe chronic liver disease and responds poorly to interferon-alpha treatment. J Viral Hepatitis 1995; 2:39–45.

5
Immunoprophylaxis of Viral Hepatitis

Jonathan M. Koff
Boston University School of Medicine, Boston, Massachusetts
Raymond S. Koff
University of Massachusetts Medical School, Worcester, Massachusetts

HEPATITIS A

General Principles

For half a century, beginning in the 1940s, passive immunization with human immune globulin (IG), subsequently shown to contain preformed IgG antibodies to HAV (IgG anti-HAV), had been the only form of immunoprophylaxis for hepatitis A. The introduction of inactivated HAV vaccines in the mid-1990s has dramatically altered the approach to immunoprophylaxis and has signaled the possibility of eventual eradication of HAV infection.

The protective efficacy of IG is due to the presence of neutralizing antibody to HAV in this material. Similarly, the protective efficacy of the HAV vaccines is a consequence of the induction of neutralizing antibodies after inoculation of the inactivated virus. Some of the characteristics of IG and the inactivated HAV vaccines are compared in Table 1. Whether a T-cell–mediated mechanism is involved in vaccine-induced or natural immunity remains to be determined. Immunity to HAV reinfection after natural infection is known to be lifelong. Although the level of circulating antibody associated with immunity has yet to be precisely defined, serum anti-HAV levels of about 10–20 mIU/mL are thought to be protective. Anti-HAV levels following natural infection are often 100- to 300-fold higher. While immunoprophylaxis of hepatitis A by administration of IG provides relatively low anti-HAV levels, administration of the currently available inactivated HAV vaccines results in the induction of anti-HAV levels that may approach those seen after natural infection. Following IG administration the duration of protection is usually short-lived, not exceeding 2–4 months. In contrast, immunity after vaccination using the two-dose schedule is likely to be prolonged; it may exceed 10 to 20 years.

Table 1 Comparison of Immune Globulin vs. Inactivated Hepatitis A Vaccine in HAV Immunoprophylaxis

	Immune globulin (IG)	Hepatitis A vaccine
Serum-derived biological	Yes	No
Passive acquisition of anti-HAV	Yes	No
Induction of anti-HAV	No	Yes
Time to first appearance of anti-HAV in serum	Immediate	1–2 weeks
Time to achieve protective levels of anti-HAV	1 day	2 weeks
Peak anti-HAV titer (GMT)	~150 mIU/mL	~4000 mIU/mL
Protective efficacy rate	<70–90%	>95–100%
Duration of protection	2–6 months	>10–20 years
Cost	$	$$$

IG in Immunoprophylaxis of Hepatitis A

Historically IG has been used for both pre- and postexposure prophylaxis. While protective efficacy rates approached 90% or better in the preexposure setting, lower rates (70–85%) have been associated with postexposure administration of IG, even when given within 2 weeks of exposure to household and other close personal contacts of an index case. IG efficacy in the control of community-wide or institutional outbreaks and in common-source epidemics has been problematic. Routine shortages in IG supplies in the United States and the concept that inactivated HAV vaccines are likely to be far more effective than IG for preexposure prophylaxis have strongly supported a shift to the use of vaccine in the preexposure setting. Furthermore, vaccine may also be far more useful in the control of community-wide outbreaks than IG.

On the other hand, the effectiveness of HAV vaccine in postexposure immunoprophylaxis has yet to be established in field trials. Experimental challenge data in nonhuman primates are very limited. Until evidence of HAV vaccine effectiveness in the postexposure setting becomes available, IG prophylaxis of household contacts of infected patients will continue to be recommended. The conventional dose of IG is 0.02 mL/kg body weight given intramuscularly within 2 weeks of exposure to the index case.

Inactivated HAV Vaccines

Because only one human serotype of HAV is known to exist, HAV vaccines produced from any single strain should prove effective against all HAV isolates, regardless of their geographic origin. The first commercially available, formalin-inactivated, whole-virus vaccine (HAVRIX) utilized the HM-175 strain of HAV propagated in tissue culture. The cumulative protective efficacy rate for this vaccine against symptomatic and asymptomatic HAV infection was 95% in an extensive field trial. Another inactivated HAV vaccine (VAQTA), produced from a different HAV strain, has also been shown to confer complete protection by 18 days after administration in an epidemic setting. In the United States, HAVRIX is given in an initial dose of 1440 ELISA units (E1.U) for adults, with a booster dose at 6–12 months. In children, age 2–18 years, a three-dose (two doses 1 month apart with a booster 6–12 months later) 360 E1.U schedule or a two-dose 720 E1.U regimen, with a time course

Table 2 Comparison of the Commercially Available Inactivated Hepatitis A Vaccines Available in the United States

	HAVRIX	VAQTA
Manufacturer	SmithKline Beecham	Merck and Co.
Strain of HAV	HM-175	CR326F
Tissue culture	MRC-5 cells	MRC-5 cells
Chemical treatment	Formaldehyde	Formaldehyde
HAV content		
Adult dose	⩾19 years: 1440 El.U	⩾18 years: 50 units[a]
Pediatric dose	2–18 years: 720 El.U	2–17 years: 25 units
Pediatric dose	2–18 years: 360 El.U	
Approved two-dose schedule		
Adults	0, 6–12 months	0, 6 months
Children (720 El.U)	0, 6–12 months	0, 6–18 months
Approved three-dose schedule		
Children (360 El.U)	0, 1, 6–12 months	
Recommended injection site	Deltoid	Deltoid
Cost	$$$	$$$

[a]1 unit = 1 ng HAV antigen.

similar to that for adults, has been approved. VAQTA is also given in a two-dose schedule (0 and 6 months for adults and 0 and 6–18 months for children), employing different concentrations of HAV protein (as shown in Table 2). The inactivated HAV vaccines are highly immunogenic and have high protective efficacy rates. Depending on the assay used, anti-HAV may be detected in serum as early as 15 days after a single dose of either vaccine in about 70–98% of vaccinees. Inactivated hepatitis A vaccine has been shown to confer readily detectable anti-HAV for at least 1 year after a single dose and, as already noted, prolonged protection for 10–20 years or longer after the booster vaccination. In HIV-positive and immunosuppressed individuals, the vaccines may be less immunogenic.

Both HAV vaccines are well tolerated. Transient soreness at the injection site has been the most frequently reported adverse reaction, seen in over half of adults. Systemic adverse events such as headache, fever, fatigue, and malaise are reported in less than 15% of vaccinees. Most adverse reactions last less than 24 h and resolve spontaneously. An unusual HAV vaccine, not currently available in the United States, incorporates immunogenic HAV proteins within reconstituted influenza virosomes. A live, attenuated HAV vaccine has been utilized in China; information about this product is very limited.

Candidates for HAV Vaccine

It seems reasonable to assume that screening for anti-HAV prior to vaccination, if limited to individuals born before 1945 and those who give a past history of hepatitis or have lived in an HAV-hyperendemic region, may save some costs depending on the actual costs of screening, vaccine prices, and the administrative costs of giving the vaccine and record keeping as well as on the prevalence of previous HAV infection. The following groups of individuals should be considered candidates for immunoprophylaxis of HAV with vaccine.

Travelers

Preexposure immunoprophylaxis with inactivated HAV vaccine should be given to travelers to HAV endemic regions: Mexico, the Caribbean, Southeast Asia, South and Central America, and Africa. Tourists, business travelers, foreign-service workers, missionaries, health-care workers, military personnel and peacekeeping forces, airline and shipping employees, and others working abroad and their accompanying family members are appropriate candidates for HAV vaccine. For travelers leaving within too short a period to be certain of vaccine-induced immunity, simultaneous administration of IG and HAV vaccine, at separate deltoid sites, may be appropriate. In this circumstance, peak anti-HAV titers may be slightly lower than after vaccine alone.

Chronic Liver Disease Patients

Because HAV infection in patients with preexisting chronic liver disease may be more severe than in patients without liver disease, HAV vaccine should be considered for all such patients who are seronegative. Inactivated HAV vaccine has been shown to be highly immunogenic in this population.

Other Candidates

Susceptible recipients of solvent/detergent-treated clotting factors are appropriate candidates for HAV vaccine, since such preparations have been reported to transmit HAV infection in the United States. HAV vaccine should also be considered for sexually active homosexual and bisexual men, users of illicit injection drugs, laboratory workers handling HAV, sewage workers, health-care workers in neonatal intensive care units, and veterinarians working with nonhuman primates. Employees of day-care centers and institutions for the developmentally disadvantaged also seem to be at increased risk and are appropriate candidates for vaccination. Vaccination of the native peoples of Alaska and the Americas in whom HAV infection is hyperendemic is also appropriate and has been recommended.

Immunization of food handlers is an unresolved question. Food handler–associated hepatitis A is relatively uncommon in the United States, accounting for no more than 5% of reported cases. Although food workers are not an especially susceptible group, HAV-infected food handlers have the potential to amplify the infection to tens or hundreds of individuals, thereby potentiating community-wide outbreaks. Frequent changes in employment and the absence of health insurance and health care for many part-time food handlers has limited adoption of this strategy.

Community-Wide Outbreaks

The use of HAV vaccine to interrupt HAV transmission during community-wide outbreaks has been supported by limited experience in Alaska; whether HAV vaccine can abort or control common-source outbreaks remains to be determined in future studies.

Future HAV Vaccination Strategies

Implementation of the targeted HAV vaccination strategy recommended above is likely to have a very limited impact on the occurrence of hepatitis A in the United States. Effective control of this enterically transmitted infection will necessitate universal early childhood immunization. Such an approach is most likely to be achieved when HAV vaccine is combined with other pediatric vaccines (hepatitis B, DPT, etc.) in polyvalent preparations, thereby permitting its incorporation into the conventional pediatric immunization schedule.

Because there is an important degree of overlap between risk factors for acquiring both HAV and hepatitis B virus (HBV) infections, a bivalent HAV and HBV vaccine would also be useful for the immunization of individuals at risk. Such a vaccine is likely to reduce the administrative costs of vaccination, aid in tracking immunization status, and possibly enhance compliance. A bivalent HAV and HBV vaccine (TWINRIX, SmithKline Beecham Pharmaceuticals) has been registered in many European countries.

HEPATITIS E

General Principles

Hepatitis E is probably the rarest form of viral hepatitis in the United States. Only a handful of cases are identified annually and virtually all occur in travelers returning from parts of the world where the disease is hyperendemic or in immigrants from those areas. This enterically transmitted infection has been documented in epidemic form and in sporadic cases in developing countries, particularly those on the Indian subcontinent, Asia, and Africa. Outbreaks of HEV infection have been reported from Mexico and may be present elsewhere in the Americas. The disease is particularly severe in pregnant women and may lead to acute liver failure: case fatality rates as high as 20% have been reported in pregnant women.

Passive Immunization

Conventional IG manufactured in the United States is unlikely to contain neutralizing anti-HEV. Hence, it is not likely to be useful in the prophylaxis of this infection. IG prepared in regions where the disease is endemic also appears to have insufficient anti-HEV levels to prevent infection. Furthermore, passive immunization of cynomolgus monkeys with anti-HEV containing convalescent serum from experimentally infected animals has not been shown to protect against challenge with live HEV.

Active Immunization

Immunization of cynomolgus monkeys with a recombinant HEV fusion protein from the second open reading frame of HEV protected animals against challenge with live HEV. While none of the immunized animals developed elevated ALT levels and histological evidence of hepatitis and viremia could not be detected, fecal shedding of HEV was detected in animals that received one dose but not two doses of this vaccine. These promising studies indicate that the development of an HEV vaccine to protect against outbreaks and sporadic cases should be possible.

Candidates for HEV Vaccine

An effective vaccine against HEV would be appropriate for pregnant women living in or traveling to hyperendemic regions as well as for other travelers to these areas. If an effective, safe, and cheap vaccine could be produced, its widespread use in developing countries where HEV is endemic might interrupt the cycle of infection that maintains HEV in the population.

HEPATITIS B AND D

General Principles

On a global basis, hepatitis B virus (HBV) infection has been the most important vaccine-preventable infectious liver disease. Active infections with this DNA-containing virus are believed to affect 300 million people. Hepatitis D virus (HDV), in contrast, is a transmissible, RNA-containing satellite virus of HBV affecting an estimated 15 million people. HDV requires the helper or rescue function of HBV for its expression, assembly, and pathogenicity.

The first hepatitis B vaccine was introduced in the early 1980s. This plasma-derived subunit vaccine was shown to induce immunity in controlled clinical trials in high-risk populations. Antibody to the hepatitis B surface antigen (HBsAg), termed anti-HBs, is the protective, neutralizing antibody elicited by the HBsAg in the vaccine and is deemed responsible for immunity to HBV infection. Seroprotective levels of anti-HBs are believed to be 10 mIU/mL or higher. After natural infection, anti-HBs persists for decades in slowly declining titers. Considerable data indicate that levels of anti-HBs also may fall to levels below this threshold figure after vaccination. In fact, anti-HBs may disappear in a substantial proportion of vaccinees on follow-up after initially successful vaccination. Nonetheless, immunity against clinical disease persists for a number of years after the loss of anti-HBs (see below). The precise duration of protection is still uncertain, but it seems likely that protection may last for well over a decade or possibly two or more in previously healthy vaccinated individuals.

Passive immunization—the administration of exogenous, preformed anti-HBs in the form of hepatitis B IG (HBIG)—is rarely used alone today. The protection it provided was incomplete and relatively short-lived. Active immunization, through the use of HBV vaccine and combined active-passive (HBV vaccine and HBIG) immunization are now the preferred approaches. HBsAg is the active immunogenic material in the yeast-derived recombinant HBV vaccines (Recombivax-HB and Engerix-B) available in the United States (see Table 3). These recombinant vaccines are safe, immunogenic, effective, and expensive. The original plasma-derived HBV vaccine is no longer available in the United States.

Immunogenicity of HBV Vaccines

The major host factors affecting vaccine immunogenicity are age and immunocompetency. Adults over 40 years of age respond less well than younger individuals. The immunogenic response may be slightly lower in neonates than in older children. Smoking and obesity have been linked to diminished responsiveness. In older individuals, smokers, the obese, and immunosuppressed populations there may some advantage in using the vaccine with higher concentrations of HBsAg protein. However, severely immunosuppressed individuals may not respond to HBV vaccination even after a second vaccination series. HBV vaccination of predialysis renal disease patients is preferable to vaccination of patients on hemodialysis. Among otherwise healthy and immunocompetent individuals in whom anti-HBs levels do not reach or exceed 10 mIU/mL after three doses of vaccine, an additional two or three doses may produce responses in no more than about half. Among a very small number of patients, nonresponsiveness persists despite multiple courses of vaccine and appears to be genetically determined and related to the presence of a specific extended HLA haplotype.

Table 3 Recombinant HBV Vaccines Available in the United States

	Engerix-B	Recombivax HB
Manufacturer	SmithKline Beecham	Merck and Co.
Yeast-cell source	*Saccharomyces cerevisiae*	*Saccharomyces cerevisiae*
Chemical treatment	None	Formaldehyde
HBsAg subtype	adw	adw
HBsAg protein content		
Adult dose	≥19 years: 20 μg	≥20 years: 10 μg
Pediatric dose	<19 years: 10 μg	≤ 10 years: 2.5 μg[a]
Adolescent dose		11–19 years: 5 μg
Approved schedule	0, 1, and 6 months 0, 1, 2, and 12 months	0, 1, and 6 months
Recommended injection site	Deltoid or (in infants) anterolateral muscle of the thigh	
Cost	$$$	$$$
Duration of immunity	>10 years	>10 years

[a]5 μg is recommended for neonates of HBsAg-positive mothers.

Duration of Protection and Booster Doses

The duration of protection due to vaccine-induced immunity remains uncertain. Anti-HBs persistence in the circulation is highly correlated with the peak titer after the final dose. At 10 years after initial vaccination of young, healthy individuals, the titer of anti-HBs may have fallen below 10 mIU/mL or may be undetectable in as many as 40%. Nonetheless, immunological memory remains intact and rapid anamnestic responses occur after exposure to HBV or HBsAg. Therefore, continued protection against clinical hepatitis and persistent HBV infection has been demonstrated despite the loss of anti-HBs. Hence, the timing and necessity for booster doses after successful vaccination remains uncertain in healthy adult populations. Immunity has persisted for at least 8–12 years after infant vaccination.

Boosters are recommended in immunosuppressed populations such as patients on maintenance hemodialysis if, on annual testing, anti-HBs levels fall below 10 mIU/mL.

HBV Vaccination Strategies

Screening of all pregnant women for HBsAg, regardless of whether or not risk factors for HBV infection are recognized, and administration of HBIG and HBV vaccine within 12 h of birth to the neonates of HBsAg-positive mothers, combined with universal vaccination of all other infants, catch-up vaccination of preteenagers (11- and 12-year-olds), and continuing vaccination of high-risk populations (see Table 4) is the current strategy for HBV control in the United States. Postexposure prophylaxis of susceptible sexual partners of HBV-infected individuals and victims of needle-stick or splashing accidents calls for HBIG and vaccine.

Unfortunately, screening of pregnant women for HBsAg remains incomplete. Poor physician awareness of the seriousness of the effects of perinatal transmission, absence of laws regulating screening in many states, and selective screening based on prior recommendations to test high-risk women may be responsible. Because adolescents visit physicians

Table 4 Current HBV Vaccination Strategies in the United States

Universal immunization with HBV vaccine of neonates-infants, household contacts of HBsAg-carriers, Alaskan natives, Pacific islanders
HBIG plus HBV vaccine for neonates of HBsAg-positive mothers
HBIG plus HBV vaccine for susceptible contaminated needle-stick victims and for sexual partners of acutely infected individuals
Immunization of adolescents
Immunization of high-risk populations
Health care workers
Public safety workers and first responders
Homosexual men and heterosexuals with multiple partners
Clients, staff of institutions for the developmentally disabled
Intravenous drug abusers
Prisoners
Maintenance hemodialysis patients
Recipients of multiple blood products
Immigrants, travelers, residents of endemic areas

infrequently, school-based HBV vaccination programs maybe the most effective means of vaccine delivery for these age groups. Individuals beginning training for careers in health care are candidates for HBV vaccine.

Global HBV Vaccine Programs

By the mid-1990s, universal infant immunization for HBV had been adopted in over seventy countries, a substantial increase from earlier years. Despite this progress, many countries in the developing world, including those with high HBV carrier rates, have such limited overall pediatric immunization coverage and weak immunization infrastructure that HBV vaccine programs have not been initiated. Also, because many developing countries are donor-dependent for vaccine supplies, the introduction of HBV vaccines has not been a high priority.

Where universal infant HBV immunization has been implemented, dramatic changes in the prevalence of infection and in the development of the HBV carrier state have been reported. The most extraordinary data, reported from Taiwan and shown in Table 5, indicate that eradication of HBV is a realistic and feasible goal.

Future HBV Vaccine Issues

A combination bivalent vaccine incorporating HBV vaccine with *Haemophilus influenzae* vaccine has recently been approved for use in the United States. A combined hepatitis A and B vaccine, shown to be highly immunogenic and well tolerated, may become available in the near future. Similarly, vaccines combining diphtheria, tetanus, pertussis, and HBV have been found to be immunogenic and safe following administration to infants.

So-called HBV vaccine-resistant escape mutants have been reported from Italy, Singapore, Japan, and Africa. The responsible mutations have been identified in the group-specific antigen of the HBsAg proteins. If the prevalence of this HBV mutant increases,

Table 5 Impact of Universal Infant Immunization in Taiwanese Children (<13 years of age)

	Prevaccine	Postvaccine	
	1984	1989	1994
HBsAg prevalence	10%	5%	1%
Anti-HBc prevalence	26%	15%	4%

it may be necessary to incorporate the mutant envelope protein into the next generation of vaccine.

One promising new approach to HBV vaccination is the use of naked-DNA encoding the gene for HBsAg as a vaccine that can be directly injected into muscle (or other antigen-processing tissues) without a delivery vector or adjuvant.

Immunoprophylaxis of HDV

Because of the intimate relationship of HDV and HBV (HDV infection requires the helper functions of HBV), HBV vaccination will prevent both infections in individuals previously susceptible to HBV. In contrast, immunoprophylaxis is not currently available for individuals actively infected by HBV and at risk for HDV. Limited experimental studies appear mildly promising, but the development of an HDV vaccine remains a long-term goal.

HEPATITIS C

General Principles

Improved donor-selection processes and blood-donor screening for antibodies to hepatitis C virus (anti-HCV) have dramatically reduced the frequency of transfusion-associated HCV infection. Similarly, solvent-detergent treatment of pooled plasma products has also reduced the risk of HCV transmission from these preparations. Nonetheless, HCV continues to be readily spread among users of illicit injecting drugs who share contaminated equipment. And although sexual and nosocomial transmission appears to be infrequent, it is still responsible for an important number of cases. Hence, effective immunoprophylaxis would be desirable for the general population.

Passive Immunization

HCV infection is now believed to induce a neutralizing antibody in the host, but it is a restricted response in the sense that it is isolate-specific. Conventional IG preparations may or may not contain neutralizing antibody. If they do contain neutralizing antibody, that antibody may or may not be directed to the viral strain in question, and whether it is present in sufficient quantities to complex and neutralize HCV is uncertain. At present prophylaxis of transfusion-associated or needle-stick–transmitted hepatitis C with IG is not recommended in the United States. In fact, there is no evidence that conventional IG provides protection against HCV infection in any setting. An anti-HCV high-titered IG is not available for use in human beings. Experimental production (in chimpanzees) of a hyperimmune serum directed against a synthetic peptide derived from the envelope region of HCV has been achieved. This material was shown to be capable of neutralizing HCV in vitro. In vivo protection by a high-titer anti-HCV containing human IG has yet to be reported.

Active Immunization

Development of an effective HCV vaccine remains on the drawing boards. Numerous obstacles to vaccine development have been identified. These include presently limited knowledge of the major immunodominant epitopes of the virus, the marked genetic heterogeneity of HCV, the occurrence of superinfections, the possible role of HCV-specific cellular immune responses, and questions about whether T-cell inducing epitopes should be a component of an HCV vaccine. HCV envelope glycoproteins, formulated with a potent adjuvant, have served as a prototype vaccine to immunize chimpanzees. Of the 7 animals challenged with low doses of the same strain of HCV, 5 appeared to be protected at the peak of the antibody response. Further studies to confirm this work—using heterologous HCV strains, higher challenge doses of the homologous strain, and challenges at different time periods after vaccination—will be necessary and are in progress.

In addition to use of the envelope proteins, the highly conserved HCV nucleocapsid protein, to which both B-cell and cytotoxic T-lymphocyte determinants have been mapped, may also be a potential immunogen for a HCV vaccine. Other approaches include the use of naked-DNA vaccines incorporating genes for the envelope and/or nucleocapsid antigens and the development of a live virus vector system—e.g., adenovirus—in which HCV envelope and nucleocapsid proteins have been incorporated.

Candidates for HCV Vaccine

Recently identified injecting drug users, renal failure patients likely to require hemodialysis, newly diagnosed hemophilia patients, and other recipients of multiple blood products as well as the sexual partners of infected individuals would be appropriate candidates for a HCV vaccine. Health-care workers and public safety personnel exposed to blood and body fluids might also be targeted, and the neonates of HCV-infected women might be considered for immunization. As with HBV vaccine (and as suggested for HAV vaccine), it seems likely that this targeted approach will have little impact on the overall risk of HCV infection in the United States. Ultimately, universal childhood vaccination against HCV will be required.

BIBLIOGRAPHY

Centers for Disease Control and Prevention. Prevention of hepatitis A through active or passive immunization: recommendations of the Advisory Committee on Immunization Practices (ACIP). MMWR 1996; 45(No. RR-15):1–30.

Chen H-L, Chang M-H, Ni Y-H, et al. Seroepidemiology of hepatitis B virus infection in children: ten years of mass vaccination in Taiwan. JAMA 1996; 276:906–908.

Choo QL, Kuo G, Ralston R, et al. Vaccination of chimpanzees against infection by the hepatitis C virus. PNAS USA 1994; 91:1294–1298.

Davis HL, Michel M-L, Mancini M, et al. Direct gene transfer in skeletal muscle: plasmid DNA-based immunization against the hepatitis B virus surface antigen. Vaccine 1994; 12:1503–1509.

Dobson S, Scheifele D, Bell A. Assessment of a universal, school-based hepatitis B vaccination program. JAMA 1995; 274:1209–1213.

Krawczynski K, Alter MJ, Tankersley DL, et al. Effect of immune globulin on the prevention of experimental hepatitis C virus infection. J Infect Dis 1996; 173:822–828.

Tokushiga K, Wakita T, Pachuk C, et al. Expression and immune response to hepatitis C virus core DNA-based vaccine constructs. Hepatology 1996; 24:14–20.

Treadwell TL, Keeffe EB, Lake J, et al. Immunogenicity of two recombinant hepatitis B vaccines in older individuals. Am J Med 1993; 95:584–588.

Tsarev SA, Tsareva TS, Emerson SU, et al. Successful passive and active immunization of cynomolgus monkeys against hepatitis E. PNAS USA 1994; 91:10198–10202.

Wang Y-F, Brotman B, Andrus L, Prince AM. Immune response to epitopes of hepatitis C virus (HCV) structural proteins in HCV-infected human and chimpanzees. J Infect Dis 1996; 173: 808–821.

Winokur PL, Stapleton JT. Immunoglobulin prophylaxis for hepatitis A. Clin Infect Dis 1992; 14: 580–586.

6
Management of Acute Viral Hepatitis

Andrew Bedford and Sanjiv Chopra
Harvard Medical School and Beth Israel Hospital, Boston, Massachusetts

INTRODUCTION

Viral hepatitis affects millions of people annually, results in substantial morbidity and occasional mortality, and has enormous economic ramifications. The yearly cost in the United States for care of patients with acute hepatitis A alone approaches $200 million. Significant advances in diagnosis and therapy for viral hepatitis have taken place in the last decade. New hepatotropic viruses have recently been described. For the clinician who encounters a patient with acute viral hepatitis, an understanding of the pathogenesis, clinical manifestations, and natural history of the disease can lead to expedient diagnosis, following which appropriate therapy can be initiated. In this chapter we summarize the important characteristics of the major hepatotropic viruses, briefly outline their pathogenesis, and discuss the clinical presentation and management of acute viral hepatitis.

GENERAL CONSIDERATIONS

The acute phase of viral hepatitis, regardless of the etiological agent, is typically an abrupt illness with malaise, fever, and anorexia with or without nausea and vomiting. Although most persons are anicteric, jaundice can be noted on examination and may coincide with an improvement in constitutional symptoms. This phase is often preceded by the passage of dark urine and clay-colored stools. Abdominal examination is commonly notable for tender hepatomegaly. Splenomegaly and low-grade cervical lymphadenopathy are noted in 10–20% of patients. A general approach to the examination of patients with acute hepatitis should include a careful documentation of mental status with attention to asterixis, constructional apraxia, and fetor hepaticus, which, if present, signify progression to fulminant hepatitis.

Plasma aminotransferases are characteristically elevated, ranging from 1000 to several thousand international units per liter (IU/L), though the degree of elevation bears little relation to hepatic histopathology or prognosis. Additional laboratory tests should include the prothrombin time, serum albumin, and plasma glucose.

Our approach is to hospitalize patients with acute viral hepatitis who have substantial prolongation of the prothrombin time (greater than 16 s), debilitating constitutional symptoms, or any features of hepatic encephalopathy. Encephalopathy, usually demands close following of the patient's mental status in an intensive care unit (ICU). Significant dehydration with ongoing nausea and vomiting are best managed with intravenous fluid supplementation, requiring hospitalization.

Other patients with acute viral hepatitis who should be admitted to the hospital include the elderly, those who are chronically debilitated, and patients with significant comorbid disease or inadequate social support. For patients presenting with mild forms of the illness who appear not to require hospital admission, close follow-up care is essential to ensure that the patient is improving.

The appropriate serological tests to establish the etiological agent in acute viral hepatitis are listed in Table 1 and are reviewed individually.

Occasionally, patients with acute viral hepatitis present with abdominal pain, fever, and jaundice, suggesting the diagnosis of obstructive cholangitis. Although only modest elevations in plasma ALT and AST are common in patients with choledocholithiasis (AST and ALT 50–300 IU/L), marked elevations are rarely noted, mimicking acute viral hepatitis. In jaundiced patients, an ultrasound of the biliary tree should help to exclude biliary obstruction.

The mainstay of therapy for acute viral hepatitis, regardless of the etiological agent, is supportive care. Considerations upon presentation include degree of activity, diet, and follow-up. The level of activity recommended for patients with acute viral hepatitis is

Table 1 Serodiagnosis of Acute Viral Hepatitis

Type	Serological reactivity	Comments
Acute hepatitis A	IgM anti-HAV (+)	Single serum specimen sufficient to make diagnosis
Acute hepatitis A in a hepatitis B chronic carrier	IgM anti-HAV (+) HBsAg (+) IgG anti-HBc (+)	Not unusual situation; millions of HBsAg carriers worldwide; many at risk for acute HAV infection
Acute hepatitis B	IgM anti-HBc (+) HBsAg (+) or (−)	Minority of patients with hepatitis B are HBsAg (−) at time of physician contact
Acute hepatitis B with acute delta infection (coinfection)	IgM anti-HBc (+) HBsAg (+) IgM anti-HDV (+)	Coinfection generally mild
Acute delta infection superimposed on HBV chronic carrier state (superinfection)	IgG anti-HBC (+) HBsAg (+) IgM anti-HDV (+)	Superinfection is severe, often fulminant; those who recover from acute bout always go on to chronic liver disease
Acute hepatitis C	Anti-HCV (+) HCV RNA PCR (+)	HCV antibody may take weeks to a few months to become (+) while HCV RNA PCR test is (+) within 2–3 weeks of illness

that which matches their energy level. This approach remained in dispute throughout the 1960s, when Nefzger and Chalmers retrospectively studied 460 military recruits with their first bout of jaundice and presumed acute infectious hepatitis. Subgroup analysis found no difference in outcome in patients assigned to strict bed rest or activity ad libitum. A high-protein diet had also been touted as beneficial in this disease, and the investigators again found no correlation between dietary intake of protein and the subsequent course of the illness. Our approach for patients with acute viral hepatitis is to encourage fluids and electrolytes orally, maintain a high-calorie diet, if possible, and continue modest activity as tolerated.

All patients with acute viral hepatitis who show signs of progressive hepatocellular dysfunction with worsening coagulopathy, encephalopathy, or hemodynamic compromise should have prompt evaluation by a liver transplantation team.

HEPATITIS A

Hepatitis A virus (HAV) is a single-stranded RNA enterovirus belonging to the Picornaviridae family; it accounts for approximately 40% of acute viral hepatitis cases reported annually in the United States. Susceptibility to HAV varies with age and socioeconomic status. In areas of the world where HAV is endemic, such as India and the Middle East, nearly 90% of adults have serological evidence of prior infection with HAV. The vast majority of childhood cases of hepatitis A infection produce a mild, self-limited illness that usually does not come to medical attention. Interestingly, as the rate of childhood cases declines worldwide with improved living conditions in endemic areas, higher rates of adult cases can be expected; these tend to be more severe. Transmission is by the fecal-oral route (waterborne, foodborne, shellfish, direct contact), which explains why epidemics of acute hepatitis A are regularly noted in areas of crowding and poor hygiene as well as among homosexual men.

The mechanism of hepatocellular injury due to HAV has not been defined in detail. The virus does not seem to have a direct cytolytic effect but probably incites a T cell–mediated inflammatory reaction generated against hepatocyte antigens.

Clinically, acute hepatitis A is indistinguishable from acute viral hepatitis due to other agents such as hepatitis B (HBV) or hepatitis C (HCV). Illness tends to be benign and self-limited, although fulminant hepatitis can occur in a small percentage of patients. However, in contrast to hepatitis B and C infection, hepatitis A never leads to chronic viral liver disease. After approximately 30 days of incubation, infected individuals will begin to show fecal HAV shedding, the titer of which peaks prior to clinically apparent hepatitis and drops steadily thereafter. In HAV infection, the IgM fraction of anti-HAV is diagnostic and appears during the acute phase of the illness. The antibody is present in serum beginning in the fourth week of infection and can persist until the twelfth week, at which point there is a shift to the IgG fraction, signifying recovery from HAV infection. It should be noted that since HAV fecal shedding has significantly diminished by the time patients with acute hepatitis come to medical attention, enteric precautions (gloves upon contact with the patient) are not necessary. Standard precautions such as handwashing and protective gloves for handling containers of bodily fluid should be taken.

Studies seeking to document an effect of steroid therapy on the natural history of acute viral hepatitis, including in those with fulminant hepatitis, have unfortunately failed to consistently demonstrate improved survival.

One subgroup of patients with HAV infection may be an exception. Cholestatic hepatitis manifesting as protracted pruritus and jaundice with serum bilirubin levels that may exceed 25 mg/dL has been described rarely with HAV. Patients will usually have a course of acute HAV infection followed by persistently elevated aminotransferases, jaundice, and occasionally debilitating constitutional symptoms. Marked centrilobular cholestasis with portal inflammatory changes is noted on liver biopsy. Corticosteroids have been utilized and may be effective in such circumstances, although the literature attesting to the benefit of corticosteroids is mostly anectodal. Gordon et al. described six patients with clinically apparent jaundice for at least 12 weeks. All were positive for IgM antibody to the hepatitis A virus and had no evidence of preexisting liver disease or exposure to hepatotoxic agents. All went on to complete recovery, although 4 of 6 with protracted cholestasis and debilitating symptoms were treated with a brief course of corticosteroids.

Some 10% of patients with acute hepatitis A will have a relapsing course with rebound elevations of aminotransferases into the range of 1000 IU/L and a recrudescence of fecal HAV shedding. Such bouts always resolve and no chronic sequelae have been noted.

An interesting potential association between hepatitis A infection and autoimmune hepatitis (AIH) has been described. Studies have demonstrated that there is an immune reaction to the hepatocyte asialoglycoprotein receptor in AIH, presumably due to a defect in suppressor T-cell function. Antibodies to this receptor have also been shown to be present in most patients with acute hepatitis A. To determine whether there might be clinical overlap between hepatitis A and AIH. Vento et al. followed 58 Italian patients considered susceptible to AIH (they each had a first-degree relative with a diagnosis of AIH) for 4 years and determined acquisition of HAV. Three patients had subclinical hepatitis A infection; and in two of these, AIH developed within 5 months. The authors hypothesize that HAV can act as a trigger for disease activity in patients susceptible to AIH. In patients who develop chronic hepatitis after acute HAV infection, a workup for AIH should be initiated.

Rarely, patients with acute HAV infection can have a fulminant course with severe coagulopathy, encephalopathy, and death unless they undergo successful liver transplantation. Patients with preexisting chronic liver disease may deteriorate rapidly in the setting of acute HAV infection, given their limited hepatocellular reserve.

Physicians following patients who are diagnosed with acute hepatitis A are frequently asked about the utility of vaccination for close contacts. An effective live attenuated vaccine is available for those at high risk for acquisition of HAV. If there is evidence that the patient and his or her close contacts are living in circumstances where HAV is endemic or the risk of acquisition is considerable, vaccination should be given according to recommended guidelines (see Chap. 5).

HEPATITIS B

Over 300 million people worldwide (approximately 5% of the world population) are infected with the hepatitis B virus (HBV), which, in its chronic form, can result in cirrhosis and primary hepatocellular carcinoma. Human HBV and similar hepatotropic viruses found in Peking ducks, Beechy ground squirrels, and the eastern woodchuck (*Marmota monax*) are double-stranded DNA viruses of the Hepadnaviridae family and, though not true retroviruses, employ an RNA intermediate for replication. Transmission of HBV occurs through parenteral routes: blood products, intravenous needle use, sexual contact, accidental contact via needle-stick or splashing accidents, and vertically from mother to child. The latter is most notable in areas where HBV is endemic, as in Southeast Asia and sub-Saharan Africa.

The mechanism of acute injury in patients with acute HBV is not entirely clear, but most evidence suggests that the virus is not directly cytopathic. Injury is thought to occur through the action of cytolytic T cells on infected hepatocytes.

Acute hepatitis A and B are largely indistinguishable at clinical presentation. Extrahepatic manifestations, though, which can be noted in HBV and HCV infection and are a result of immune complex–induced tissue damage, can be a clue. Approximately 10% of patients will develop a serum sickness–like syndrome with an urticarial rash, peripheral arthritis, and angioedema, which occurs during the prodrome of acute hepatitis B.

Diagnosis of acute HBV hinges on detection of serological markers of recent infection. About 7–70 days after exposure, patients can be shown to have circulating hepatitis B surface antigen (HBsAg), which precedes the acute phase of illness. Some 50–150 days after exposure, signs and symptoms of acute HBV with marked elevation in plasma ALT and AST may develop, which are clinically indistinguishable from acute HAV infection. Along with the enzyme-linked immunosorbent assay (ELISA) for HBsAg, all patients with acute hepatitis should have serum assays for antibody to HBV core antigen (antiHBc). The presence of the IgM fraction of core antibody (antiHBc IgM) signifies recent acquisition and remains the "gold standard" for the diagnosis of acute HBV, especially when HBsAg levels have waned (the "gap" or "window" period). Antibody to HBsAg (Anti-HBs) becomes detectable in over 90% of patients with acute HBV at 24–28 weeks postexposure and signifies effective clearance of the virus.

The hepatitis B viral e antigen (HBeAg) is a measure of viral replication and infectivity; it is not a necessary test to diagnose HBV infection but rather can help to assess candidacy for interferon therapy in chronic disease. HBV precore mutants—viruses that have substitutions in the gene upstream from the gene encoding core antigen—also have a mutation that prevents translation of the gene encoding HBeAg. These mutants have been associated with sporadic and epidemic fulminant hepatitis, although this association has been challenged. Liang et al. carried out studies to detect mutations in HBV isolates from 40 patients in the United States with fulminant hepatitis and found no predominance of mutant over wild-type HBV strains. The authors argue that host or virulence factors other than precore mutations influence the severity of acute hepatitis B.

The vast majority of patients with acute hepatitis B infection go on to complete recovery. The fundamental difference between HAV and HBV is the ability of the latter to incorporate itself into the host genome and lie dormant. Thus, while nearly all adult patients show complete clinical recovery, approximately 5% will remain HBsAg-positive and will not have generated anti-HBs. The host factors that predispose these patients to incomplete clearance of HBV are unclear, although higher rates of chronicity are noted in immunocompromised patients, those on hemodialysis, and infants. It is important, therefore, to document the clearance of HBsAg from the serum after clinical resolution of acute HBV in all patients. Chronic carriers remain at some risk for chronic hepatitis, cirrhosis, and primary hepatocellular carcinoma and are infectious (see Chaps. 7 and 22).

Treatment for acute HBV infection is identical to that for HAV. Supportive care and patient education are the cornerstones of management. A small percentage of patients will show evidence of progressive liver dysfunction with encephalopathy, coagulopathy, and complications of portal hypertension (see Chap. 25). Steroids have not been shown to be efficacious in attenuating the clinical course of HBV or decreasing the likelihood of developing the chronic carrier state. While there is evidence for benefit of interferon and nucleoside analogues in chronic HBV, there is no clear role for adjunctive medical therapy in acute hepatitis B.

Physicians managing patients with hepatitis B should also be aware of indications for vaccination. The currently available HBV vaccine is a recombinant vaccine with components of HBsAg; it is widely available and extremely effective. Close contacts of patients with hepatitis B, including children and spouses, should undergo serological testing for HBV and be vaccinated if they are susceptible (see Chap. 5).

HEPATITIS D (DELTA AGENT)

The hepatitis D (delta) virus (HDV) is a double-shell particle coated with HBsAg containing a single-stranded RNA genome. HDV requires the presence of HBV for expression; HDV infection can occur only in patients with hepatitis B infection. It is estimated that approximately 5% of HBV-infected patients worldwide also carry HDV. HDV has an unusual epidemiological pattern, which comes in two forms. Infection occurs throughout the world but is endemic in certain areas of the Mediterranean where the route of transmission seems to be by close personal contact affecting primarily children and young adults. In contrast, a nonendemic form occurs in patients in the United States and Europe and is transmitted via the percutaneous route, either through blood products or intravenous drug use.

HDV can cause acute and chronic liver disease (see Chap. 8). The clinical course may vary from an asymptomatic carrier state to fulminant hepatitis in a patient with prior HBV infection (superinfection) to cirrhosis. Superinfection with HDV can be associated with a virulent course and overt fulminant hepatitis and frequently leads to chronic HDV infection. Alternatively, coinfection can occur whereby HBV and HDV are transmitted simultaneously. Chronic HDV infection in this setting will develop only if the patient becomes an HBV carrier.

Regardless of the mode of transmission, acute HDV infection is self-limited and may be indistinguishable from other forms of acute viral hepatitis. Diagnosis is based upon demonstrating an elevation in total anti-HDV, which may become positive only late in the clinical course of acute hepatitis (see Chap. 4), especially in immunocompromised individuals. There is no utility in requesting this assay unless HBsAg is positive. HDV infection needs to be ruled out in patients with chronic hepatitis B who present with unexplained severe acute hepatitis or rapidly deteriorating liver disease or when a patient with acute HBV shows signs of delayed recovery or progression to fulminant hepatic failure.

Although interferon has effects on suppression of viral replication in patient with chronic HDV hepatitis, no specific treatment is available for acute HDV infection. Therapy remains largely supportive. Prevention of delta virus infection can be achieved most effectively through prevention of HBV infection. Patients at risk for acquisition of HBV should be vaccinated using standard schedules (see Chap. 5).

HEPATITIS C

Acute viral hepatitis not due to HAV or HBV (non-A, non-B hepatitis) can largely be ascribed to the family of HCV. HCV is a single-stranded RNA virus probably belonging to the Togaviridae family and accounts for 20% of sporadic hepatitis in the United States. Prior to 1991, when screening of blood products for HCV became standard, the vast majority of cases of posttransfusion acute hepatitis, which occurred in up to 5–10% of transfused individuals, was caused by HCV. Despite a drastic decrease in the incidence of transfusion-associated hepatitis, the burden of HCV infection has not decreased. Currently, the most common modes of transmission include intravenous drug use, percutaneous needle-sticks, and extensive body piercing. Cocaine snorting has recently been identified as a potential risk factor. The risk of sexual transmission of HCV appears to be low. Vertical transmission from mother to neonate is also an infrequent event, showing distinctly different biological behavior from HBV. Unfortunately, there remains a significant subgroup of patients with HCV infection, perhaps 20–30%, in whom the source of infection remains unknown. It is conceivable that many of these patients in the United States, in subsequent candid discussions with their physicians, will reveal a history of remote drug use.

The presentation of acute hepatitis C virus infection is clinically indistinguishable from that due to HAV or HBV. The incubation period ranges from 15–160 days. Acute fulminant hepatitis due to HCV remains rare in western countries. This is in contrast to areas where HBV and HAV are endemic, as in Taiwan, where HCV may account for nearly half the cases of non-A, non-B fulminant hepatitis. It is important to note that, as with HBV infection, the real clinical burden of HCV lies in its proclivity to produce chronic hepatitis and primary hepatocellular carcinoma. In contrast to HBV, an astounding 75–80% of patients who acquire HCV by any route will go on to chronic infection. Hepatitis C is the most common cause of nonalcoholic chronic liver disease in the United States, with up to 1.8% of the general population being infected (see Chaps. 9 and 10).

The diagnosis of HCV infection relies on the detection of antibodies to hepatitis C virus by immunoassay (see Chap. 4). The ELISA has become sufficiently specific that, in patients with an identifiable risk factor and abnormal plasma ALT levels, further confirmatory tests are not necessary. In contrast to anti-HBs, however, hepatitis C virus antibody is not an effective neutralizing antibody and does not confer protection. Quantitative measures of HCV RNA are used in assessing viral burden and the response of chronic HCV to therapy (see Chaps. 4 and 9).

The treatment of acute hepatitis due to HCV is largely supportive, with patient education as a cornerstone of the treatment plan. Recently several small trials have suggested that alpha interferon may have a role in the management of acute transfusion-associated hepatitis C. Four randomized, controlled trials examined the role of interferon in treatment of acute HCV and in preventing progression to chronic infection. In these studies, patients with transfusion-acquired HCV within 7 to 10 weeks of the onset of their illness were evaluated (see Table 2). In three of the four studies, diagnosis was confirmed by PCR assay for HCV RNA. Interferon at the dose of 3 million units three times per week for a total duration of 3 months was given to those randomized to treatment (one study differed in that beta interferon was used in a front-loaded regimen). Significant differences were noted between the treatment and control groups, including a higher rate of complete normalization of ALT at the end of treatment (69 vs. 29% in the control groups), and a higher sustained ALT response 12 months after treatment (53 vs 32% in the control group). Moreover, in the three trials that followed HCV RNA levels, substantially higher rates of disappearance of serum HCV RNA were noted in the group treated with interferon when compared with controls (41% HCV RNA disappearance versus 4% among the controls). The findings are summarized in Figure 1.

Table 2 Characteristics of Four Trials Comparing Interferon with Controls in Patients with Acute Hepatitis C[a]

Author	IFM schedule	Follow-up (months)	Arms[b] (interferon/control)
Lampertico	3 MU tiw[c] × 3 months	15	27/21
Omata	3 MU/day × 5 days then 3 MU tiw	12	11/14
Vladomiu	3 MU tiw × 3 months	9	15/13
Hwang	3 MU tiw × 3 months	12	17/16

[a]In 57 of the 60 interferon recipients, the mode of acquisition was via transfusion.
[b]Size of treated and control groups.
[c]tiw = three times a week.
Source: Modified from Poynard et al., Hepatology 1996; 24: 784.

Thus, in patients with acute transfusion-acquired HCV who, after comprehensive medical and psychosocial evaluation, have no contraindications to therapy, we recommend initiating a course of alpha interferon 3 million units, three times per week for 6–12 months. Preliminary data by Dr. Juan Estaban utilizing this treatment regimen have shown most encouraging results (personal communication).

Unfortunately, despite significant advances in the detection of early hepatitis C infection, only a small percentage of these patients are diagnosed at or near the time of acquisition.

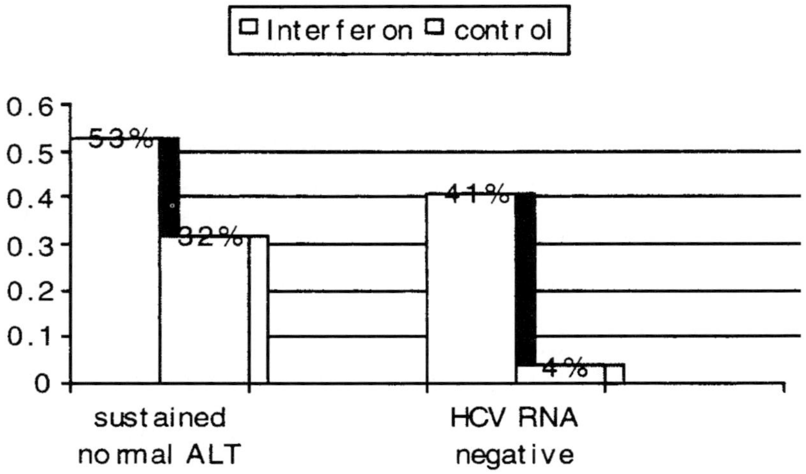

Figure 6 Interferon for acute hepatitis C, biochemical and serological response. Response measured 12 months after completion of therapy.

HEPATITIS E

Morphologically and clinically similar to HAV, the hepatitis E virus (HEV) is a single-stranded RNA virus that has been labeled the enterically transmitted non-A, non-B virus. Epidemics of acute hepatitis in Central America, the Indian subcontinent, and Central and Southeast Asia have been tracked to contamination of water supplies after floods or monsoons. Some 30,000 cases of icteric hepatitis were noted, for example, in Delhi in 1955–1956 after flooding of the Yamuna River. Sporadic cases have also been noted in endemic areas as well or in patients who have traveled to other countries from endemic areas. Clinically, HEV infection is indistinguishable from other forms of acute viral hepatitis and, like HAV, has no proclivity toward a chronic carrier state. An inordinately high mortality rate has been noted in pregnant women in virtually all large-scale outbreaks. Diagnosis can be confirmed through serological tests of antibodies to HEV available through the Centers for Disease Control in the United States.

HEPATITIS G/GBV-C

In the mid-1960s, Friedrich Deinhart and colleagues conducted seminal work in infectious hepatitis using primates as an animal model. One particular finding was that serum from a patient with acute hepatitis (a surgeon, "G.B.") transmitted severe hepatitis to tamarins. This was initially thought to be the hepatitis A virus, but subsequent assays revealed that the GB virus was unique. Studies using nucleic acid sequencing of the GB virus revealed three different strains, designated GBV-A, GBV-B, and GBV-C. GBV-A and GBV-B were not infective in humans; only GBV-C was isolated in patients with non–A-E hepatitis. Concurrent work at the National Institutes of Health yielded a new non–A-E hepatitis blood-borne virus designated hepatitis G virus. The GBV-C and hepatitis G virus are now considered variants of the same virus.

HGV, found throughout the world, is an RNA virus resembling HCV and belongs to the family of Flaviviridae. Some 10–20% of patients with chronic non–A-E hepatitis will harbor HGV, and a high prevalence has been noted among those with risk factors for exposure to blood products (hemodialysis patients, intravenous drug abusers). Although a great deal of interest was initially focused on HGV as a hepatotropic virus with the ability to cause acute post-transfusion and chronic hepatitis, this has been called into question. HGV, for example, is as common in blood donors with abnormal ALT as it is in those with normal ALT. Only 17% of patients with acute non–A-E posttransfusion hepatitis are infected with HGV, the same frequency found in community-acquired non–A-E hepatitis. In addition, HGV can commonly be found by PCR in patients with HCV; among patients with HCV, 10–20% will be positive for HGV RNA. However, there is no evidence that infection alters the clinical course of HCV. One study evaluated 189 patients with chronic HCV, 21% of whom were positive for HGV RNA. The course of disease and response to interferon was not affected by the presence of HGV/GBV-C. In contrast to other hepatotropic viruses, HGV has not been shown to replicate in the liver.

In summary, HGV is a viral infection that has yet to be clearly established as an etiological agent in human non–A-E viral hepatitis. At the present time we do not recommend testing for HCV RNA by PCR in the clinical setting. Further investigation in this field is ongoing.

BIBLIOGRAPHY

Chu CM, Sheen IS, Liaw YF. The role of hepatitis C virus in fulminant viral hepatitis in an area with endemic hepatitis A and B. Gastroenterology 1994; 107:189.

DiBisceglie AM. Hepatitis G virus infection: a work in progress. Ann Intern Med 1996; 125:772.

Gordon S, Reddy KR, Schiff L, Schiff E. Prolonged intrahepatic cholestasis secondary to acute hepatitis A. Ann Intern Med 1984; 101:635.

Hwang SF, Lee SC, Chan CY, Lu RH, Lo KJ. A randomized controlled trial of recombinant interferon alpha-2b in the treatment of Chinese patients with acute post-transfusion hepatitis C. J Hepatol 1994; 21:861.

Karayiannis P, McHarvey MJ. The GB hepatitis viruses. J Viral Hepatitis 1995; 2:221.

Lampertico P, Rumi M, Romeo R, Craxi A, Soffredini R, Blassoni D, Colombo M. A multicenter randomized controlled trial of recombinant interferon alpha 2b in patients with acute transfusion-associated hepatitis C. Hepatology 1994; 19:19.

Liang T, Hasegawa N, Rimon N, Wands JR, Ben-Porath E. A hepatitis B virus mutant associated with an epidemic of fulminant hepatitis B. N Engl J Med 1991; 324:1705.

Liang TJ, Hasegawa K, Munoz S, Shapiro C, Yoffe B, McMahon B, Feng C, Bei H, Alter MJ, Dienstag JL. Hepatitis B virus precore mutation and fulminant hepatitis in the United States. J Clin Invest 1994; 93:550.

Omata M, Yokasura O, Takano S, Kato N, Hosoda K et al. Resolution of acute hepatitis C after therapy with natural beta I interferon. Lancet 1991; 338:914.

Petruff CA, Bedford A, Gordon F, Chopra S. Hepatitis vaccines. Dig Dis 1997; 15:1.

Poynard T, Leroy V, Cohard M, Thevenot T, Mathurin P, Opolon P, Zarski J. Meta-analysis of interferon randomized trials in the treatment of viral hepatitis C: effects of dose and duration. Hepatology 1996; 24:778.

Rizzetto M, Ponzetto A, Forzani I. Epidemiology of hepatitis delta virus; an overview. Prog Clin Biol Res 1991; 354:1.

Takano S, Satamura Y, Omata M, Japan Acute hepatitis Cooperative Study Group. Effect of interferon beta on non-A non-B acute hepatitis; a prospective, randomized, controlled-dose study. Gastroenterology 1994; 107:805.

Vento S, Garofano T, Di Perri G, Dolci L, Concia E, Bassetti D. Identification of hepatitis A virus as a trigger for autoimmune chronic hepatitis type I in susceptible individuals. Lancet 1991; 337:1183.

Vladomiu L, Genesca J, Esteban JI, Allende H, Gonzalez A, Lopez-Talavera JC, Esteban R, et al. Interferon-alpha in acute post-transfusion hepatitis C: a randomized, controlled trial. Hepatology 1992; 15:767.

7
Management of Chronic Hepatitis B

Helma P. Cotrim
Universidade Federal de Bahia, Salvador, Brazil

Gabriel Garcia
Stanford University School of Medicine, Palo Alto, California

GENERAL PRINCIPLES

Patients with chronic hepatitis B are generally discovered when abnormal aminotransferases are noted during a routine medical exam, or as part of a screening evaluation for individuals at high risk for hepatitis B. This is not an unusual event since hepatitis B is relatively common: 300,000 new infections are estimated to occur in the United States each year, and chronic hepatitis B affects as many as 5% of the world's population. It is also an important disease from a public health perspective, accounting for significant morbidity and mortality from cirrhosis and hepatocellular carcinoma. Patients may be unaware of the presence of their infection, of their particular risk for infection, or of their ability to transmit hepatitis B to others.

Health care workers need to take advantage of a newly diagnosed case of chronic hepatitis B as an opportunity to educate the patient, to screen the patient's family and sexual contacts for the presence of hepatitis B infection and vaccinate those still at risk, and to establish a management strategy (Table 1). The key components of a management strategy for patients with chronic hepatitis B are screening for hepatocellular carcinoma and antiviral therapy. Essentially all patients with chronic hepatitis B should be considered for hepatocellular carcinoma screening. In contrast, antiviral therapy or liver transplantation are only appropriate for selected patients.

INITIAL EVALUATION

The purpose of the initial evaluation is to confirm the diagnosis of chronic hepatitis B, characterize the patient both clinically and virologically so that the prognosis can be estimated, and determine whether the patient is a candidate for antiviral treatment, liver

Table 1 Initial Evaluation of the Patient with Chronic Hepatitis B

Clinical and virological staging
Patient education
Risk of transmission
Prognosis
Screening of contacts
Family and sexual
Vaccination of all at risk
Establish management strategy
Hepatocellular carcinoma surveillance
Antiviral therapy
Transplantation

transplantation, or hepatocellular carcinoma surveillance. The elements of the medical evaluation that are critical to establish the baseline data are as follows.

Medical History

The route of transmission of the patient's infection should be determined so that high-risk behaviors are recognized and avoided and further person-to-person or parenteral spread does not occur. In areas of high endemicity of hepatitis B infection, most hepatitis B transmission occurs from mother to child in the perinatal period (Asia) or among young children in a household with a young HBsAg carrier (West Africa). In areas of moderate to low endemicity, adults with hepatitis B may have the previously stated risk factors but must also be screened for a history of blood transfusion, parenteral drug use, or needle-stick injury, promiscuity, and sexual activity in the absence of barrier contraception. An unusual case of nosocomial transmission from a surgeon to a patient during an invasive procedure has been documented this possible route of transmission must be kept in mind in patients with past invasive surgical or dental procedures and no other risk factors.

In addition, the history should establish the presence of any family members with hepatitis B, and determine who may be still be at risk of infection so that they may be vaccinated. It may be difficult to distinguish the onset of the disease, since most children and young adults have asymptomatic initial presentations. Furthermore, a history of jaundice may represent the initial infection with hepatitis B virus, acute infection with another hepatitis virus, a nonviral liver injury, or clinical exacerbation of established chronic liver disease. This makes it difficult to determine precisely how long the patient has placed his or her contacts at risk, and argues for a universal vaccination approach to prevention.

Finally, the medical history will determine whether there have been any signs of decompensated liver disease, such as variceal bleeding, ascites, spontaneous bacterial peritonitis, or hepatic encephalopathy. The majority of patients will be asymptomatic or have nonspecific symptoms unless they have progressed to cirrhosis or advanced chronic hepatitis.

Physical Examination

The value of the physical examination is to look for evidence of high-risk behavior (homemade tattoos, sites of injection drug use) not volunteered by the patient, and for signs of advanced liver disease. Although the latter are not frequently found in cirrhotic patients, the presence of spider angiomas and ascites has been well established as a sign of advanced liver disease and a poor prognosis. Similarly, the presence of jaundice, signs of malnutrition, firm hepatomegaly, splenomegaly, asterixis, or impaired intellectual function may identify the patient with cirrhosis not previously diagnosed.

Laboratory Studies

The presence of an abnormal aminotransferase (usually ALT greater than AST, in contrast to alcoholic liver disease) is the usual laboratory sign of chronic hepatitis B. The levels may range from minimal elevations to as high as twenty times the upper limit of normal. However, the laboratory measurements most useful in determining the severity of the underlying liver disease are the complete blood count, prothrombin time, and serum albumin and bilirubin levels. The presence of a low platelet count,with or without a low white blood cell count, can signal the presence of portal hypertension and hypersplenism, although recent studies have highlighted the importance of thrombopoetin deficiency in the pathogenesis of the thrombocytopenia in advanced liver disease. Liver synthetic dysfunction may be suggested by finding a prolonged prothrombin time or a low serum albumin and may signal the presence of cirrhosis.

A serum alpha-fetoprotein is a reliable test for the presence of hepatocellular carcinoma, its widespread availability makes it an important part of the initial evaluation. Any level greater than the upper limit of normal should be considered suspect for hepatocellular carcinoma and further evaluation should be performed. Depending on the degree of abnormality, this may involve merely repeat testing within 4–8 weeks, hepatic imaging test studies, or a guided liver biopsy (see Chap. 23).

Virological Studies

The development of diagnostic virologic studies allow the clinician to precisely diagnose and characterize hepatitis B virus infection (see Chap. 4). Given a patient with a positive HBsAg who presents asymptomatically or has a known or presumed chronic infection, it is important to classify the patient by the use of the HBeAg, HBV DNA assay and aminotransferase levels into one of the four categories listed in Table 2, as they may impart both prognostic information and establish candidacy for antiviral therapy.

Chronic HBsAg carriers are clinically well patients with normal aminotransferases and evidence of HBsAg in serum for at least 6 months. Their prognosis over time is excellent unless they show evidence of clinical or laboratory exacerbations, which may place them at risk for the development of cirrhosis. In the few studies in which liver biopsies were performed in this group, there were either no histological abnormalities or minimal

Table 2 Classification of Hepatitis B Virus Infection

Classification	HBsAg	HBeAg	HBV DNA	ALT
HBsAg carrier	+	+ or −	+ or −	Normal
Chronic hepatitis, wild type, active replication	+	+	+	Elevated
Chronic hepatitis, wild type, no active replication	+	−	−	Elevated
Chronic hepatitis, precore mutant	+	−	+	Elevated

changes, and progression of the histological changes was unusual. They are not felt to be candidates for antiviral therapy given their good prognosis. However, they are at risk for hepatocellular carcinoma, albeit at a much lower rate than those patients with chronic hepatitis and cirrhosis. They should be considered for hepatoma surveillance (serum alpha-fetoprotein) along with a basic clinical and laboratory evaluation (CBC, liver function studies, prothrombin time, and HBV DNA level) on a yearly basis or at any time that symptoms suggestive of liver disease are present.

If the aminotransferase levels are persistently abnormal for greater than 6 months, then chronic hepatitis can be presumed to be present, and further virological evaluation should be aimed at determining the level of viral replication and the presence of a pre-core mutant. Patients with a wild-type HBV infection that are actively replicating virus will be identified by the presence in serum of both HBeAg and HBV DNA. Seroconversion of HBeAg to anti-HBe and loss of serum HBV DNA (by non-PCR-based methods) may occur spontaneously in about 10% of patients yearly or as a result of antiviral therapy. This seroconversion may be clinically silent or be accompanied by a clinical exacerbation. It results in a patient without active viral replication, decreased infectivity, lower aminotransferase levels, and less inflammation on the liver biopsy.

A minority of patients with chronic hepatitis B have an infection with a precore mutant virus, first described in a report of patients with chronic hepatitis B in whom serum anti-HBe was present simultaneously with high levels of HBV DNA. These mutant viruses, unable to synthesize HBeAg because of a mutation in the precore reading frame, represent on average 15% of chronic infections, although the geographic prevalence of precore mutant viruses varies widely. These mutants may arise during the natural course of wild-type chronic HBV infection and influence the clinical manifestations of the disease; although they have been linked to patients with a greater degrees of histological injury and to an initial fulminant presentation, there is as yet no direct proof of greater pathogenicity of these mutants. The relative amount of circulating precore mutant virus, rather than its absolute absence or presence, may be important in determining the clinical course.

Liver Biopsy

Traditionally, a liver biopsy has been performed in all patients to stage the degree of histological damage, evaluate for any other coexisting liver disease, and establish whether the patient is a candidate for antiviral therapy. We believe that the liver biopsy is important as a prognostic tool in patients with chronic hepatitis B. However, one must take into account that the degree of histological injury is not static over time. In addition, studies that have specifically looked at survival in chronic hepatitis B have established the following prognostic factors not dependent on a liver biopsy: age, presence of spider angiomas or ascites, level of viremia, and serum bilirubin. Progression from chronic hepatitis to cirrhosis in hepatitis B has also been most often seen in patients with frequent clinical exacerbations, with or without clinical decompensation, or virological reactivations.

The availability of precise and reliable diagnostic tests for possible coexisting liver diseases has improved over time. This is particularly true given the availability of accurate diagnostic tests for hepatitis C infection, and reliable screening tests for hemochromatosis, Wilson's disease, alpha-1 antitrypsin deficiency, and autoimmune hepatitis. The liver biopsy offers only limited additional diagnostic information once a complete noninvasive diagnostic evaluation has been performed. Uncertainty regarding the predominant liver disease may arise in the patient in whom alcoholic liver disease or nonalcoholic fatty liver is suspected. The contribution of the coexisting disease may become clear after a period of alcohol withdrawal or weight loss, respectively. Similarly, if autoimmune liver disease is suspected because of high level autoantibody titers or marked hyperglobulinemia, it will be difficult to distinguish one liver disease from another.

Finally, the clinician needs to decide who is a candidate for treatment. This is a setting in which the liver biopsy has been used either to establish a minimal degree of liver injury above which one would be willing to use antiviral therapy or the absence of cirrhosis which had been an exclusion criterion. We now have studies that suggest that antiviral therapy of patients with well-compensated cirrhosis is possible and safe and has significant efficacy. Other studies have shown that the presence of abnormal aminotransferases in chronic hepatitis B viral infection in general predicts the presence of at least a minimal histological injury that would make the patient a candidate for antiviral therapy.

Thus, we believe that it is important to perform a liver biopsy in the patient in whom the diagnosis of a coexisting disease is in question, in whom the initial noninvasive evaluation suggests the presence of advanced liver disease despite the absence of clinical signs of decompensation, or who is participating in a clinical trial in which the degree of histological damage is an entry criterion or an endpoint of therapy. However, in the more common situation of a well-compensated patient with wild-type, viremic chronic hepatitis B infection and no clinical or laboratory signs of decompensated liver disease, the additional information available from the liver biopsy does not necessarily establish whether antiviral therapy is appropriate and may not change the management of that particular patient. A liver biopsy will always be of prognostic value and physicians must decide whether this is a sufficient reason to expose the patient to the small but real morbidity and mortality of a liver biopsy.

SCREENING FOR HEPATOCELLULAR CARCINOMA

Hepatocellular carcinoma is one of the most common malignancies worldwide, especially in Africa and Asia (see Chap. 22). Its incidence mirrors the prevalence of hepatitis B viral infection, and it is almost always associated with chronic underlying liver cirrhosis. It causes 1.25 million deaths a year worldwide, predominantly in men of ages 40–70. When hepatocellular carcinoma is discovered in a patient as a result of symptoms due to the tumor, median survival is 4 months after diagnosis. It follows that the purpose of screening should be to detect the tumor at a treatable stage. Patients with hepatocellular carcinomas that are discovered incidentally when they are small (less than 3–5 cm), single, and not spread beyond the capsule of the liver or into the blood vessels have a much better prognosis than those discovered at a later stage. In order to diagnose a tumor at a treatable and potentially curable stage, it is important that appropriate screening measures be adopted.

An ideal screening test would be easy to administer and interpret, inexpensive, safe, and sensitive, with good positive and negative predictive values. Although no test available today fits all these criteria, the serum alpha fetoprotein and the abdominal ultrasound have been used in most screening programs for hepatocellular carcinoma. The sensitivity of a serum alpha-fetoprotein test for the presence of a hepatocellular carcinoma is approximately 75%. Similar data for screening with abdominal ultrasound are not available from a field study; however, in other settings an abdominal ultrasound exam has a sensitivity of about 80%. Other imaging studies such as the abdominal CT scan and magnetic resonance imaging do not appear to be appropriate for screening examinations due to their expense and limited availability; they have not been proven to be more sensitive than the ultrasound for initial screening. Although the efficacy of screening for hepatocellular carcinoma has not yet been proven to be useful, tumors of the liver discovered by screening appear to be smaller, less often multiple, and less often invasive of nearby vessels.

As stated previously, all patients with chronic hepatitis B should be considered candidates for hepatocellular carcinoma screening. Although most hepatocellular carcinomas occur in patients with cirrhosis, many population-based studies and consecutive series have documented the presence of hepatocellular carcinomas in noncirrhotic individuals. Patients at the highest risk for hepatocellular carcinoma are those with cirrhosis, an elevated alpha fetoprotein, a family history of hepatocellular carcinoma, a previously resected hepatocellular carcinoma, age greater than 50, and male gender. Patients who would not be considered candidates for treatment of their hepatocellular carcinoma because of advanced age or frailty will not benefit from screening.

The average doubling times of hepatocellular carcinoma is between 3–6 months. Thus, patients at highest risk of hepatocellular carcinoma are usually screened every 3 months with serum alpha-fetoprotein determinations and every 6 months with an abdominal ultrasound. Current recommendations for noncirrhotic patients are not well delineated; yearly screening has been proposed.

ANTIVIRAL THERAPY

The purpose of antiviral therapy in patients with chronic hepatitis B is to eradicate the infection and prevent further spread of the infection and progression of the liver disease. Resolution of the infection has traditionally been defined as loss of serum HBsAg and development of anti-HBs. This definition describes a person who is felt to be no longer infectious, not likely to have abnormal aminotransferases, and not prone to further progression of their liver disease. It is for practical purposes, correct; however, there have been many well-characterized exceptions to it. For example, livers used in a transplant operation from donors who are HBsAg-negative and anti-HBc-positive have been responsible for transmitting typical HBsAg positive hepatitis B infection to the recipient. In addition, patients who have had prior acute viral hepatitis B and are HBsAg negative and anti-HBc positive have been shown to have small amounts of circulating HBV DNA in their peripheral blood. Last, a minority of patients with prior chronic hepatitis B who are HBsAg-negative and anti-HBc-positive may present with either decompensated liver disease or hepatocellular carcinoma.

Keeping the above caveats in mind, the measures of success of antiviral therapy that have been proposed in clinical studies are outlined in Table 3. Both complete and partial

Table 3 Types of Response to Antiviral Therapy Based on Serological Tests Following Therapy

Response	HBeAg	HBV DNA	HBsAg	Interpretation
Complete	Negative	Negative	Negative	Resolution of infection
Partial	Negative	Negative	Positive	Loss of active viral replication
Transient or none	Positive	Positive	Positive	No significant response

responses have been associated with lesser infectivity, fewer and less severe symptoms, reduced aminotransferase levels, and improvement in the amount of inflammation seen in a liver biopsy following therapy. In addition, follow-up studies of patients who achieved a partial response suggest that they lose HBsAg at a more rapid rate than patients who lose markers of rapid viral replication spontaneously. Thus, either a complete or partial response is felt to be of benefit to the patient.

In evaluating the results of clinical trials, it is important to determine whether treatment actually led to an improvement in the baseline spontaneous loss of viremia. This can best be determined by placebo-controlled, randomized clinical trials, since spontaneous loss of HBeAg and/or HBV DNA from blood occurs in about 10% of patients with chronic hepatitis B yearly. Many agents are active against the hepatitis B virus and cause a fall in viremia during drug administration, but it is important to limit the clinical use of these drugs to those shown to have effects that are sustained after treatment has ceased or that are safe and persistently effective over chronic long-term use.

Interferon

Clinical trials of interferon treatment in patients with chronic hepatitis B have usually been performed in immunocompetent patients with adult-acquired wild-type (HBeAg-positive) virus infection, abnormal aminotransferases, and well-compensated liver disease. However, the majority of patients with chronic hepatitis B are individuals who acquired hepatitis B viral infection as neonates or infants, have normal aminotransferases, and are immune-tolerant. The results in the former group are not necessarily applicable to the latter, and may not reflect the outcome of therapy in other special settings—i.e., immunosuppressed patients (HIV or other comorbid conditions), patients with decompensated cirrhosis, transplant recipients, and precore mutant infections (HBeAg negative, anti-HBe-positive and HBV DNA-positive). Results of interferon therapy in each of these groups are analyzed below.

Immune-Competent Adults with Adult-Acquired Wild-Type HBV Infection

Initial treatment studies with interferon used a human leukocyte preparation and were able to demonstrate a dose-related reduction of serum HBV DNA polymerase (a marker of viremia) in patients with chronic hepatitis B. Subsequently, synthetic interferon preparations became available and tested. A multicenter, randomized, controlled study of interferon-alpha-2b treatment showed that approximately 36% of patients treated with 5 million units subcutaneously daily for 16 weeks responded to treatment with loss of HBV DNA and HBeAg from serum. This response occurred most often in patients with elevated ALT levels (above 100 IU/L) and low levels of viremia (serum HBV DNA levels below 200 pg/mL). A less significant response occurred in patients given 1 million units of interferon alpha-2b daily, suggesting a dose related response to treatment. This study showed that therapy with interferon alpha-2b results in a sustained suppression of viral replication in a significant minority of patients treated. The addition of a 6-week period of prednisone treatment or "immunological priming" prior to interferon-alpha-2b therapy did not improve the overall response rate; however, there was a suggestion that patients with low levels of aminotransferases may have benefited from pretreatment with prednisone. A dosing interval of 10 million units three times weekly can achieve similar efficacy and is equally well-tolerated. A subsequent meta-analysis of 15 randomized clinical trials of interferon therapy in chronic hepatitis B showed an overall benefit to interferon therapy,

Table 4 Interferon Treatment of Chronic Hepatitis B: Outcome Variables

Host	Viral	Treatment
Aminotransferase level	Viral titer	Dose
Gender	Viral mutations	Type
Age at onset		Duration
Duration of infection		
Immune status		

with a loss of serum HBeAg in 33% of treated patients versus 12% of controls. Variables that predict loss of HBeAg and HBV DNA are outlined in Table 4. The most significant are HBV DNA levels greater than 200 pg/mL, ALT levels greater than 100 IU/L, and dose of interferon. Most studies show that only a small minority of patients who lose HBeAg and HBV DNA with interferon-alpha-2b treatment reactivate their infection over time. Retreatment of interferon failures, or increasing the dose or length of treatment, has not been shown to significantly improve the overall response to treatment.

Data from four small, randomized, controlled trials in children with chronic hepatitis B suggest that interferon therapy is as efficacious in HBeAg positive children with abnormal aminotransferases as in adults. Factors predictive of response (elevated aminotransferases and low levels of serum HBV DNA) were similar, and pretreatment with prednisone did not improve the overall response rate. Results of a large multicenter, multinational, randomized, controlled study are pending.

Treatment with interferon may result in a flare, a transient twofold or greater increase in aminotransferase levels, usually during the second or third month of therapy. This flare is felt to represent an interferon-induced activation of the immune system and a rapid lysis of hepatocytes infected with hepatitis B virus. This flare is seen twice as commonly in patients who respond to interferon treatment than in nonresponders.

During the flare, patients may experience symptoms or signs of liver disease. Patients with advanced stages of liver disease may experience decompensation and life-threatening complications (hepatic encephalopathy, sterile or infected ascites, variceal bleeding, or death). During a flare, interferon therapy should be continued as tolerated and the patient should be monitored more frequently. Treatment with interferon should cease if significant adverse effects or evidence of decompensation occur during a flare.

Adverse effects of interferon are common. They include fevers chills, myalgias, headache, and anorexia, which occur soon after the first injection. They occur in nearly all patients treated with regimens that have been proven effective. Bone marrow suppression, hair loss, depression, irritability, and confusion can occur after days to weeks of therapy, as can immune adverse effects such as thyroiditis, arthritis, and hepatitis. Despite the many adverse effects, interferon is relatively well tolerated, and over 90% of patients do not need dose adjustments or discontinuation of therapy. In order to monitor the patient for drug-related adverse effects, it is customary to evaluate the patient at the start of therapy and weeks 2, 4, 8, 12, and 16. At each evaluation, a review of symptoms, physical evaluation, complete blood count, general chemical survey panel, and prothrombin time should be performed. A TSH level to test thyroid function should be performed at baseline and every 8 weeks during treatment. Efficacy should be tested with HBeAg and HBV DNA levels at the end of therapy and in 6 months, as some patients have a delayed response to therapy. If a patient loses HBeAg and HBV DNA during therapy, repeat tests for HBsAg should be performed on each subsequent yearly evaluation to test for delayed loss of HBsAg.

Immune-Tolerant and Immunosuppressed Patients

Asian patients with chronic hepatitis B who have normal aminotransferases do not respond well to treatment with interferon, both because of poor initial responses and frequent relapses. This is assumed to be due to immunological tolerance to the hepatitis B virus because of infection in the neonatal period, at a time when the immune system is immature. Attempts to increase responses to antiviral therapy by the use of immune priming strategies such as pulse prednisone pretreatment have not proven to be of significant benefit. Other immunostimulants have not yet been extensively evaluated.

It would be difficult to generalize the effect of interferon therapy in a group of immunosuppressed patients with chronic hepatitis B because they are heterogeneous in their etiologies and defects in immunity. However, certain general characteristics can be found in patients in this group. They circulate large amounts of HBV DNA and have defects in cell-mediated immunity. Their comorbid conditions (HIV infection, organ transplantation, disorders that are inherently immunosuppressive or require immunosuppressive therapy) may be the ultimate determinants of their quality of life or their ultimate prognosis, although death from complications of end-stage liver disease is not uncommon in immunosuppressed patients. However, studies have shown that patients with HIV infection can respond to alpha interferon with loss of HBeAg and HBV DNA, albeit at a much lower rate than patients without HIV coinfection. Whether the outcome of an immunosuppressed patient will be different as a result of antiviral therapy is unclear at this time.

Patients with Decompensated Cirrhosis

In general, patients with decompensated liver disease (those having blending from portal hypertension, ascites, hepatic encephalopathy, or jaundice) have not been considered candidates for treatment with alpha interferon and have been referred for liver transplantation. They have been systematically excluded from most large treatment studies. In the limited studies available, it was observed that standard doses of interferon were not well tolerated and frequently led to treatment-related adverse effects such as bacterial infections or flares that caused further decompensation and death. When reduced doses of interferon were used, fewer patients flared and sustained losses of serum HBV DNA were seen. In a rare patient awaiting liver transplantation, this resulted in stabilization of disease and indefinite postponement of the transplant but no changes in overall survival or reinfection rates following transplantation.

In the largest study to date, 36 patients with histological evidence of cirrhosis and evidence of liver synthetic dysfunction or fluid retention were treated with low dose (0.5–3 MU SC qid) alpha interferon up to 24 weeks. A sustained loss of HBV DNA was seen in all Child's class A patients, in 5 of 15 (33%) Child's B, subjects and in none of 6 Child's C subjects. Adverse effects severe enough to require dose modifications occurred in 17 (65%) of patients, and 7 (21%) did not complete therapy. This approach may be considered for patients with stable Child's class A cirrhosis. We believe that patients with cirrhosis who are considered for interferon therapy should undergo simultaneous liver transplant evaluation, as this may prove to be lifesaving if the patient decompensates during therapy.

Patients with Non–Wild-Type Hepatitis B Virus Infection

Data on interferon treatment of patients with non–wild-type hepatitis B virus infection are available only for patients who are simultaneously anti-HBe and HBV DNA positive and are presumed to have a predominant infection with a precore mutant virus. In general, the response of the anti-HBe/HBV DNA positive patient to a standard course of alpha interferon, as measured by sustained loss of serum HBV DNA, is not as good. In the largest series reported, 53 patients were treated with either interferon alpha-2a or lymphoblastoid interferon at doses of 6–18 million units two or three times daily for 4–6 months. Although 34 (60%) achieved loss of HBV DNA at the end of the treatment period, only 5 (10%) achieved a sustained loss of viremia. The other 29 relapsed, with a biochemical flare and recurrence of viremia within 6 months of their last injection. Increasing the length of therapy may improve the response rate.

Other Therapeutic Agents

Most patients with chronic hepatitis B do not respond to standard therapy with alpha interferon. Retreatment is rarely useful and not recommended. There are no other treatments that have been proven to be of long-term benefit to patients with chronic hepatitis B. However, there are many agents for which pilot studies suggest activity against hepatitis B virus that may become important management options or the basis for combination therapy in the future. The two most important classes of agents appear to be immunomodulators and nucleoside analogues.

Immunomodulators

Although most patients with chronic hepatitis B viral infection have no known immune deficiency, the outcome of patients with chronic hepatitis B infection has been frequently linked to the inability of the patient to generate an immune response to promote clearance of HBV infected cells by cytotoxic T lymphocytes. This is exemplified in patients with chronic hepatitis B who received a bone marrow transplant from a patient immune to hepatitis B and showed loss of HBeAg and eventually HBsAg following successful marrow engraftment. Therapy with thymic extracts, cytokines such as IL-12, prostaglandins, and T-cell vaccines have been proposed. Thymosin alpha, a highly purified thymic extract, has been shown to have activity in chronic hepatitis B in small clinical trials. It may have an equal effect to interferon alpha in anti-HBe positive patients. It may be best used in combination with interferon alpha. Therapy with IL-12 has been shown in a transgenic mouse model to suppress HBV gene expression and is currently in clinical trials; trials with IL-2 in the past did not show a benefit. A pilot study of prostaglandin PGE2 resulted in a sustained loss of HBeAg and HBV DNA in 47% of patients. T-cell peptide vaccines have been shown to enhance HBcAg specific T-cell responses in experimental animals and healthy subjects, and pilot studies are under way in patients with chronic hepatitis B.

Nucleoside Analogues

The replication strategy of HBV involves reverse transcription via an RNA intermediate using the viral-encoded DNA polymerase. A series of nucleoside analogues that inhibit the action of the viral DNA polymerase have been found to have activity against HBF in cell cultures and animal models and are now undergoing clinical evaluation.

The best studied is lamivudine, a 2′,3′-dideoxy cytosine analogue. Short-term therapy (25, 100, or 300 mg daily for 12 weeks) has been associated with a profound suppression of HBV replication of rapid onset, which was sustained for the length of the study and associated with loss of HBeAg in 12% of study subjects. Cessation of therapy was generally accompanied by return of serum HBV DNA to pretreatment levels, although a small number of patients had a sustained loss of HBV DNA (19%) or HBeAg (12%) and normalization of ALT. Subsequent pilot studies have confirmed these observations. A randomized controlled trial with 6 or 12 months of therapy with either 25 mg or 100 mg of lamivudine daily documented improvement in histology in 66 and 58% of treated patients versus 30% of placebo recipients. Drug-resistant mutants were isolated from 15% of treated patients, their appearance usually accompanied by a rise in serum HBV DNA levels. Patients with HIV infection on combination nucleoside analogue and protease inhibitor therapy and immunosuppressed organ-transplant recipients can respond to lamivudine with loss or marked fall of detectable serum HBV DNA. The drug is well tolerated and rapidly absorbed after oral administration; serious side effects are rare and may include anemia, neutropenia, elevated aminotransferases, and peripheral neuropathy.

Famciclovir, a guanine analogue, is rapidly absorbed after oral administration and converted to the active drug penciclovir. Prior studies in patients infected with herpesviruses have shown it to be well tolerated; adverse effects are infrequent and include headache, diarrhea, nausea, fatigue, dizziness and abdominal pain. Studies in primary duck hepatocytes and ducks infected with duck hepatitis B virus showed a reversible reduction in serum and liver DHBV titers. A randomized, controlled trial of famciclovir 125–500 mg three times daily has been performed in 333 patients with chronic hepatitis B; the HBeAg seroconversion rate was 14% in the treated group and 3% in the placebo group, and improvement in aminotransferase levels was seen. A similar agent, ganciclovir, has also been shown to reduce serum levels of HBV DNA in liver transplant candidates with cirrhosis due to hepatitis B. Oral ganciclovir has also been studied and was similarly active in reducing HBV DNA titers in patients with chronic hepatitis B. In all studies, however, the effect was transient and limited to the duration of therapy.

Adefovir dipivoxil and lobucavir have also been shown to have a dose-dependent suppression of serum HBV DNA levels, and further studies are underway on these drugs. This class of antivirals may alter our expectations regarding the results of therapy. If continuous therapy with these agents is well tolerated and results in not only prolonged suppression of viremia but improved aminotransferases and findings on liver biopsy, then extended and perhaps lifelong administration of these agents may be useful. However, the emergence of viral mutants resistant to drug therapy has been documented, similar to that seen in the use of nucleoside analogues in HIV infection, and may limit this approach.

Liver Transplantation

Prior to 1993, liver transplantation had been avoided in patients with chronic hepatitis B. Studies from the University of Pittsburgh showed nearly universal HBV recurrence and an accelerated postoperative injury frequently resulting in liver failure and death. A 20% excess mortality attributable to HBV recurrence was seen, and a frequently lethal fibrosing cholestatic syndrome was described. However, a multicenter study in France suggested that postoperative high dose HBIG infusion can prevent recurrence of infection and disease in $>$ 80% of patients, independent of the presence or initial level of serum HBV DNA. Based on this study, transplantation for patients with end-stage liver disease due to HBV became feasible. Patients are treated with 45 mL (10,000 IU) or HBIG IV during the anhepatic phase, daily for the first 7 postoperative days, and every 4 weeks or as required to maintain an anti-HBs titer greater than 1:150. Patients with infections with precore mutants have a higher rate of recurrent disease and graft loss (7 of 10) than patients with wild type infection (1 of 10) or HBV DNA negative patients (0 or 4). How to manage the patients in whom HBV recurs posttransplant is still unclear; pilot studies with oral nucleoside analogues and interferon suggest limited efficacy.

BIBLIOGRAPHY

Barbera C, Bortolotti F, Crivellaro C, Coscia A, Zancan L, Cadrobbi P, Nebbia G, Pillan MN, Lepore L, Parrella T, et al. Recombinant interferon alpha 2a hastens the rate of HBeAg clearance in children with chronic hepatitis B. Hepatology 1994; 20:287–290.

Bartholomew MM, Jansen RW, Jeffers LJ, Ready KR, Johnson LC, Bunzendahl H, Condreay LD, Tzakis AG, Sxhiff ER, Brown NA. Hepatitis B virus resistance to lamivudine given for recurrent infection after orthotopic liver transplantation. Lancet 1997; 349:20–22.

Benhamou Y, Dohin E, Lunel-Fabiani F, Poynard T, Huraux JM, Katlama C, Opolon P, Gentilimi M. Efficacy of lamivudine on replication of hepatitis B virus in HIV infected patients. Lancet 1995; 345:396–397.

Dienstag JL, Perrillo RP, Schiff ER, et al. A preliminary trial of lamivudine for chronic hepatitis B infection. N Engl J Med 1995; 333:1657–1661.

Farhat BA, Marinos G, Daniels HM, Naoumov NV, Williams R. Evaluation of safety and efficacy of thymus humoral factor gamma 2 in the management of chronic hepatitis B. J Hepatol 1995; 23:21–27.

Garcia G, Smith CI, Weissberg JI, Eisenberg M, Bissett J, Nair PV, Mastre B, Rosno S, Roskamp D, Waterman K, Pollard RB, Tong MJ, Brown BW, Robinson WS, Gregory PB, Merigan TC. Adenine arabinoside (vidarabine phosphate) monophosphate in combination with human leukocyte interferon in the treatment of chronic hepatitis B: a randomized, double-blinded, placebo-controlled trial. Ann Intern 1987; 107:278–285.

Gish RG, Lau JY, Brooks L, Fang JW, Staedy SL, Imperial JC, Garcia-Kennedy R, Esquivel CO, Keeffe EB. Ganciclovir treatment of hepatitis B virus infection in liver transplant recipients. Hepatology 1996; 23:1–7.

Gregorio GV, Jara P, Hierro L, Diaz C, de la Vega A, Vegnente A, Iorio L, Bortolotti F, Crivellaro C, Zancan L, Daniels H, Portmann B, Mieli-Vergani G. Lymphoblastoid interferon alfa with or without steroid pretreatment in children with chronic hepatitis B: a multicenter controlled trial. Hepatology 1996; 23:700–707.

Hoofnagle JH, Di Bisceglie AM, Waggoner JG, Park Y. Interferon alfa for patients with clinically apparent cirrhosis due to chronic hepatitis B. Gastroenterology 1993; 104:1116–1121.

Lai CL, Liaw YF, Leung NWY, Chang TT, Guan R, Tai DI, Ng KY, Wu PC, Dent JC, Gray DF. 12 months of lamivudine (100 mg od) therapy improves liver histology: results of a placebo controlled multicenter study in Asia. J Hepatol 1997; 26:79.

Marcellin P, Samuel D, Areias J, Loriot MA, Arulnader JL, Gigou M, David MF, Bismuth A, Reynes M, Brechot C, Benhamou JP, Bismuth H. Pretransplantation interferon therapy and recurrence of hepatitis B virus infection after liver transplantation for hepatitis B-related end-stage liver disease. Hepatology 1994; 19:6–12.

Niederau C, Heingtges T, Longe S, Goldmann G, Niederau CM, Mohr L, Haussinger D. Long-term follow-up of HBeAg-positive patients treated with interferon alfa for chronic hepatitis B. N Engl J Med 1996; 334:1422–1427.

Papakonstantinou A, Manesis E, Hadziyannis S. Oral ganciclovir in HBeAg positive and negative chronic hepatitis B. J Hepatol 1997; 26:91.

Perrillo R, Tamburro C, Regenstein F, Balart L, Bodenheimer H, Silva M, Schiff E, Bodicky C, Miller B, Denham C, et al. Low-dose, titratable interferon alfa in decompensated liver disease caused by chronic infection with hepatitis B virus. Gastroenterology 1995; 109:908–916.

Perrillo RP, Schiff ER, Davis GL, Bodenheimer H, Lindsay K, Payne J, Dienstag JL, O'Brien C,

Tamburro C, Jacobson MI, Sampliner R, Lefkowich J, Kuhns M, Meschievitz C, Sanghv B, Albrecht J, Gibas A. A randomized, controlled trial of interferon alfa-2b alone and after prednisone withdrawal for the treatment of chronic hepatitis B. Hepatitis Intervention Therapy Group. N Engl J Med 1990; 323:295–301.

Samuel D, Muller R, Alexander G, et al. Liver transplantation in European patients with the hepatitis B surface antigen. N Engl J Med 1993; 329:1842–1847.

Sokal EM, Wirth S, Goyens P, Depreferre A, Cornu C. Interferon alfa-2b therapy in children with chronic hepatitis B. Gut 1993; 34 (suppl 2):87–90.

Trepo C, Jezek P, Atkinson GF, Boon RT. Longterm effects of famciclovir in chronic hepatitis B. Results of a phase IIB study. J Hepatol 1997; 26:74.

8

Management of Chronic Hepatitis D (Delta)

Philippe Merle and Philippe Chossegros
Hôtel-Dieu Hospital and INSERM U271, Lyon, France

Christian Trepo
Claude Bernard University and INSERM U271, Lyon, France

HISTORICAL PERSPECTIVE

Hepatitis D (delta) antigen (HDAg) was first described by Rizzetto in 1977. This nuclear antigen, distinct from HBs and HBc antigens, was present in hepatocyte nuclei of Italian patients infected by the hepatitis B virus (HBV). Antibodies directed against it were also present in the serum of patients with severe B hepatitis. Experimental transmission to chimpanzees confirmed its pathogenicity and transmissibility. Following this first description, the epidemiology of hepatitis D virus (HDV) has shown its worldwide distribution. A geographic variability of HDV infection prevalence is observed among different countries and even within the same country between geographically and ethnically distinct groups, whatever the level of endemicity of HBV. The causes of these variations are unknown.

The most common transmission of HDV is through blood and blood products, leading to a high prevalence among intravenous drug addicts in all populations studied in developed countries. The low perinatal transmission may reflect the uncommon perinatal transmission of HBV in countries where HDV is endemic. Sexual transmission may represent a major risk of transmission. A study of familial transmission, conducted in Italy, independently associated HDV superinfection with female sex and infection in index HBsAg carriers. In the Amazon basin, children are infected before the age of 10. Thus, in areas of high endemicity, a transmission through person-to-person contact is possible. Open skin lesions have been considered.

NATURAL HISTORY OF HEPATITIS D

Since infections with HDV can develop only in the presence of ongoing HBV replication, clinical presentations can occur as simultaneous coinfections with HBV or as superinfections of preexisting chronic HBsAg carriers.

In acute coinfections, incubation duration, studied in chimpanzees, ranged from 6 weeks to 6 months and seemed dependent on the viral load of the inoculum. Clinical symptoms do not differ significantly from other acute viral infections apart from a biphasic illness, which is more often present than with HBV infection alone. The occurrence of fulminant hepatitis is the other distinctive characteristic of coinfections with HDV and HBV. The evolution to a chronic HBsAg carrier state is observed in less than 5% and does not differ between cases of HBV-HDV coinfection and those of HBV infection alone. A rapid progression toward cirrhosis in patients who did not clear HBsAg has been suggested. However, since few cases have been reported and many cohorts consisted mostly of intravenous drug addicts with a possible influence of hepatitis C virus (HCV) coinfections, generalization of that conclusion is still questionable.

In HDV superinfections, the shorter incubation period observed in animal models could be related to the ongoing HBV replication, which may allow a more rapid dissemination of HDV. Superinfections can be clinically symptomatic in more than 50% of cases. Acute superinfections suppress HBV replication, which can lead in some cases to HBsAg clearance. However, in most cases, a chronic carrier state of HDV is observed. Superinfection can also lead to fulminant evolution. A peculiar clinicopathological form is observed in children and young adults in Amazonian regions and central Africa and could be related to more cytopathic strains of HDV.

Conflicting results have been reported concerning the natural history of HDV infections. All the earlier studies concerned patients with a rapid progression to cirrhosis in 2–6 years. In these patients, usually referred to liver centers for clinical an/or biological features of chronic hepatitis, progression to cirrhosis was significantly more rapid in cases coinfected by HBV and HDV than in those infected by HBV alone. However, progression to severe liver disease has not always been present, and investigations conducted in Greece and Samoa have shown that, in areas endemic for HDV, the majority of carriers of HDV and HBV had no biological or histological signs of liver disease.

HEPATITIS DELTA VIRUS: STRUCTURE AND DISEASE EXPRESSION

The average diameter of the HDV particle is about 38–41 nm. The virion is composed of a lipid envelope containing the RNA genome and the proteins of HDV, the two forms of delta antigen. No core or nucleocapsid structure has as yet been specifically identified within HDV particles. The envelope of HDV contains the same surface proteins as HBV, but the relative amounts of these proteins differ between the two viruses, as the HDV envelope contains essentially the smallest S protein, while the larger proteins are much more enriched in HBV particles.

The genome is a very small (about 1700 nucleotides) single-stranded circular RNA of negative polarity. It is able to fold onto itself by base-pairing to form an unbranched rodlike structure. A significant sequence heterogeneity, as high as 39%, has been found among the various HDV isolates sequenced, and a classification by genotypes has been proposed.

The replication occurs in the nucleus of infected cells, probably via cellular RNA polymerase II. First, antigenomic strand RNA is synthesized, and a polyadenylation signal enables the production of a subgenomic mRNA, which is translated into HDAg in the cytoplasm. Second, transcription continues in a rolling-circle fashion. Multimeric antigenomic RNA is synthesized and then cleaved to produce monomeric antigenomic RNA. Third, this antigenomic RNA acts as a matrix for genomic RNA synthesis.

An open reading frame for HDAg is present on the HDV antigenomic strand. However, some HDV RNA encodes a 195–amino acid delta antigen while others encode a longer 214–amino acid delta antigen because of a change in the termination codon of the small antigen. The input genome encodes the small HDAg, which enables genome replication to start. Because of an RNA editing reaction in the nucleus, some of the antigenomic RNAs are specifically altered. These newly formed RNAs engender the synthesis of the larger form of the HDAg. This leads to the assembly of new delta particles. Small HDAg enhances genome replication. The large protein can interfere with the ability of the small HDAg to support genome replication, acting as a dominant negative inhibitor of replication and as a promoter of viral particle assembly.

HDV requires sequences of the envelope encoding region of the coinfecting HBV to exit from the initially infected cell and spread from cell to cell. In vitro and in vivo, HDV infection inhibits HBV replication. Small HDAg may block RNA transcription of HBV. However some degree of HBV activity is required by HDV to exert its pathogenic potential. If HBV is further suppressed by interferon (IFN), HDV can be cleared itself or enter a nonpathogenic phase, possibly sustained by overexpression of the noncytotoxic HDAg. In vivo in humans, evaluation of HBV replication suggests that it represents the main prognostic factor. In two studies, histological findings and disease activity were related to the presence of active HBV replication.

Clinically, HDV infection is associated with an array of presentations ranging from the asymptomatic healthy carrier to end-stage cirrhosis. These variations in pathogenicity may depend on viral factors and possibly on sequence heterogeneity, which occurs extensively for HDV. The virus could be directly hepatotoxic by interaction between numerous HDV-RNA copies and the host nuclear contents. HDV replication might interfere with the physiological functions of the cellular RNA polymerases or with DNA replication and cell division. Also, host immune responses may influence pathogenesis. Interactions between the immune system and delta antigens are unknown. The two pathogenic pathways may coexist in a mutual balance throughout the natural history of the infection, but the precise mechanisms are still poorly understood. In addition, autoimmune reactivity is found in a significant proportion of HDV infections, as indicated by an antibody reacting against the liver kidney microsomes-3 (anti-LKM-3), specifically against UDP glucuronosyltransferases.

DIAGNOSIS OF DELTA VIRUS INFECTION

Methods

Serological tests for detection of IgG and IgM anti-HD are available. The first test was a competitive inhibition radioimmunoassay (RIA). Subsequently, an enzyme immunoassay (EIA) was developed, whose sensitivity was intermediate between those of immunofluorescence (IF) and RIA. More recently, specific tests for IgM anti-HD, a capture RIA and an EIA, were developed.

Detection of delta antigens is possible in serum by immunoblot (IB), RIA, or EIA, which is more sensitive and can detect HDAg for a much longer time. Detection of HDAg in liver by immunohistochemistry (IF or immunoperoxidase) of biopsy material, consisting of frozen or paraffin-embedded sections from patients, is used for diagnosis of current

HDV infection. HDAg can also be found in infected liver by Western blot, using high-titered anti-HD serum and iodine-125 (^{125}I)-labeled protein A.

Detection of HDV-RNA genome by nucleic acid hybridization or reverse-transcriptase polymerase chain reaction (RT-PCR) in serum represents an additional tool for diagnosis of HDV infection and to measure viremia levels. RT-PCR is much more sensitive than traditional hybridization. Also, it enables the analysis of genetic variability of the HDV-RNA genome. It is therefore a potentially useful method for therapeutic monitoring in chronic HDV infection. A direct in situ hybridization method has been described to detect HDV-RNA in routinely frozen or formalin-fixed liver. This method is not more sensitive than direct immunofluorescence for HDAg. This test can be used in cases where HDAg cannot be stained in liver tissue.

Diagnostic Strategies

In HDV-infected patients, the timing of the appearance and the levels of the above markers allows discrimination between the different phases of the natural course of infection (see Table 1). Because of the dependence of HDV on HBV, detection of some markers of HBV infection, especially detection of HBsAg, is usually necessary before considering HDV infection. Serum HDV-RNA or HDAg are primarily tested in cases of very early infections or in cases of a coinfection with human immunodeficiency virus (HIV). In other cases, anti-HDV antibodies are tested. Detection of antibodies may be transient and does not necessarily indicate ongoing or active HDV infection. The specific diagnosis of active HDV infection is usually made by detection of HDV-RNA and HDAg in serum and liver, or by detection of specific IgM antibodies. A transient IgM anti-HD activity is observed only in HBV/HDV coinfection, whereas a prolonged IgM anti-HD activity is seen in superinfections. IgM anti-HD activity persists at high levels in patients with unremitting or progressive liver disease, whereas it decreases or disappears in case of improvement or resolution of disease. Serological HDV markers should be used whenever a suspicion of acute or chronic hepatitis is present and especially in fulminant hepatitis. The diagnosis of acute coinfection is made on the presence of high titers of anti-HBc IgM. HDAg can be detected in the serum for a short duration often less than 2 weeks, at the onset of clinical symptoms. Levels of serum HDAg are variable during the course of acute delta infection and are rarely detected in chronic delta hepatitis. The most reliable and sensitive tests for active HDV infection are those based on molecular hybridization techniques. Detection of HDAg and

Table 1 Markers of the Different Phases of the Natural Course of HDV Infection

	IgG anti-HD	IgM anti-HD	HDAg in serum	HDAg in liver	HDV RNA in serum
Early acute infection	±	±	++	++	+
Acute infection	++	++	+	++	++
Postacute infection	±	±	−	−	−
Active chronic infection	+++	++	+	++	++
Inactive chronic infection	++	−	−	−	−

Key: + = present; − = absent; ± = inconsistent.

HDV RNA in serum or liver are useful in monitoring the clinical course of patients treated for chronic HDV infections.

THERAPEUTIC MANAGEMENT

The past decade has considerably increased the understanding of hepatitis B and hepatitis D virus infection. Various antivirals have been used to treat chronic viral infection, and at this time interferons (IFNs) were the most used agents. IFNs are considered useful in HBV or HDV infection by their antiviral and immunomodulatory activities.

In Vitro Results and Mechanisms of IFN Action on HDV Infection

These mechanisms are largely unknown. A variety of cell culture systems and animal models are presently available to study HBV and/or HDV replication and the effects of different antivirals. The cell culture experimental model provides insights into the function of the IFN system and may help to define future therapeutic strategies on a preclinical level. An in vitro model system has been used to assay for an antiviral effect of IFN on HDV genome replication. IFN-α and -γ did not affect the rate of replication of the HDV genome. Thus, in the absence of HBV, it appears that HDV is resistant to IFN-α. In vitro experiments contrast with the in vivo results, wherein IFN reduces ALT and HDV-RNA levels, evoking a direct antiviral property. But patients are always coinfected by HBV, which could represent a potential target for IFN. The HDV genome forms double-stranded RNA (dsRNA) by intramolecular base pairing, which can be an inducer of endogenous IFN synthesis and may activate two IFN-inducible enzymes that provide antiviral activity. These enzymes are 2′,5′ A synthetase and a dsRNA-dependent protein kinase. The 2′,5′ A synthetase activates endogenous ribonuclease, leading to the breakdown of RNA. In vitro, levels of HDV-RNA are not affected by IFN, suggesting that the synthetase or the ribonuclease is inhibited in cell lines or that HDV-RNA does not exist in a form able to induce 2′,5′ A synthetase. A circular form of HDV RNA may be responsible for the resistance to ribonuclease. It is conceivable that IFN activity against HBV plays a crucial role. Potent new anti-HBV agents such as lamivudine and famciclovir may allow clarification of this point, since they are more potent anti-HBV molecules they are likely to be of promise for HBV/HDV coinfection.

Ribavirin and suramin showed an antiviral effect in primary woodchuck hepatocytes. Suramin is too toxic for long-term use in humans, and ribavirin has shown no biochemical or virological benefit in small clinical trials in humans. In vitro, trisodium phosphonoformate (foscarnet) enhances the synthesis of HDV-RNA rather than inhibiting it.

Therapy of Acute Hepatitis D

Traditionally no therapy has been attempted in acute hepatitis D. In rare fulminant cases, trisodium phosphonoformate (foscarnet) has been claimed to have enabled patients to recover. This drug is an inhibitor of the HBV DNA polymerase and was used at a bolus dose of 20 mg/kg over 30 min followed by an infusion of 0.16 mg/kg/min for 4–14 days. Since this drug was tested on only a very small number of patients, it is impossible to draw conclusions about its possible beneficial effect on severe acute HDV infections. Theoretically, because of its severity, superinfection of asymptomatic HBV carriers by HDV should be considered as an indication for therapy without waiting for complications to occur. The question remains as to which modalities to use.

Therapy of Chronic Hepatitis D

Current treatment remains somewhat experimental and not very efficacious in chronic hepatitis D. Nucleoside analogues such as adenine arabinoside or immunomodulatory drugs such as corticosteroids, azathioprine, and levamisole tested in the early 1980s were of no benefit. Ribavirin has demonstrated in vitro but not in vivo efficacy. The availability of large doses of molecularly engineered IFN and the demonstrated efficacy of this cytokine against DNA and RNA viruses prompted investigators to try IFN-α in chronic HDV hepatitis. IFN-α is at present the treatment of choice for chronic viral hepatitis, but the results obtained in chronic hepatitis D are the least satisfactory.

First Retrospective and Pilot Studies

IFN-α therapy used in the mid-1980s showed a transient efficacy in hepatitis D control, with an improvement of the disease, inducing normalization of alanine aminotransferase (ALT) level in 0–60% of patients at the end of therapy. It was associated with a decrease of HDV-RNA and HDAg levels in serum and HDAg in liver. Nevertheless HBsAg and antibody to HDV persisted in serum. An improvement in liver histology was present in about 50% of cases. However, the benefit was transient. Types of IFNs used included lymphoblastoid or recombinant α-2b administered at variable doses of 2.5–7.5 million units (MU)/m^2 for 2–4 months.

Further Trials

Those preliminary observations led to many small, uncontrolled trials and a few randomized controlled trials in which higher doses of IFN were administered for longer periods of time; the rate of response in these tended to be proportional to the IFN doses. A dose of 9 MU thrice a week (tiw) produced better results than 3 MU tiw, with a biochemically complete response of 71 versus 28%, and a virological complete response of 71 versus 36% at the end of treatment. But only 36% versus 0% achieved a sustained biochemical response at the end of the follow-up. A virological relapse occurred in all patients after the end of treatment, whatever the dose of IFN. In a small study, half of the patients treated with 9 MU whose ALT became normal retained a biochemical response with a normalization of ALT that persisted for up to 4 years. Attempts to decrease the dose of IFN from 5 MU/m^2 to 3 MU/m^2 were followed by a breakthrough. Virological data have not indicated a clear effect on HDV, since in most studies HDV-RNA in serum was not diminished by therapy. The efficacy of IFN in chronic hepatitis D may be related to dose, but the lack of a consistent antiviral effect argues against a true curative effect of high doses of IFN. DiBisceglie et al. showed that a daily administration of 5 MU IFN could be beneficial. More complex schedules and combination with other antiviral drugs such as acyclovir have not been found more successful.

In patients treated with 9 MU, the normalization of ALT was associated with a marked improvement in histological findings. Histologically, IFN led to an improvement both at the end of treatment and during the follow-up. All treated patients had significant improvement in periportal necrosis, portal inflammation, and lobular inflammation compared with untreated groups. Those treated with higher doses of IFN had a significantly greater improvement in periportal necrosis than those treated with lower doses.

Efficacy of Therapy in Chronic HBV Infection

In vitro and in vivo results focus on HBV as a potential target for IFN in chronic HDV infection, suggesting the use of deoxynucleotide analogues. Therapy with IFN-α for chronic hepatitis B does not prevent HDV superinfection. Many patients with concomitant active HBV replication who cleared HBV-DNA and HBeAg from serum and seroconverted to anti-HBe had no additional change in liver chemistry, and their liver histology did not improve. However, such a turn does represent a positive event in the long term, since associated infections with a replicative phase of HBV infection engenders a worse prognosis. Patients who respond to IFN with a persistent normalization of ALT may ultimately clear HBsAg. In patients presenting a clearance of HBsAg and a seroconversion to anti-HBs, HDV-RNA and HDAg are no longer detectable in serum and liver. Other patients, however, enter a prolonged phase of biochemical and histological remission, despite persistence of active HDV replication and latent HBV infection. Thus IFN seems to act on HBV but not on the HDV replication itself, which, however, when it remains isolated, does not seem to generate much harm to the liver. This fact is of major relevance in favor of the potential benefit of the new potent anti-HBV drugs, including lamivudine, famciclovir, lobucorvin, and adefovin.

Treatment Overview

IFN-α is currently the only prescribed treatment, although existing information concerning its benefit remains unclear. A graphical presentation of the odds ratios and of their 95% confidence of the four controlled trials comparing treated to untreated patients is impossible. The odds ratios range from 2.5–32.5, with confidence intervals ranging from 2.81–1512. These huge variations were mainly related to the small size of the trials. However, when exact tests were used to account for this small size, the results were homogeneous. The comparison of treatment to no treatment gave a very significant overall odds ratio ($p < 0.0001$) of HDV-RNA negativation of 3.916 (95% confidence interval:1.948–8.122) and of ALT normalization of 15.67 (95% confidence interval:5.862–56.68). These differences disappeared in every trial as soon as injections were discontinued. These results provide a good argument for treatment continuation until the occurrence of HBsAg/anti-HBs seroconversion or perhaps HBeAg/anti-HBe seroconversion, but additional data are required.

Predictive Factors of Response to IFN Therapy

The only factor which has been identified to predict response to IFN therapy in HDV infection is short duration of disease. In one study, a few patients which chronic hepatitis D was acquired 6–20 months prior to therapy were treated with 10 MU IFN tiw during 4 months, followed by 6 MU tiw for another 8 months. Some 71% of patients normalized ALT level and cleared viremia at the end of the therapy. A sustained biochemical and virological remission was observed in 43% of patients during a 12-month post-therapy follow-up.

Good results have also been described in patients infected by intravenous drug abuse, probably because they have harbored their infection for a relatively short period of time, as opposed to patients in endemic areas who frequently acquire infection early in life.

In pediatric cases, IFN is again less efficient in HBV/HDV coinfections than in HBV infections alone. Clinical and histological improvement is rare, even after 1 year of treatment. Furthermore, the appearance of decompensated cirrhosis has been reported during IFN therapy, with severe biochemical exacerbation leading to liver failure.

Side Effects

Flu-like symptoms, fatigue, and weight loss are universally present, their intensity being dependent on the dose. These side effects may become an important problem with the prolonged 9-MU dose. Poor and intermittent use of IFN may increase the incidence and the severity of side effects. Self-injection of IFN can trigger a specific psychological stress in previous drug abusers, leading to an intermittent reuse of addictive drugs.

Major side effects, including severe flares, have been reported in only a few patients. Most patients with anti-LKM-3 antibodies completed cycles of IFN therapy without complications. However, thyroid disease and suicide have been reported.

Liver Transplantation

Liver transplantation remains the only effective therapy for terminal disease. A high level of graft reinfection was reported in the initial series of transplantation. Since the first reports, our ability to detect HBV and HDV infections has improved. In most cases where it has been searched for, HBV-DNA, reflecting HBV replication, could be detected in the serum by PCR when HDV reinfection was found in the absence of detectable HBsAg. Liver histological activity was directly related to the level of HBV replication. HBeAg and HBV DNA detected by dot-blot hybridization were present in the two cases of fulminant evolution 3 and 4 months after transplantation, as reported by Ottobrelli et al. On the contrary, our patients with HDAg in their liver and no sign of hepatitis had no detectable serum HBsAg; the return of liver disease in the 11 patients where it was observed was invariably preceded by HBV reactivation. Anti-HBs specific immunoglobulins were found effective in preventing HDV as well as HBV recurrence. Thus, liver transplantation seems an acceptable solution in the presence of terminal HDV liver disease. Since the post-transplantation prognosis is directly related to HBV reinfection, lowering and, if possible, abrogating HBV replication through aggressive antiviral therapy should be attempted in the pretransplantation period.

CONCLUSIONS

In fulminant hepatitis caused by coinfection of HDV and HBV, it will be necessary to perform randomized controlled trials to demonstrate the benefit of anti-HBV drugs such as famciclovir, lamivudine, lobucorvin, and adefovin. Most of the time, treatment of HDV/HBV simultaneous coinfections is not necessary. Treatment should be considered in cases of superinfection of asymptomatic HBV chronic carriers by HDV. Since HDV superinfection runs a chronic course in over 90% of cases and early administration of IFN may improve the response rate, treatment should be initiated in such cases. The optimal timing of IFN treatment remains to be determined. Patients with no history of overt acute hepatitis and no sign of decompensated liver cirrhosis should be treated as soon as the diagnosis is made. IFN is more likely to be effective if administered to patients with a recent infection (within 1 year) at high doses (9–10 MU tiw) and for a prolonged length of time (at least 12 months). IFN needs to be administered for at least 1 year before defining a patient as a nonresponder, since HDV infection response can take up to 10 months.

Apart from the clearance of HBsAg and seroconversion to anti-HBs, no other biochemical or virological marker can predict a sustained response. Loss of serum HDV-RNA and HDAg does not always reflect the clearance of the virus. Patients presenting with these features may often relapse after the end of the therapy. The gradual disappearance of IgM anti-HD in patients responding to IFN with the normalization of ALT probably also indicates that HDV infection may be eradicated. Treatment can be safely interrupted if HBsAg is cleared. Otherwise, therapeutic management should be guided by histological and HDV detection in the liver. If HDV is undetectable in the liver, IFN can be stopped and the patients monitored. If HDV is still detectable but histological features are improved, IFN should be continued until HDV disappearance is maintained.

FUTURE THERAPY

In vitro and in vivo results indicate that HBV remains at this time the best potential target for conventional antiviral therapy in chronic hepatitis D, prompting the testing of new anti-HBV drugs such as lamivudine and famciclovir and others for this form of viral hepatitis.

Some RNA molecules exhibit specific self-cleavage sites in the absence of proteins, depending on the secondary and tertiary structures, themselves determined by the primary RNA sequence. Such RNAs are named *ribozymes*. The HDV-RNA sequence has sites with ribozyme activity (ribozyme delta), working by transesterification. Those potential targets for pharmacological attack open future possibilities for treatment. Since the self-cleavage of genomic and antigenomic HDV-RNAs is essential to the viral replication cycle, pharmacological blocking of the ribozymic sites should lead to inhibition or termination of HDV synthesis. The delta ribozyme also has potential in gene therapy. It is massively produced in cells and is functional in hepatocytes and other cell types. Modification of the RNA primary structure can be achieved without altering nucleotides important for catalysis. An artificial ribozyme could recognize a specific target such as a viral RNA and inactive it by cleavage. A successful separation of the genomic and antigenomic delta ribozymes has been achieved, and they both cleave HDV-RNAs. These encouraging preliminary results are confronted by the problem of ribozyme recycling. At present, one ribozyme molecule cleaves only one target RNA molecule.

VACCINATION

No specific vaccine is yet available to specifically prevent HDV infection. The HBV vaccines do prevent HBV infection and therefore prevent infection with HDV, which requires the hepatitis B virus helper function to exert its pathogenic potential. However, up to 300 million people are chronically infected by HBV, so a vaccine specifically protective against HDV would be helpful for these individuals.

The major problem is represented by a lack of humoral immune protection against HDV. In chronic delta infections with active replication, specific anti-delta antibodies are present. They do not block HDV and can coexist with viral replication. The cellular immune response could be of interest. Chimpanzees infected by HBV and superinfected by HDV had mild hepatitis when rechallenged by HDV. Protection through cellular immune response was thought to operate when vaccinating with the core antigen of HBV. In those cases, animals did not develop any anti-HBs antibody, while they were partially protected against infectious challenges.

Several vaccines against HDV infection have been tested. Different kinds of HDAg have been employed, including liver extract, recombinant proteins, and synthetic peptides. Liver-derived HDAg failed to protect animals challenged with inoculum of very high titer. Recombinant proteins and synthetic peptides provided more promising results. However, in most cases, infection could not be prevented, although the severity and duration of the disease as well as viremia were markedly reduced. DNA vaccination with the gene encoding for HDAg under control of a vaccinia virus construct failed to prevent HDV superinfection of chronic WHV infected woodchucks, possibly because of insufficient levels of HDAg expression.

ACKNOWLEDGMENT

We would like to thank A. Kay for helpful discussions and critical review of the manuscript.

BIBLIOGRAPHY

Caselmann WH. HBV and HDV replication in experimental models: effect of interferon. Antivir Res 1994; 24:121–129.

Farci P, Mandas A, Coiana A, Eliana M, Desmet V, Van Eyken P, Gibo Y, Caruso L, Seaccabarozzi S, Cricuolo D, Ryff JC, Balestrieri A. Treatment of chronic hepatitis D with interferon alfa-2a. N Engl J Med 1994; 330:88–94.

Gaudin JL, Faure P, Godinot H, Gerard F, Trepo C. The French experience of treatment of chronic type D hepatitis with 12-months course of interferon alpha-2b: results of a randomized controlled trial. Liver 1995; 15:45–52.

Negro F, Rizzetto M. Diagnosis of hepatitis delta virus infection. J Hepatol 1995; 22(suppl 1):136–139.

Ottobrelli A, Marzano A, Smedile A, Recchia S, Salizzoni M, Cornu C, Lamy ME, Otte JB, De Hemptinne B, Geubel A, Grendele M, Colledan M, Galmarini D, Marinucci G, Di Giacomo C, Agnes S, Bonino F, Rizzetto M. Patterns of hepatitis delta virus reinfection and disease in liver transplantation. Gastroenterology 1991; 101:1649–1655.

Perrotta AT, Been MD. A pseudoknot-like structure required for efficient self-cleavage of hepatitis delta virus RNA. Nature 1991; 350:434–436.

Polish LB, Gallagher M, Fields HA, Hadler SC. Delta hepatitis: molecular biology and clinical and epidemiological features. Clin Microbiol Rev 1993; 211–229.

Ponzetto A, Eckart M, D'Urso N. Towards a vaccine for the prevention of hepatitis delta virus superinfection in HBV carriers. Prog Clin Biol Res 1993; 382:207–210.

Rosina F, Cozolongo R. Interferon in HDV infection. Antivir Res 1994; 24:165–174.

Smedile A, Rosina F, Saracco G, Chiaberge E, Lattore V, Fabiano A, Brunetto MR, Verme G, Rizzetto M, Bonino F. Hepatitis B virus replication modulates pathogenesis of hepatitis D virus in chronic hepatitis D. Hepatology 1990; 13:413–416.

Taylor J, Negro F, Rizzetto M. Hepatitis delta virus: from structure to disease expression. Rev Med Virol 1992; 2:161–167.

9
Management of Chronic Hepatitis C

Scott J. Cotler and Donald M. Jensen
RUSH-Presbyterian–St. Luke's Medical Center, Chicago, Illinois

HISTORY OF HEPATITIS C TREATMENT

The use of purified fibroblast and leukocyte interferon for chronic hepatitis first underwent clinical testing for hepatitis B in the mid-1970s. These agents, though effective, were associated with a high frequency of side effects, high cost, and lack of standardization. Recombinant interferon entered clinical trials in the early 1980s, following successful use in oncology. The first U.S. clinical trial of recombinant interferon-alpha(α) 2b for chronic non-A, non-B hepatitis was published in 1987 from the National Institutes of Health (NIH). Although relatively low doses of interferon were used, a reduction in serum ALT could be demonstrated. The first multicenter trial in the United States was published in 1989. This study demonstrated efficacy of 3 million units (MU) administered three times a week (tiw) for 6 months in improving ALT values in 54% of treated patients. Although many of these patients suffered biochemical relapses over the ensuing 6 months of follow-up, this study formed the basis for FDA approval of interferon in 1991.

INTERFERON ACTIONS

Natural interferon-α consists of a group of proteins produced by leukocytes in response to viral infection. These proteins bind to a 110-kDa cell-surface receptor, leading to modulation of numerous biochemical pathways with antiviral, immunoregulatory, antiproliferative, and antifibrotic effects. Single-species human interferon-α is synthesized commercially by recombinant DNA techniques for therapeutic use.

Antiviral Activity

Interferon-α induces enzymes in virus-susceptible cells including Mx proteins, 2′,5′-oligoadenylate synthetase (2,5 OAS), and eIF-2α protein kinase, which interfere with viral replication and protein synthesis. Mx proteins have not been fully characterized but seem to interfere with transcription of viral RNA. Double-stranded RNA present in virally infected cells activates 2,5 OAS which polymerizes adenosine triphosphate into adenosine oligomers. The oligoadenylates activate a cellular endoribonuclease that degrades viral RNA, blocking protein synthesis. Viral double-stranded RNA also activates the eIF-2α protein kinase, which phosphorylates a protein important in initiating translation of viral proteins. Other proposed antiviral actions of interferon include promoting glycosylation of viral proteins, which may interfere with virus packaging and function.

Immune Regulation

Interferon has immunomodulatory properties and may function in part to enhance the efficacy of immune-mediated processes directed against the hepatitis C virus (HCV). Interferon therapy facilitates cytotoxic T-cell (CTL) recognition and lysis of virally infected hepatocytes by enhancing major histocompatibility (MHC) class I antigen expression. Furthermore, T-helper (Th) 1–like cells are stimulated to produce cytokines relative to Th2-like cells. Thl-like cells produce cytokines including interferon-γ and interleukin 2 (IL-2), which activate CTL responses, whereas Th2-like cells produce cytokines including IL-4 and IL-10, which facilitate humoral (B-cell) responses. Other immunoregulatory processes include stimulation of macrophages and natural killer cells. Interferon exerts anti-inflammatory effects through induction of IL-1 receptor antagonist and suppression of IL-8, which may potentially limit HCV-related liver damage to uninfected bystander hepatocytes.

Antiproliferative Effects

Interferon-α has activity against a number of hematological malignancies and solid tumors. Deletion of interferon genes has been identified in some patients with acute lymphoblastic leukemia. Preliminary data suggest that successful interferon therapy may slow progression to hepatocellular cancer in hepatitis C–infected cirrhotic patients. Possible tumor suppressor effects include cell-cycle slowing and/or arrest in the resting phase (G_0) and regulation of cell growth factors including the oncogene c-*myc*. Interferon may block tumor growth and metastasis by inhibiting ornithine decarboxylase, resulting in depletion of essential metabolites, and by interfering with angiogenesis. Interferon also affects cell motility and adhesion molecules important in tumor metastasis.

Immunoregulatory mechanisms may contribute to the antineoplastic properties of interferon. Increased MHC class I expression improves the efficacy of immune surveillance and clearance of malignant cells by CTL. Stimulation of natural killer cells and macrophages may also promote tumor-cell killing.

Antifibrotic Effects

Interferon inhibits fibrogenesis in vitro, suppressing collagen synthesis by fibroblasts. In patients with hepatitis C, response to interferon therapy is associated with a reduction in serum markers of hepatic fibrogenesis. This observation may be related to the antifibrotic effects of interferon or may be secondary to an improvement in hepatic inflammation. While most studies have not shown improvement in established hepatic fibrosis with interferon therapy, some investigators have detected a reduction in fibrosis when each portal zone of liver biopsies is examined separately to generate a fibrosis score.

INTERFERON PHARMACOLOGY

Recombinant α-interferons are produced in bacterial cells through molecular techniques. Interferon-α2b (Intron) has a molecular mass of 19,271 Da and a specific antiviral activity of 2×10^8 IU/mg protein (a 3-MU dose contains 15 μg of interferon). Animal data suggest that the kidney is the major site of interferon degradation in the body. In human volunteers given 5 MU/m^2 of interferon-α2b, peak serum levels (18–116 IU/mL) were obtained 3 to 12 h following IM or SC injection. The elimination half-lives were calculated to be 2–3 h, with no interferon detectable after 16 h. Following IV administration, higher peak levels were observed (135–273 IU/mL), with an elimination half-life of 2 h (Fig. 1).

Interferon-α2a (Roferon) differs from interferon-α2b by a single amino acid substitution (lysine for arginine) at position 23. A 3-MU dose of interferon-α2a contains 11 μg of interferon protein. The terminal half-life of subcutaneously administered interferon-α2a is 2.1 h with serum levels undetectable after 12 h. Both preparations are now available as human serum albumin (HSA)–free formulations.

Interferon alfacon-1 (Infergen) is a non–naturally occurring, synthetic α-interferon produced by assigning the most frequent amino acid at each of the 166 sites from the more than 14 natural α-interferons. It has a molecular mass of 19,600 Da and differs from interferon-α2a at 20 amino acid sites. This formulation is associated with greater in vitro activity in antiproliferative and antiviral assay systems than either interferon-α2b or interferon-β.

Leukocyte interferon-α (Alferon) is purified from a culture medium of stimulated leukocytes, while lymphoblastoid interferon N-α (Wellferon) is produced from a culture medium of stimulated, immortalized B lymphocytes.

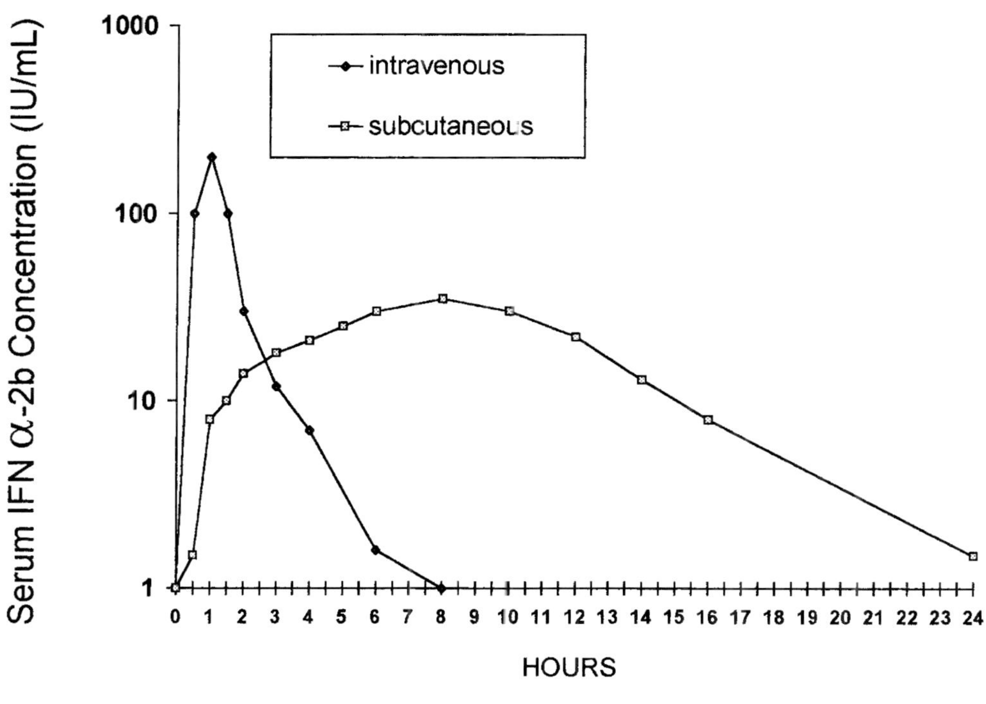

Figure 1 Interferon-α2b pharmacokinetics.

ENDPOINTS OF INTERFERON THERAPY

Interpretation of clinical trials requires careful attention to the response criteria used, which may include biochemical and/or virological parameters. Biochemical response is defined as normalization of serum alanine aminotransferase (ALT), while virological response is defined as undetectable HCV RNA in serum. At the end of therapy, patients are classified as biochemical or virological complete responders or nonresponders. Complete responders are designated as biochemical or virological sustained responders or responders with relapse, depending on their status at 6 to 12 months of follow-up.

Qualitative reverse-transcriptase polymerase chain reaction (RT-PCR) provides a highly sensitive method to detect HCV RNA in serum and is used to determine virological response. The lower limit of detection of qualitative PCR is less than a thousand viral copies per milliliter in most commercial assays and less than a hundred copies per milliliter in some research laboratories. Quantitative tests for HCV RNA, including branched chain DNA (bDNA), and quantitative PCR provide important information regarding viral load, but are less sensitive in determining the presence or absence of HCV RNA in serum. Virological testing requires careful specimen handling to avoid HCV RNA degradation and false-negative results. Furthermore, care should be taken in choosing a reliable laboratory if PCR testing is to be used. PCR methodology for the detection of hepatitis C is not standardized and there can be substantial variability in proficiency among laboratories.

Biochemical Response

Studies performed before testing for HCV RNA became widely available based response solely on normalization of serum ALT. Approximately 40–50% of patients with a biochemical response to 6 months of interferon therapy relapse during follow-up, indicating that end-of-therapy normalization of ALT is not a sensitive indicator of successful treatment. Furthermore, persistent viremia is found in up to 25–50% of patients who achieve a sustained biochemical response, depending on the sensitivity of the PCR assay used to detect HCV RNA. It is not known whether sustained biochemical response significantly changes the natural history of hepatitis C in patients who remain viremic. Liver biopsies of sustained biochemical responders with persistent viremia show a reduction in necroinflammatory activity, although some inflammatory changes may persist. Subsequent biochemical relapse is frequently observed in this group of patients.

Virological Response

Similar to the findings regarding biochemical responders, 60–75% of virological responders to 6 months of interferon therapy relapse during follow-up. However, sustained virological response seems to indicate long-term efficacy. In one small series, 100% (12/12) of sustained virological responders (6 months after a 60-week course of interferon) remained HCV RNA–negative and had persistent histological improvement at 2 years of follow-up. A subsequent study confirmed these findings, providing follow-up on patients treated with 6 to 12 months of interferon. While some patients relapsed 6 to 12 months after treatment, those who were HCV RNA–negative at 12 months posttreatment remained so for as long as 4 years. Whether hepatitis C is truly eradicated in these patients or whether it remains present at very low levels, posing a risk for future disease recurrence, remains to be determined.

In most instances, virological response is accompanied by biochemical response. However, in a small number of patients treated with interferon, ALT levels increase while

HCV RNA becomes undetectable. Biochemical abnormalities are due to interferon-related hepatotoxicity in some of these cases and tend to resolve when interferon is discontinued.

HCV RNA in Liver and Extrahepatic Sites

The high frequency of recurrent viremia in responders to interferon therapy has led to interest in identifying sites of HCV persistence. HCV RNA is present in the livers of some complete responders, providing evidence that clearance of HCV from serum does not necessarily indicate hepatic viral clearance. As would be expected, the absence of detectable HCV RNA in liver following interferon therapy is associated with sustained response. However, recurrent viremia can occur in patients with undetectable HCV RNA in both serum and liver at the completion of therapy. Positive- and negative-stranded HCV RNA has been identified in peripheral blood mononuclear cells (PBMC), and extrahepatic HCV replication may account for recurrent viremia in some cases. Unfortunately, PBMC status alone is not a reliable indicator of HCV clearance, as viremia can recur in virological responders with undetectable HCV RNA in PBMC at the end of therapy.

A more complete assessment of end-of-therapy response may consist of testing serum, liver, and PBMC for HCV RNA, although even this approach cannot exclude very low levels of HCV RNA that are below the limits of detection of PCR assays. In one small study, HCV RNA was undetectable in all three sites following interferon therapy in sustained responders, whereas the virus was detectable in liver or PBMC in responders who later relapsed.

Interim Biochemical and Virological Measurements and Response

Sustained response to 6 months of interferon is rare in patients with persistently elevated ALT and/or detectable viremia 3 months into therapy. Consequently, failure to normalize ALT by 3 months of treatment is often considered an indication to discontinue interferon. Dose escalation and intensification of daily dosing have been evaluated in such cases and can lead to end-of-treatment responses in up to 20% of patients. However, these strategies have not been successful in achieving sustained response. It is not known whether persistently elevated ALT or detectable HCV RNA 3 months into therapy will predict failure to respond to longer courses of interferon or to the combination of interferon and ribavirin.

Documenting the absence of detectable viremia during therapy potentially may be useful in directing length of treatment in complete responders to accomplish a sustained response. Reduced relapse rates in patients receiving 12–18 months of interferon as compared to 6 months of treatment suggest that therapy should be continued for a period of time after HCV RNA is no longer detectable in serum in order to achieve viral clearance. Identification of a treatment interval needed to consolidate a complete response into a sustained response would provide a means to maximize treatment efficacy while minimizing excess days of interferon therapy.

SIDE EFFECTS

Incidence

The most frequently reported adverse events associated with interferon-α administration are flu-like symptoms occurring 2–8 h after injection, which typically improve even with

Table 1 Frequency of Adverse Events Reported in Trials of Interferon-α2b 3 mU tiw

Adverse reaction	Frequency
Flu-like symptoms	
Fever	50%
Headache	49%
Myalgias	45%
Fatigue	37%
Chills/rigors	34%
Arthralgias	24%
Asthenia	17%
CNS/psychiatric	
Depression	11%
Irritability	13%
Sleep disturbance	5%
Dizziness	14%
Gastrointestinal complaints	
Nausea	25%
Diarrhea	14%
Anorexia	15%
Skin disorders	
Alopecia	17%

continued therapy (Table 1). Injection-site inflammation occurs in up to 10–15% of patients. Due to the antiproliferative effects of interferon, a reversible bone marrow suppression may be observed in 7–19% of patients. However, severe leukopenia (< 500 granulocytes per cubic millimeter) occurs in less than 1% of patients.

Perhaps one of the more disconcerting aspects of interferon therapy is its ability to induce or aggravate psychiatric disturbances. Depression and/or irritability may be observed in 11–13% of patients. Depression is the most common adverse experience, leading to withdrawal of treatment; it occurs in 6% of patients treated with 3 MU tiw and 11% of those treated with 6 MU tiw. Malaise and fatigue are common, though many patients report improvements in these symptoms during treatment (36% initial to 18% end).

Thyroid abnormalities occur in approximately 5% of patients. These may manifest as either hypo- or hyperthyroidism. Although some cases are irreversible, many subjects will return to a euthyroid state with time.

Fatal or life-threatening side effects are fortunately rare. In a retrospective study by Fattovich et al. of 11,241 interferon-treated patients, the incidence of fatal side effects was 0.04% (liver failure, 4; sepsis, 1), while life-threatening side effects occurred in 0.07% (suicide attempt, 2; severe bone marrow suppression, 6).

With doses of 3 MU tiw, less than 5% of patients require discontinuation of treatment due to adverse events and 9% require dose reductions. The use of higher doses or for longer than 6 months is associated with a higher incidence of side effects. However, even with doses of 5–6 MU tiw for up to 12 months, only 5% of patients require withdrawal from treatment, although 22% require dose reductions.

Managing Side Effects

Most of the side effects of interferon are mild and manageable. Careful education of patients about possible side effects and their management can be extremely helpful in minimizing concern and apprehension. Flu-like symptoms occur within hours of the first few injections and typically dissipate by 6–8 h. Administering the injections in the evening and premedicating with acetaminophen may allow the patient to sleep through much of this annoyance. Advising patients to allow for increased rest during the first few weeks and to increase their daily fluid intake (to at least 2 L) is also helpful.

Monitoring of blood counts during the first few weeks will allow prompt recognition of potentially severe cytopenias. In general, a temporary 50% interferon dose reduction is indicated if platelet counts drop below 50,000/mm^3, hemoglobin declines to 10 g, or granulocytes decrease below 1000/mm^3.

A prior history of depression necessitates psychiatric evaluation prior to initiating treatment. Mild depression occurring during treatment usually responds to antidepressant therapy. If there is doubt, however, psychiatric consultation is suggested, as suicides have occurred in patients on interferon.

A TSH level is obtained prior to therapy with interferon and at 3- to 6-month intervals during treatment. This is a sensitive indicator of thyroid dysfunction, and any TSH abnormalities uncovered should prompt further endocrinological evaluation. Other metabolic disorders may also occur during interferon treatment. These include hyperlipidemia and diabetes mellitus.

Certain side effects should mandate at least temporary discontinuation of treatment. These include severe depression, other severe psychological side effects (psychosis, delirium, paranoia, coma), sepsis or other severe infection, cardiac abnormalities (arrhythmias, congestive heart failure), hyperthyroidism, hypothyroidism, severe peripheral cytopenias, seizures, renal disease, and exacerbation of liver disease.

In summary, interferon's side effects are generally mild and easily managed. Nonetheless, adequate patient education and monitoring are essential if more severe problems are to be avoided.

INTERFERON TREATMENT TRIALS

Interferon dosing in the initial U.S. and European treatment trials for hepatitis C consisted of 3 MU tiw for 6 months. More recently, investigators have compared standard dosing with prolonged duration of therapy, higher doses, and daily dosing of interferon.

Standard Interferon Dosing

The end-of-therapy biochemical response rate for patients treated with 3 MU tiw of interferon for 6 months is 40–50%. Relapse occurs in approximately half of these cases at 6 months of follow-up, yielding a sustained biochemical response rate of 20–25%. Large series have reported a sustained virological response rate of 10%, measured 6 months after the completion of interferon therapy. Histological necroinflammatory changes improve in 50–70% of treated patients, including patients who do not achieve biochemical or virological response. In a recent study, improvements in necroinflammatory activity were found to persist for 6 months after the completion of interferon in virological responders with relapse and nonresponders. In another report, histological improvement regressed to baseline in responders with relapse by 1 year of follow-up. The serum HCV RNA level may rise acutely in relapsers and nonresponders when interferon is discontinued, although it tends to return toward the pretreatment baseline over time.

Effects of Dose and Duration of Interferon on Treatment Response

A lack of response to treatment in more than 50% of subjects receiving interferon-α, 3 MU tiw for 24 weeks, could suggest that host or viral resistance factors might be amenable to higher dose or longer duration therapy. Indeed, body weight and high viral load are examples of negative treatment predictors that might respond to higher initial interferon doses or longer treatment duration.

Poynard showed that improvements in sustained biochemical and virological responses to interferon-α could be obtained by extending the period of treatment to 12–18 months from the usual 6 months. Although the extended duration of treatment was not associated with a greater percentage of initial interferon responders, it was associated with a lower relapse rate after interferon was discontinued. The beneficial effect of 12–18 months of therapy on treatment response has now been demonstrated by a meta-analysis of published treatment trials (Fig. 2).

Chemello and colleagues demonstrated comparable sustained biochemical and virological responses in patients treated with 3 MU tiw for 12 months (31%) or with 6 MU tiw for 6 months (28%). However, the primary ("induction") response after 3 months was higher in those treated with 6 MU tiw (74 vs. 56%). Patients treated with the higher initial doses did report a higher frequency of flu-like syndrome (63 vs. 33%). When higher initial doses (6 MU tiw decreasing to 3 MU tiw based upon ALT normalization) were combined with longer treatment duration (12 months), a 49% sustained biochemical response rate was observed. In a meta-analysis by Poynard, there was indeed a significant dose effect (6 MU vs. 3 MU tiw) upon the sustained response at 12 months, with a mean 18% increase (28 to 46%, $p < 0.001$), which was not observed at 6 months. Lam et al. have provided further

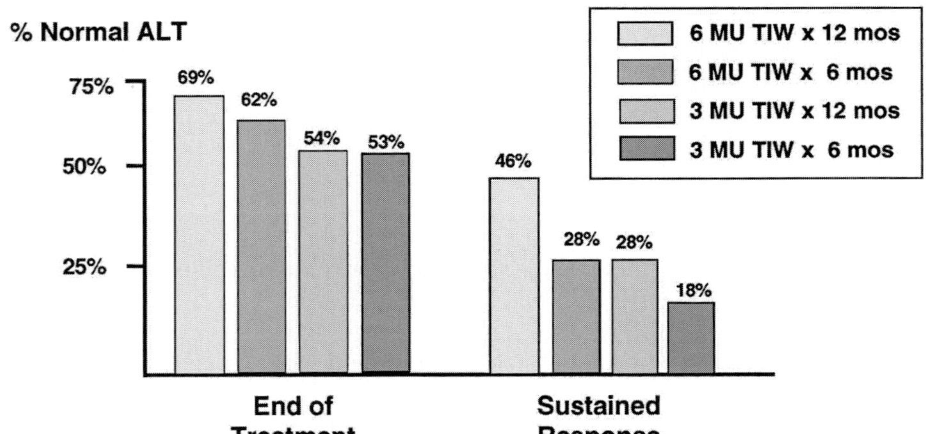

Figure 2 Biochemical response to different interferon-α treatment schedules.

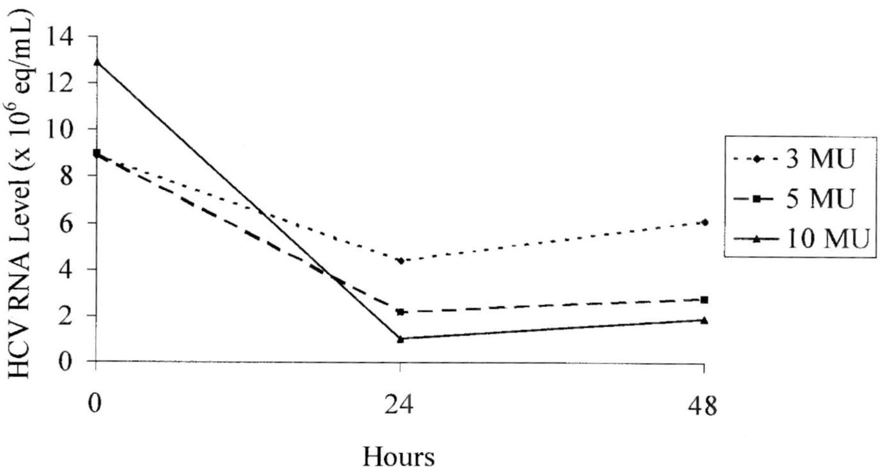

Figure 3 Dose response relations for interferon-α2b.

evidence for a dose effect in showing a greater mean reduction in serum HCV RNA level 24 h after a single 10-MU dose of interferon, as compared with doses of 5 and 3 MU (86 vs. 64 vs. 41% respectively) (Fig. 3). Hepatitis C virus RNA levels rose in all patients at 48 h, suggesting that thrice-weekly dosing may not be optimal.

Daily Interferon Dosing

The use of relatively low doses of interferon on an intermittent schedule to treat the rapidly replicating hepatitis C virus raises theoretical concerns about promoting the development of resistant quasispecies variants. This consideration has prompted trials of daily therapy and daily induction therapy followed by thrice-weekly dosing. Induction regimens are designed to maximize treatment intensity at the outset of therapy when levels of viral turnover are highest. In one uncontrolled trial, treatment with 5 MU of interferon daily for 6 months led to a relatively high sustained virological response rate (39%). Similarly, a sustained virological response rate of 25% was reported in an uncontrolled study in which 6 MU of interferon was given daily for 2 weeks followed by thrice-weekly dosing for 22 weeks. Randomized trials comparing daily interferon dosing and induction regimens to 12 months of thrice-weekly therapy are needed. Any potential benefit gained by more aggressive dosing strategies will have to be weighed against toxicity.

PREDICTORS OF RESPONSE TO INTERFERON THERAPY

The effect of viral and host characteristics on response to interferon therapy has been evaluated primarily in 6-month treatment trials. As reviewed by Davis, a large number of factors have been associated with response by univariate analysis, although only HCV RNA quantity in serum, viral genotype, and liver histology have been identified repeatedly as independent predictors of response by multivariate methods. Low pretreatment HCV

RNA level, defined as undetectable by the first generation bDNA assay ($< 0.35 \times 10^6$ genome equivalents per milliliter), or alternatively less than 1.0×10^6 genome equivalents per milliliter, has been associated with sustained response. However, this finding may have been confounded by underestimation of viral quantity for genotypes 2 and 3 by the first-generation bDNA assay. Some studies that have corrected HCV RNA level for genotype or measured virus level by quantitative PCR have not confirmed a relationship between viral quantity and response to interferon therapy. Infection with HCV genotype 2 or 3 is associated with higher sustained response rates to interferon than genotype 1 (1a or 1b). With regard to host factors, patients without cirrhosis on pretreatment liver biopsy are more likely to respond to interferon than cirrhotics.

Factors associated with reduced response rates to interferon provide prognostic information but are not highly accurate in predicting the outcome of therapy. In a retrospective analysis of data from a large interferon treatment trial, Davis et al. found that excluding patients with cirrhosis, genotype 1 infection, and high levels of viremia would have denied therapy to 60% of those who had a sustained response. Consequently, therapy should not be withheld based on presence of these factors or a significant proportion of potential responders will be excluded.

There are insufficient data to determine whether response predictors identified in 6-month interferon treatment trials are relevant to prolonged courses of interferon or to combination therapy with interferon and ribavirin. Preliminary data suggest that the addition of ribavirin to interferon may diminish the associations between HCV genotype and response and between HCV RNA level and response. If this pattern of results is confirmed, predictive factors may prove to be useful in guiding choices among therapeutic options in patients with hepatitis C.

Less information is available regarding other potentially important host and virological features. Increased hepatic iron content has recently been identified as a negative predictor of response to interferon. Quasispecies heterogeneity may also affect response to interferon therapy, as sustained responders have been found to have significantly less genetic heterogeneity in HCV than nonresponders and responders who relapse. Enomoto et al. have identified a portion of the NS5A region of HCV genotype 1b (interferon sensitivity-determining region, Fig. 4) in which mutations are associated with sensitivity to interferon therapy in Japan, although this association has not been found in European isolates. Attempts are being made to characterize other HCV RNA sequences that may predict response to interferon therapy.

Interferon therapy for hepatitis C should be deferred in patients actively abusing

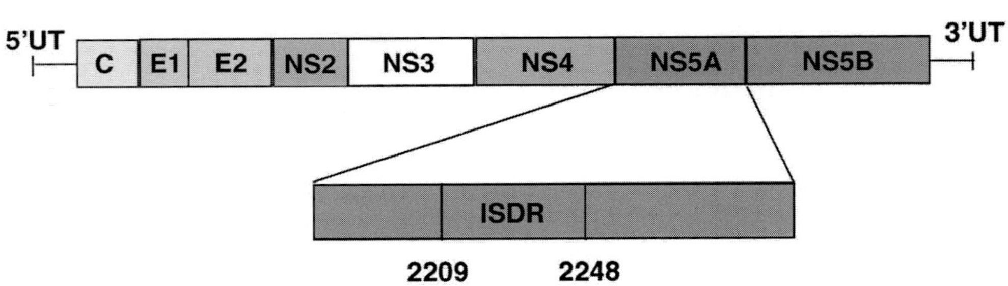

Figure 4 Interferon sensitivity-determining regions.

alcohol or using intravenous drugs until a period of abstinence has been achieved. Patients who continue to drink heavily until the time of interferon therapy have a reduced response rate. Furthermore, in one report, habitual drinkers who were abstinent from alcohol for a minimum of 6 months prior to starting interferon were more likely to respond than patients who continued to drink until the time of treatment. Ongoing intravenous drug use poses theoretical risks, including superinfection with additional strains of HCV and infection with other viruses that may cause liver injury.

INTERFERON ANTIBODIES

Although interferon-α is a natural biological compound, the prevalence of interferon-α2a and interferon-α2b varies considerably in populations. These variations in natural occurrence led to the speculation that prolonged treatment with recombinant interferon-α could give rise to the production of neutralizing antibodies that might decrease the therapeutic effectiveness. Although neutralizing anti-interferon antibodies have been reported in patients treated with interferon (approximately 15%), there has been an inconsistent relationship to clinical response. This may be partially explained by the time course of antibody development, which typically occurs after 6 or more weeks of therapy. In summary, there is insufficient reason to implicate interferon antibodies in clinical response rates using current formulations of recombinant or natural interferon.

SPECIAL TREATMENT CONSIDERATIONS

Normal Aminotransferases

It is estimated that up to one-third of patients persistently infected with the hepatitis C virus will have normal serum aminotransferases. Most of these patients will have disease activity if a liver biopsy is performed, although liver injury tends to be mild. Therefore, treatment of patients with persistently normal aminotransferases should be determined on a case-by-case basis.

Cirrhosis

HCV-infected patients with cirrhosis comprise a group with a poor long-term prognosis who would most benefit from a treatment strategy that could arrest or delay the progression of their disease. Unfortunately, cirrhotic patients respond poorly to conventional interferon treatment schedules (3 MU tiw × 6 months) and rarely demonstrate sustained biochemical improvement (approximately 0–5%). In addition, the presence of hypersplenism may potentiate the deleterious effect of interferon on peripheral cell counts; decompensation during treatment is at least a theoretical possibility.

On the other hand, a virological response in cirrhotic patients may be associated with improvements in serum albumin levels and prothrombin time, suggesting functional improvement. Preliminary studies from Japan and Europe suggest that interferon treatment of cirrhotic HCV patients may be associated with a lower incidence of subsequent hepatocellular carcinoma irrespective of the response to therapy. However, Fattovich et al. recently reported a large series in which 5-year survival rates were similar for treated and untreated cirrhotic patients.

In summary, suitably selected cirrhotic subjects may be appropriate candidates for interferon therapy. These should be compensated individuals; they require close observation and monitoring to prevent complications. In addition, because of the relatively high relapse rate in responders, consideration should be given to extending the treatment duration beyond 6 months.

Relapse

Subjects who suffer a biochemical and/or virological relapse after achieving a complete response during interferon therapy represent 20–40% of treated individuals. Lower relapse rates are observed with longer treatment duration (12–18 months). Retreatment with a second course of interferon is associated with an 80–90% complete biochemical response rate, suggesting that the first treatment course did not induce virological resistance. Retreatment of relapsed patients with a more aggressive schedule has been found to improve the subsequent sustained response rates. For example, an overall 58% sustained virological response rate was reported in relapsed patients treated with interferon alfacon-1, dosed at 15 μg tiw for 48 weeks. Response for genotypes 2 and 3 were greater than those for genotype 1. It would appear, therefore, that patients who relapse after an initial course of interferon therapy are suitable candidates for retreatment. The best retreatment strategy has yet to be determined. It is anticipated that the number of relapse patients will decline as improved therapeutic strategies are developed for the initial course of treatment.

Nonresponse

The most frustrating group of subjects are those in whom there is no apparent biochemical or virological response to therapy. These account for more than 50% of patients treated with interferon-α, 3 MU tiw for 6 months. The reason for nonresponse is likely to be multifactorial, including both virus and host factors (Table 2).

Very few studies have reported successful retreatment of nonresponders. Iron depletion followed by a more aggressive interferon schedule has been successful in some patients. Substituting interferon alfacon-1 for the retreatment has also been demonstrated to improve virological and biochemical responses.

Perhaps the best approach to nonresponders is to induce a sustained response to the initial course of treatment. Early identification of individuals who are likely to be non-

Table 2 Possible Reasons for Interferon Nonresponse

Viral factors	Host factors
Genotype 1	Iron
Quasispecies	Obesity
Treatment factors	Alcohol
Inadequate dose	Cirrhosis
Inadequate duration	Autoimmunity
Noncompliance	Age
Interferon antibodies	

responders may allow for the development of more aggressive treatment strategies for clinical trials.

Acute Hepatitis C

In a 1996 meta-analysis, four controlled interferon treatment trials were evaluated. Three of these trials used interferon-α2b at 3 MU tiw for 3 months and one utilized interferon-β with an induction schedule of 3 MU daily for 5 days followed by 3 MU tiw. A complete ALT response at the end of treatment was observed in 69% of treated patients, compared with 29% of controls ($p < 0.001$). A sustained ALT after 12 months was observed in 53% of treated subjects (versus 32% in controls, $p = 0.02$). Perhaps most striking was the 12-month sustained disappearance in HCV RNA with treatment in 41 versus 4% in the controls ($p < 0.001$). It appears, therefore, that a 3-month course of interferon at a dose of 3 MU tiw is effective in providing a sustained biochemical and virological response in acute hepatitis C.

OTHER THERAPIES

The modest success of interferon in the treatment of hepatitis C has led to a search for other agents. To date, interferon remains the only compound found to have significant antiviral activity when used as monotherapy for HCV infection. There are data to suggest that ribavirin may be useful when combined with interferon. Other therapeutic approaches of interest include combining interferon with iron reduction, amantadine, and thymosin. Ursodeoxycholic acid, nonsteroidal anti-inflammatory drugs (NSAID), and corticosteroid priming have been tried for hepatitis C but have shown little efficacy.

Ribavirin

Ribavirin is an orally administered guanosine analogue with activity against RNA and DNA viruses. While the mechanism of action of ribavirin in the treatment of HCV remains unknown, both direct antiviral and immunomodulatory effects have been proposed. Therapy with ribavirin alone reduces serum ALT levels but does not lead to clearance of HCV RNA from serum or to significant improvement in hepatic inflammation on liver biopsy. Initial controlled studies comparing 6 months of interferon and ribavirin with interferon alone have found combination therapy to be superior. In a study of noncirrhotic patients, Lai et al. reported a 43% sustained virological response rate with interferon and ribavirin versus 6% with interferon alone (follow-up, 96 weeks). Similarly, Reichard et al. reported a 45% sustained response rate in patients treated with combination therapy, compared with 23% in patients treated with interferon alone. There are also preliminary data suggesting that some responders with relapse to interferon therapy may benefit from retreatment with interferon and ribavirin. Large multicenter trials are under way to further evaluate the efficacy of combination therapy with interferon and ribavirin. Whether combination therapy is more effective than a 1-year course of interferon alone remains to be determined.

The main side effect of ribavirin is hemolytic anemia, which tends to be mild with doses of 1000–1200 mg daily, commonly used to treat hepatitis C. However, hemoglobin levels drop precipitously in some cases, posing a risk to patients with coronary artery disease. Ribavirin is also associated with hepatic iron deposition, presumably as a consequence of hemolysis. It is not known whether this process will render patients less responsive to further treatment with interferon. Efforts are under way to minimize ribavirin-related hemolysis by identifying the lowest dose of ribavirin that is effective in combination with interferon for the treatment of hepatitis C.

Iron Reduction Therapy

A number of clinical observations have been made regarding iron and hepatitis C, although the mechanisms of interaction between iron and HCV remain unclear. Phlebotomy significantly reduces ALT levels but not HCV RNA quantity in HCV infected patients. In some studies, responders to interferon have lower hepatic iron concentrations than nonresponders. Other investigators have observed that portal iron deposition is inversely correlated with response to interferon, suggesting that the distribution of iron in the liver may affect the response to therapy. These findings have led to interest in using iron reduction as an adjunct to interferon in treating hepatitis C. Preliminary reports indicate that achieving iron reduction with phlebotomy prior to interferon therapy may improve biochemical response rates. Multicenter trials are under way to evaluate this issue.

Amantidine

Preliminary data have been reported regarding amantidine monotherapy for the treatment of previous nonresponders to interferon. In one study, HCV RNA levels were reduced by at least 50% in half of the patients treated with amantidine. Controlled trials are planned to test the efficacy of combination therapy with interferon and amantidine.

Thymosin Alpha-1

Thymosin is an immunomodulatory agent which does not appreciably affect ALT levels when used alone to treat hepatitis C. In a randomized controlled trial, the combination of thymosin and interferon led to a more rapid decline in HCV RNA level than interferon monotherapy. However, by 24 weeks of treatment, HCV RNA levels were similar in the two groups. Whether thymosin may enhance the efficacy of interferon therapy in the treatment of hepatitis C is not known.

Ursodeoxycholic Acid

Ursodeoxycholic acid is a hydrophilic bile salt that improves serum ALT levels in a number of chronic liver diseases, including hepatitis C. While some clinicians prescribe ursodeoxycholic acid for patients with hepatitis C, it has not been found to have antiviral activity. The combination of ursodeoxycholic acid and interferon has been compared with interferon alone in a randomized controlled trial. There was no significant difference in end-of-treatment or sustained virological response in the two groups. Patients treated with combination therapy did show an improvement in portal inflammation at the end of treatment, which was not present in patients treated with interferon alone.

Additional Approaches

NSAID have been tried in combination with interferon based on in vitro data suggesting that inhibition of prostaglandin E2 may increase interferon-induced production of antiviral proteins. Preliminary reports showed biochemical improvement in previous nonresponders to interferon treated with indomethacin or ketoprofen and interferon. However, the absence of virological data make these findings difficult to interpret. Corticosteroid priming prior to interferon administration increases the response rate in hepatitis B–infected patients with low ALT levels and has been evaluated in the treatment of hepatitis C. This strategy transiently increases HCV RNA levels but does not have an impact on virological response. Granulocyte colony stimulating factor (G-CSF), has also been used as an adjunct to interferon therapy. G-CSF is a cytokine with immunomodulatory properties, including induction of leukocyte proliferation. It is effective in increasing granulocyte counts in cirrhotic patients treated with interferon and may facilitate therapy in patients with leukopenia. However, G-CSF has not been found to enhance the antiviral activity of interferon.

FUTURE OF HEPATITIS C THERAPY

During the past decade, therapy for chronic hepatitis C has evolved from low-dose interferon (2–3 MU tiw) monotherapy administered for 6 months to combination therapy administered for 12–18 months. Along with these more aggressive treatment schedules have come improved and sustained virological responses. It would appear that the treatment of HCV is recapitulating the treatment strategies for HIV infection—i.e., aggressive induction therapy with multiple agents targeted to attack the virus at different points in its cycle. The development of HCV-specific protease inhibitors in conjunction with ribavirin and improved interferon formulations and administration strategies should offer the best hope for long-lasting control of chronic hepatitis C.

REFERENCES

Antonelli G, Currenti M, Turriziani O, Dianzani F. Neutralizing antibodies to interferon-α: relative frequency in patients with different interferon preparations. J Infect Dis 1991; 163:882–885.

Baron S, Tyring SK, Fleischmann WR, Coppenhaver DH, Niesel DW, Klimper GR, Stanton J, Hughes TK. The interferons: mechanisms of action and clinical applications. JAMA 1991; 266:1375–1383.

Blatt LM, Davis JM, Klein SB, Taylor M. The biologic activity and molecular characterization of a novel synthetic interferon-alpha species: consensus interferon. J Interferon Cytokine Res 1996; 16:489–499.

Bonetti P, Diodati G, Drago C, Casarin C, Scaccabarozzi S, Realdi G, Ruol A, Alberti A. Interferon antibodies in patients with chronic hepatitis C virus infection treated with recombinant interferon alpha-2a. J Hepatol 1994; 20:416–420.

Camps J, Garcia-Granero M, Riezu-Boj JI, Larrea E, de Alava E, Civeira MP, Castilla A, Prieto J. Prediction of sustained remission of chronic hepatitis C after a 12 month course of alfa interferon. J Hepatol 1994; 21:4–11.

Chemello L, Bonetti P, Cavalletto L, Talato F, Donadon V, Casarin P, et al. Randomized trial comparing three different regimens of alpha-2a-interferon in chronic hepatitis C.

Chemello L, Cavalletto L, Casarin C, Bonetti P, Bernardinello E, Pontisso P, et al. Persistent hepatitis C viremia predicts late relapse after sustained response to interferon-alpha in chronic hepatitis C. Ann Intern Med 1996; 124:1058–1060.

Davis GL, Lau JYN. Predictive factors for a beneficial response. NIH Consensus Development Conference: Management of Hepatitis C. Hepatology 1997; 26:113–117.

Davis GL, Balart LA, Schiff ER, et al. Treatment of chronic hepatitis C with recombinant interferon alfa: a multicenter randomized, controlled trial. N Engl J Med 1989; 321:1501–1505.

Enomoto N, Sakuma I, Asahina Y, Kurosaki M, Murakami T, Yamamoto C, et al. Mutations in the nonstructural protein 5A gene and response to interferon in patients with chronic hepatitis C virus 1b infection. N Engl J Med 1996; 334:77–81.

Fattovich G, Giustina G, Degos F, Tremolada F, Diodati G, Almasio P, Nevens F, Solinas A, Mura D, Brouwer JT, Thomas H. Morbidity and mortality in compensated cirrhosis type C: a retrospective follow-up study of 384 patients. Gastroenterology 1997; 112:463–472.

Fattovich G, Giustina G, Favarato S, Ruol A. A survey of adverse events in 11,241 patients with chronic viral hepatitis treated with alfa interferon. J Hepatol 1996; 24:38–47.

Gutterman JU. Cytokine therapeutics: Lessons from interferon alpha. Proc Natl Acad Sci USA 1994; 91:1198–1205.

Heathcote EJL, Keefe EB, Lee SS, et al. Re-treatment of chronic hepatitis C with consensus interferon. Hepatology 1998; 27:1136–1143.

Kanazawa Y, Hayashi N, Mita E, Li T, Hagiwara H, Kasahara A, Fusamoto H, Kamada T. Influence of viral quasispecies on effectiveness of interferon therapy in chronic hepatitis C patients. Hepatology 1994; 20:1121–1130.

Hoofnagle JH, Mullen KD, Jones DB, Rustgi V, DiBisceglie A, Peters M, Waggoner JG, Park Y, Jones EA. Treatment of chronic non-A, non-B hepatitis with recombinant human alpha interferon: a preliminary report. N Engl J Med 1987; 315:1575–1578.

Lam NP, Neumann AU, Gretch DR, Wiley TE, Perelson AS, Layden TJ. Dose-dependent acute clearance of hepatitis C genotype 1 virus with interferon alfa. Hepatology 1997; 26:226–231.

Poynard T, Bedossa P, Chevallier M, Mathurin P, Lemonnier C, Trepo C, Couzigou P, et al. A comparison of three interferon α2b regimens for long-term treatment of chronic non-A, non-B hepatitis. N Engl J Med 1995; 332:1457–1462.

Poynard T, Leroy V, Cohard M, Thevenot T, Mathurin P, Opolon P, Zarski J. Meta-analysis of interferon randomized trials in the treatment of viral hepatitis C: effect of dose and duration. Hepatology 1996; 24:778–789.

Radwanski E, Perenteses G, Jacobs S, Oden E, Affrime M, Symchowicz S, Zampaglione N. Pharmacokinetics of interferon a-2b in healthy volunteers. J Clin Pharmacol 1987; 27:432–435.

Reichard O, Norkans G, Fryden A, Braconier JH. Randomized, double-blind, placebo-controlled trial of interferon α-2b with and without ribavirin for chronic hepatitis C. Lancet 1998; 351:83–87.

Zaaijer HL, Cuypers HTM, Reesink HW, Winkel IN, Gerken G, Lelie PN. Reliability of polymerase chain reaction for detection of hepatitis C virus. Lancet 1993; 341:722–724.

10

Management of Cryoglobulinemia in Chronic Hepatitis C

Ira M. Jacobson
New York–Presbyterian Hospital (Cornell Campus), New York, New York

Edward L. Parrish
Hospital for Special Surgery–Cornell University Medical College, New York, New York

INTRODUCTION

The remarkable advance in medical knowledge resulting from the discovery of hepatitis C virus (HCV) is not limited to the liver disease we once called non-A, non-B hepatitis. It is now accepted that most patients with the syndrome of what was once called "essential" mixed cryoglobinemia (EMC) have chronic hepatitis C as the underlying cause. Estimates of the prevalence of HCV infection in patients with EMC have ranged from 50 to over 90%. In addition to this striking prevalence, evidence for a causative role for HCV infection in EMC is provided by the finding that cryoglobulins in affected patients contain concentrations of HCV RNA and HCV antibodies exceeding those in serum by up to a thousandfold. Deposition of cryoglobulins in blood vessels and tissues leads to an inflammatory response and the overt organ involvement comprising the clinical syndrome of EMC.

Mixed cryoglobulinemia is the most prominent of a group of extrahepatic manifestations of HCV infection to have been elucidated. Other disorders currently associated with HCV include porphyria cutanea tarda, lichen planus, Mooren's corneal ulcers, salivary gland lesions resembling those seen in Sjögren's syndrome, and lymphoma. With suitable assays, cryoglobulins can be demonstrated in 30–55% of patients with chronic hepatitis C. However, clinical manifestations of cryoglobulinemia are apparent in only about 2%. In such patients, the complications produced by the cryoglobulinemia, particularly when there is renal involvement or neuropathy, may be disproportionate to the degree of liver disease and dominate the clinical picture.

With recognition of the association between HCV and EMC has come a fundamental shift in our concept of therapy in EMC. The mainstay of treatment for EMC prior to the recognition of its association with chronic hepatitis C was immunosuppressive therapy, but such treatment enhances viral replication. Therefore, therapy for HCV-associated EMC now focuses predominantly on antiviral therapy in these patients. As might be expected in light of the causative role of HCV in this setting, the fate of the cryoglobulinemia appears to be inextricably linked with that of the virus in patients treated with antiviral therapy. The additional role of plasmapheresis in these patients is discussed below.

Hepatitis C virus is known to infect peripheral blood mononuclear cells. This has led to speculation that it is infection and subsequent proliferation of B lymphocytes that leads to abnormal production of rheumatoid factor in HCV-infected patients with cryoglobulinemia. An alternative explanation is that B-cell proliferation occurs in response to chronic antigenic stimulation. The recent recognition of a link between HCV infection and non-Hodgkin lymphomas has led to additional speculation that malignant transformation may occur in patients with previously benign B-cell expansion in response to HCV infection.

DEFINITION OF CRYOGLOBULINEMIA

Cryoglobulins are immunoglobulins that precipitate at cool temperatures and redissolve when warmed. There are three major types. Type I cryoglobulins are monoclonal IgG immunoglobulins (i.e., not rheumatoid factor). In most cases, type I cryoglobulinemia occurs in patients with lymphoproliferative malignancies, multiple myeloma, and Waldenström's macroglobulinemia.

Types II and III cryoglobulinemia are the mixed cryoglobulinemias strongly associated with HCV. In type II cryoglobulinemia, there is polyclonal IgG and monoclonal IgM rheumatoid factor, while type III features polyclonal IgG and polyclonal IgM rheumatoid factors. Most EMC associated with HCV is type II, though this has not been noted by all investigators. The immune complexes within the cryoglobulins are central to the causation of tissue damage and contain virions bound to IgG antibodies that are cross-linked by IgM with rheumatoid factor activity. The rheumatoid factor is usually the WA type, a germline gene-encoded product. In most patients with type II cryoglobulinemia, the monoclonal rheumatoid factor contains kappa rather than lambda light chains. Thus, genetic factors may play a role in the predisposition to cryoglobulin formation. Another feature of these cryoprecipitable immune complexes is their propensity to activate complement via the classical pathway, which may play a role in the pathogenesis of the disease.

CORRELATIONS WITH VIRAL FACTORS AND LIVER DISEASE

In most studies, the distribution of HCV genotypes in patients with cryoglobulinemia has mirrored that in the general population of HCV-infected persons. Thus, cryoglobulinemia does not seem strongly tied to any particular genotype. In one study from Italy, however, 41% of patients with hepatitis C–associated cryoglobulinemia were infected with genotype 2a, compared with 15% of "control" patients with hepatitis C but without cryoglobulinemia. In another study, cryoglobulinemia was significantly less prevalent in patients infected with genotype 1a. In yet another report, genotype 1b correlated significantly with the presence of peripheral neuropathy. A correlation between cryoglobulinemia and quantitative titer of virus in serum has not been reported.

The preponderance of published evidence suggests that cirrhosis is more prevalent in patients with HCV-associated cryoglobulinemia than in those without. Cryoglobulinemia may occasionally be seen in other liver diseases, perhaps due to impaired clearance of immune complexes. Thus, the apparent association of HCV-related cirrhosis and cryoglobulinemia may be a nonspecific effect of the liver disease present in chronic HCV infection, such as impaired hepatic clearance of circulating immune complexes. Moreover, it is difficult to exclude duration of infection as a contributing factor in these studies. Finally, it is clear that despite the advanced histological state of the liver disease in some patients with cryoglobulinemia, others may have clinically overt cryoglobulinemia with only mild liver disease histologically.

CLINICAL FEATURES OF CRYOGLOBULINEMIA

The most common manifestations are cutaneous; visceral involvement is less frequent. Cutaneous manifestations include palpable purpura, which is most commonly seen as red papules on the lower extremities. Other dermatological features include urticaria, Raynaud's phenomenon, livedo reticularis, and frank ulcerations. The underlying pathology is almost always a leukocytoclastic vasculitis, but cases of necrotizing arteritis have been reported, with palpable purpura or livedo reticularis as the presenting cutaneous manifestations accompanying visceral organ involvement.

Fatigue and weakness are common systemic symptoms of cryoglobulinemia. Patients may complain of arthralgias or myalgias. Frank arthritis is uncommon. Peripheral neuropathy with paresthesias and numbness in the hands or feet may be sufficiently severe as to be disabling. Mononeuritis multiplex and brain infarction have been reported in association with necrotizing arteritis. There are increasing anecdotal reports of inflammatory myopathy occurring in the setting of hepatitis C. Demonstrable weakness should be distinguished from fatigue.

Approximately 50% of patients with cryoglobulinemic vasculitis develop renal involvement. Often this is manifest as microscopic hematuria and proteinuria, which may be in the nephrotic range, as well as hypoalbuminemia and renal insufficiency or even frank renal failure. Renal biopsy almost always reveals membranoproliferative glomerulonephritis (MPGN) in these patients. Distinctive features may include (1) eosinophilic, PAS-positive intraluminal deposits filling the glomerular capillary lumen (intraluminal thrombi); (2) glomerular infiltration with monocytes and lymphocytes, resulting in endocapillary hypercellularity; and (3) diffusely thickened, double-contour–appearing glomerular basement membrane.

In patients with hepatitis C, there is a particularly strong association between MPGN and type II cryoglobulinemia. For several years after this association was recognized, it was presumed in the absence of definitive evidence that virus-containing immune complexes were directly responsible for the kidney damage in this syndrome. Recently, viral proteins have, in fact, been detected in deposits along glomerular capillary walls, mesangial cells, and in tubulointerstitial blood vessels. Moreover, deposits of IgM, IgG, and C3 are found in the same distribution as viral antigens at sites of glomerular damage. As in a few patients with cutaneous vasculitis, there have been reports of vasculitis of small and medium-sized arteries in up to one-third of patients with hepatitis C and acute renal disease.

Cryoglobulinemia may be exacerbated or even appear de novo after liver transplantation for hepatitis C. Nearly all patients transplanted for this indication become viremic again postoperatively, and the immunosuppressive therapy results in higher levels of viremia than were present before operation. The adverse permissive effect on viral replication appears to predominate over any amelioration of tissue damage that one might have expected from immunosuppressive therapy. In one recent report of three patients, two developed MPGN—one with renal failure, and one died of multiorgan failure 5 months after transplantation. Although reported in some patients with hepatitis C–related cryoglobulinemia, lymphoma has not, at least yet, been associated with hepatitis C post-transplantation.

LABORATORY FEATURES

An assay for serum cryoglobulins should be performed whenever there are clinical features consistent with vasculitis in a patient with hepatitis C. A qualitative assay will reveal whether cryoglobulins are present or not, while a quantitative assay determines the cryocrit (the percent of precipitate per volume of serum, similar to a hematocrit).

Quality controls are important in assaying for cryoglobulinemia. False-negative tests are common and often related to improper handling of the specimen. The serum must be kept at 37 °C until it is separated and placed at 0–4 °C. False-positive tests occur when other cryoprecipitates (nonimmunoglobulin) are present.

Some patients with chronic hepatitis C and features of immune complex disease lack detectable cryoglobulins even with properly performed assays. This is a particularly important consideration in patients with hepatitis C–associated MPGN, because in some reports up to one-third of such patients lack cryoglobulins or other clinical features of cryoglobulinemia, such as palpable purpura or arthritis. In patients suspected of hepatitis C–associated immune complex disease, rheumatoid factor may be present even in the absence of detectable cryoglobulinemia and should be sought routinely.

It is felt that a central component in the pathogenesis of the disease is the fixation of complement by immune complexes along the vascular endothelium and subsequent generation of inflammatory mediators. Thus, additional laboratory features of hepatitis C–associated cryoglobulinemia include hypocomplementemia, with reduced levels of C1q, C4, and CH50. C3 is slightly low or normal and late components tend to be normal or high. Although some patients with chronic hepatitis C have low levels of autoantibodies, such as smooth muscle or antinuclear antibodies, these are not more prevalent in patients with cryoglobulinemia.

TREATMENT OF HCV-ASSOCIATED CRYOGLOBULINEMIA

The traditional therapy for essential mixed cryoglobulinemia consisted of immunosuppressive therapy, which was intended to decrease the inflammatory response to immune complex deposition within affected tissues. Therapeutic agents included steroids, azathioprine, methotrexate, cyclophosphamide, chlorambucil, and colchicine. In addition, plasmapheresis offered the theoretical potential to diminish the cryoglobulin load within the blood, thereby decreasing the deposition of cryoglobulins within tissues. This was particularly important in patients with glomerulonephritis, neuropathy, and skin ulcers.

With recognition of the central role of HCV in many patients with EMC, attention has shifted toward antiviral therapy. Since cryoglobulins consist of complexes of virus and antibodies, it was theorized that a reduction in viral load would translate into reduced levels of cryoglobulins. For the most part, this expectation has been substantiated. However, the success of this approach to cryoglobulinemia is subject to the substantial limitations of antiviral therapy in achieving long-term eradication or sustained reductions in viral load.

A pivotal randomized study demonstrating the correlation between efficacy in reducing viral load and in treating cryoglobulinemia in Italian patients by Misiani et al. was published in 1994. Twenty seven patients with HCV infection and EMC were randomized to treatment with interferon alpha-2a at a dose of 3 MU thrice weekly, while 26 control patients received no treatment. Of the 25 evaluable patients receiving interferon, 15 had undetectable HCV RNA at end of treatment, while all control patients remained viremic. In comparison with control patients, those who lost detectable RNA had significant reductions in cryoglobulin levels, rheumatoid factor, cutaneous vasculitis and palpable purpura, and serum creatinine. With virological relapse following cessation of therapy, which occurred in all the end-of-treatment responders, cryoglobulinemia and its accompanying clinical manifestations recurred.

The correlation between response to interferon and resolution of cryoglobulinemia has been upheld in other studies. In a series of 36 patients, reported by Casaril, for example, cryoglobulinemia disappeared in 11 of 21 responders to interferon but in 0 of 15 nonresponders. Although not as consistently responsive as cutaneous symptoms, neuropathy may improve when there is a successful virologic response to interferon. We have seen a sculptor with disabling neuropathy improve dramatically with effective suppression of HCV. However, there have been reports of lack of improvement or even exacerbation of peripheral neuropathy with interferon therapy.

The response to interferon of the renal disease that occurs with cryoglobulinemia warrants particular attention. In the randomized study by Misiani discussed above, responders to interferon had a slight but significant reduction in serum creatinine, from 1.3 to 1.15. The urinary protein-creatinine index fell from 0.81 to 0.55, but this did not reach the level of statistical significance.

In another series by Johnson et al. with somewhat different conclusions, 19 patients received interferon. In two patients, therapy was discontinued because of worsening neuropathy or the development of erythema multiforme. In a third patient with a baseline creatinine of 5.2 mg/dL, renal disease progressed rapidly on treatment and dialysis was required. Of the remaining 16 patients, 14 received interferon for 6 or more months. Urine protein excretion decreased from a mean of 5.8 g/day to 2.0 g posttreatment; in seven cases to less than 1 g/day, and in four of these to less than 500 mg/day. In 11 of 14 patients, serum creatinine improved 0.2 mg/dL or more, but the overall reduction of the mean in the group, 2.0–1.5 mg/dL, did not reach statistical significance.

Virological response correlated with a better response of the renal disease. Of 11 patients tested for HCV RNA during therapy, 6 became negative while 5 remained viremic. Of the 6 whose RNA cleared, daily urinary protein excretion fell from 6.1 to 1.3 g, while in the other 5 the drop was only from 6.1–4.2 g. All 5 patients who cleared RNA and stopped interferon had virological relapse within 3 months, with recurrence of nephrotic syndrome in 3.

In contrast to the failure of interferon to be effective in the aforementioned patient with severe renal failure, another report by Moses et al. highlighted successful treatment of two such patients with standard doses of interferon-alpha-2b.

There are relatively few reports of immunosuppressive therapy in HCV-associated cryoglobulinemia. Johnson et al. observed no improvement in renal function in five patients treated with oral prednisone, although purpura did improve in two of them. Pulse steroids (1 g daily for 3 days, followed by tapering doses of oral prednisone) were given to two patients. Both had improvement in renal function, and in one, who had required dialysis prior to treatment, the creatinine fell to 2.4 mg/dL. Five patients received prednisone and cyclophosphamide with or without plasma exchange. Three died from infections (an outcome similar to that of a patient so treated by our group), while two others had improvement in renal function. In a separate case report of a single patient, MPGN responded to cyclophosphamide with an improvement in creatinine clearance from 59 to 89 mL/min within 3 months of treatment. Therapy was continued for a year, and 14 months after cessation of cyclophosphamide the creatinine clearance was 105 mL/min despite persistence of HCV RNA.

The potential role of immunosuppressive therapy combined with interferon for EMC was evaluated in a randomized study by Dammacco et al. There were 65 patients divided into four treatment groups: natural interferon-alpha alone at a dose of 3 MU three times weekly for 48 weeks, 6-methyl prednisolone alone at 16 mg/day, natural interferon-alpha plus 6-methyl/prednisolone 16 mg on non-IFN days, and controls who received no therapy. Approximately 80% of the patients in each group had HCV infection with detectable viral RNA. Complete response was defined as a reduction of cryocrit to less than 50% of its initial value associated with one or more of the following: disappearance of purpura, improvement in neuropathy, or improvement in kidney function. A partial response was a 10–50% reduction in cryocrit with improvement in one or more clinical features.

Complete response occurred in half of the interferon and combination groups but in only 17% of those given prednisone alone and 7% of controls. Partial response occurred in 13 and 18% of the first two groups and 6 of each of the other two groups. Purpura, weakness, and arthralgias improved in the majority of the treated patients. The data on renal function and neuropathy were incomplete but did improve in some patients. (Significant improvement in renal disease was stated to occur in 1 of 3 and 2 of 5 patients in the IFN and combination groups, respectively, but a larger number of patients had renal disease and are unaccounted for in the results.)

Response to therapy correlated with a decrease in HCV titers. (The authors could draw "no obvious conclusions" about the RNA-negative patients.) Clearance of HCV RNA preceded reductions in the cryocrit. The majority of patients relapsed following cessation of therapy, with accompanying recurrence of clinical signs of cryoglobulinemia. Relapse was significantly delayed in the patients who had received combination therapy with interferon and prednisone as opposed to interferon alone (5 months versus 2 months), but ultimate relapse rates were similar. Despite this advantage, the authors concluded that combination therapy is not warranted.

RECOMMENDATIONS FOR MANAGEMENT

There is now an overwhelming preponderance of evidence that, in patients with HCV-associated cryoglobulinemia, "wheresoever goes the virus, so go the cryoglobulins." Therefore, the emphasis on treating these patients should be on antiviral rather than immunosuppressive therapy. For most patients with this syndrome, including those with chronic, stable renal involvement, treatment should consist of interferon or other antiviral regimens that may come into use.

As in patients in whom liver disease from HCV infection is the major consideration, treatment decisions in those with EMC should be individualized. Some clinicians have argued that patients with long-standing HCV infection whose liver biopsies reveal minimal damage may legitimately be followed conservatively, while further therapeutic developments in the field are awaited. In contrast, in light of data indicating optimal response rates in patients with mild disease, others treat such patients aggressively with antiviral therapy, hoping for a response before more advanced fibrosis supervenes.

It would be an overstatement to suggest that the presence of even mild clinically overt cryoglobulinemia constitutes an absolute indication for treatment. However, the presence of symptomatic EMC, even if limited to mild purpura or arthralgias, does constitute an additional argument for therapy even if there is only minimal liver disease. Moreover, the presence of neurological or renal involvement warrants treatment of all such patients regardless of the status of the liver.

As for patients with hepatitis C in general, we favor liver biopsy prior to initiation of therapy even when it has been decided that treatment will, in fact, be offered. The small risk of the biopsy is well offset by the potential value of the histological data at baseline in formulating future management decisions. Examples of situations in which knowledge of the patient's liver histology is important include patients with significant side effects of interferon calling further therapy into question or patients with relapse after completion of successful treatment. Moreover, a biopsy may be critical in formulating therapeutic plans several years later, as a repeat biopsy reveals whether significant histological progression has occurred. These considerations are as relevant to patients with HCV who have associated cryoglobulinemia as they are to patients who do not.

We do not recommend routine assay for serum cryoglobulins in patients with hepatitis C in the absence of clinical features of EMC. Cryoglobulins are highly prevalent in chronic hepatitis C; in asymptomatic patients, they have not been shown to have prognostic significance.

Immunosuppressive therapy should be considered in patients with severe or rapidly progressive nephritis. Occasionally, severe neurological disease may also prompt consideration of immunosuppressive therapy. Although such therapy will, if anything, augment the degree of HCV replication, it may reduce the inflammatory activity causing tissue injury. Oral prednisone at standard doses appears to be ineffective, but a regimen of pulse steroids followed by maintenance doses is more promising, based on anecdotal reports. Cyclophosphamide offers additional therapeutic potential in addition to or instead of steroids. Plasmapheresis may also be useful in reducing serum cryoglobulin levels and stabilizing or improving renal function.

In patients with severe renal involvement, interferon may exacerbate renal dysfunction, but reports of improvement with interferon alone make it difficult to proscribe its initial use entirely. Our preference in these patients is to attempt to stabilize them with immunosuppressive therapy and plasmapheresis, following it with antiviral therapy after stabilization or maximal improvement has been achieved. If virological studies then reveal significant reduction or clearance of HCV RNA, immunosuppressive therapy can be tapered or eventually discontinued. In this context, recent studies have consistently shown that patients destined to respond to interferon have dramatic reductions in RNA levels within 1 month and even sooner. Thus, in patients with severe EMC in whom immunosuppressive therapy is being used, aggressive monitoring of HCV RNA levels may help to formulate treatment decisions early in the course of interferon therapy.

CONCLUSIONS

The striking association between HCV infection and cryoglobulinemia has dramatically refined our concept of the etiology of EMC in most affected patients. The virus and associated IgG antibodies are linked by rheumatoid factor to form immune complexes, which deposit in various tissues to produce the clinical features of EMC. These features include purpura, weakness, arthralgias, and neuropathy. Renal involvement in the form of membranoproliferative glomerulonephritis is generally the most severe manifestation of EMC.

Antiviral therapy is the cornerstone of treatment for patients with HCV-associated cryoglobulinemia. The fate of the cryoglobulinemia is linked inextricably with that of the virus. Thus, virological responders can be expected to have reduction or clearance of cryoglobulins and improvement in the clinical manifestations of EMC. Immunosuppressive therapy should, in general, be considered only in patients with severe nephritis or, occasionally, severe neurological involvement. Plasmapheresis is a useful adjunct in such patients. Once significant improvement occurs in such patients, we recommend that a trial of antiviral therapy be initiated.

ACKNOWLEDGMENT

The authors thank Stuart Saal, M.D., Rogosin Kidney Institute, New York, for his helpful review and comments on the manuscripts.

REFERENCES

Apartis E, Leger JM, Musset L, et al. Peripheral neuropathy associated with essential mixed cryoglobulinemia; a role for hepatitis C virus infection? J Neurol Neurosurg Psychiatry 1996; 60: 661–666.

Casaril M, Capra F, Gabrielli GB, et al. Cryoglobulinemia in hepatitis C virus chronic active hepatitis: effects of interferon-alpha therapy. J Interferon Cytokine Res 1996; 16:585–588.

D'Amico G, Fornasieri A. Cryoglobulinemia gomerulonephritis: a membranoproliferative glomerulonephritis induced by hepatitis C virus. Am J Kidney Dis 1995; 25:361–369.

Dammacco F, Sansonno D, Han JH, et al. Natural interferon-alpha versus its combination with 6-methyl-prednisolone in the therapy of type II mixed cryoglobulinemia: a long-term, randomized, controlled study. Blood 1994; 84:3336–3343.

Dupin N, Chosidow O, Lunel F, et al. Essential mixed cryoglobulinemia: a comparative study of dermatologic manifestations in patients infected or noninfected with hepatitis C virus. Arch Dermatol 1995; 131:1124–1127.

Frangeul L, Musset L, Cresta P, et al. Hepatitis C virus genotypes and subtypes in patients with hepatitis C, with and without cryoglobulinemia. J Hepatol 1996; 25:427–432.

Gournay J, Ferrell LD, Roberts JP, et al. Cryoglobulinemia presenting after liver transplantation. Gastroenterology 1996; 110:265–270.

Johnson RJ, Gretch DR, Couser WG, et al. Hepatitis C virus–associated glomerulonephritis. Effect of alpha-interferon therapy. Kidney Int 1994; 46:1700–1704.

Johnson RJ, Wilson R, Yamabe H, et al. Renal manifestations of hepatitis C virus infection. Kidney Int 1994; 46:1255–1273.

Karlsberg PL, Lee WM, Casey DL, et al. Cutaneous vasculitis and rheumatoid factor positivity as presenting signs of hepatitis C virus–induced mixed cryoglobulinemia. Arch Dermatol 1995; 131:1119–1123.

Lunel F, Musset L, Cacoub P, et al. Cryoglobulinemia in chronic liver diseases: role of hepatitis C virus and liver damage. Gastroenterology 1994; 106:1291–1300.

Misiani R, Bellavita P, Fenili D, et al. Interferon alfa-2a therapy in cryoglobulinemia associated with hepatitis C virus. N Engl J Med 1994; 330:751–756.

Moses PL, Krawitt EL, Aziz W, Corwin HL. Renal failure associated with hepatitis C virus infection:

improvement in renal function after treatment with interferon-alpha. Dig Dis Sci 1997; 42: 443–446.

Quigg RJ, Brathwaite M, Gardner DF, et al Successful cyclophosphamide treatment of cryoglobulinemia membranoproliferative glomerulonephritis associated with hepatitis C virus infection. Am J Kidney Dis 1995; 25:798–800.

Sansonno D, Gesualdo L, Manno C, et al. Hepatitis C virus–related proteins in kidney tissue from hepatitis C virus-infected patients with cryoglobulinemic membranoproliferative glomerulonephritis. Hepatology 1997; 25:1237–1244.

Zignego AL, Ferri C, Giannini C, et al. Hepatitis C virus genotype analysis in patients with type II mixed cryoglobulinemia. Ann Intern Med 1996; 124:31–34.

11

Management of Autoimmune Hepatitis

Ian G. McFarlane
King's College Hospital, London, England

Edward L. Krawitt
University of Vermont College of Medicine, Burlington, Vermont

Autoimmune hepatitis (AIH) is a chronic, progressive, sometimes fluctuating, necroinflammatory liver disease of unknown etiology presumed to have a basis in aberrant autoreactivity. It is characterized by elevation of serum transaminases, hypergammaglobulinemia, circulating autoantibodies, and destruction of the hepatic parenchyma, often with progression to cirrhosis. In severe cases, it carries a high mortality if untreated, but it usually responds to immunosuppressive therapy, even if cirrhosis is already established. The disease predominantly (4:1) affects females and may present at any age (median, 40 years), but it is usually more aggressive in younger patients. It often presents insidiously, but it is now well recognized that AIH can also have an acute (occasionally fulminant) presentation. AIH may also be discovered in asymptomatic individuals. The majority of cases relapse when treatment is withdrawn. Thus, many patients require maintenance therapy to improve quality of life, prolong survival, and defer liver transplantation.

DIAGNOSIS

Classification

Classification of AIH can be based on a number of features including histology, genetics, pathogenesis, and clinical manifestations. The system which is currently most widely used subdivides AIH into types 1 and 2 on the basis of autoantibody specificities (Table 1).

Type I Autoimmune Hepatitis

The form of AIH presently identified as type 1, or classic AIH, was originally known as active chronic hepatitis and subsequently as lupoid hepatitis, plasma cell hepatitis, and, most frequently, as autoimmune chronic active hepatitis. It is characterized by circulating antibodies to nuclei (antinuclear antibodies, ANA) or to smooth muscle (smooth muscle antibodies, SMA); the latter were thought to be reflective of more specific antibodies to actin.

Table 1 Classification of Autoimmune Hepatitis

Disorder	Autoantibody
Type I (classic) AIH	Antinuclear (ANA) Smooth muscle (SMA) Antineutrophil cytoplasmic (ANCA) Anti-asialoglycoprotein receptor (anti-ASGPR) Anti-soluble liver antigen (anti-SLA) Anti-liver cytosolic antigen (anti-LC-1)
Type 2 AIH	Anti-liver/kidney microsome-1 (ALKM-1) Anti-LC-1 Anti-ASGPR
Overlap syndromes	a. Antimitochondrial (AMA) without histological evidence of PBC b. ANA ± any of the above, together with histological evidence of biliary disease

Type 2 Autoimmune Hepatitis

A second type of AIH, almost always seen in children or young females and characterized by the presence of antibodies to cytochrome P-450 IID6 (anti-liver/kidney microsome antibodies, ALKM-1), is referred to as type 2 or ALKM-1–positive AIH.

Nonetheless, up to 20% of patients may not have ANA, SMA, or ALKM-1 when they first present, although these autoantibodies may appear later in the course of the disease, particularly during relapses. However, the majority of patients (whether or not they have ANA, SMA, or ALKM-1) have one or more of a range of other autoantibodies, most notably those reacting with the hepatic asialoglycoprotein receptor (anti-ASGPR), a soluble liver antigen (anti-SLA), a liver-specific cytosolic antigen (ALC-1), and neutrophil cytoplasmic antigens (ANCA). But, apart from ANCA, tests for these are not widely available.

Overlap Conditions

In addition to types 1 and 2 AIH, there are conditions in which features of AIH occur together with those of either primary biliary cirrhosis (PBC) or primary sclerosing cholangitis (PSC). In the so-called AIH/PBC overlap syndrome, serological findings in some cases are those of PBC, characterized by antimitochondrial antibodies (AMA) directed toward enzymes in the 2-oxoacid dehydrogenase family, but with histological findings (periportal, or interface, hepatitis) of AIH. Other cases are seronegative for AMA but have circulating ANA, SMA, or other autoantibodies associated with AIH, together with histological and/or cholangiographic changes suggestive of PBC or PSC. These overlap conditions have been variously described as autoimmune cholangitis, immune cholangitis, or autoimmune cholangiopathy. Some patients appear to respond to glucocorticoid treatment, and a trial of immunosuppressive therapy in these cases is reasonable.

Associated Conditions

There is often a history of other autoimmune disorders in patients and/or their first-degree relatives. Endocrinopathy is common, with a significant proportion of females experiencing amenorrhea or oligomenorrhea and up to 20% of patients having thyroid disease

(Hashimoto's or Graves'). Juvenile-onset insulin-dependent diabetes (IDDM) is very rare in type 1 AIH, but up to 30% of the older patients develop late-onset diabetes (possibly triggered or unmasked by corticosteroid therapy) and some require insulin. IDDM is more common (but still relatively rare) in type 2 AIH. A further 10–20% of AIH patients have any one of a wide range of other disorders, including Coombs-positive hemolytic anemia, fibrosing alveolitis, glomerulonephritis, idiopathic thrombocytopenia, myasthenia gravis, pernicious anaemia, rheumatoid arthritis, Sjögren's syndrome, and ulcerative colitis.

Presenting Features

Symptoms and Signs

Onset is typically insidious but may be acute and mimic the presentation of viral or toxic hepatitis. A history of other autoimmune conditions in patients or first-degree relatives is suggestive. In 10–20% of cases, however, the underlying liver disease may be revealed only during routine health screening or during investigation of another condition. Symptoms vary widely and often do not immediately suggest the diagnosis. Some patients may be entirely asymptomatic. The commonest complaints are lethargy (often extreme fatigue), general malaise, nausea, anorexia (with consequent weight loss), and upper abdominal discomfort (sometimes with intermittent pain). Other symptoms include oligomenorrhea, mild pruritus, skin rashes (various, but often maculopapular), arthralgia with or without myalgia, and, occasionally, persistent pyrexia. Any of these symptoms may occur alone or in combination with any or all of the others.

Signs of liver disease also vary widely. About 75% of patients are either icteric at presentation or give a recent history of jaundice. This may be associated with pale stools and/or dark urine. Up to 50% of patients have hepatomegaly, while splenomegaly and/or cutaneous stigmata of liver disease occur in about 25%; up to 20% may present with ascites and/or peripheral edema. Many patients are cirrhotic at presentation (reflecting the fact that the disease can remain asymptomatic for long periods before it reveals itself). Occasionally patients present with hematemesis or melena as the first sign of their liver disease.

Serum Biochemistry

The pattern of biochemical liver test abnormalities is typically one of elevated serum aminotransferase (AST/ALT) activities and bilirubin concentrations but normal or only moderately raised alkaline phosphatase levels. However, AST/ALT and bilirubin levels vary widely. Hyperglobulinemia is a characteristic feature and is due to selectively increased IgG levels, which may be elevated even if occasionally total globulin concentrations are within the normal range.

Histology

Histologically, AIH cannot be distinguished from other forms of chronic hepatitis, although generally the ductopenic disorders, PBC and PSC, can be ruled out. AIH is characterized by a portal-periportal infiltrate of mononuclear cells, which may be accompanied by fibrosis and/or cirrhosis. Although rosettes of hepatocytes, multinucleated cells, and an exuberant plasma cell infiltrate are frequently present, there is no absolute correlation of the clinical presentation with the pathological appearance. Thus, although patients with a severe clinical presentation often have advanced histopathological findings, the asymptomatic patient may also have severe disease, even established cirrhosis. The histological picture in patients with a spontaneous or a pharmacologically induced remission may revert to that of

Table 2 Scoring System for Diagnosis of Autoimmune Hepatitis[a]

Parameter		Score
Gender		
Female		+2
Male		0
Serum biochemistry		
Ratio of elevation of serum alkaline phosphatase vs. aminotransferase[b]	>3.0	−2
	<3.0	+2
Total serum globulin or γ-globulin or IgG		
Times upper normal limit	= >2.0	+3
	= 1.5–2.0	+2
	= 1.0–1.5	+1
	= < 1.0	0
Autoantibodies (titers by IF on rodent tissues)		
Adults: ANA, or SMA or LKM-1	= >1:80	+3
	= 1:80	+2
	= 1:40	+1
	= <1:40	0
Children: ANA or LKM-1	= > 1:20	+3
	= 1:10 or 1:20	+2
	= <1:10	0
or SMA	= >1:20	+3
	= 1:20	+2
	= <1:20	0
Antimitochondrial antibody	= Positive	−2
	= Negative	0
Seronegative for above but positive for any other defined "liver autoantibody"[d]		+2
Viral markers		
IGM anti-HAV, or HBsAg or IgM anti-HBc positive		−3
Anti-HVC positive by ELISA and/or RIBA		−2
or HVC RNA seropositive		−3
Positive test for active infection with any other virus		−3
Seronegative for all of the above		+3

Parameter			Score
Other etiological factors			
History of recent hepatotoxic drug use or parenteral exposure to blood	Yes		−2
	No		+1
Alcohol (average intake, g/day)			
	Males <35	Females <25	+2
	35–50	25–40	0
	50–80	40–60	−1
	>80	<60	−2
Histology			
Periportal necroinflammation			
With lobular involvement/bridging necrosis			+3
Without lobular involvement/bridging necrosis			+2
Rosetting of liver cells			+1
Predominantly plasma cell infiltrate			+1
Biliary changes			−1
Any other change(s), e.g., granulomas, siderosis, copper deposits, steatosis, etc., suggestive of a different etiology			−3
Genetic factors			
Other autoimmune diseases in patient or first-degree relatives			+1
HLA B8-DR3 or DR4 phenotype			+1
Response to therapy[c]			
Complete response			+2
Partial response			0
Treatment failure			0
No response (in terms of disease activity)			−2
Relapse during or after treatment withdrawal following "complete" initial response			+3

Before treatment	After treatment	Diagnosis
>15	>17	"Definite" AIH
10–15	12–17	"Probable" AIH[a]
<10	<12	Not diagnostic

[a]There are sufficient points allocated to allow for a diagnosis to be made without all of the parameters, but a diagnosis of "Definite" AIH should not be made without histology.

[b]Calculation of ratio of elevation of serum alkaline phosphatase (AP) vs. aminotransferase (AST) relates to the degree of elevation above the upper normal limits (unl) of these enzymes, i.e., = (AP/unl ÷ AP)/(AST/unl ÷ AST).

[c]Scores for response to therapy are to be added to scores for findings at initial presentation, for confirmation of diagnosis.

[d]A defined "liver autoantibody" is one for which there is published information relating to methodology of its detection and its relevance to AIH.

strictly portal inflammation or, if cirrhosis has already ensued, to that of an inactive cirrhosis.

"Definite" and "Probable" AIH

Against the above background, the International AIH Group recommended that a diagnosis of AIH should be considered in any patient (particularly female) who presents with an unexplained acute or chronic hepatitic illness or biochemical liver test abnormalities in the absence of signs or symptoms of liver disease, especially if there is a history of other autoimmune disorders in the patient or first-degree relatives, and that such patients should be classified as having "definite" or "probable" AIH according to the scoring system in Table 2. As with any scoring system, the specifications are not absolute. The utility of this system, now that methods to measure hepatitis C virus by polymerase chain reaction or branched DNA are widely available and the increasing recognition of overlap syndromes, is undergoing reevaluation.

MANAGEMENT

Background

Almost all patients with AIH will respond to immunosuppressive therapy, and remission can be maintained for very long periods on low doses of immunosuppressive drugs by careful adjustment of such therapy. Prednisone (or prednisolone) and azathioprine are the drugs of choice and are standard therapy.

Opinion is somewhat divided over whether to treat "mild" AIH—i.e., those patients who are asymptomatic—with aminotransferases less than twice upper normal limit and whose liver biopsy reveals activity without fibrosis or cirrhosis. One approach is to offer some form of immunosuppressive therapy in all cases of AIH, even those with minimal histological activity. An alternative approach would be to withhold treatment while monitoring carefully, including periodic biopsy for evidence of progression of disease. AIH can enter long periods of treatment-induced or spontaneous remission, only to flare (sometimes acutely) later.

Treatment Strategies

The pressure to reduce (and withdraw) steroid therapy as quickly as possible is the major factor in designing a treatment strategy for this condition. Obviously, long-term steroid therapy is associated with an increased risk of serious side effects (diabetes, cataracts, osteoporosis, hypertension, and psychoses), and many patients who have been successfully maintained in complete remission for long periods question the need to continue on treatment, especially those who suffer the cosmetic side effects (weight gain, Cushingoid facies, acne, emotional lability) of steroids. However, up to 90% of patients will relapse (the majority within 1 year) if all treatment is withdrawn—even if they have been in complete remission for several years on maintenance therapy. The remainder require continuous follow-up, because relapses can occur at any time (even many years after stopping treatment). In other words, it is doubtful if a complete cure can ever be achieved.

In recent years, based on more than 25 years of experience with different therapeutic regimens, several of the major centers where significant numbers of AIH patients are seen have independently evolved similar treatment strategies that approach a consensus. The

Table 3 Treatment of Autoimmune Hepatitis[a]

	Single-drug therapy	Combination therapy
Initial regimens	Prednisone, 20–40 mg daily	Prednisone, 20–30 mg daily, and azathioprine, 50–100 mg daily
Maintenance regimens	Prednisone, 5–15 mg daily, or azathioprine, 100–200 mg daily	Prednisone, 5–10 mg daily, and azathioprine, 50–150 mg daily

[a]Prednisolone may be substituted for prednisone.

objective is to achieve complete remission as quickly as possible on glucocorticoid or combination therapy (if azathioprine is tolerated) and then maintain the patient on the lowest possible dose of prednisolone or prednisone (± azathioprine) for at least 1 year before contemplating any major change in therapy. There are two main variations of these regimens, each with several minor modifications:

1. *Lifetime immunosuppression*—either on low-dose (5–10 mg/day) prednisone with or without azathioprine, or on azathioprine (1–2 mg/kg/day) alone. The advantage of this variation is that once the maintenance regimen is established, patients require less frequent monitoring. A disadvantage relates to the possibility of development of some of the more serious side effects of the drugs in the longer term. However, at the doses used, this risk seems to be relatively low. Also, many patients who have experienced relapses following withdrawal of all treatment prefer to continue on some form of maintenance therapy. Thus, if there are no complications and the patient is comfortable with the regimen, this is a reasonable approach.
2. *Symptomatic treatment*—i.e., only when the patient is symptomatic and/or has abnormal biochemical liver tests or histological evidence of active disease, with treatment being reintroduced when symptoms appear and/or liver tests become abnormal again. This approach reduces the risk of development of adverse side effects but has the disadvantage that many (if not most) patients will repeatedly relapse and will therefore require frequent monitoring, including repeat biopsies. Relapses can be severe (even fulminant) and deaths have occurred in cases where immunosuppression has not been reintroduced sufficiently early. Also, common sense dictates that the more often a patient relapses, the greater the likelihood of permanent liver damage (cirrhosis).

A third approach involves the use of alternating doses of prednisolone (± azathioprine) or the same dose on alternate days or pulses of high doses at intervals of 1 or 2 weeks. However, controlled trials have shown that, perhaps because of the relatively short half-lives of these drugs, this form of intermittent therapy is not effective for controlling the disease. We recommend the treatment regimens in Table 3 as the basis for initial and maintenance treatment strategies.

TREATMENT PROTOCOL

Initial Induction of Remission

Initial treatment with prednisone or prednisolone, alone or in combination with azathioprine, should be instituted in all patients in whom the histological appearance is that of a severe hepatitis with or without fibrosis or cirrhosis. In those patients in whom a mild hepatitis is present on biopsy, the decision to treat is often determined by symptoms. Asymptomatic patients and those with mild changes may be observed without institution of treatment, but their clinical status and liver biopsy appearance should be monitored carefully for evidence of progression of disease, keeping in mind the sometimes undulant nature of this disease. In order to avoid the effects of steroid treatment, particularly in patients with diabetes mellitus and in postmenopausal women, some physicians elect to treat initially with a combination of prednisone and azathioprine (Table 3).

In most patients, treatment is initiated with 20–30 mg of prednisone or prednisolone a day. Higher doses may sometimes be needed, especially in younger patients with severe disease, but this increases the risk of major side effects. The use of lower doses (10–15 mg/day) initially, with subsequent incremental increases if there is not a satisfactory response, may not control the disease adequately in many cases and may prolong the period during which there is ongoing liver damage. In children, the usual starting dose is 2 mg/kg/day up to a maximum of 60 mg/day.

The AST or ALT, total globulins (or gamma globulin or IgG) and full blood count should be monitored at least monthly initially. When the AST/ALT has fallen by at least 50%, steroid dose may be reduced to 15 mg/day in decrements of 5 mg/day fortnightly or monthly. Alternatively, at this point azathioprine may be introduced at 1 mg/kg/day (50–100 mg/day) while reducing steroid dose to 15 mg/day in decrements of 5 mg/day fortnightly.

If the AST/ALT and globulins/IgG continue to fall, steroids are reduced toward 15 mg/day. If not, the dose is held at the nadir of the AST/ALT. If transaminases rise, steroids should be increased by 5 mg/day increments weekly until AST/ALT fall again with subsequent attempts to reduce steroids as above.

When AST/ALT and globulins/IgG are normal, steroids should be maintained for 1 or 2 months at 15 mg/day prednisolone and 50–75 mg/day azathioprine. Then prednisolone can be reduced to 12.5 mg/day for 3 months and then to 10 mg/day for 3 months.

If remission is sustained on 10 mg/day of prednisolone in combination with azathioprine, consideration may be given to reducing the steroids further to a final maintenance dose of 7.5 or 5 mg/day. In practice, it is advisable to use the highest dose within this range that the patient will tolerate. The patients can be maintained on that dose with azathioprine for at least 1 year (and preferably 2 years), unless complications develop (see below). Liver function tests and blood counts should be monitored at 3-monthly intervals during this period.

Long-Term Management

Opinion varies about how to proceed after clinical and biochemical remission has been sustained for 1 or 2 years on maintenance therapy. Most authorities agree, however, that further changes in treatment should not be contemplated until remission is confirmed histologically.

For the patient who has sustained complete clinical, biochemical, and histological remission for 1 or 2 years on maintenance therapy, there are three possible long-term options:

Long-Term Immunosuppression

If there are no complications and the patient is happy to continue on treatment, it is not unreasonable to continue with maintenance therapy (perhaps with a small further reduction in the steroid dosage) almost indefinitely.

Withdrawal of All Treatment

If a decision is taken to withdraw all treatment, this should be done slowly and carefully. Begin by withdrawing the azathioprine in decrements of 25 mg/day at monthly intervals. Maintain the patient for 3 months on their maintenance dose of prednisolone alone for a further 3 months, then withdraw the steroids in decrements of 2.5 mg/day monthly. Monitor at monthly intervals for the next 6 months, 3-monthly for the following year and 6-monthly thereafter. Most patients who relapse after treatment withdrawal do so within the first year.

Maintenance on Azathioprine Alone

Many patients can be successfully maintained in remission on azathioprine alone. If white cells (WBCs) are $> 4.0 \times 10^9$/L and platelets are $> 100 \times 10^9$/L, it is usually safe to proceed. If either WBCs or platelets are below these values, *proceed with caution*. Note that lymphopenia is common in AIH but seems to be a feature of the disease rather than any specific effect of azathioprine, because it occurs as frequently in those receiving this drug as in those treated with prednisolone alone. Macrocytosis of red blood cells commonly occurs with this regimen, but anemia is rarely a problem.

If there are adequate WBCs and platelets, begin by increasing the azathioprine dose to the nearest approximation to 2 mg/kg/day that is possible with 25-mg tablets. Monitor FBC fortnightly for 1 or 2 months to ensure that myelosuppression is not developing on this higher dose (see "Problems and Complications," below). If the patient reports no adverse effects of the higher azathioprine dose and the FBC is satisfactory, begin withdrawing the steroids in decrements of 2.5 mg/day monthly while monitoring AST/ALT, globulins/IgG, and blood counts monthly. If either AST/ALT or globulins/IgG begin to rise, hold at the current dose of prednisolone and continue to check these parameters at fortnightly intervals (sometimes the AST and/or the globulins give a slight "blip" when steroids are being withdrawn). If AST/ALT and globulins/IgG remain normal, continue to withdraw steroids as above while monitoring laboratory values monthly at first and then every 3 months.

If the patient is still in *complete clinical, biochemical, and histological* remission after *2 years* on the higher dose of azathioprine alone, reduction to 1 mg/kg/day may be considered. In that event, reduce the azathioprine to 1.5 mg/kg/day for 1 month, then to 1 mg/kg/day. Liver tests should be monitored fortnightly for 1 month, monthly for 3 months, three-monthly for 6 months, and then at 6-month intervals. It should be noted that up to 25% are likely to relapse within 2 years on this lower dose.

Tips on Successful Management

- Treat each patient as an individual. A modest rise in AST/ALT or globulin/IgG levels may be of little consequence in one patient but highly significant and a herald of relapse in another. Furthermore, because of genetic variations in the metabolism of, and response to, the drugs used, each patient will require a particular dose regimen, which needs to be carefully titrated.
- Try to control the disease as quickly as possible initially without using very high doses of steroids.
- Remember that it may take 3–6 months for azathioprine to be fully effective.
- Do not panic over low WBC or platelet counts. True myelosuppression needs to be distinguished from the leukopenia and thrombocytopenia due to hypersplenism. In myelosuppression, there is usually a fairly rapid and progressive fall in cell counts, whereas in hypersplenism the counts remain fairly stable, albeit at low levels.

- Never stop treatment suddenly. Withdraw drugs gradually and monitor at frequent intervals. Remember that azathioprine is used for its "steroid-sparing" effects so, if this drug has to be discontinued, most patients will require a compensatory increase in the steroid dose to maintain remission.
- The AST/ALT is conventionally used for monitoring but it is not unusual for patients to have values within the normal range while still having histologically active disease. Autoantibody (ANA, SMA, LKM) titers are not useful in this regard, but the total globulin or IgG may be a sensitive indicator. A rise in serum IgG, even within the normal range, almost always indicates that the disease is not fully under control, even if the AST/ALT is normal.

Induction of Remission After Relapse

The first indication of relapse may only be increasing fatigue, anorexia, and general malaise, with or without arthralgia/myalgia (other than that associated with steroid withdrawal—see below), with little or no change in the biochemical liver tests. On the other hand, some patients can continue to be asymptomatic despite increases in AST/ALT. Early diagnosis is very important because, without intervention, relapses can become severe, even uncontrollable, and deaths can occur when appropriate treatment is not given promptly.

A sudden rise in the AST/ALT to greater than twice the upper normal limit must set alarm bells ringing, particularly if this is accompanied by signs or symptoms of relapse. However, as noted above, there is often a slight "blip" in the transaminase and/or globulin levels during reduction or withdrawal of steroids. Such "blips" may also occur during or after common viral infections which, as noted, are often accompanied by similar symptoms. Conversely, patients can have quite severe underlying liver damage with only modest increases in AST/ALT (less than twice upper normal limit). It is therefore often difficult to know initially whether a slight rise in AST/ALT is significant in terms of impending relapse.

The problem is compounded by the variability between individual patients. Thus, a rise in AST/ALT to 50 IU/L in a patient whose "normal" level is usually within the range of 35–40 IU/L may just be normal fluctuation, but such an increase is probably significant in a patient whose AST/ALT has previously been consistently under 30 IU/L. When there is any rise in transaminase in a patient who has previously been in complete remission, it is wise to repeat the liver tests at least fortnightly to determine whether there is a consistent upward trend.

Once relapse has been diagnosed, precise management will depend on how severe it seems to be and what treatment the patient was receiving at the time. In cases of severe relapse, it will be necessary to again use levels high enough to attempt to induce remission as before. In less severe cases, lower doses of steroids may be adequate. For the patient receiving azathioprine alone, reintroduce prednisone or prednisolone at 15 mg/day initially and continue azathioprine. If the AST/ALT continues to rise, increase the prednisolone by increments of 5 mg/day weekly until both the AST/ALT and globulin/IgG levels begin to fall. Hold at that dose for at least 1 month after these parameters have normalized, then begin to reduce the prednisone or prednisolone by 5 mg/day decrements monthly to whatever level is adequate to maintain the patient in remission.

Patients who relapse while on azathioprine alone will probably require maintenance on combination therapy for life. Those patients who relapse after complete withdrawal of all therapy should subsequently be treated as though they were presenting for the first time.

In these cases, it may still be possible to later wean steroids and maintain remission with azathioprine alone.

Problems and Complications

"Steroid Nonresponsiveness"

Although it has been generally accepted that a small proportion of patients in most series seem to have "steroid unresponsive" AIH, this term is really a contradiction of one of the defining criteria for the disease—namely, that it is responsive to immunosuppressive therapy. Furthermore, the term needs to be qualified in relation to adequacy of immunosuppression. Some centers use a standard dose of 15 or 12.5 mg/day of prednisolone as the initial therapy in all patients, regardless of severity or body weight, which may be inadequate for initial control.

Other than the rare cases presenting with fulminant hepatic failure (when the disease may be too severe or manifest itself too late for standard therapy to be effective), most of these "unresponsive" patients will show an initial fall in the AST/ALT after starting steroids. In some, the AST/ALT then plateaus or may even rise again. In others, the AST/ALT may become normal, only to rise again some weeks or months after maintenance therapy has been established.

Careful questioning may reveal that many such patients are either unwittingly taking the wrong dosages of the drugs or (particularly the younger patients) defaulting therapy intermittently. In most of the remainder, further investigations may uncover other underlying causes, including unsuspected or undisclosed heavy alcohol consumption or occult HCV infections. Additionally, retrospective analysis has revealed that there is a group who, by all criteria, have AIH but who (sometimes many years) later are found to have an overlap syndrome. In other words, it is doubtful if there are many patients with definite AIH who are truly "steroid unresponsive."

When difficulty is experienced in inducing or maintaining remission:

1. Carefully ascertain that the patient is taking the correct dose of medication.
2. Consider whether viral hepatitis, PSC or an overlap syndrome may be present.
3. Consider the possibility of malabsorption, in particular celiac sprue.
4. Consider alcohol and/or medications as playing a role.
5. Consider alternative immunosuppression.

Alcohol or HCV Complicating AIH

As noted above, the diagnosis of AIH in patients who consume excessive amounts of alcohol or who have evidence of HCV infection can be difficult, and these agents may also be occult causes of "steroid unresponsiveness."

Patients with hepatitis C will show a response to corticosteroid therapy in terms of marked reduction (and even normalization) of serum aminotransferases and gamma globulins. HCV RNA by sensitive polymerase chain reaction should be performed in all patients with AIH to exclude chronic hepatitis C.

Myelosuppression

Myelosuppression is an ever-present risk with azathioprine, particularly at the higher doses, but needs to be distinguished from cytopenia related to hypersplenism. Lymphopenia, with lymphocyte counts of $0.5–1.5 \times 10^9/L$, and thrombocytopenia due to sequestration of cells in the spleen are common in AIH, even in those maintained on prednisolone alone.

In our experience, azathioprine-induced myelosuppression is not a major problem in the majority of patients treated with 1 or 2 mg/kg/day of azathioprine. However, it does occasionally occur, usually within a few months of first introducing azathioprine at conventional doses and rarely in those who have been on the drug for a year or more. About 5% of patients tolerate azathioprine at 1 mg/kg/day but develop myelosuppression on higher doses. Blood counts must be monitored every 3–6 months in all patients receiving azathioprine. Patients with WBCs of $< 3.0 \times 10^9$/L and platelet counts $< 100 \times 10^9$/L should be treated with particular caution. If there is a sustained downward drift in the WBC and platelet counts, urgent consideration needs to be given to reducing or withdrawing the azathioprine.

Withdrawal of Azathioprine

Reduction in dosage or withdrawal of azathioprine should always be approached with extreme caution. Occasionally patients have had their azathioprine precipitously reduced or withdrawn because of concerns about low WBC and/or platelet counts or development of symptoms that might be related to the drug. Almost all such cases relapse within a few months.

When reduction or withdrawal of azathioprine is contemplated, the reasons for doing so should be carefully considered. If it is because of cytopenia, it should be firmly established that the low cell counts are indeed due to myelosuppression and not simply to hypersplenism. The azathioprine should be reduced cautiously, at a rate not greater than 25 mg/day fortnightly, and consideration must be given to the need to reintroduce or increase the dose of prednisolone to compensate for the loss of the immunosuppressive effect of the azathioprine, particularly in the patient who has had previous relapses while on maintenance therapy. If there is an urgent need to stop azathioprine because of severe myelosuppression, the steroid dose should be increased to 0.5 mg/kg/day for 1 or 2 weeks and then tapered to the appropriate maintenance dose.

On the other hand, as noted above, withdrawal or reduction of the drug may be contemplated in patients who have been maintained in complete remission on 2 mg/kg/day of azathioprine alone (see "Treatment Protocol" above). Whatever the reason for reducing or withdrawing the azathioprine, liver function tests and blood counts should be monitored every 2 weeks during the period of reduction and monthly for the subsequent 6 months, and every 3 months thereafter.

Azathioprine Toxicity/Intolerance

There is evidence that, at high doses, azathioprine can induce cholestatic liver injury. Other reported complications include pancreatitis and venoocclusive disease and, in the liver transplant setting, nodular regenerative hyperplasia (NRH). However, the drug appears to be relatively safe at the doses used in AIH. Even after many years on 2 mg/kg/day, patients show at most only very mild elevations in serum bilirubin (which may be due to the natural progression of their disease rather than to the drug). Paradoxically, serum alkaline phosphatase or gamma-glutamyl transpepetidase activities drift downward in most patients.

Occasionally, patients report adverse side effects such as rashes, general malaise, and nausea/vomiting when first started on azathioprine, but it is not at all clear whether these are drug-related or are coincidental symptoms due to some other cause. Nevertheless, in such cases, it is wise to discontinue the azathioprine and try it again after a few months—starting at a low dose (25 mg/day) and gradually increasing it while carefully monitoring the patient to see if the symptoms recur.

The major problem in patients maintained on azathioprine alone is the development of arthralgia affecting mainly the hinged joints. This occurs in about 50% of cases soon after the steroids are withdrawn. It is a noninflammatory arthropathy that does not seem to be due to the azathioprine but rather is an effect of steroid withdrawal. It varies in severity from simple early morning stiffness, lasting a few weeks, to occasionally very severe, incapacitating joint pain lasting a year or more. Most patients seem to prefer to persevere with their arthralgia rather than restart steroid therapy. In 80% of these cases, the arthralgia will last less than 6 months and symptomatic relief can be obtained with acetaminophen, but total dosage should not exceed 2000 mg/day. The remaining patients require nonsteroidal anti-inflammatory drugs. Very occasionally, the arthralgia may persist and be so severe that it becomes necessary to reintroduce prednisolone at a low dose (2.5 or 5 mg/day), which brings immediate relief.

Azathioprine Carcinogenicity/Teratogenicity

Evidence that azathioprine may be carcinogenic is based mainly on the finding of an increased incidence of lymphomas and squamous carcinomas of the skin in transplant patients receiving the drug. Azathioprine at 1 mg/kg/day has been used for more than 25 years in AIH patients, and in some centers at 2 mg/kg/day for more than 10 years; there have been few reports of major problems with respect to malignancies.

Pregnancy

There seems no good reason why the majority of younger females with well-controlled AIH should not become pregnant if they so desire, but caution is advised. Each case should be considered individually and should be monitored carefully during the pregnancy and for 6 months postpartum. The natural immunosuppression that is a part of the gestation process seems to benefit the condition in some cases and the patient may do well during pregnancy, only to relapse soon after giving birth. Conversely, some patients have exacerbations of their disease during their pregnancies. In the patient with advanced cirrhosis with portal hypertension and gastric or esophageal varices, however, pregnancy must be considered inadvisable because of the risk of variceal haemorrhage.

Planned Pregnancy. In patients maintained on combination therapy or on azathioprine alone, the azathioprine should be carefully withdrawn and prednisolone reintroduced or increased in dosage to compensate. Patients should be advised not to attempt to become pregnant until at least 1 month after azathioprine has been withdrawn. Liver function tests should be carefully monitored during the pregnancy and for at least 6 months thereafter. When the mother has stopped breast-feeding, azathioprine may be reintroduced and the prednisolone reduced or withdrawn as before.

Unplanned Pregnancy. Amenorrhea is often a feature of the disease, and contraceptive precautions are often not taken. In this setting, when pregnancy arises, a woman is often unaware for several months that she is pregnant. This generally occurs in those whose disease is well controlled.

This situation presents a dilemma. Any teratogenic effects of azathioprine are likely to have already occurred, but the possibility that such effects may be exerted later during gestation must also be considered, along with the possible immunosuppressive effects of the drug on the baby after birth (which are unknown). Adverse effects on children born to mothers taking azathioprine have not yet been reported. it is also necessary to balance the health of the baby against that of its mother. The risk to the fetus of a relapse of AIH is probably greater than that due to azathioprine. However, most authorities feel that the safety of the drug during pregnancy is not proven and it is best to attempt to withdraw the azathioprine as quickly as possible. It may be reintroduced when the mother has stopped breast-feeding.

REFERENCES

Batts KP, Ludwig JP. Histopathology of autoimmune hepatitis, primary biliary cirrhosis, and primary sclerosing cholangitis. In: Krawitz EL, Wiesner RH, Nishioka M, eds. Autoimmune Liver Diseases, 2d ed. Amsterdam: Elsevier Science Publishers. In press.

Ben-Ari Z, Dhillon AP, Sherlock A. Autoimmune cholangiopathy: part of the spectrum of autoimmune chronic active hepatitis. Hepatology 1993; 18:10–15.

Boberg KM, Fausa O, Haaland T, Holter E, Mellbye OJ, Spurkland A, Schrumpf E. Features of autoimmune hepatitis in primary sclerosing cholangitis: an evaluation of 114 primary sclerosing cholangitis patients according to a scoring system for the diagnosis of autoimmune hepatitis. Hepatology 1996; 23:1369–1376.

Czaja AJ. Low-dose corticosteroid therapy after multiple releases of severe HBsAg-negative chronic active hepatitis. Hepatology 1992; 11:1044–1049.

Czaja AJ, Manns MP. The validity and importance of subtypes in autoimmune hepatitis: a point of view. Am J Gastroenterol 1995; 90:1206.

Czaja AJ, Cassani F, Cataleta M, Valentini P, Bianchi FB. Frequency and significance of antibodies to actin in type 1 autoimmune hepatitis. Hepatology 1996; 24:1068.

Davis PA, Leung P, Manns M, Kaplan M, Munoz SJ, Gorin FA, Dickson ER, Krawitt E, Coppel R, Gershwin ME. M4 and M9 antibodies in the overlap syndrome of primary biliary cirrhosis and chronic active hepatitis: epitopes of epiphenomena? Hepatology 1992; 16:1128–1136.

Gough A, Chapman S, Wagstaff K, Emery R, Elias E. Minocycline induced autoimmune hepatitis and systemic lupus erythematosus-like syndrome. Br Med J 1996; 312:169–172.

Gregorio GV, Portmann B, Reid F, Donaldson PT, Doherty DG, McCartney M, Mowat AP, Vergani D, Mieli-Vergani G. Autoimmune hepatitis in childhood: a 20-year experience. Hepatology 1997; 25:541–547.

Krawitt EL. Autoimmune hepatitis. N Engl J Med 1996; 334:897–903.

Johnson PJ, McFarlane IG. Meeting report: international autoimmune hepatitis group. Hepatology 1993; 18:998–1005.

Johnson PJ, McFarlane IG, Williams R. Azathioprine for long term maintenance of remission in autoimmune hepatitis. N Engl J Med 1995; 333:958.

Pratt DS, Flavin DP, Kaplan MM. The successful treatment of autoimmune hepatitis with 6-mercaptopurine after failure with azathioprine. Gastroenterology 1996; 110:271–274.

Roberts SK, Therneau TM, Czaja AJ. Prognosis of histological cirrhosis in type 1 autoimmune hepatitis. Gastroenterology 1996; 110:848.

Ruiz-Moreno M, Rua JM, Carreño V, Quiroga JA, Manns M, Meyer zum Buschefeldde K-H. Autoimmune chronic hepatitis type 1 manifested during interferon therapy in children. J Hepatol 1991; 12:265–266.

Sanchez-Urdazpal LS, Czaja AJ, van Hoek B, Krom RAF, Wiesner RH. Prognostic features and role of liver transplantation in severe corticosteroid-treated autoimmune chronic active hepatitis. Hepatology 1992; 15:215–221.

Targan S, Landers C, Vidrich A, Czaja AJ. High titer antineutrophil cytoplasmic antibodies in type-1 autoimmune hepatitis. Gastroenterology 1995; 108:1159–1166.

Treichel U, McFarlane BM, Seki T, Krawitt EL, Alessi N, Stickel F, McFarlane IG, Kiyosawa K, Futura S, Freni MA, Gerken G, Meyer zum Buschenfelde K-H. Demographics of anti-asialoglycoprotein receptor autoantibodies in autoimmune hepatitis. Gastroenterology 1994; 107:799–804.

12
Management of Primary Biliary Cirrhosis

Young-Mee Lee and Marshall M. Kaplan
New England Medical Center, Boston, Massachusetts

INTRODUCTION

Primary biliary cirrhosis is a chronic, progressive cholestatic liver disease that occurs predominantly in middle-aged women. The disease is characterized by the destruction of small intralobular bile ducts, causing a progressive impairment of bile flow with retention of potentially toxic substances such as bile acids within the liver. Ultimately, there is destruction of liver cells, progressive portal fibrosis, the development of cirrhosis, and liver failure. The exact etiology is unknown but appears to be related to some abnormality of immune regulation. Estimates of its incidence range from 3.9–15 cases per million population per year. Although primary biliary cirrhosis is uncommon, it is one of the leading indications for liver transplantation.

CLINICAL FEATURES

Fatigue and pruritus are the most common presenting symptoms. Approximately 25–50% of patients have skin hyperpigmentation due to the increased deposition of melanin. Jaundice is usually a later manifestation but may be seen at presentation in some patients. Other manifestations of primary biliary cirrhosis include osteoporosis, hypercholesterolemia with xanthoma and xanthelasmas, and an association with other autoimmune disorders such as sicca syndrome, hypothyroidism, CREST (calcinosis, Raynaud's phenomenon, esophageal motility disorders, sclerodactyly, and telangiectasia) syndrome, and arthritis.

The diagnosis of primary biliary cirrhosis should be considered in all patients with unexplained cholestatic liver function tests. The diagnosis is based on clinical features and characteristic elevations of liver function tests, particularly elevations of alkaline phosphatase levels. Antimitochondrial antibody is positive in approximately 95% of patients with primary biliary cirrhosis. Many patients have elevations of serum IgM. Mechanical bile duct obstruction should be excluded with imaging tests such as ultrasonography. Computed tomography is rarely needed, and endoscopic cholangiography is helpful in the patient with a negative antimitochondrial antibody test.

The diagnosis should be confirmed by percutaneous liver biopsy. The biopsy also allows for histological staging and is useful for prognosis. Histologically, primary biliary cirrhosis has been divided into four stages. In stage I, there are florid bile duct lesions, which are characterized by the infiltration and degeneration of small bile ducts by lymphocytes. Inflammation is confined to portal triads. Granulomas are most likely seen at this stage. In stage II, the lesion is more widespread. There is bile duct degeneration with the absence of bile ducts in some portal triads and atypical bile duct proliferation in others. Inflammation extends from the portal triads into the surrounding parenchyma, a process termed *piecemeal necrosis*. In stage III, there is progression of scarring with linkage of adjacent portal triads by fibrous septa. Stage IV is characterized by frank cirrhosis which is often indistinguishable from other types of cirrhosis except that there is usually a decreased number of normal appearing bile ducts in the areas of scarring.

PROGNOSIS

The course of primary biliary cirrhosis is variable but is usually slowly progressive. Median survival or referral for liver transplantation in untreated symptomatic patients is approximately 7 years. Survival in asymptomatic patients with primary biliary cirrhosis is longer than in symptomatic patients.

MANAGEMENT

There are two goals in the medical management of primary biliary cirrhosis: (1) treatment of the symptoms and complications that result from chronic cholestasis and (2) specific therapy targeting the underlying pathogenic process.

Management of Symptoms and Complications

Pruritus

One of the most distressing symptom in primary biliary cirrhosis is pruritus. It is worse at night and in hot weather. It can be severely debilitating, causing extensive excoriations, and may be exacerbated by a high dietary fat intake. The pathogenesis of pruritus is unknown. There is no correlation between pruritus and concentration of bile acids in serum or sequestration in skin. However, there is recent evidence suggesting a role of endogenous opioids in the pathogenesis of pruritus (see Chap. 39).

Various agents have been evaluated in the management of pruritus. Antihistamines at bedtime may be used to treat mild pruritus. However, for the treatment of moderate or severe pruritus, the bile acid–binding resins cholestyramine and colestipol are effective first-line agents. They must bind an unidentified pruritogenic substance in bile and promote its elimination in feces. The usual starting dosage of cholestyramine is 4 g three times per day. Cholestyramine takes 2 to 4 days from the initiation of treatment to bring about a remission of the itching. If itching fails to respond to the usual dose of cholestyramine after 4 days, the dose should be increased in 4-g increments up to 24 g/day. The major limitation is its taste and consistency. Its palatability may be improved by mixing with fruit juice or blended fruits. Cholestyramine may cause severe constipation, which is readily treated with laxatives or bulking agents, and it can interfere with the absorption of many medications. Thus, medications should be taken as far apart from the cholestyramine as possible, at least 2 h before or after cholestyramine is taken. Blood levels of fat-soluble vitamins A, D, E, and K should be monitored periodically or replacement therapy given, since patient requiring cholestyramine may malabsorb fat-soluble vitamins. Cholestyramine has also been associated with folic acid deficiency. Serum folate should be monitored or concomitant treatment with folic acid 1 mg/day is recommended. For those patients who cannot tolerate cholestyramine, colestipol hydrochloride, another nonasorbed anion-exchange resin, may be an alternative therapy. Its efficacy and side effects are similar to those of cholestyramine. The usual dose is 5 mg three times a day orally.

In rare patients who are unresponsive to cholestyramine or colestipol hydrochloride, there are reports of varying success with ursodeoxycholic acid (600–1800 mg/day), phenobarbital, rifampin (150–300 mg twice a day), testosterone, phototherapy with ultraviolet light, glucocorticoids, *S*-adenosyl-L-methionine, ondansetron, and naloxone (see Chap. 39). For those patients with intractable pruritus unresponsive to medications, large-volume plasmapheresis may be effective. Its beneficial effects usually last 2–4 weeks, but its great expense makes it impractical.

Bone Disease

Hepatic osteodystrophy or osteopenia with diffuse bone pain and spontaneous bone fractures is a serious complication occurring in some patients with primary biliary cirrhosis. Osteoporosis is the most commonly associated metabolic bone disease in patients with primary biliary cirrhosis. Osteomalacia occurs rarely and only in patients with advanced disease. Low bone mineral densities of the lumbar spine occur in 30–50% of patients with primary biliary cirrhosis. Patients with osteoporosis may present with bone pain and spontaneous fractures, usually of the vertebral bodies and ribs. The exact pathogenesis of osteoporosis is not well understood. Patients with primary biliary cirrhosis rarely have low serum levels of 25-hydroxy vitamin D but may have normal serum levels of the most active vitamin D metabolite, $1,25(OH)_2$ vitamin D. Recent data suggest that osteoblast inhibitors in cholestatic serum may play a role in the pathogenesis of osteoporosis.

There is no proven therapy for osteoporosis in patients with primary biliary cirrhosis. Vitamin D and calcium supplementation, 1.0–1.5 g/day, may be given, since there is little risk. Its safety can be monitored by measuring serum calcium levels and maintaining 24-h urinary calcium excretion at less than 200 mg/day. If serum levels of 25-hydroxy vitamin D are low, supplementation with 25-hydroxy vitamin D_3, 20 μg/day, may be given to maintain its level in the high-normal range. Treatment with 25-hydroxy vitamin D will correct or prevent the osteomalacia that occurs in patients with advanced disease. A preliminary study with fluoride (50 mg/day orally) was encouraging, as the fluoride appeared to prevent bone loss in seven patients. Medications used to treat postmenopausal osteoporosis, such as calcitonin or alendronate, have not been fully evaluated. Liver transplantation is associated with improvement in bone density, usually 6–12 months after surgery.

Malabsorption

Patients with primary biliary cirrhosis who are clinically jaundiced may develop diarrhea and weight loss due to steatorrhea. The steatorrhea is due primarily to decreased concentrations of bile acids within the small intestinal lumen. Pancreatic insufficiency may also contribute to steatorrhea in patients with concomitant sicca syndrome. This may be detected with the bentiromide test and treated with oral pancreatic extract. The steatorrhea may be clinically significant and cause nocturnal diarrhea, weight loss, and muscle wasting. Symptomatic steatorrhea can be partially corrected by restricting dietary fat and adding medium-chain triglycerides. Each milliliter of medium-chain triglyceride oil has 7.5 calories. Most patients can tolerate 60 mL/day without difficulty. The medium-chain triglyceride oil may either be taken directly by the teaspoon or be used as a substitute in cooking.

Patients with primary biliary cirrhosis may malabsorb the fat-soluble vitamins A, D, and K. Vitamin A deficiency occurs in approximately 30% of patients but rarely causes symptoms. Vitamin A deficiency may be prevented by monitoring serum levels and with dietary supplements of vitamin A, 15,000 U/day (three times the recommended daily allowance). Vitamin E deficiency occurs rarely except in patients with end-stage disease awaiting liver transplantation. Clinically significant vitamin K deficiency is uncommon except in the patient who is taking cholestyramine on a regular basis and is deeply jaundiced. The prothrombin time is normal in most patients until an advanced stage, when there are signs of liver failure. Vitamin K is rarely required except in these patients.

Hypothyroidism

Approximately 20% of patients with primary biliary cirrhosis have or will develop hypothyroidism. Routine tests for thyroid function, such as total T_4 or free T_4 index, may be normal due to elevated concentrations of thyroid-binding globulin. Hypothyroidism is most accurately evaluated by measuring the serum thyroid-stimulating hormone (TSH). Patients with hypothyroidism respond to thyroid hormone replacement.

Xanthomas

Hypercholesterolemia and hyperlipidemia are common in patients with primary biliary cirrhosis. Xanthomas—which are cholesterol deposits in tendon sheaths, over bony prominences, and at peripheral nerves—occur in less than 10% of patients with primary biliary cirrhosis. Xanthomas may occur on the palms and soles, cause pain, and interfere with manual dexterity and walking. They are usually associated with plasma cholesterol levels above 600 mg/dL for greater than 3 months. If xanthomas become symptomatic, large-volume plasmapheresis at 1- to 2-week intervals are usually effective. The goal of plasmapheresis is to remove cholesterol from the body; each session will lower the serum cholesterol level by approximately 50%. Xanthomas usually resolve once the serum cholesterol level approaches normal.

Portal Hypertension

The development of portal hypertension and bleeding from esophageal varices or congestive gastropathy may be seen in patients with early histological stages of primary biliary cirrhosis. Although the reason for development of portal hypertension early in the course of primary biliary cirrhosis is unknown, some have ascribed it to nodular regenerative hyperplasia. Survival after distal splenorenal shunt is not adversely affected and is similar to that predicted by the Mayo prognostic model.

In patients with iron-deficiency anemia, a thorough search for a site of gastrointestinal blood loss should be done. Chronic intermittent blood loss from congestive gastropathy or esophageal varices is a possible cause. If treatment with oral iron is not adequate, modalities such as beta blockers, sclerotherapy, and variceal band ligation should be considered. If these measures fail, distal splenorenal shunting is the preferred treatment for patients with early stages of primary biliary cirrhosis. For patients with advanced primary biliary cirrhosis, transjugular intrahepatic portosystemic stent shunt and liver transplantation are indicated.

Liver Failure

Patients with advanced primary biliary cirrhosis, like patients with other types of end-stage cirrhosis, develop symptoms of liver failure such as ascites, encephalopathy, spontaneous bacterial peritonitis, and bleeding esophageal varices. The management is similar to that in liver failure due to other causes.

The efficacy of liver transplantation in prolonging survival in primary biliary cirrhosis is proven. Liver transplantation is recommended in cirrhotic patients with impending liver failure, bleeding from portal hypertension, or jaundice. It is best not to delay transplantation until patients have advanced liver failure with recurrent hepatic encephalopathy, intractable ascites, or severe muscle wasting.

TREATMENT OF THE UNDERLYING PROCESS

Although there is no proven medical treatment for the underlying disease process in primary biliary cirrhosis, the management of these patients has been evolving rapidly. Various immunosuppressive, antifibrotic, cupruretic, and choleretic agents have been evaluated, as shown in Table 1. However, the evaluation of treatment efficacy has been difficult due to the chronic course of the disease, with great variation in severity and rate of progression among individual patients. Studies of azathioprine, glucocorticoids, cyclosporine, and D-penicillamine have shown little benefit. Results with ursodeoxycholic acid, colchicine, and methotrexate are encouraging. There have been some improvements in the biochemical tests of liver function as well as in liver histology in some patients. Because specific therapy targeting the underlying process of primary biliary cirrhosis is still evolving, relevant clinical data are reviewed in this section.

Azathioprine

Azathioprine, an immunosuppressive drug, has been used in autoimmune diseases and transplantation. In doses of 1–2 mg/kg/day, azathioprine was initially shown to be of no therapeutic benefit in two prospective, controlled trials. On reanalysis of the larger randomized study of 248 patients—to correct for the fact that patients who received azathioprine had more advanced disease—there was a beneficial effect on survival and stabilization of clinical symptoms. The effects of azathioprine on biochemical tests and histology were not given in this report and presumably were not positive. In addition, more than one-third of the patients in this study were either lost to follow-up or withdrew. Azathioprine is rarely used now to treat primary biliary cirrhosis.

Table 1 Drug Treatment of PBC

Ineffective and/or toxic	Promising/in trial
Azathioprine	Colchicine
Glucocorticoids	Ursodiol
Cyclosporine	Methotrexate
D-Penicillamine	

Glucocorticoids

In early uncontrolled trials, glucocorticoid therapy was associated with improvement of pruritus but also with acceleration of osteoporosis. In controlled trials, the drug was associated with decreased symptoms, improvement in serum immunoglobulins and alkaline phosphatase levels, but worsening osteoporosis. The predictable complications seemed to outweigh the short-term improvement in some biochemical tests. There is little enthusiasm for the use of glucocorticoid therapy.

Cyclosporine

Cyclosporine, an inhibitor of T-cell function, is an effective immunosuppressive agent in preventing and treating allograft rejection and autoimmune diseases. Cyclosporine has been evaluated in several controlled trials. In a large trial of 349 patients, cyclosporine 3 mg/kg/day was associated with improvements in serum bilirubin, alkaline phosphatase, alanine aminotransferase, and albumin. However, there were significant side effects of hypertension and worsening of renal function. Cyclosporine did not improve symptoms or liver histology. There was no effect on survival unless survival was corrected with the Cox multiple hazards model because cyclosporine-treated patients had more advanced disease at baseline. Cyclosporine has predictable toxicity with limited efficacy and is rarely used to treat primary biliary cirrhosis.

D-Penicillamine

D-Penicillamine was evaluated because of its beneficial effect as a cupruretic agent in patients with Wilson's disease. Primary biliary cirrhosis, like Wilson's disease, is characterized by increased hepatic copper stores. In addition to its cupruretic effect, D-penicillamine has anti-inflammatory effects and can impair the maturation of collagen, a process that might slow the development of cirrhosis.

Unfortunately, the theoretical promise of D-penicillamine has not been fulfilled. Seven prospective, controlled trials of D-penicillamine have been conducted in primary biliary cirrhosis. Although the drug was associated with decreased hepatic copper levels, there were no beneficial effects on symptoms, biochemical tests of liver function, liver histology, or survival. Furthermore, D-penicillamine was associated with a high incidence of serious side effects, up to 46% in some studies. Thus, D-penicillamine is not recommended in the treatment of primary biliary cirrhosis.

Colchicine

Colchicine has been evaluated for treatment of primary biliary cirrhosis based on its anti-inflammatory and antifibrotic properties. It has been used in the treatment of acute gouty arthritic and familial Mediterranean fever. It inhibits intracellular microtubule assembly, decreases collagen synthesis, increases collagenase activity in vitro, and decreases the expression of selectins on endothelial and inflammatory cells.

In one prospective double-blind trial, colchicine 0.6 mg twice daily significantly improved levels of serum albumin, bilirubin, alkaline phosphatase, aminotransferases, and cholesterol after 2 years when compared with those levels of patients on placebo. More importantly, colchicine appeared to decrease the risk of death from liver failure after 4 years. The cumulative mortality from liver disease was 21% in colchicine-treated patients and 47% in patients taking placebo. However, there was no improvement in liver histology or symptoms. Several patients developed diarrhea, which disappeared when the dose was lowered to 0.6 mg once a day. Overall, there was little toxicity.

Colchicine showed variable biochemical benefit in two similar studies. There was no improvement in histology and symptoms in any of these trials. Patients in one study were followed for up to 8 years, at which time biochemical tests were stable but survival benefit was lost. One placebo-controlled trial of 90 patients evaluated colchicine and ursodiol. Both drugs improved pruritus. Colchicine improved biochemical tests modestly, whereas ursodiol decreased serum alkaline phosphatase and aminotransferase activities significantly as compared with placebo and colchicine. Ursodiol also lowered serum bilirubin levels. In another study, 12 patients received ursodiol and colchicine together for 2 years. There appeared to be a synergistic effect on biochemical tests and liver histology.

Ursodeoxycholic Acid

Ursodoxycholic acid has been widely used to treat patients with primary biliary cirrhosis. Recently, it has been approved by the medical advisory board of the Food and Drug Administration for the treatment of patients with primary biliary cirrhosis. It is a naturally occurring hydrophilic dihydroxy bile acid with choleretic properties. In vivo, ursodeoxycholic acid decreases serum levels of endogenous bile acids; in vitro, it stabilizes liver cell membranes exposed to toxic concentrations of the naturally occurring bile acid.

The results of treatment with ursodeoxycholic acid have been encouraging. A pilot study demonstrated that patients with primary biliary cirrhosis had a significant decrease in symptoms and improvement in serum alkaline phosphatase and aminotransferases. The use of ursodiol has been evaluated in four randomized prospective double-blind trials. Usodiol, 13–15 mg/kg/day, improved the serum levels of bilirubin, alkaline phosphatase, gamma glutamyl transpeptidase, alanine and aspartate aminotransferase, and IgM. It was safe and well tolerated. Diarrhea occurred in less than 2% of patients. In some patients, ursodiol has been associated with decreased serum cholesterol levels, relief of pruritus, and delayed formation of varices. There were no benefits with regard to osteoporosis. Most encouraging, compared with placebo, it prolonged the interval before liver transplantation or death after 4 years. When data from three of these studies were pooled, ursodiol significantly prolonged survival "free of liver transplantation" compared with placebo, 3.66 versus 3.45 years ($p = 0.014$). Ursodiol decreased the probability of liver transplantation or death at 4 years by 32%. These results suggest that ursodeoxycholic acid is safe and effective.

The effect of ursodiol on liver histology is less clear. There was a beneficial effect on liver histology with decreased inflammation in one study but not in three other studies. Ursodiol appears to be more effective in patients with early disease. In one trial, 12 of 65 patients had complete normalization of biochemical tests after 2 years of treatment. Compared with the patients whose tests did not normalize, responders had earlier histological stages of disease and lesser elevations of serum bilirubin and alkaline phosphatase. Most of the beneficial biochemical effects of ursodeoxycholic acid occur within 2–3 months of initiating therapy. Ursodiol is less effective in patients with advanced disease. In one study, ursodiol worsened symptoms and blood tests in some patients with stage III and IV disease. Further long-term observations are required to determine how long the beneficial effects of ursodiol are sustained.

Methotrexate

Methotrexate at low dose of 15 mg/week orally was initially used in nine patients with precirrhotic primary biliary cirrhosis. There was improvement in serum levels of alkaline phosphatase, the aminotransferases, cholesterol, and bilirubin, while serum albumin remained stable.

Methotrexate is currently being evaluated alone and in combination with ursodiol and colchicine. In a randomized, prospective trial of 89 patients comparing methotrexate to colchicine, there was an improvement in biochemical tests and symptoms of pruritus and fatigue in those receiving methotrexate. There was an encouraging improvement in liver histology, with decreased portal inflammation and bile duct necrosis. There was a transient increase in aminotransferase levels 2 weeks to 8 months after methotrexate was initiated, followed by a decrease in aminotransferase activity. Worsening aminotransferase levels appear to be a marker of an ultimately good response to methotrexate. In contrast to the ursodeoxycholic acid response, which occurs within 2–3 months of initiating therapy, the response to methotrexate occurs slowly and is often not obvious until 6–10 months after starting methotrexate and may continue slowly for several years. Patients with advanced primary biliary cirrhosis, particularly those with cirrhosis and jaundice and/or portal hypertension, do not respond to methotrexate or any other medical treatment.

We have recently reported the sustained remission in five women with well-established primary biliary cirrhosis, stages I to III, all antimitochondrial antibody–positive, who have now been on methotrexate for 6–8 years and followed on some medical treatment for 7–15 years. All had florid bile duct lesions at onset, striking inflammation within portal triads, and granulomas within the liver. Biochemical tests of liver function returned to normal and pruritus and fatigue remitted in all. Mean serum alkaline phosphatase decreased from 620 IU (range, 231–1245) to 73 IU (range, 64–102), ALT from 145 U/L (range, 40–251) to 19 U/L (range, 8–25), and serum bilirubin from 18.1 UM/L (range, 6.8–32.5) to 9.2 UM/L (range, 8.5–10.3). Of note, serial biopsies demonstrated progressive improvement. After 5 years of treatment, liver biopsies showed no feature of primary biliary cirrhosis and were normal in two patients. Mean histological stage decreased from 2.5 to 1.

The major side effect of methotrexate is an allergic pneumonitis, which may occur in up to 15% of patients with primary biliary cirrhosis. It resolves rapidly after cessation of methotrexate and use of glucocorticoids. Oral aphthous ulcers, hair loss, fatigue, anorexia, and bone marrow suppression occur rarely in our experience.

Not all patients with primary biliary cirrhosis respond to treatment with one agent. Based on the diverse mechanism of action of ursodiol, colchicine, and methotrexate, the use of a combination of these drugs is a logical approach. The effects of methotrexate and ursodiol were additive in two studies in which methotrexate was given to patients who had responded incompletely to ursodeoxycholic acid. In these studies, of nine and eight patients respectively, the addition of methotrexate improved both symptoms and biochemical tests more completely than ursodiol alone. In another study of 32 patients who received methotrexate and ursodiol together, no additive effects on biochemical tests of liver function were observed when this group was compared with patients who were part of an earlier study of ursodiol alone. Because biochemical tests may become normal or improve greatly in many patients receiving ursodiol alone, it is possible that an additive effect of methotrexate was missed in some patients because of the study design.

Liver Transplantation

Liver transplantation has improved the survival of patients with primary biliary cirrhosis and liver failure. It is the treatment of choice in patients with symptomatic advanced liver disease. One-year survival after liver transplantation is 85–90% at most transplant centers. The survival thereafter resembles that of a control population matched for age and sex. One question is whether primary biliary cirrhosis will occur in the transplanted livers. In one report, 5 of 60 patients had minor histological lesions on liver biopsy which resembled early primary biliary cirrhosis. However, these patients were clinically asymptomatic and had normal liver function tests. There are close histological similarities between patients with primary biliary cirrhosis and those with rejection of transplanted livers. As a result, histology is difficult to evaluate. A clinicopathological study in long-term survivors showed that clinically important primary biliary cirrhosis does not recur if appropriate immunosuppression is used.

CONCLUSIONS

Progress has been made in our efforts to treat primary biliary cirrhosis. The guidelines for specific therapy are rapidly evolving and still unresolved. Primary biliary cirrhosis is a progressive disease in most patients. When cirrhosis and portal hypertension develop, the disease is irreversible and therefore untreatable. Treatment with ursodeoxycholic acid, colchicine, and methotrexate along has been moderately effective and safe. Treatment with these drugs is better than no treatment, with the eventual development of liver failure and the need for liver transplantation. A combination of these agents may be more effective than treatment with only one. Studies employing multidrug therapy are currently in progress.

REFERENCES

Buscher HP, Zietzchmann Y, Gerok W. Positive responses to methotrexate and ursodeoxycholic acid in patients with primary biliary cirrhosis responding insufficiently to ursodeoxycholic acid. J Hepatol 1993; 18:9–14.

Combes B, Carithers RL, Jr., Maddrey WC, Lin D, McDonald MF, Wheeler DE, Eigenbrodt EH, Munoz SJ, Rubin R, Garcia-Tsao G, Bonner GF, West AB, Boyer JL, Luketic VA, Schiffman ML, Mills AS, Peters MG, White HM, Zetterman RK, Rossi SS, Hofmann AF, Markin RS. A randomized, double-blind, placebo-controlled trial of ursodeoxycholic acid in primary biliary cirrhosis. Hepatology 1995; 22:759–766.

Heathcote EJ, Cauch-Dudek K, Walker V, Bailey RJ, Blendis LM, Ghent CN, Michieletti P, Minuk GY, Pappas SC, Scully LJ, Steinbrecher UP, Sutherland LR, Williams CN, Witt-Sullivan H, Worobetz LJ, Milner RA, Wanless IR. The Canadian multicenter double-blind randomized controlled trial of ursodeoxycholic acid in primary biliary cirrhosis. Hepatology 1994; 19:1149–1156.

Kaplan MM. Primary biliary cirrhosis. N Engl J Med 1996; 335:1570–1580.

Kaplan MM, DeLellis RA, Wolfe HJ. Sustained biochemical and histological remission of primary biliary cirrhosis in response to medical treatment. Ann Intern Med 1997; 126:682–688.

Kaplan MM, Alling DW, Zimmerman HJ, Wolfe HJ, Sepersky RA, Hirtsch GS, Elta GH. A prospective trial of colchicine for primary biliary cirrhosis. N Engl J Med 1986; 315:1448–1454.

Lombard M, Portmann B, Neuberger J, Williams R, Tygstrup N, Ranek L, Ring-Larsen H, Rodes J, Navasa M, Trepo C, Pape G, Schou G, Badsberg JH, Andersen PK. Cyclosporin A treatment in primary biliary cirrhosis: results of a long-term placebo controlled trial. Gastroenterology 1993; 104:519–526.

Ludwig J. New concepts in biliary cirrhosis. Semin Liver Dis 1987; 7:293–301.

Poupon RE, Poupon R, Balkau B. Ursodiol for the long-term treatment of primary biliary cirrhosis. N Engl J Med 1994; 330:1342–1347.

Shibata J, Fujiyama S, Honda Y, Sato T. Combination therapy with ursodeoxycholic acid and colchicine for primary biliary cirrhosis. J Gastroenterol Hepatol 1992; 7:277–282.

13
Management of Primary Sclerosing Cholangitis

Russell H. Wiesner
Mayo Clinic, Rochester, Minnesota

Primary sclerosing cholangitis (PSC) is a chronic cholestatic syndrome of unknown etiology, characterized by chronic cholestasis and diffuse inflammation and fibrosis, that involves the entire biliary tree. The pathological process obliterates intrahepatic and extrahepatic bile ducts, ultimately leading to biliary cirrhosis, portal hypertension, and hepatic failure. PSC may occur alone, but it is commonly (>75%) associated with inflammatory bowel disease, usually chronic ulcerative colitis (CUC). Today, PSC is among the foremost common indications for liver transplantation in adults in the United States. Approximately 70% of patients with PSC are male and the mean age at the time of diagnosis is usually under 40 years. PSC most commonly occurs in patients with previously diagnosed inflammatory bowel disease; nearly 90% of patients with PSC who have associated inflammatory bowel disease have CUC, with approximately 10% having Crohn's colitis. On the other hand, approximately 5% of patients with CUC have or will develop PSC.

SYMPTOMS AND SIGNS

PSC usually begins insidiously, which makes it difficult to determine the onset of the disease accurately. Nevertheless, most patients have had symptoms for an average of 24 months before the diagnosis is made. The gradual onset of progressive fatigue and pruritus followed by jaundice is the most frequent symptoms complex leading to the diagnosis of PSC. Clinical evidence of cholangitis (right-upper-quadrant pain associated with fever and jaundice) is uncommon unless previous bile duct reconstructive surgery has been performed. More recently, totally asymptomatic patients with PSC are being diagnosed because of abnormalities found on routine blood tests that prompt further workup, including liver biopsy and cholangiography. Although some patients with PSC may have a normal physical examination, most have some type of abnormality, most commonly hepatomegaly, jaundice, or splenomegaly.

BIOCHEMICAL TESTING

Virtually all patients with PSC have a cholestatic biochemical profile. The serum alkaline level is almost always abnormal, although it may fluctuate and, in rare instances, may even normalize. The vast majority of patients have an increase in serum aspartate aminotransferase levels, but usually to a mild degree. Approximately one-half of patients will have a modest increase in their total serum bilirubin level at the time of diagnosis. Autoantibodies—including the antimitochondrial antibody, antinuclear antibody, and anti-smooth muscle antibody—are absent in 80% of cases. Recently, we and others have described the presence of antibodies to as yet unidentified antigens present in the cytoplasm of neutrophils in approximately 70% of PSC patients. Investigators have described anti-colon and neutrophil cytoplasmic antibodies in patients with PSC alone, CUC alone, and both PSC and CUC. However, to date, no specific serological marker has been diagnostic of PSC.

Tests related to copper metabolism are virtually always abnormal in patients with PSC. For example, hepatic copper levels are elevated in approximately 90% of patients, while urine copper levels are increased in two-thirds. These copper levels are increased to the same degree seen in patients with primary biliary cirrhosis, Wilson's disease, and Indian childhood cirrhosis. Similarly, serum copper and ceruloplasmin levels are usually increased in patients with PSC, as is commonly noted in patients with primary biliary cirrhosis. These abnormalities in copper metabolism appear to be related to chronic cholestasis and do not seem to play a role in the primary pathogenesis of PSC.

RADIOLOGICAL FEATURES

Early articles, based largely on findings at surgery, emphasized the extrahepatic location of the ductal changes in PSC. Many surgeons describe the extrahepatic bile duct as a "fibrotic cord." In more recent times, however, improved cholangiographic techniques have allowed evaluation of the intrahepatic ducts, which are usually involved radiologically, often to a greater degree than the extrahepatic ducts. Endoscopic retrograde cholangiopancreatography showed diffusely distributed strictures of the intrahepatic and extrahepatic bile ducts in virtually all PSC patients. Most commonly, the strictures are short (1–2 cm long) and annular, with intervening segments of apparently normal or dilated ducts, producing the characteristic "beaded" appearance. Focal dilatation of bile ducts between strictures is also a common finding, but diffuse nonsegmented dilatation is unusual. In a minority of patients, the cholangiogram may be normal because the disease may be limited to the small intrahepatic ducts; this condition is often referred to as *small-duct PSC*.

LIVER HISTOLOGY

In virtually all patients with PSC, histological abnormalities are present on liver biopsy specimens. The characteristic features include bile duct proliferation, periductal fibrosis, periductal inflammation, duct obliteration, and eventually loss of bile ducts (ductopenia). Most commonly, the disease begins with enlargement of portal areas (stage I), characterized by edema, connective tissue and proliferation of intralobular bile ducts, and inflammatory infiltrates limited to the portal areas. With progression, tongues of inflammatory infiltrates with or without connective tissue grow into the periportal parenchyma (stage II), again, usually with mild cellular inflammation. This process leads to the formation of fibrosepta (stage III) and eventually biliary cirrhosis with ductopenia (stage IV). The pathognomic histological changes on liver biopsy specimens occur in the early stages and are characterized by fibro-obliterative cholangitis, leading to replacement of duct segments by solid cords of connective tissue and complete loss of interlobular and adjacent septal bile ducts. The finding of a fibro-obliterative bile duct lesion in the context of a patient with CUC is nearly diagnostic of PSC.

PATHOGENESIS

The cause of PSC remains unknown; however, genetic factors, acquired factors, or both may be involved (Table 1). Several recent observations are consistent with an important role for genetic factors in the pathogenesis of PSC. For example, the frequency of HLA-B8 is significantly higher in patients with PSC (60%) as compared to control subjects (25%). In addition, a familial occurrence of both PSC and CUC provide further evidence suggesting a genetic component to the disease.

Important acquired factors could theoretically include toxins, infectious agents, or altered immunity. Although elevated hepatic copper levels were initially thought to be an important potential toxin in the initiation and/or perpetuation of the disease, recent negative results from a controlled trial with D-penicillamine, which leads to decreased hepatic copper levels, make it unlikely that elevated hepatic copper levels are pathogenically important. Recently, extrahepatic biliary tract disease closely mimicking PSC has been described following infusion of the hepatic artery with chemotherapeutic agents such as 5-floxuridine. This drug apparently causes small vessel arteriopathy, which likely leads to bile duct fibrosis and destruction. This syndrome, however, represents a type of secondary sclerosing cholangitis rather than primary sclerosing cholangitis.

To date, no infectious agent has been shown to play a role in the etiopathogenesis of PSC. Results of several studies have excluded hepatitis A, B, and C as causative agents. While cytomegalovirus infection can affect both intrahepatic and extrahepatic bile ducts, serological studies have not shown a correlation between cytomegalovirus infection and PSC. In addition, the histological picture in PSC differs vastly from that of acute cytomegalovirus infection.

Reo-type 3 virus has also been associated with neonatal biliary atresia, which, like PSC, is characterized by obliterative cholangitis. However, Reo-type 3 virus infection has

Table 1 Potential Etiopathogenic Factors

Portal bacteremia
Absorbed colon toxins
Toxic bile acids
Copper toxicity
Viral infection
Genetic predisposition
Ischemic arteriolar injury
Immunological (autoimmune) mechanisms

not so far been directly linked to the development of PSC, and a preliminary report indicates that elevated antibody titers of Reo-type 3 virus are no more prevalent in patients with PSC than in the general population.

Currently, the pathogenesis of PSC is most closely linked with alteration in the immune system. Although serological markers for autoimmunity are generally absent, other data strongly support disturbed alterations in immunity. For example, PSC is associated with HLA-B8 and DR3, and there is a secondary association with DR2. Other more direct lines of evidence supporting an immunological basis include the inhibition of leukocyte migration by biliary antigens, elevated IgM levels, presence of circulating immune complexes, decreased clearance of immune complexes, and increased complement metabolism. In addition, cells involved in the destruction of bile ducts in PSC have recently been shown to be T lymphocytes, and abnormalities in lymphocyte subsets in peripheral blood have also been demonstrated. Furthermore, patients with PSC consistently experience hypergammaglobulinemia, with an increase in serum IgM, anticolon epithelial autoantibodies, perinuclear antineutrophil cytoplasmic antibodies, and associations with other autoimmune diseases, such as inflammatory bowel disease, thyroiditis, and type I diabetes. Finally, enhanced autoreactivity of suppressor/cytotoxic T lymphocytes from peripheral blood of patients with PSC has been reported. All these studies support alterations in the immune system as being pathogenically related to the development and/or perpetuation of PSC, although the exact mechanisms are not understood. It is possible that many of these immunological abnormalities are secondary manifestations of chronic cholestatic liver disease. Furthermore, recent studies reveal that smoking may be a preventive factor; however, little is known about its potential mechanism of action.

One of the major reasons for the inadequate understanding of the pathogenesis of PSC relates to inadequate models for this disease. Recently, we and others have reported on an animal model of immunological cholangitis with some features resembling both PSC and primary biliary cirrhosis. Others have described a model associated with intestinal bacterial overgrowth. It seems likely as these models are further developed and evaluated additional insights into the pathogenesis of PSC will be forthcoming.

Natural History

Based on prospective follow up of large numbers of PSC patients, there appears to be growing evidence that PSC is most often a progressive syndrome leading to significant complications related to chronic cholestasis (Fig. 1). Investigators at several institutions have published studies on the natural history of PSC, suggesting disease progression and a poor prognosis in most patients. Our own experience indicates that (1) PSC patients have a median survival of approximately 12 years from the time of diagnosis; (2) both symptomatic and asymptomatic patients have reduced survival relative to a control population based on age, sex, and race; and (3) one-third of patients with disease will die from PSC or a complication such as cholangiocarcinoma.

One of the main purposes of analyzing the natural history of PSC is to determine the rate of disease progression more accurately and to be able to estimate survival for the individual patient at any point in the course of the disease. Predicting survival based on clinical, biochemical, and histological features of PSC at any point in time is also very important for the timing of liver transplantation. Attempts to evaluate prognosis and estimate survival have applied both univariate and multivariate approaches. We first reported an

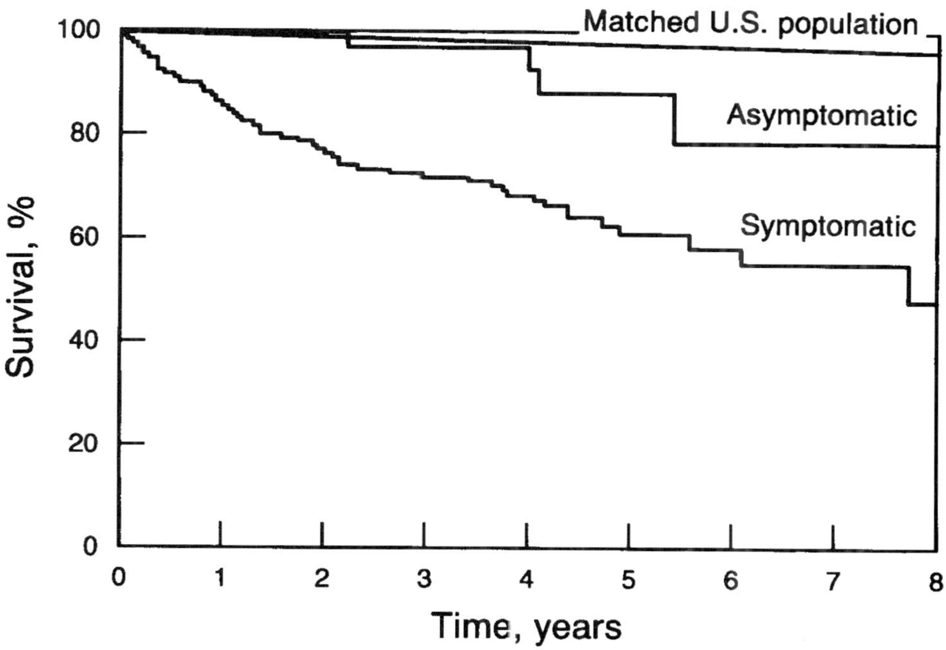

Figure 1 Kaplan-Meier estimated survival curves for asymptomatic and symptomatic patients with primary sclerosing cholangitis. For comparison, survival curves in the United States population matched for age, sex, and race to asymptomatic patients are also shown. Difference in survival: asymptomatic versus control subjects, $p < 0.001$; symptomatic versus asymptomatic patients, $p < 0.003$. (From Wiesner et al. Hepatology 1989; 10:430–436.) Reproduced with permission of W.B. Saunders Company.

association between increased hepatic and urinary copper levels and diminished survival, an example of the univariate approach. The multivariate approach, while more demanding of sophisticated statistics, most notably the Cox multiple regression analysis, is more appropriate in a disease like PSC, which has a fluctuating course. The first report using this analysis was by Helzberg et al., who found that the presence of hepatomegaly and a serum bilirubin level of >1.5 mg/dL were independent predictors of a poor prognosis in patients with PSC. More recently, we developed a prognostic model based on five independent variables in which a risk score could be calculated and translated into a survival function to estimate survival for the individual patient at any time in the course of the disease. Variables identified included age, serum bilirubin, hepatic histological stage, and splenomegaly. The need for histological data in this model was a major limiting factor; therefore, further development of the model was undertaken. The new Mayo model for PSC includes the variables of age; serum levels of bilirubin, albumin, and aspartate aminotransferase; and the presence or absence of variceal bleeding. Others have used the Child-Pugh classification with success. While these and other models do provide some objective evidence of disease severity and estimation of survival, none have been cross-validated and their general application to all PSC patients remains speculative.

MANAGEMENT OF COMPLICATIONS OF PSC

The management of complications of PSC can be divided into three categories: (1) complications of chronic cholestasis, (2) complications of decompensated cirrhosis and portal hypertension, and (3) treatment of specific complications of PSC.

Chronic Cholestasis

Complications associated with chronic cholestatic liver disease include fatigue, pruritus, steatorrhea, and deficiencies of fat-soluble vitamins and their consequences (Table 2). Fatigue, although a nonspecific symptom, is a frequent complaint of patients with PSC. Fatigue of notable severity can be present early in the course of the disease and parallels the progression of liver disease. Little is known about what causes fatigue in cholestatic liver disease; thus, no specific therapy is available to treat this symptom. It can, however, on rare occasions contribute to a marked decreased quality of life and can be an indication for liver transplantation alone in rare instances.

Pruritus, another common and often debilitating symptom of PSC, can lead to severe excoriations and diminished quality of life. The etiology of this condition remains unknown. The effects of retained bile acids in the skin or in hepatocytes have been incriminated in the pathogenesis of pruritus, but the evidence is inconsistent. Several observations support the contention that an opiate agonist pathway stimulating central opiate receptors may be involved. Patients with chronic cholestasis may have increased plasma levels of endogenous opiate peptides and may react to opiate antagonists, causing opiate withdrawal symptoms. Exogenous opiate agonists are known to induce pruritus, which can be treated with the opiate antagonist naloxone. The severity of pruritus does not tend to parallel disease progression in PSC.

Various therapies may be helpful in treating pruritus in patients with PSC. These include the use of cholestyramine, phenobarbital, ursodeoxycholic acid, antihistamines, rifampin, plasmapheresis, charcoal hemoperfusion, ultraviolet light, and even liver transplantation in severe cases (see Chap. 34). Recently, opiate receptor antagonists have shown the most promise in controlling cholestatic pruritus. Rifampin has also been helpful in a number of patients who have failed cholestyramine therapy.

Steatorrhea associated with fat-soluble vitamin deficiency has also been described in patients with PSC. As in primary biliary cirrhosis, fat malabsorption in PSC is probably related to diminished intestinal concentrations of bile acids. Steatorrhea in PSC, however,

Table 2 Treatment for Complication of Cholestasis

Pruritis	Steatorrhea and fat-soluble vitamin deficiency	Osteoporosis
Cholestyramine	Low-fat diet	Calcium
Naloxone (opiate antagonists)	Medium-chain triglycerides	Vitamin D
Rifampicin	Elemental diet	Estrogen (females)
Phenobarbital	Vitamins A, D, E, and K supplements	Bisphosphonates
Plasmapheresis		Fluoride
Phototherapy		

can be caused by concurrent chronic pancreatitis, celiac disease, or both, which should be considered in the differential diagnosis, particularly if steatorrhea occurs in a PSC patient who is not jaundiced and has early histological stage disease on liver biopsy.

Recent studies have shown that PSC patients frequently develop fat-soluble vitamin deficiency. Vitamin A deficiency was found in approximately 40% of patients, and deficiencies in vitamins D and E were reported in 14 and 2%, respectively. Fat-soluble vitamin deficiencies seem to parallel disease progression and are most prominent in PSC patients with cirrhosis who are undergoing liver transplantation evaluations.

Metabolic bone disease associated with compression fractures of the spine has also been shown to occur with increased frequency in PSC patients. Bone biopsies reveal that osteoporosis, rather than osteomalacia, is the most common form of bone disease in patients with PSC. It also appears that corticosteroid therapy exacerbates bone disease associated with PSC and should be avoided or used with caution only in controlled clinical trials.

Finally, vitamin K deficiency related to malabsorption of vitamin K from the gastrointestinal tract or to severe hepatic parenchymal damage can occur in PSC. A trial of parenteral vitamin K is reasonable to attempt to correct a prolonged prothrombin time. If this prolonged prothrombin time is related to vitamin K malabsorption, a marked improvement in prothrombin time is noted within 2 days. If the prolonged prothrombin time is related to severe hepatic parenchymal damage, vitamin K therapy will have no effect.

Decompensated Cirrhosis and Portal Hypertension

The end-stages of PSC are associated with complications of portal hypertension, such as esophageal variceal bleeding, ascites, spontaneous bacterial peritonitis, and hepatic encephalopathy (Table 3). As in other forms of chronic liver disease, esophageal variceal bleeding is best managed by variceal band ligation or sclerotherapy. Another option to obliterate varices is the creation of a transvenous intrahepatic portosystemic shunt. If possible, surgical shunting procedures should not be performed to avoid the risks associated with a subsequent liver transplantation if indicated. Ascites is best treated with large volume paracentesis and diuretic therapy. Administration of albumin should be considered in patients who have serum albumin levels below 2.8.

In PSC, spontaneous bacterial peritonitis is a complication often related to biliary sepsis and cholangitis. In this situation, the use of oral selective bowel decontamination solution or chronic antibiotic therapy would be especially appropriate to prevent recurrence of this severe life-threatening complication.

Table 3 Management for Complications of Portal Hypertension

Esophageal variceal bleeding	Bacterial peritonitis
Beta blockers, nitrates	Antibiotics (prophylactic and therapeutic)
Banding, sclerotherapy	Hepatic encephalopathy
Transjugular intrahepatic portosystemic shunt	Lactulose
Ascites	Dietary protein restriction
Sodium restriction	Neomycin
Large-volume paracentesis	Peristomal varices
Diuretics	Transjugular intrahepatic portosystemic shunt

Treatment of Specific Complications of PSC

Complications specific to PSC include (1) gallbladder and biliary stones, (2) dominant bile duct strictures and recurrent bacterial cholangitis, (3) cholangiocarcinoma, and (4) peristomal varices (Table 4).

Cholelithiasis and choledocholithiasis occur in up to 30% of patients with PSC. Chronic cholestasis predisposes patients to the formation of cholesterol gallstones, and bacterial cholangitis predisposes patients to the formation of pigment stones. Indeed, if patients with PSC who have intact gallbladders are surveyed by ultrasonography, gallstones will be found in between 25 and 30%. Because most of these patients are young men, this high incidence of gallstone disease probably represents an increased frequency of cholelithiasis in PSC patients. We have shown that choledocholithiasis can cause bacterial cholangitis as a complication of PSC. This diagnosis can be extremely difficult in patients with PSC, since bacterial cholangitis may occur in the absence of biliary stones. A cholangiogram to exclude choledocholithiasis superimposed on PSC should be considered, particularly in patients who have not had biliary surgery and who have recently experienced the onset of one or more episodes of bacterial cholangitis or who have recently become jaundiced.

In PSC, a dominant stricture of the biliary tract develops in between 15 and 20% of patients at some time during the course of the disease. These high-grade strictures most often occur at the biliary hilus, but they also can occur in the common bile duct and the common hepatic duct. This complication typically is associated with the onset of jaundice, pruritus, and fever related to bacterial cholangitis. If a patient with PSC should develop these clinical symptoms, cholangiography should be performed. If a dominant stricture is found, cytological studies should be performed to exclude cholangiocarcinoma and balloon dilatation should be performed by either a transhepatic or endoscopic retrograde approach, depending on the location of the stricture and the expertise available at the institution. Balloon dilatation of dominant strictures with removal of biliary sludge in patients with PSC can be quite effective in alleviating jaundice and pruritus as well as in decreasing the frequency and severity of bacterial cholangitis. These procedures appear to be most effective in patients whose symptoms are of recent onset and less effective in those with long-standing jaundice or those who have experienced recurrent episodes of bacterial cholangitis. Results of dilatation of dominant strictures frequently depend on the severity of stricturing and disease obstruction of the intrahepatic bile ducts. Patients with PSC and

Table 4 Treatment for Complications Specific to Primary Sclerosing Cholangitis

Gallbladder and biliary stones
Cholecystectomy
Endoscopic retrograde cholangiopancreatography (sphincterotomy/biliary flushing)
Dominant stricture
Balloon dilatation
Surgery (biliary resection)
Cholangiocarcinoma
No effective therapy
Experimental protocols
Peristomal varices
Transjugular intrahepatic portosystemic shunt

severe intrahepatic disease benefit less from balloon dilatation of a dominant stricture of the common bile duct compared to those who have only minimal changes involving the intrahepatic biliary system.

Approximately 50% of patients with PSC who undergo balloon dilatation of dominant strictures have improvement in symptoms for up to 2 years. About one-third of patients will require repeat balloon dilatation for recurrent stricturing. In recent studies, stenting of the strictured area has been associated with improvement of biochemical liver tests; 57% of patients remained asymptomatic with a median follow up of 29 months. However, early postprocedure–related complications occurred in one-third of patients, of which bacterial cholangitis was the most common.

Another approach to the dominant stricture in PSC is direct surgical intervention. Because most dominant strictures can be dilated using either a radiological or endoscopic approach, our opinion has been that surgical intervention should be avoided because of an increased risk of bacterial cholangitis and the potential for causing technical difficulties if a liver transplant is indicated at a later time. However, a recent study has suggested that carefully selected noncirrhotic patients with PSC may benefit from biliary resection and long-term stenting; such a surgical procedure may diminish the risk for developing cholangiocarcinoma. These findings are in need of confirmation by other investigators.

Bacterial cholangitis is an unusual presenting symptom in patients with PSC but commonly occurs in patients who have undergone biliary surgery or in whom an obstructing dominant stricture of the large bile ducts has developed. Episodes of bacterial cholangitis are best treated with broad-spectrum antibiotics, and many patients appear to benefit from prophylactic antibiotic therapy to prevent recurrent bouts of cholangitis. We presently use ciprofloxacin for prophylaxis of bacterial cholangitis because it achieves high biliary concentrations and has a broad spectrum of action against both gram-positive and gram-negative aerobic bacteria. The ability of long-term ciprofloxacin therapy to reduce the frequency and severity of bacterial cholangitis remains to be studied at this time.

It is now established that cholangiocarcinoma may develop during the course of the disease in up to 30% of patients with PSC. The patients who appear to be at the highest risk for development of cholangiocarcinoma are those with long-standing CUC and cirrhotic-stage PSC on liver biopsy. Indeed, we consider PSC to be a premalignant condition of the biliary tree, just as CUC is a premalignant condition of the colon. Bile duct carcinoma has been difficult to diagnose early in the setting of PSC, since there are no diagnostic serological markers and biliary cytology has been insensitive for the early diagnosis of cholangiocarcinoma. The difficulty in making the diagnosis of cholangiocarcinoma in PSC is supported by a report from the University of Pittsburgh, in which 10% of patients with PSC undergoing liver transplantation were found to have an unsuspected cholangiocarcinoma. Recent efforts have focused on the identification of serum and biliary markers for the early detection of cholangiocarcinoma. In one study, the serum glycoprotein CA 19-9 was found to be 89% sensitive and 86% specific for detecting cholangiocarcinoma when present in PSC patients. Another study involving 74 patients revealed that an index combining two serum markers (CA 19-9 and CEA) provided an accuracy of 86% in the diagnosis of cholangiocarcinoma.

Recently, a study from our institution showed that human cholangiocarcinoma expressed somatostatin receptors and responded in vitro to somatostatin and its analogue with growth inhibition. The data suggest the use of somatostatin or its analogue as a potential clinical tool for the localization and treatment of cholangiocarcinoma. In another report, the overexpression of p53 protein in cholangiocarcinoma tissue from PSC was demonstrated. However, none of these techniques have been shown to detect cholangiocarcinoma at its earliest stages and thus are less valuable for screening patients with PSC for the development of cholangiocarcinoma.

Operative management, chemotherapy, and radiation therapy have not been shown to be useful in treating cholangiocarcinoma (see Chap. 23). In patients with PSC and concomitant cholangiocarcinoma undergoing liver transplantation, recurrence of bile duct carcinoma has almost been universal. Hoping for a better outcome in these patients, experimental protocols combining radiation therapy and chemotherapy (5-fluorouracil) before orthotopic liver transplantation are currently being studied.

A special complication of portal hypertension in PSC is the development and bleeding from peristomal varices in patients who have undergone proctocolectomy for underlying CUC and who have an ileal stoma. Bleeding from peristomal varices can be severe, and local measures to control bleeding, including ileostomy revision and local injection of sclerosants, are usually unsuccessful. Peristomal variceal bleeding can be controlled by surgical shunt and by transjugular intrahepatic portosystemic shunt procedure. The surgical shunt procedure should be avoided in potential liver transplant candidates because of the long waiting times to receive a donor liver. However, the transjugular intrahepatic portosystemic shunt procedure appears to be the best alternative in those patients in whom severe peristomal bleeding occurs.

PRIMARY THERAPY FOR PSC

Primary therapy for PSC can be subdivided into medical, radiological (see above), and surgical approaches (Table 5).

Medical Therapy

Over the last 20 years, various medical treatments have been used in PSC patients with the hope of improving the natural history of the hepatobiliary disease and improving survival.

Table 5 Treatment Aimed at Retarding Disease Progression

Medical	Radiological
1. Cupruretic	1. Cholangioplasty
D-Penicillamine	2. Biliary infusion therapy
2. Immunosuppressive	Surgical
Prednisone	1. Reconstructive biliary surgery
Azathioprine	2. Proctocolectomy
Cyclosporine	3. Liver transplantation
Methotrexate	
Tacrolimus	
3. Antifibrotic	
Colchicine	
4. Choleretic	
Ursodeoxycholic acid	

The diversity of medical therapies includes the use of cupruretic, immunosuppressive, antifibrogenic, and choleretic agents, which suggests their ineffectiveness and reveals a lack of complete understanding of the etiopathogenesis of the disease.

Cupruretic Therapy

The evidence of increased hepatic copper in PSC provided the main rationale for evaluating D-penicillamine as a therapeutic agent for PSC. In a prospective randomized, double-blind, placebo-controlled trial, D-penicillamine had no favorable effect on PSC progression and patient survival. This was determined after 36 months of follow-up based on careful analysis of clinical and biochemical profiles, radiological findings, liver histology, and survival data between the two groups of PSC patients. Furthermore, major adverse effects of D-penicillamine, including proteinuria and thrombocytopenia, led to the discontinuation of the drug in 20% of treated patients.

Immunosuppressive Therapy

The use of immunosuppressive agents in the therapy of PSC was based on the concept that PSC is an autoimmune disease. In uncontrolled observations, oral corticosteroids have been shown to improve the biochemical profile in PSC patients; however, long-term or controlled studies of corticosteroids are lacking. In a small controlled study in PSC patients, topical corticosteroid application in the biliary tree via nasobiliary lavage provided no advantage over placebo. Other immunosuppressive agents that have been employed in the treatment of PSC include (1) azathioprine the experience has been mostly anecdotal; (2) cyclosporine: the results were negative; (3) methotrexate: in a randomized, double-blind, placebo-controlled trial, showed no benefit in the treatment group; and (4) tacrolimus: a small open-label study showed only improvement in liver enzymes leading to the conclusion that further studies are needed to define the immunosuppressive effects in PSC patients. In addition, an open trial of prednisone and colchicine in PSC patients demonstrated no benefit on progression of hepatic histology and liver biochemical tests over a 2-year period. A pilot study combining ursodeoxycholic acid and methotrexate for the treatment of PSC was associated with toxicity and without improvement in liver function tests compared with ursodeoxycholic acid therapy alone.

Antifibrotic Therapy

Because PSC leads to liver cirrhosis, antifibrotic agents such as colchicine were suggested as therapeutic options for PSC. Recently, in a prospective, double-blind study, 84 PSC patients were randomized to received 1 mg of colchicine versus placebo daily for a period of 3 years. The results of the multicenter study revealed that colchicine had no beneficial effect on patient symptoms, liver biochemistry, hepatic histology, or survival.

Choleretic Therapy

The enthusiasm for the use of ursodeoxycholic acid, a hydrophilic bile acid, in the treatment of PSC emerged from favorable data on its use for primary biliary cirrhosis and from promising clinical and biochemical improvement reported in PSC patients receiving ursodeoxycholic acid in small uncontrolled studies. Subsequently, a small prospective, randomized, double-blind, placebo-controlled trial was performed to further examine the efficacy of ursodeoxycholic acid. These authors conclude that PSC patients treated with ursodeoxycholic acid at 13–15 mg/kg/day for 1 year demonstrated marked improvement in serum liver tests and histology on liver biopsy. The proposed benefit of orally administered ursodeoxycholic acid in cholestatic patients is thought to be related to (1) its accumulation in the endogenous bile pool, which leads to replacement of endogenous potentially toxic bile acids in the cholestatic liver; (2) its protective effect at the cellular and subcellular levels of the hepatocyte and cholangiocyte; (3) its hypercholeretic activity; and (4) its immunomodulatory effect.

In the recently published largest randomized, double-blind, placebo-controlled trial of ursodeoxycholic acid treatment for PSC, however, no clinical benefit was found. The study included 105 patients with well-established PSC given ursodeoxycholic acid 13–15 mg/kg/day compared with placebo. The mean follow up was 2.2 years. In this study, ursodeoxycholic acid, but not placebo, demonstrated improvement in liver function tests at 1 and 2 years of treatment. Nevertheless, the primary outcome (time to treatment failure), as defined by the authors, and survival were not significantly different in the two groups of PSC patients (Fig. 2). In another randomized, controlled study involving 59 PSC patients treated for 2 years with either ursodeoxycholic acid (300 mg twice a day) or colchicine (0.6 mg twice a day), the outcome was not better in the treated group than in the untreated control group.

Summary of Medical Therapy

To date, effective pharmacological treatment for the underlying hepatobiliary disease in PSC is lacking. The data do not support use of any mentioned agent except in the context of well-designed experimental studies. Future therapeutic trials for PSC must be centered

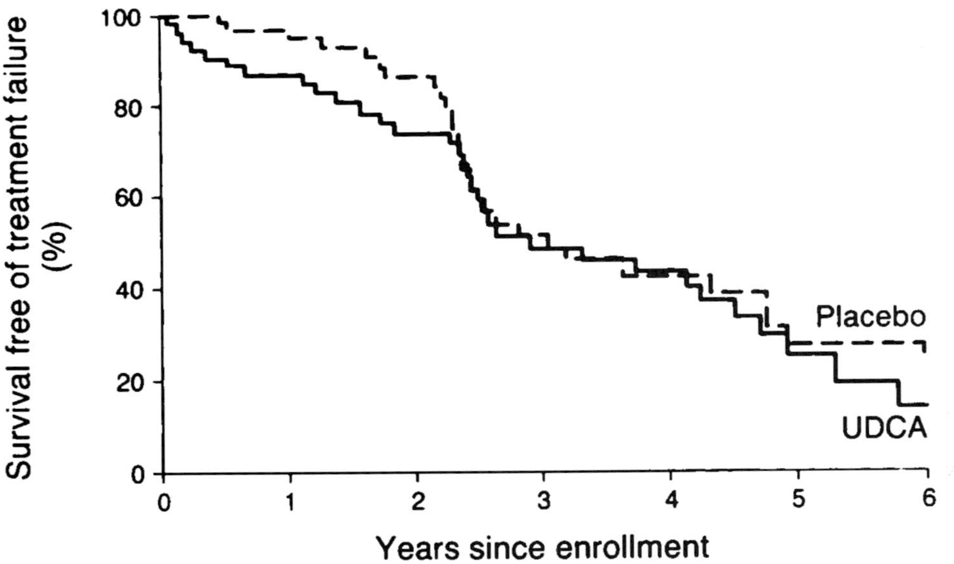

Figure 2 Kaplan-Meier analysis of survival free of treatment failure among study patients. Treatment failure was defined as one or more of the following: (1) death, (2) liver transplantation, (3) histologic progression by two stages, (4) progression to cirrhosis, (5) development of esophageal varices, (6) development of ascites or encephalopathy, (7) sustained quadrupling of the serum bilirubin concentration, (8) marked worsening of fatigue or pruritus, (9) inability to tolerate the drug, (10) voluntary withdrawal from the study. (Lindor KD. N Engl J Med 1997; 336:691–695.) Reproduced with permission of The New England Journal of Medicine.

on the asymptomatic patient, because when ductopenia occurs, the disease appears to be irreversible, since bile duct epithelial cells are unable to regenerate.

Surgical Therapy

Until the advent of liver transplantation, surgical therapy for PSC was focused on alleviation of pruritus and jaundice, excluding cholangiocarcinoma, and prevention of colonic adenocarcinoma by performing a proctocolectomy in patients with concurrent PSC and CUC.

Biliary Surgery

Since PSC is a progressive disease, biliary surgery was introduced primarily to improve symptoms. Biliary enteric anastomoses with biliary stenting and reconstruction of the hepatic duct bifurcation with long-term transhepatic stents have been performed. In two retrospective studies evaluating biliary tract reconstructive surgery, the cirrhotic group of PSC patients showed a significantly higher mortality rate compared to the noncirrhotic group. Thus, it is now widely accepted that biliary surgery should be avoided in PSC patients with cirrhosis or severe, diffuse intrahepatic disease. Instead, these patients should be considered for liver transplantation.

Although biliary reconstruction may benefit noncirrhotic PSC patients with extrahepatic disease, the lack of prospective, controlled data makes it impossible to assess the long-term effects of this procedure on the natural history of PSC and the subsequent risk of developing cholangiocarcinoma. In our view, the value of biliary surgery is limited to select PSC patients without cirrhosis who are not candidates for liver transplantation when extrahepatic dominant strictures are not amenable to endoscopic or transhepatic dilatation.

Proctocolectomy

In patients with both PSC and CUC, proctocolectomy is frequently performed due to indications relevant to inflammatory bowel disease. The possible effect of proctocolectomy on the natural history of PSC was examined in a retrospective analysis involving 45 patients with coexisting PSC and CUC, where almost half had undergone proctocolectomy and the rest had not. This study revealed that the clinical signs, biochemical profile, histological progression on liver biopsy, and survival were not different in the two groups. Moreover, the fact that PSC can occur years after proctocolectomy argues against any beneficial effect of this procedure on the progression of PSC. Nonetheless, patients with both PSC and CUC remain at high risk for the development of adenocarcinoma of the colon; thus, an annual surveillance colonoscopy is strongly indicated, particularly in patients with PSC who have undergone liver transplantation. Proctocolectomy should be performed for intractable symptoms of inflammatory bowel disease not amenable to medical treatment and for colonic dysplasia and malignancy. In patients with PSC and CUC, if proctocolectomy is indicated, an ileal pouch anal anastomosis is the procedure of choice, since this procedure prevents the development of peristomal varices. Of note, a complication of the ileal pouch anal anastomosis is pouchitis, a nonspecific inflammation of the ileal reservoir that occurs more frequently in patients with coexisting PSC and CUC than in those with CUC alone. Frequently, treatment with metronidazole (Flagyl) or other antibiotics will effectively control this condition.

Orthotopic Liver Transplantation

Currently, the only suitable lifesaving treatment for patients with end-stage PSC is orthotopic liver transplantation. The initially reported data for the outcome of liver transplantation for PSC were disappointing. However, during the last decade, the outcome of liver transplantation in PSC patients with end-stage disease has improved significantly, and liver transplantation has emerged as the treatment of choice for these patients. Indeed, retrospective analysis of PSC patients using the Mayo PSC natural history model has shown that liver transplantation significantly improve the survival rate at all risk stratifications compared with the estimated survival and the absence of liver transplantation. Recently, the 1- and 5-year patient survival after liver transplantation for PSC has been reported to be between 90 and 97% and 85 and 88%, respectively.

Based on independent studies of patients with end-stage PSC from three major liver transplant centers, one of the major clinical challenges is selecting the ideal time for liver transplantation. It is known that patients with high Mayo PSC risk scores have an increased risk of death after orthotopic liver transplantation compared with patients with low Mayo risk scores. In addition, risk factors specific to PSC that affect the outcome of liver transplantation have been recognized. Recently, a prognostic model to predict the post–liver transplant morbidity in PSC and primary biliary cirrhosis has been described. In PSC patients, the guidelines for liver transplantation should include intractability of symptoms, signs, and complications of portal hypertension. However, careful consideration of each patient's needs and quality of life remain important in this disease.

Despite a favorable outcome, liver transplantation for PSC is associated with specific complications. In PSC patients, post–liver transplant complications include an increased incidence of acute and chronic rejection, frequently leading to graft loss, biliary strictures and leakage, hepatic artery thrombosis, and lymphoproliferative disease. The recurrence of PSC after liver transplantation has been controversial, primarily due to the lack of "gold standard" criteria for the diagnosis of recurrent PSC. Recently, a cohort of PSC patients from the Mayo Clinic were evaluated for recurrent disease based on biochemical, cholangiographic, and histological criteria as well as the timing rof the event. In these patients, with a mean follow up of 55 months, 20% were found to have evidence of recurrent disease following liver transplantation. A number of these patients have required retransplantation, and the impact of the recurrence of PSC is yet to be determined.

It is also important to point out that in patients with concurrent PSC and CUC, liver transplantation and immunosuppressive therapy do not appear to affect the natural history of CUC, and the development of colorectal adenocarcinoma after liver transplantation continues to be a major risk. Thus, PSC patients who have undergone liver transplantation should continue to have annual surveillance colonoscopies for detection of colonic dysplasia and carcinoma and must undergo total proctocolectomy if these findings are identified.

SUMMARY AND CONCLUSION

PSC is a chronic cholestatic disease of unknown cause characterized by progressive inflammation and fibrosis of the entire biliary tree. PSC affects primarily young men and displays a strong association with CUC. The hallmark of diagnosis is cholangiography; however, the presence of the obliterative duct lesion on liver biopsy is nearly diagnostic. The most serious complications of PSC are bile duct and colon adenocarcinoma in patients with concurrent PSC and CUC. Annual surveillance colonoscopy for the detection of early-stage colon cancer is strongly indicated. To date, medical therapy has been totally ineffective in altering the natural history of disease; the only effective treatment is orthotopic liver transplantation. Future treatment strategies will rely heavily on defining the etiopathogenesis of the disease.

BIBLIOGRAPHY

Ahrondt SA, Pitt HA, Kallou AN, et al. Primary sclerosing cholangitis: resect, dilate, or transplant? Ann Surg 1998; 227:412–423.

Bergasa NV, Jones EP. The pruritus of cholestasis. Semin Liver Dis 1993; 13:319–327.

Bergquist A, Glauman H, Persson B, et al. Risk factors and clinical presentation of hepatobiliary carcinoma in patients with primary sclerosing cholangitis: a case-control study. Hepatology 1998; 27:311–316.

Hay JE, Lindor KD, Wiesner RH. Metabolic bone disease in primary sclerosing cholangitis. Hepatology 1991; 14:257–261.

Jorgenson RA, Lindor KD, Wiesner RH, et al. Serum lipid and fat-soluble vitamin levels in primary sclerosing cholangitis. J Clin Gastroenterol 1995; 20:215–219.

Knox TA, Kaplan MM. A double-blind controlled trial of oral pulse methotrexate therapy in the treatment of primary sclerosing cholangitis. Gastroenterology 1994; 106:494–499.

Lee YM, Kaplan MM. Primary sclerosing cholangitis. N Engl J Med 1995; 332:924–933.

Loftus EV Jr, Aguilar H, Sandborn WJ, et al. Risk of colorectal neoplasia in patients with primary sclerosing cholangitis and ulcerative colitis following liver transplantation. Hepatology 1998; 27:685–690.

Loftus EV Jr, Sandborn WJ, Tremaine WJ, et al. Primary sclerosing cholangitis is associated with nonsmoking: a case control study. Gastroenterology 1996; 11:1658–1662.

Mayo PSC Study Group. Ursodiol for primary sclerosing cholangitis. N Engl J Med 1997; 336: 691–695.

Narumi S, Roberts JP, Emond JC, et al. Liver transplantation for sclerosing cholangitis. Hepatology 1995; 22:451–457.

Olsson R, Broome U, Danielson A, et al. Colchicine treatment for primary sclerosing cholangitis. Gastroenterology 1995; 108:1199–1203.

Rosen CA, Nagorney DM, Wiesner RH, et al. Cholangiocarcinoma complicating primary sclerosing cholangitis. Ann Surg 1991; 213:21–25.

Wiesner RH. Primary sclerosing cholangitis. In: Schiff L, Schiff ER, eds. Diseases of the Liver, 7th ed. Philadelphia: Lippincott, 1993:411–426.

Wiesner RH. Current concepts in primary sclerosing cholangitis. Mayo Clinic Proc 1994; 69: 969–982.

Wiesner RH. Etiopathogenesis of primary sclerosing cholangitis. In: Gentilini P, Arias IM, McIntyre N, Rodes J, eds. Cholestasis. Amsterdam: Excerpta Medica, 1994:153–160.

Wiesner RH, Grambsch PM, Dickson ER, et al. Primary sclerosing cholangitis: natural history, prognostic factors, and survival analysis. Hepatology 1989; 10:430–436.

Wiesner RH, Porayko MK, Hay JE, et al. Liver transplantation for primary sclerosing cholangitis: impact of risk factors on outcome. Liver Transplant Surg 1996; 5(suppl):99–108.

14
Management of Overlap Syndromes

Martin Black
Temple University Hospital, Philadelphia, Pennsylvania

Thomas D. Schiano
University of Chicago Hospitals, Chicago, Illinois

INTRODUCTION

Autoimmune liver diseases are differentiated on the basis of particular clinical, serological, biochemical, and histological hallmarks. Specific diagnoses are based on particular combinations of these features, though no specific immunoserological finding or laboratory pattern is pathognomonic of any one autoimmune liver disease. The occurrence of shared clinical and histopathological features in these disorders has fueled speculation that these disease processes may represent different manifestations of a single autoimmune disorder. Definitive diagnosis is difficult at times, since the course of autoimmune liver disease is variable, both in terms of progression and potential change in pattern of disease. In addition, the autoantibodies that accompany these disorders are diverse and can occur in various combinations, thus further obscuring the diagnosis. The term *overlap syndrome* initially was introduced into clinical hepatology to describe patients with features of both primary biliary cirrhosis (PBC) and autoimmune hepatitis (AIH). An expanded definition would make the term applicable to a greater number of patients with liver disease in whom a specific diagnosis is difficult to establish or in whom the pattern of disease appears to change with time.

Various overlap syndromes have been described, including hepatitis C-AIH, PBC-AIH, autoimmune cholangitis, and primary sclerosing cholangitis (PSC)-AIH. Since these overlap syndromes occur infrequently, much of the experience in their management and treatment has been gathered through case series involving small numbers of patients. For this reason, many of these syndromes remain obscure or not well characterized, and information on optimal treatment is modest at best. This chapter provides background into the diagnosis and management of overlap syndromes.

Autoimmune Hepatitis and Its Subtypes

AIH classically affects a variably symptomatic patient (often with arthralgias, fatigue, menstrual irregularity, etc.), abnormal liver biochemistries (increased serum bilirubin, moderately increased alkaline phosphatase, aminotransferases in the 300–600 IU/L range), hypergammaglobulinemia (e.g., greater than 2.5 g/dL) and positive antinuclear (ANA) and/or smooth muscle antibodies (SMA) with titers in excess of 1:640. However, an enlarged spectrum of AIH (sometimes referred to as the autoimmune chronic hepatitis variants) (see Fig. 1), includes patients without positive ANA or SMA, some with positive anti-LKM (liver/kidney microsomal) antibody, and some with positive soluble liver antibody (SLA). Although these subtypes of AIH serve to group patients into a more logical format, they do not appear to signify important etiological differences and do not influence approaches to therapy. Administration of prednisone with or without azathioprine is the cornerstone of therapy. Those who fail to achieve substantial remission on steroids do not appear to represent a pretreatment-identifiable subgroup.

Primary Biliary Cirrhosis—Autoimmune Hepatitis

PBC is usually easily distinguished from AIH since each disorder has characteristic laboratory and immunoserological profiles with distinctly different liver histopathology. Clinical

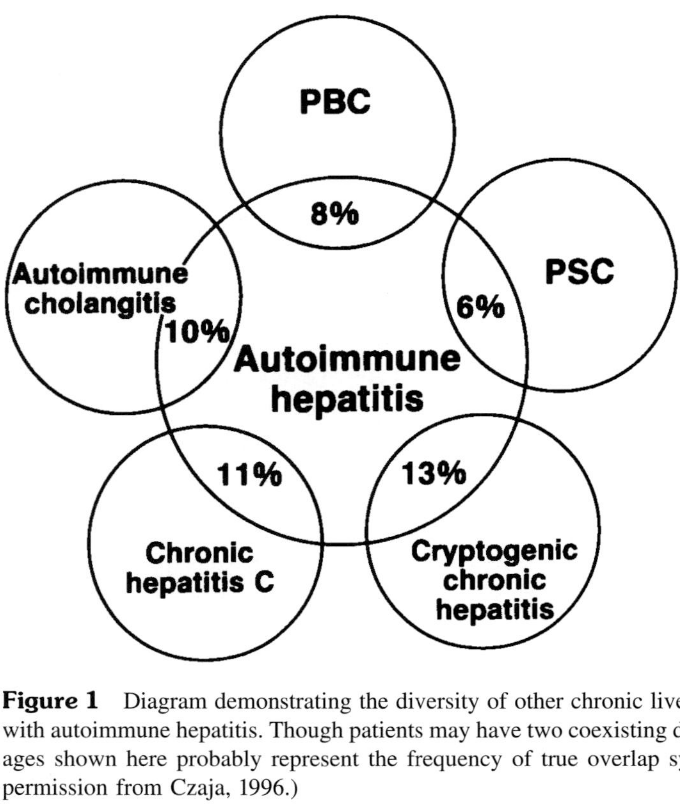

Figure 1 Diagram demonstrating the diversity of other chronic liver diseases that share features with autoimmune hepatitis. Though patients may have two coexisting disease processes, the percentages shown here probably represent the frequency of true overlap syndromes. (Reproduced with permission from Czaja, 1996.)

and biochemical features of cholestasis are present in many patients with AIH but predominate in less than 10%. When appreciable cholestasis is present, patients may represent true overlap syndromes of AIH and PBC. Autoimmune cholangitis, the recently described syndrome, may be part of this spectrum of PBC or may represent a separate disorder.

Antimitochondrial antibodies (AMA) are found in 95% of PBC cases but may be found in up to 20% of patients with AIH, mostly at a titer of 1:160 or less. Low-titer AMA may also be present as a background epiphenomenon in a variety of other autoimmune diseases. Surveys of antibodies to M_2 autoantigens (a more specific finding in PBC) have shown that no more than 8% of patients with AIH have antibodies to the E2 subunits of the pyruvate dehydrogenase complex; these may, in fact, be found in AMA-negative PBC. Attempts to utilize other subtypes of AMA to differentiate PBC, AIH, and "overlap syndrome" have generally proved unsuccessful. In addition, false-positive AMA may also occur; AMA may be confused with antibodies to liver/kidney microsome type I (anti-LKM-1) on indirect immunofluorescence. ANA is detected in 24–31% of patients with PBC. IgM and IgG may be elevated in both AIH and PBC, but IgG tends to be higher in the former and IgM in the latter. Kenny et al. found 20% of 187 patients with AIH to have AMA, 88% with a titer $\leq$ 1:40, when compared with a group of patients with liver biopsies typical of PBC. Liver histopathology differentiated PBC from AMA-positive autoimmune hepatitis in 91% of cases. AMA levels $\geq$ 1:160, IgM concentrations $\geq$ 6.0 mg/mL, $\geq$ 4-fold elevations of alkaline phosphatase, and serum cholesterol $\geq$ 300 mg/dL were laboratory features that separated the disorders in 92% of cases. Though PBC and AIH typically have quite different clinical presentations, clinical features are often not helpful in alerting the clinician to the possibility of an overlap syndrome.

Though liver histopathology can often differentiate PBC from AIH, similar features may be found in both disorders—i.e., the florid duct lesion of PBC is occasionally seen in AIH and eosinophilic portal tract inflammation may frequently be seen in early-stage PBC. Abnormal bile duct epithelium may be found in 30–40% of patients with AIH. The true overlap syndromes that have been described have shown highly active periportal inflammation in association with considerable bile duct damage. Interlobular bile ducts are often infiltrated and surrounded by variable mixtures of polymorphonuclear leukocytes, eosinophils, lymphocytes, and plasma cells. The ducts themselves are injured and there is irregularity of the epithelial cells, disruption of the basement membrane and, at times, inflammatory cells within the duct lumen. There may also be areas of bridging necrosis. Comparative analysis of bile duct lesions in patients with PBC and those with AIH with cholestatic features demonstrated that only in the former are the bile ducts actually destroyed, often by granuloma. This may not always be readily apparent because of sampling error and because nondestructive bile duct lesions are sometimes seen in AIH. Hepatic copper deposition, which is typical of cholestasis, is present in 19% of AMA-positive patients with clinical features of AIH.

A typical example of PBC-AIH overlap is an abnormal liver chemistry test profile with disproportionate cholestatic enzyme elevations or cholestasis and bile duct destruction on liver biopsy in a patient with clinical features of autoimmune hepatitis and a high titer of SMA. On physical examination, xanthelasmata (indicative of cholestasis-related hypercholesterolemia) may rarely be present. Other patients may have high-titer AMA and SMA with cholestasis, bile duct destruction or hepatocellular necrosis, with plasma cell portal inflammation on liver biopsy. Rarely, patients with PBC or AIH may develop features of the other during the course and treatment of their initially diagnosed illness. Repeat serological evaluation and liver biopsy may be necessary.

Concomitant use of certain prescription medications by a patient with autoimmune hepatitis (i.e., chlorpromazine) may confuse the histological picture, so these should be discontinued. Before consideration of a PBC-AIH overlap syndrome, appropriate evaluation to rule out other causes of chronic liver disease (i.e., viral hepatitis, PSC) should be undertaken. A full immunoserological workup—including AMA, SMA and, when available, anti-M_2 autoantigens—should be performed. Review by an experienced liver pathologist of a liver biopsy specimen (deemed to contain an adequate number of portal tracts and bile ducts) is essential. In cases where definitive diagnosis is unclear, liver biopsy is helpful if it shows a preponderance of piecemeal or bridging necrosis or granulomas and bile duct destruction. Overall, histological features appear more reliable than laboratory findings in differentiating PBC and AIH, but they may not be as clear-cut in diagnosing an overlap syndrome. A cholangiogram to rule out PSC may be necessary.

Patients with AIH and PBC-autoimmune hepatitis overlap appear to respond well to steroid therapy or therapy with cyclosporine. Geubel et al. studied 125 patients, 15 (12%) of whom had features of both AIH and PBC on liver biopsy. Treatment with prednisone and azathioprine normalized biochemical and morphological features of disease activity, including pruritus. Analysis of initial biochemical and histological findings correlated failure of response with PBC-like features. Ben-Ari et al. treated four patients that they considered to have autoimmune cholangitis (see below) having overlapping features of PBC and AIH with prednisolone. These patients were AMA- and M_2-negative with high-titer ANA, positive SMA, elevated alkaline phosphatase and gamma glutamyl transpeptidase, with liver biopsies typical of PBC but with marked cellular infiltration and bile duct damage; intralobular inflammation and piecemeal necrosis were mild. Serial liver biopsies showed decreased inflammation and cholestasis with prednisolone therapy, but the bile duct lesions persisted. The patients relapsed on lower doses of prednisolone. Other authors have used steroids and azathioprine in small numbers of patients and found them to be ineffective.

It appears that if patients have all the clinical, biochemical, and histological features of AIH in the presence of positive AMA or cholestasis, immunosuppressive therapy is indicated and, in general, is effective. Responsiveness to corticosteroids (as defined by the International Autoimmune Hepatitis Group) justifies the presumption that AIH is the predominant disease. Concurrent use of ursodeoxycholic acid or use after a failed corticosteroid trial may be warranted. The clinician should be vigilant to monitor these overlap patients for the myriad of other autoimmune illnesses that are associated with either PBC or autoimmune hepatitis (e.g., thyroid disease) and those more typical of one or the other (e.g., CREST syndrome with PBC). Appropriate management of osteoporosis, which can be accelerated with corticosteroid use is essential. In considering these patients for liver transplantation, surgeons should be aware of the possibility of PBC-AIH as they may wish to perform a Roux-en-Y bile duct anastomosis, as they do in patients with PBC and PSC.

Case History

JMK, a 40-year-old woman, was seen for the first time in February 1983 following a recent onset of jaundice. She denied pruritus, had no travel history, was on no regular medications or the birth control pill, consumed very little alcohol, and offered no additional risk factors for hepatitis. Physical examination was unremarkable except for jaundice. Laboratory testing revealed normal CBC, bilirubin 15.0 mg/dL, alkaline phosphatase 3250 u/L, 5′ nucleotidase 130 u/L, AST 285 IU/L, ALT 339 IU/L, cholesterol 1285 mg/dL, AMA 1:640, ANA 1:320, SMA 1:40. Quantitative immunoglobulins were IgG 949 mg/dL, IgM 294 mg/dL, IgA 238 mg/dL. Liver biopsy revealed lymphocytic portal tract inflammation, modest piecemeal necrosis, and few identifiable bile ducts; it was signed out as probable PBC.

In light of the atypical presentation for PBC, it was decided to institute a "trial of steroids." Prednisone, started at 40 mg daily, led to a rapid fall in serum bilirubin to 1.8 mg/dL at the end of 2 months. The prednisone was progressively tapered and discontinued after another 5 months, but this was followed by early reappearance of jaundice, with bilirubin reaching 11.5 mg/dL. Reintroduction of steroids led to clearance of the jaundice but little change in the aminotransferase levels for the first year of therapy. Thereafter, these levels declined progressively. Alkaline phosphatase and cholesterol levels also changed little over the first year but then similarly declined. Xanthelasmata and palmar lipid deposits gradually disappeared over an approximately 10-year follow-up period. Autoantibody levels fluctuated over time, with the AMA declining over the first year of treatment, while the ANA titer rose to 1:1280.

In late follow-up, the prednisone dose was tapered to 2.5 mg daily and azathioprine was instituted in a dose of 50 mg/day. Laboratory testing reveals normal values for bilirubin, alkaline phosphatase, AST, and ALT. ANA is negative, SMA 1:20, AMA 1:640. The most recent follow-up biopsy obtained in 1990 showed a near normal appearance with normal-size portal areas containing normal-appearing bile ducts.

Commentary

This patient presented with jaundice of abrupt onset, which is distinctly unusual for PBC. Thus, despite the strongly positive antimitochondrial antibody, markedly cholestatic liver biochemistries, and liver biopsy—appearances that favored the diagnosis of PBC over AIH—therapy with corticosteroids was initiated. Such an approach has been recommended previously in recognition of the overlap of these syndromes. That this patient benefited from the steroid therapy appears incontrovertible. Nevertheless, it is noteworthy that treatment had little early effect on aminotransferase levels (unlike typical AIH), and AMA remained detectable in high titer 15 years after presentation.

Primary Sclerosing Cholangitis—Autoimmune Hepatitis

Patients with PSC and AIH have similar HLA-related risk factors (HLA-B8, HLA-DR3, HLA DRB1*0301, HLA DRB3*0101). Cholangiography may demonstrate changes of PSC in up to 40% of patients diagnosed as having AIH and ulcerative colitis; they are frequently clinically and biochemically indistinguishable from those with typical AIH. Boberg et al. assessed 114 ERCP-documented PSC patients for features of AIH as classified by the scoring system of the International Autoimmune Hepatitis Group. Some 2% of patients satisfied diagnostic criteria for definite AIH and 33% could be classified as probable. Hypergammaglobulinemia was noted in 60% of cases and 22% had positive ANA or AMA. About 33% had histological features of AIH, including periportal piecemeal necrosis. Five patients had been initially diagnosed with AIH several years before PSC was confirmed on endoscopic retrograde cholangiopancreatography (ERCP).

In patients with AIH, the findings suggesting an overlap syndrome are inflammatory bowel disease, features associated with cholestasis, histological bile duct injury, and poor response to corticosteroid therapy. Though mild alkaline phosphatase elevations are common in autoimmune hepatitis, a more than twofold increase is unusual. Histopathology can often differentiate the two. Ductopenia, fibrous or obliterative cholangitis, and bile stasis are uncommonly seen in AIH. These findings occurring in a patient with AIH, cholestasis, and concurrent inflammatory bowel disease suggest an overlap syndrome. Histological evidence of bile duct injury is more common in patients with AIH and ulcerative colitis than in those with AIH and no colitis. The cholangiographic changes of PSC are absent in about 15% of patients with typical histological disease, suggesting that overlap syndromes are likely to be encountered when the disease involves only the smaller intrahepatic bile ducts.

In patients with AIH and cholestatic features, a full immunoserological workup and liver biopsy should be performed. In the absence of AMA and the presence of chronic cholestasis, PSC must be considered. Though p-ANCA lacks high diagnostic specificity, it may be present in up to 70% of patients with PSC. Particularly in children, PSC may present with features of autoimmune hepatitis. In children, there appears to be significant difficulty in differentiating the two without cholangiography.

In best-documented cases of PSC-AIH overlap, the development of PSC followed the diagnosis of AIH by 2–8 years. There have only been rare instances of PSC preceding AIH or the coexistence of both diseases at the time of initial diagnosis. In these patients corticosteroids with or without azathioprine may result in clinical and biochemical improvement, but treatment failure is not uncommon. Furthermore, among patients with AIH, those with ulcerative colitis experience more treatment failures, undergo remission less frequently, and progress to cirrhosis more often than those without colitis. Demonstration of characteristic PSC cholangiographic features in patients not responding to corticosteroids justifies discontinuation of therapy. Corticosteroids do not appear to prevent the evolution of PSC. In children with AIH and cholestatic features, a poor response to corticosteroids should prompt a workup for PSC. Empirical therapy with ursodeoxycholic acid is warranted if cholestatic symptoms are marked. Clinicians should be watchful for the development of typical complications of PSC (i.e., bacterial cholangitis, osteoporosis, fat-soluble vitamin malabsorption). Roux-en-Y biliary anastomosis should be performed at the time of liver transplantation.

Case History

A 29-year-old African-American women presented in June 1991 with acute-onset bloody diarrhea, leading to a diagnosis of ulcerative colitis. She has subsequently suffered continuing low-grade colitis for which she has received prednisone, azathioprine, and olsalazine sodium (Dipentum). She also experienced one episode of pyoderma gangrenosum. At the time of her presentation, abnormal liver function tests were recognized, and within 2 months clinical jaundice had appeared. At that time, laboratory tests revealed serum bilirubin 10 mg/dL, alkaline phosphatase 155 U/L, AST 980 U/L, ALT 543 U/L, GGT 31 U/L, ANA 1:1280, SMA 1:320, gamma globulins 5.8 g/dL. ERCP examination was interpreted as showing normal extrahepatic bile ducts but abnormalities of the intrahepatic ducts, "with beading suggestive of early sclerosing cholangitis." Repeat studies in 1996 and February 1998 demonstrated progression of the intrahepatic changes but continued normal appearances of the extrahepatic bile ducts.

Liver biopsies in January 1992, February 1996, and December 1997 were reported as showing changes suggestive of AIH, although the pathologist interpreting the February 1996 specimen did offer the following caveat: "This specimen has features of both autoimmune hepatitis and primary sclerosing cholangitis."

Presently, she is receiving prednisone 10 mg, azathioprine 50 mg, and Dipentum 500 mg b.i.d. and is progressing reasonably well apart from sporadic diarrhea. Laboratory testing reveals serum bilirubin 1.7 mg/dL, alkaline phosphatase 221 U/L, AST 68 U/L, ALT 44 U/L, GGT 71 U/L, gamma globulins 2.7 g/dL. Titers of ANA and SMA have tended to decline over the years.

Commentary

This patient has evidence to justify diagnosis of either PSC or AIH. It is conceivable that she has both conditions. However, unlike previously reported patients, she has not demonstrated involvement of extrahepatic bile ducts, which suggests that she will not manifest as rapidly progressive a course as is typical of PSC. The benefit she receives from the steroids with respect to her ulcerative colitis has discouraged discontinuation of the medication.

Autoimmune Cholangitis

A small subset of patients with a clinical presentation of otherwise typical PBC are negative for AMA. These patients have been referred to over the years as having AMA-negative PBC and account for 5–10% of most PBC study populations. In recent times it has been noted that most such patients have positive tests for ANA and/or SMA, and those antibodies may be present in high titer. Furthermore, a recent study has shown that antibodies directed against a subtype of carbonic anhydrase (CA-II), an enzyme present in bile duct epithelium, may be present, but their specificity is not known. There has followed a groundswell argument that these patients be accorded the diagnosis of "autoimmune cholangitis" as opposed to the more negative description "AMA-negative PBC." As mentioned, the clinical presentation of such patients is similar to that of PBC, and no major differences in histopathology or natural history have been reported.

It should be recognized that the original reports on "autoimmune cholangitis," "autoimmune cholangiopathy," and "immune cholangiopathy" described patients whose clinical characteristics were more like those of patients with PBC-AIH overlap syndrome rather than typical PBC. While this serves to gather all such patients under a common umbrella, with autoimmunity representing the force linking these infrequently encountered hepatic disorders, it does not imply that decisions regarding therapy and natural history concerns are easily resolved. Thus, Taylor et al. evaluated 9 patients with autoimmune cholangitis; the median ANA titer was 1:1280 and 6 of the 9 were negative for anti-M2 mitochondrial autoantigens. Liver biopsies showed marked paucity of interlobular bile ducts, bile ductular proliferation at the periphery of portal tracts, and chronic portal tract inflammation, including plasma cells and eosinophils. Of the 9 patients treated with corticosteroids and azathioprine, 7 had no clinical benefit. During a 1–5 year follow-up, the disease progressed and 5 patients developed new autoimmune diseases. ERCP was normal in 3 patients.

Other small case series have demonstrated some improvement of clinical and laboratory features with corticosteroid therapy. Heathcote has pointed out the dangers of using corticosteroids in a setting of chronic cholestasis and encouraged the use of ursodeoxycholic acid. Others have voiced similar concerns and reached similar conclusions. We suspect that this debate will not soon be resolved, given the small numbers of patients with autoimmune cholangitis, which makes it unlikely that a randomized controlled trial of any therapy will be conducted.

Autoimmune cholangitis should be suspected in patients with clinical and histological features of PBC who are AMA-negative. Many of these individuals will have positive SMA or high-titer ANA. Liver histopathology may be suggestive of PBC-AIH overlap syndrome in the presence of more extensive bile duct injury. Though granulomatous cholangitis and bile ductular proliferation may be present, the degree of bile duct loss may be dysynchronous with early-stage PBC. Cholangiography is always unremarkable.

The natural history of autoimmune cholangitis appears to parallel that of PBC. Patients with autoimmune cholangitis seem predisposed to developing other autoimmune disorders. There are variable responses to corticosteroids and ursodeoxycholic acid. Patients with autoimmune cholangitis share many characteristics of patients with AMA-positive or AMA-negative PBC and seem to have a response to biochemical treatment with ursodeoxycholic acid similar to that of PBC patients.

Primary Biliary Cirrhosis and Primary Sclerosing Cholangitis

PBC and PSC share many clinical, biochemical, and histopathological features. They are usually differentiated on the basis of cholangiography. Other than the pruning of proximal intrahepatic biliary radicles, which is typical of cirrhosis in general, no cholangiographic abnormalities are seen on ERCP in PBC. The AMA titer is rarely greater than 1:100 in sclerosing cholangitis. Liver histopathological features are usually able to distinguish the two entities, but occasionally they lack characteristic appearances. Rapid elevations in the serum bilirubin are more often related to sclerosing cholangitis and its related biliary stricturing than to PBC. Rare patients may have features of both PBC and sclerosing cholangitis; in such patients both diseases may be present or a true overlap syndrome may exist. Several case reports have described patients with high titer AMA and the typical nonsuppurative cholangitis of PBC on liver biopsy, but with a strictured intrahepatic biliary system on ERCP, typifying sclerosing cholangitis (see Fig. 2). The clinical features and intrahepatic cholestasis seen in these patients were typical of both PBC and sclerosing cholangitis, and ERCP was performed as part of the initial diagnostic workup. In a patient with PBC, an episode of cholangitis, new ductal dilatation on radiological studies or fluctuating levels of total serum bilirubin may alert the clinician to the possibility of an overlap syndrome with sclerosing cholangitis. Patients with PBC can have choledocholithiasis; however, that may result in similar symptoms. There are no data on the medical management of these patients, but treatment with ursodeoxycholic acid is appropriate. In patients with PBC–sclerosing cholangitis overlap syndrome, vigilance must be maintained in watching for the development of cholangiocarcinoma and sepsis related to bile duct strictures. Appropriate timing of referral for liver transplantation remains important.

Primary Biliary Cirrhosis and Sarcoidosis

Sarcoidosis is a multisystem granulomatous disorder that most often affects the lungs, lymph nodes, eyes, skin, and liver. Some 75% or more of patients with sarcoidosis are found to have granulomas on liver biopsy. Bile duct loss may occur due to a large number of granulomas clustering in portal areas and destroying the ducts as a secondary phenomenon. As in PBC, portal hypertension and intrahepatic cholestasis may be early features of hepatic sarcoidosis; hepatic synthetic dysfunction is usually preserved until the disease is quite advanced. The majority of patients with sarcoidosis and hepatic granulomas, however, have no clinical evidence of hepatic disease, and laboratory abnormalities are commonly mild and nonspecific.

In general, sarcoidosis and PBC have distinctive characteristics that permit accurate differentiation between the two. For example, the coexistence of other autoimmune phenomena (i.e., thyroiditis) is unusual in sarcoidosis. Though extrahepatic granulomas have been reported to occur in PBC, they are almost always localized to the abdominal lymph nodes. AMA are rarely seen in sarcoidosis; elevated levels of angiotensin-converting enzyme occur in up to 50% of patients with sarcoidosis but much less often in PBC and other

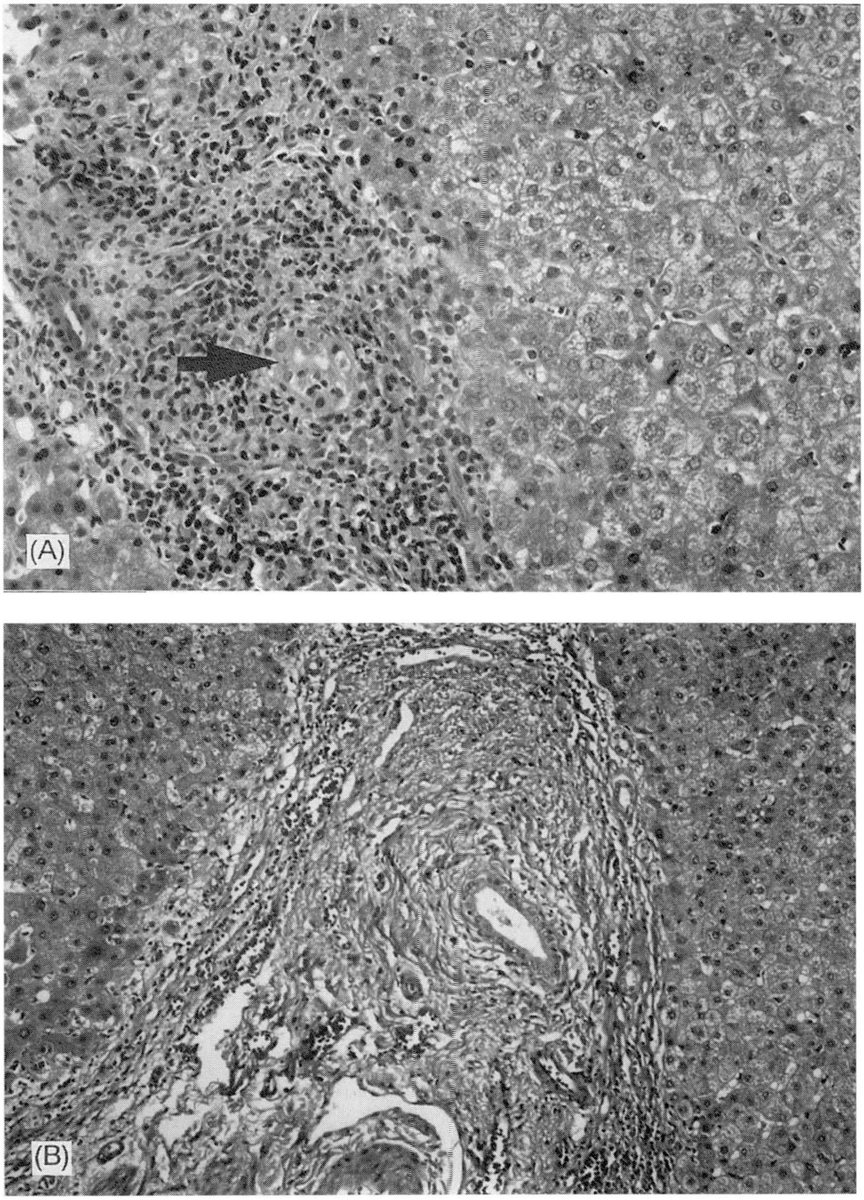

Figure 2 Liver biopsy from a 45-year-old woman with low-titer positive AMA, positive SMA and negative ANA, and liver chemistries notable for moderately raised aminotransferases and an alkaline phosphatase level of 350 IU/L. (A) Note florid duct lesion with bile duct injury (arrow); lymphocytes are present infiltrating the bile ducts. (B) Concentric fibrosis surrounding a medium-sized bile duct in a morbidly fibrotic portal tract. (Hematoxylin and eosin stain, magnification ×400.) (*Note*: ERCP demonstrated typical changes of PSC in intrahepatic biliary tree only.)

granulomatous diseases. Last, in PBC, there is a predominant elevation of serum IgM, while it is of IgG in sarcoidosis.

Several cases of coexistent PBC and sarcoidosis have been described and have blurred the distinctions between the two, suggesting they may be a single entity with a spectrum of clinical manifestations. Clinical and laboratory features of both may be present in the same individual as an overlap syndrome. There have been multiple reports of women initially presenting with lung disease, with cholestasis developing later in the clinical course. These patients had high titer AMA, hepatic granulomas, and, in some cases, even a positive Kveim test. In addition, there are multiple reports of pulmonary fibrosis occurring in PBC especially in the setting of coexisting Sjögren's syndrome.

True overlap syndromes between PBC and sarcoidosis are rare. A patient with systemic sarcoidosis who develops chronic cholestasis more likely has hepatic sarcoidosis than AMA-negative PBC. Laboratory evaluation can almost always differentiate between PBC and sarcoidosis. A search for other autoimmune diseases should be undertaken. Liver histology will often be helpful. Nonsuppurative destructive cholangitis is typical of PBC. Sarcoid granulomas are often large and noncaseating, containing eosinophils. Hepatic granulomas can be seen in many conditions, especially with the use of various medications (i.e., quinidine, allopurinol, sulfonamides); therefore drug-induced granulomatous hepatitis must always be considered in the differential diagnosis. Rarely, histological patterns of both disease entities may be found in the same liver. There is little experience in the treatment of these patients with steroids, ursodeoxycholic acid, or liver transplantation. Appropriate ophthalmological referrals should be made to rule out the uveitis associated with sarcoidosis. Long-term steroid use for sarcoidosis may further accelerate bone loss in patients with coexistent PBC and chronic cholestasis.

Autoimmune Hepatitis and Chronic HCV Infection

The existence of overlap between these two entities has emerged as one of the more controversial issues in contemporary hepatology. Several investigators have documented the presence of positive tests for ANA and/or SMA in patients with chronic hepatitis C (HCV); on occasion, these occur in high titer. Conversely, studies in patients with steroid-responsive AIH have found some who were anti-HCV positive, with a smaller number being positive for HCV RNA. These findings have fueled speculation that HCV might be capable of triggering an immune-mediated reaction involving the liver.

Geographic differences have been recognized in some reports, and those same factors might explain the rarity of positive results for anti-LKM-1 testing in U.S. patients with chronic hepatitis with or without chronic HCV infection.

While the demonstration of autoantibodies in the serum of otherwise typical cases of chronic hepatitis C is of limited importance, the occurrence of circulating autoantibodies, hypergammaglobulinemia, and histopathological features typical of AIH, together with positive HCV RNA, raises practical questions regarding the optimal approach to management. Interferon therapy is known to lead to deleterious effects (including liver failure) in patients with autoimmune diseases. Thus, selection of the correct approach to therapy is of considerable importance. In this spirit, a number of groups have reported on the effects of corticosteroids in patients with overlap features. We have reported the results of steroid administration in two patients with overlap syndromes, both of whom displayed clinical, laboratory and histopathologic benefit from the therapy.

As shown in Table 1, we have to date treated a total of 9 patients in whom features of

Table 1 Response to Corticosteroids in Patients with AIH/Chronic Hepatitis C "Overlap Syndrome"

Patient	Sex	Age	Race	Risk factor for HCV	HVC RNA–positive	Laboratory features of AIH	Liver biopsy	Response to corticosteroids
ET	F	72	AA	0	Yes	Gamma globulins 2.3, ANA 1:640, SMA 1:1280	Severe chronic hepatitis with autoimmune features	Resolution of syndrome
SL	F	38	C	IVDA	Yes	Gamma globulins 2.1, ANA 1:640	Moderately severe chronic hepatitis	Resolution of syndrome
OM	F	69	AA	BT[b]	Yes	Gamma globulins 4.5, ANA 1:640, SMA 1:640	Severe chronic hepatitis with autoimmune features	Resolution of syndrome
GI	F	51	AA	BT[b]	Yes	Gamma globulins 3.4	Severe chronic hepatitis with cirrhosis and with autoimmune features	No response
LT	M	64	AA	0	Yes	Gamma globulins 3.2, ANA 1:640, ANA 1:640	Chronic hepatitis with autoimmune features	Resolution of syndrome
EM	F	52	AA	0	No	Gamma globulins 3.2, ANA 1:640, SMA 1:160	Chronic hepatitis with autoimmune features	Resolution of syndrome
EJ	F	54	AA	BT[b]	Yes	Gamma globulins 2.9	Severe chronic hepatitis with cirrhosis	No ALT response, gamma globulins to normal
RA	M	47	AA	BT[b]	Yes	Gamma globulins 1.8, ANA 1:1280, SMA 1:160	Exacerbation of AIH	Responded to cyclosporine and prednisone
AM	M	46	AA	0	Yes	Gamma globulins 1.8, SMA 1:640	Mild chronic hepatitis	Resolution of syndrome

[a]Also had bone marrow transplant for promyelocytic leukemia.
[b]BT = blood transfusions.

AIH were encountered in combination with chronic HCV infection. Eight were treated with prednisone in doses ranging from 20–40 mg/day while the remaining patient was treated with cyclosporine and prednisone. Six showed the characteristic AIH response with prompt decline in amino-transferase levels and gamma globulins, and follow-up liver biopsies were often dramatically improved (see Fig. 3). Anti-HCV tests remained positive, and HCV RNA titers remained stable or increased. In one patient (GI), prednisone treatment failed to lower aminotransferase levels or improve the hypergammaglobulinemia; she had a well-established cirrhosis and did not benefit from subsequent interferon therapy. In another patient (EJ), treatment with interferon had proved unsuccessful before prednisone was tried. She showed a prompt fall in her gamma globulin values following initiation of prednisone treatment, but little change in the aminotransferase levels.

Successful treatment with corticosteroids of other patients with chronic hepatitis C and features of an autoimmune chronic hepatitis has been reported by others. The feasibility of eradicating the accompanying HCV infection once the autoimmune component has been treated is largely unexplored. Czaja et al. performed retrospective examination of HCV infection in patients thought to have AIH in the prehepatitis C–testing era who had responded to steroids and found several who were positive for hepatitis C. Similar findings were reported by Nishiguchi et al. This does not appear to be a nonspecific response to steroids in HCV-infected patients, even though one study demonstrated moderate declines in serum aminotransferase levels in an unselected cohort of hepatitis C patients. In his recent assessment of this phenomenon, Czaja proposed use of the phrases *autoimmune-predominant* and *viral-predominant* to describe patients with features of combined disease in whom the diagnosis was based upon points accrued according to a scoring system devised by the International Autoimmune Hepatitis Group. Response to corticosteroids was accorded special priority with respect to its usefulness as a diagnostic tool.

Most of our patients and other steroid-treated patients of similar type demonstrate a rapid and complete response to therapy as judged clinically, biochemically, and histopathologically. However, viral levels tended to increase even as evidence of hepatic injury lessened. Furthermore, remission was maintained only as long as steroid therapy was continued, unlike the case in other patients with AIH. Although dramatic improvement in clinical, laboratory, and histopathological features of the chronic hepatitis has been observed, it is uncertain whether this has an impact on the later risk of development of hepatocellular carcinoma. We assume that this would be the case, since transition to cancer usually occurs in the setting of an established cirrhosis from HCV infection, and none of our responders had histopathological evidence of cirrhosis when they started therapy. In occasional patients (e.g., patient GI) steroid therapy produced no benefit. Curiously, switching these patients to interferon was equally ineffective. Other therapeutic options for these overlap patients who fail both steroid and interferon therapy have yet to be identified.

Case History

A 65-year-old African-American woman with a remote history of blood transfusion (at the time of hysterectomy) was found to have abnormal liver chemistry tests on routine laboratory testing. Examination revealed firm hepatomegaly with the liver edge palpable just below right costal margin. Laboratory data included total serum bilirubin 3.3 mg/dL, AST 466 IU/L, ALT 245 IU/L, alkaline phosphatase 163 U/L and GGT 347 U/L. Anti-HCV and PCR for HCV RNA were positive. Additional testing disclosed ANA-positive in titer 1:640, SMA-negative, and gamma globulin fraction 4.8 g/dL. Liver biopsy (Fig. 3A) revealed severe chronic hepatitis with prominent plasma cell infiltration, piecemeal necrosis, and rosette formation; fibrosis was abundant, with features suggestive of cirrhosis. Treatment with prednisone 40 mg/day was initiated and azathio-

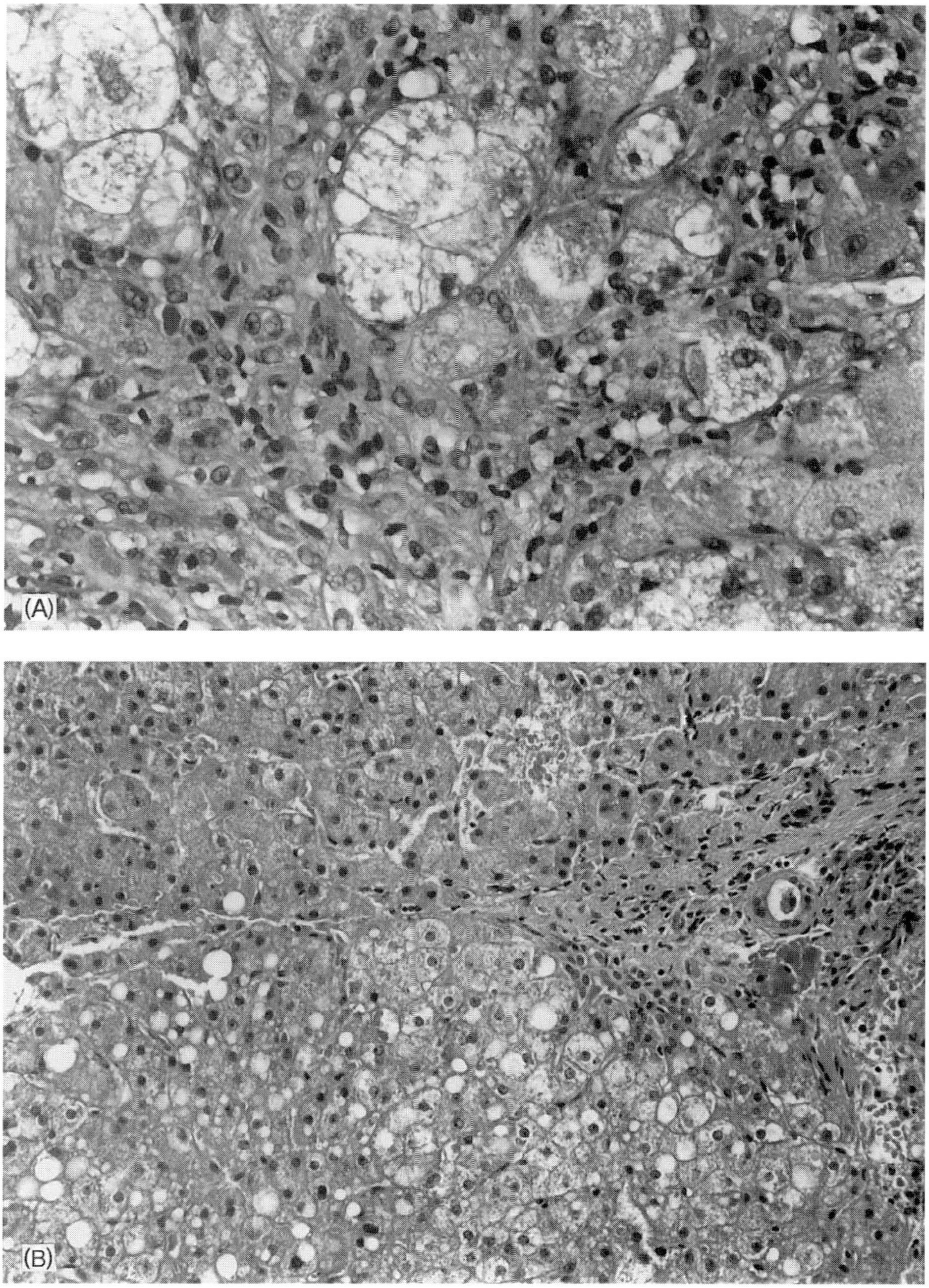

Figure 3 Liver biopsies from a patient with features of AIH and circulating HCV RNA. (A) Initial biopsy obtained following presentation. (Hematoxylin and eosin–stained section, magnification ×400.) Ballooned hepatocytes with prominent lobular and piecemeal activity. (B) Follow-up liver biopsy obtained after periods of steroid therapy. (Hematoxylin and eosin–stained section, magnification ×200.) Fibrous portal expansion with minimal portal inflammation and no significant lobular or piecemeal activity; mild macrovesicular steatosis. (Dr. Rebecca Thomas interpreted the biopsy material and prepared the photomicrographs.)

prine 50 mg/day added 2 months later. AST and ALT promptly fell to normal, gamma globulins returned to normal levels in 2 months, and HCV RNA levels rose slightly. Follow-up liver biopsy 2 years after initiation of therapy revealed dramatic improvement in terms of reduced portal tract inflammation, piecemeal necrosis, rosette formation, and bridging fibrosis (see Fig. 3B). The patient has remained asymptomatic throughout treatment and is currently receiving prednisone 2.5 mg daily and azathioprine, 50 mg daily. Liver chemistries and serum protein electropheresis remain within normal limits.

Commentary

Despite the clear-cut documentation of chronic HCV infection, the presence of laboratory and histopathological features of AIH persuaded us to initiate treatment with corticosteroids. The patient responded promptly to this intervention, in analogous fashion to other patients with AIH. She remains in remission despite the persistence of chronic HCV infection. We interpret her beneficial response to the corticosteroids as evidence that autoimmune processes (possibly triggered by HCV infection) were the principal factors in progression of her liver disease.

Autoimmune Chronic Hepatitis and Chronic HBV Infection

Patients with features of AIH and chronic HBV infection have been described. In a cohort of patients with "severe chronic active liver disease" recruited to a trial of various therapies at the Mayo Clinic in the late 1960s/early 1970s, several were recognized retrospectively to have chronic hepatitis B. Patients later diagnosed with chronic hepatitis B were sometimes noted to have immunoserological markers (i.e., LE cell, ANA, SMA, AMA) present and several achieved a clinical, biochemical, and histological remission with corticosteroids (± azathioprine). Thus, this analysis demonstrated a modest overlap between AIH and chronic hepatitis B and suggested that in occasional patients with overlap features, corticosteroids can be effective therapy.

Although seemingly occurring in fewer numbers than with chronic HCV infection, these patients appear to have a comparable disorder to that described in patients with HCV infection. There are insufficient data to ascertain whether overlap cases are more likely to occur with chronic hepatitis B in its replicative or nonreplicative phases of infection. In fact, cases of autoantibody induction have appeared to follow initiation of alpha-interferon or gamma-interferon therapy for replicative disease or for chronic hepatitis C. However, each of these publications emphasized the absence of features of AIH (or other autoimmune diseases) in association with the appearance of the autoantibodies.

HCV Infection and Cholestatic Liver Diseases

Although early reports linked PBC with HCV infection, this seems likely to reflect shortcomings of the original anti-HCV enzyme-linked immunosorbent assay (ELISA) and has not been supported by subsequent investigations. An aspect of overlap between the two syndromes is provided by the long-time observation that some patients with chronic hepatitis (termed *chronic persistent hepatitis* in the past and likely to include patients with chronic HCV infection) may have lesions simulating PBC—the "florid-duct lesion." These changes were named the "Poulsen lesion," after the original reporter of the change. In virtually all instances, the absence of clinical or biochemical evidence of PBC allowed for a straightforward separation of the two entities. However, HCV patients are now being recognized with complaints of severe pruritus—often as their major presenting feature—

and occasionally with cholestatic liver chemistries. Curiously, in the author's experience, it has been distinctly unusual for such patients to benefit clinically from therapies that are often helpful in patients with traditional cholestatic liver disease. They have, however, benefitted from antiviral medication.

Differentiation of HCV from PBC is usually easily achieved by testing for the AMA (negative in HCV). Differentiation from primary sclerosing cholangitis requires performance of cholangiography.

CONCLUSIONS

Appropriate management of overlap syndromes is based on certain basic principles. These are as follows:

Provisional diagnosis of a specific entity should be made on the presence of customary diagnostic features.

Treatment strategies should be planned for defined periods of time and be subject to review at specified times.

Treatment should be with medications that have a high degree of safety and are inexpensive.

Endpoints of treatment must be identified at the beginning of treatment and should be simply obtainable, amenable to ready interpretation, and consistent with customary expectations of the goals of therapy.

Differentiation of syndromes should be pursued when it means that different medications are required for treatment and/or the prognosis of the conditions is not the same.

One approach to management of some of these overlap syndromes is offered by Czaja in Table 2.

Table 2 Empirical Treatments for Some Variants of Autoimmune Hepatitis[a]

Variants	Treatment strategy
Autoimmune hepatitis and primary biliary cirrhosis	Prednisone 20 mg/day for 3–6 months Ursodeoxycholic acid 13–15 mg/kg per day for 3–6 months if prednisone is ineffective
Autoimmune hepatitis and primary sclerosing cholangitis	Prednisone 20 mg/day for 3–6 months if autoimmune predominant Investigational protocols if prednisone is ineffective or empirical trial with ursodeoxycholic acid 13–15 mg/kg daily for 3–6 months Therapy for symptoms only
Autoimmune hepatitis and chronic viral hepatitis	Prednisone 20 mg/day or 10 mg/day, azathioprine 50 mg/day for 3–6 months if autoimmune-predominant Recombinant interferon, 3 million U three times weekly for 6 months if viral-predominant Prednisone 20 mg/day for 3–6 months
Autoimmune cholangitis	Prednisone 20 mg/day for 3–6 months Ursodeoxycholic acid 13–15 mg/kg daily for 3–6 months if prednisone is ineffective

[a]Overlap syndromes of PBC–sclerosing cholangitis and PBC-sarcoid are so exceedingly rare that management options should be individualized for each patient.
Source: From Czaja, 1996.

BIBLIOGRAPHY

Bellary S, Schiano T, Hartman G, Black M. Chronic hepatitis with combined features of autoimmune chronic hepatitis and chronic hepatitis C: favorable response to prednisone and azathioprine. Ann Intern Med 1995; 123:32–34.

Ben-Ari Z, Dhillon AP, Sherlock S. Autoimmune cholangiopathy: part of the spectrum of autoimmune chronic active hepatitis. Hepatology 1993; 18:10–15.

Boberg KM, Fausa O, Haaland T, Holter E, Mellbye OJ, Spurkland A, Schrumpf E. Features of autoimmune hepatitis in primary sclerosing cholangitis: an evaluation of 114 primary sclerosing cholangitis patients according to a scoring system for the diagnosis of autoimmune hepatitis. Hepatology 1996; 23:1369–1376.

Cassani F, Cataleta M, Valentini P, et al. Serum autoantibodies in chronic hepatitis C: comparison with autoimmune hepatitis and impact on the disease profile. Hepatology 1997; 26:561–566.

Clifford BD, Donohue D, Smith L, et al. High prevalence of serological markers of autoimmunity in patients with chronic hepatitis C. Hepatology 1995; 21:613–619.

Colombato LA, Alvarez F, Cole J, Huet PM. Autoimmune cholangiopathy: the result of consecutive primary biliary cirrhosis and autoimmune hepatitis. Gastroenterology 1994; 107:1839–1843.

Czaja AJ, The variant forms of autoimmune hepatitis. Ann Intern Med 1996; 125:588–598.

Davis PA, Leung P, Manns M, et al. M4 and M9 antibodies in the overlap syndrome of primary biliary cirrhosis and chronic active hepatitis: epitopes or epiphenomena. Hepatology 1992; 16:1128–1136.

Duclos-Vallée J-C, Hadengue A, Ganne-Carrié N, et al. Primary biliary cirrhosis—autoimmune hepatitis overlap syndrome. Dig Dis Sci 1995; 40:1069–1073.

Garcia-Buey L, Garcia-Mouzon C, Rodriguez S, et al. Latent autoimmune hepatitis triggered during interferon therapy in patients with chronic hepatitis C. Gastroenterology 1995; 108:1770–1777.

Gohlke F, Lohse AW, Dienes HP, et al. Evidence for an overlap syndrome of autoimmune hepatitis and primary sclerosing cholangitis. J Hepatol 1996; 24:699–705.

Goodman ZD, McNally PR, David DR, Ishak KG. Autoimmune cholangitis: a variant of primary biliary cirrhosis. Clinicopathologic and serologic correlations in 200 cases. Dig Dis Sci 1995; 40:1232–1242.

Gordon SC, Quattrociocchi-Longe TM, Khan BA, et al. Antibodies to carbonic anhydrase in patients with immune cholangiopathies. Gastroenterology 1995; 108:1802–1809.

Heathcote EJ. Autoimmune cholangitis. Clin Liver Dis 1998; 2:303–311.

Invernizzi P, Crosignani A, Battezzati PM, et al. Comparison of the clinical features and clinical course of antimitochondrial antibody-positive and -negative primary biliary cirrhosis. Hepatology 1997; 25:1090–1095.

Ludwig J, Batts KP. Histopathology of autoimmune liver disease. In: Krawitt EL, Wiesner RH, Nishioka M, eds. Autoimmune Liver Diseases, 2d ed. Amsterdam: Elsevier Science Publishers, 1998.

McNair ANB, Moloney M, Portmann BC, et al. Autoimmune hepatitis overlapping with primary sclerosing cholangitis in five cases. Am J Gastroenterol 1998; 93:777–784.

Perrillo RP, Mason AL, Jacob S, et al. Hepatitis and cholestasis in a middle-aged woman. Hepatology 1996; 24:730–734.

Reddy KR, Krawitt EL, Homberg J-C, et al. Absence of anti LKM-1 antibody in hepatitis C viral infection in the United States of America. J Virol Hepatitis 1995; 2:175–179.

Taylor SL, Dean PJ, Riely CA. Primary autoimmune cholangitis: an alternative to antimitochondrial antibody-negative primary biliary cirrhosis. Am J Surg Pathol 1994; 18:91–99.

Vento S, Cainelli F, Renzini C, Concia E. Autoimmune hepatitis type 2 induced by HCV and persisting after viral clearance. Lancet 1997; 350:1298–1299.

15
Management of Alcoholic Liver Disease

Anne M. Larson and Robert L. Carithers, Jr.
University of Washington, Seattle, Washington

OVERVIEW

Approximately 25–40% of patients hospitalized in the United States have medical problems resulting from alcohol abuse. Alcoholic hepatitis and cirrhosis, the most common liver diseases encountered in the United States, result in 10,000–20,000 deaths annually and together are the fourth leading cause of death among middle-aged Americans. The 5- and 10-year survival rates of patients with alcoholic cirrhosis range from 20–50% and 0–30%, respectively.

Despite these rather frightening figures, the pathogenesis of alcoholic liver disease remains an enigma. In addition, specific treatments are less than satisfactory. However, the clinical features and prognostic markers of alcoholic hepatitis and cirrhosis have been well characterized and liver transplantation now offers hope to many patients with otherwise untreatable alcoholic liver disease. In this chapter we review current concepts of the pathogenesis, clinical features, prognosis, important coexistent diseases, and management of patients with alcoholic liver disease.

ALCOHOLISM

Although many cases are sporadic, there is increasing evidence for a genetic predisposition to alcoholism. Alcoholism tends to run in families, a phenomenon first observed by ancient Greek scholars. Many studies show that as many as one-third of male alcoholics have at least one alcoholic parent, and sons of alcoholic fathers face a 25–30% risk of becoming alcoholics. This is true whether they are reared by their biological parents or by nonalcoholic foster families. In addition, the concordance of alcoholism is over twice as high among monozygotic twins than among dizygotic twins. However, despite extensive research, no specific biochemical abnormality has been found to explain the familial risk of alcoholism, and the precise genetic component remains to be determined. Nevertheless, alcoholism appears at an earlier age, dependency is more severe among familial cases, and patients with a family history of alcohol abuse nearly always have a poorer prognosis than other alcoholics.

THE SPECTRUM OF LIVER DISEASE

Alcohol abuse can result in a spectrum of liver injury ranging from fatty liver to cirrhosis with end-stage liver disease (Fig. 1). Fatty liver can occur even after moderate weekend drinking but usually resolves quickly with abstinence. Much more ominous is the development of necroinflammatory hepatocellular injury, commonly called alcoholic hepatitis. This pattern of injury appears to be an important step in the evolution of progressive liver injury and is a direct precursor of cirrhosis in many if not all patients. Perisinusoidal fibrosis, most commonly involving the central portions of the hepatic lobule, can progress to form small, well-circumscribed nodules, the histological hallmark of micronodular or Laennec's cirrhosis. With time, dense bands of fibrosis circumscribing large nodules may develop, which are indistinguishable from the macronodular cirrhosis of other forms of liver disease. Although alcoholic liver disease has been conveniently separated into fatty liver, alcoholic hepatitis, and cirrhosis, many patients have a spectrum of histological features, including fat accumulation, hepatocellular injury and inflammation, and fibrosis. However, even among the most incorrigible alcoholics, severe liver disease is the exception rather than the rule. This observation underlies the enigma of the pathogenesis of alcoholic liver disease.

PATHOGENESIS

Earlier in this century, it was popularly held that alcoholic liver disease was simply due to poor nutrition. However, numerous animal and human studies support the concept that excessive alcohol ingestion is a major force in the development of alcoholic liver disease. Nevertheless, cirrhosis occurs in only 20–50% of patients who drink excessively for years, providing convincing evidence that the pathogenesis of liver injury cannot be explained simply by the toxic effects of alcohol ingestion. Rather, it appears that liver injury in alcoholics is a complex process including hepatotoxicity, immunological injury, and stimulation of fibrogenesis. In addition, genetic susceptibility and gender appear to influence the risk of developing severe alcoholic liver disease.

Alcohol Metabolism

Over 90% of ingested alcohol is metabolized in the liver. Ethanol is readily absorbed from the gastrointestinal tract, predominantly in the small intestine. Once it has entered the portal venous system, ethanol is carried to the liver, where it is oxidized first to acetaldehyde and then to acetate. Two families of enzymes facilitate the conversion of ethanol to acetaldehyde: (1) alcohol dehydrogenases (ADH) within the hepatic cytosol and (2) enzymes of the microsomal ethanol oxidizing system of the endoplasmic reticulum, particularly cytochrome P-450IIE1 and cytochrome P-450 reductase (Fig. 2). By far the greatest fraction of ethanol is metabolized via the ADH pathway. Acetaldehyde, the by-product of ethanol oxidation, is further metabolized to acetate by mitochondrial acetaldehyde dehydrogenase

(ALDH). ALDH is an extremely efficient enzyme. As a result, only about 1% of the acetaldehyde produced by the liver actually enters the bloodstream.

Heterogeneity of Enzymes Involved in Alcohol Metabolism

Since each step in the alcohol oxidation pathway contributes to the overall rate of ethanol metabolism, genetic variants in ADH cytochrome P-450IIE1, and ALDH could potentially alter the pharmacokinetics of alcohol. Five classes of alcohol dehydrogenases with over twenty isoenzyme forms have been identified. The enzymes in each class differ considerably in their ability to metabolize alcohol. However, despite numerous studies, neither qualitative nor quantitative differences in ADH isoforms identify patients with a unique susceptibility to alcoholic liver disease. This may be due to the fact that NADH reoxidation, rather than the level of ADH activity, appears to be the rate-limiting step in the ADH pathway of ethanol metabolism. Genetic polymorphisms have also been identified in the CYPIIE1 isoenzymes but do not appear to be associated with the severity of alcoholic liver disease. Mitochondrial acetaldehyde dehydrogenase is the most important enzyme influencing acetaldehyde metabolism. A polymorphic variant of this ALDH is catalytically inactive because of a single amino acid substitution. Approximately 50% of Chinese, Japanese, and South American Indians express this aberrant enzyme. Individuals with this "deficient" phenotype who drink develop uncomfortable symptoms of flushing, resulting from excessive accumulation of acetaldehyde in the serum, which triggers systemic release of catecholamines. This may explain why these ethnic groups have a low incidence of alcoholism. However, with this exception, studies of polymorphisms of the enzymes involved in alcohol metabolism have not helped to explain the pathogenesis of either alcoholism or alcoholic liver disease.

Effects of Alcohol Metabolism on the Pathogenesis of Alcoholic Liver Disease

Although ethanol does not appear to cause hepatic injury directly, its metabolism triggers a variety of intracellular events, many of which are thought to culminate in profound metabolic changes in the hepatocyte and make it unusually susceptible to injury. In addition, by-products of ethanol metabolism may well initiate a cascade of injurious events that result in hepatocellular necrosis and hepatic fibrosis, the hallmarks of alcoholic liver disease. The following events occur during the metabolism of alcohol: (1) marked changes in the redox state of the hepatocyte; (2) hypoxia, especially in the central zones of the liver; (3) generation of superoxide and other potentially toxic radicals; and, (4) formation of aldehyde adducts. Each of these events combines to destroy the integrity of hepatocytes, ultimately resulting in cellular necrosis. In addition, these intracellular derangements appear to stimulate immune responses, which further enhance hepatocellular destruction and also promote the development of hepatic fibrosis.

Altered Redox State. Conversion of ethanol to acetaldehyde by alcohol dehydrogenase results in intrahepatic generation of $NADH^+$ (Fig. 2). Because of a paucity of cytoplasmic substrates and the impermeability of the inner mitochondrial membrane to $NADH^-$, the hydrogen and electrophilic by-products of ethanol metabolism must be shuttled to the respiratory chain of the mitochondria. There, NAD is regenerated through utilization of oxygen and generation of ATP. ATP generation is the rate-limiting step in this process, and ultimately, in the metabolism of ethanol. The net result of this rather cumbersome process is the accumulation of $NADH^+$ and an altered redox state of the hepatocyte. This altered redox state exerts profound effects on both carbohydrate and lipid metabolism

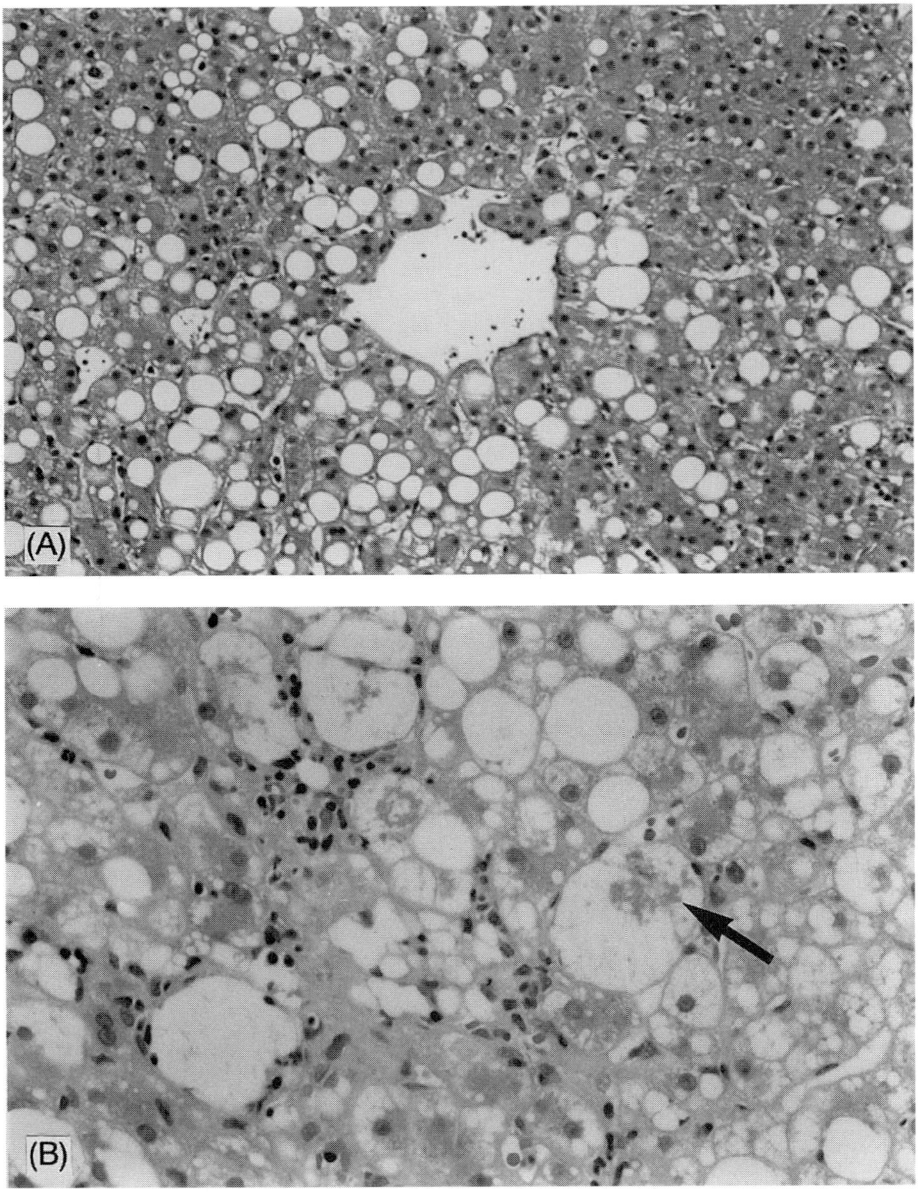

Figure 1 The spectrum of alcoholic liver disease. (A) Fatty liver (steatosis) with macrovesicular fatty changes. (B) Alcoholic hepatitis with fatty changes, inflammation, and Mallory's hyaline (arrow). (C) Laennec's cirrhosis with small, well-circumscribed nodules (micronodular cirrhosis). (D) Macronodular cirrhosis.

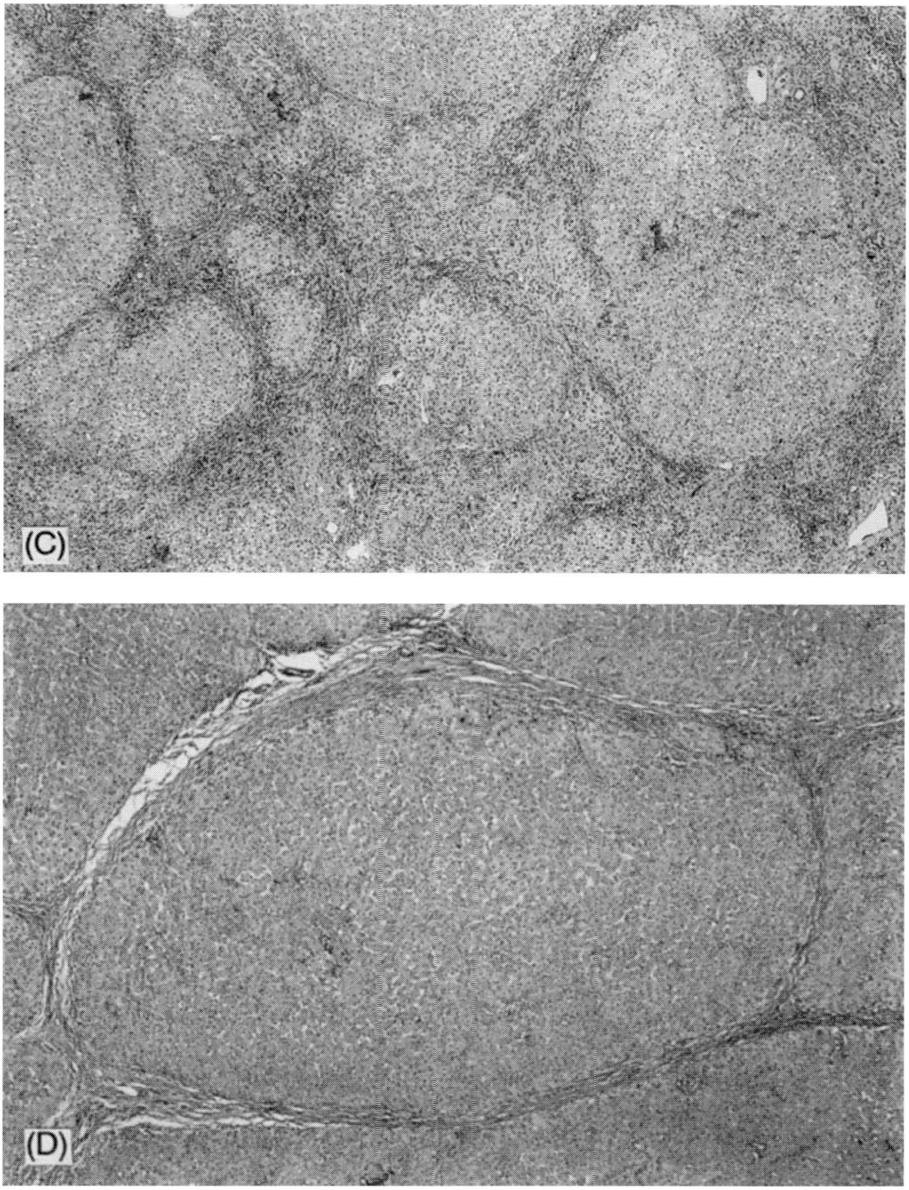

and results in many of the biochemical changes characteristic of alcohol abuse including hypoglycemia, lactic acidosis, interference with fatty acid oxidation, and stimulation of triglyceride synthesis. The latter two alterations are thought to be primary factors leading to fatty liver. However, changes in the redox state alone do not lead to hepatocellular necrosis. Other factors must be invoked to explain the pathogenesis of alcoholic hepatitis and cirrhosis.

Hypoxia and Hypermetabolic State. Ethanol metabolism increases hepatic oxygen consumption, inducing a hypermetabolic state, particularly in the centrilobular portion of

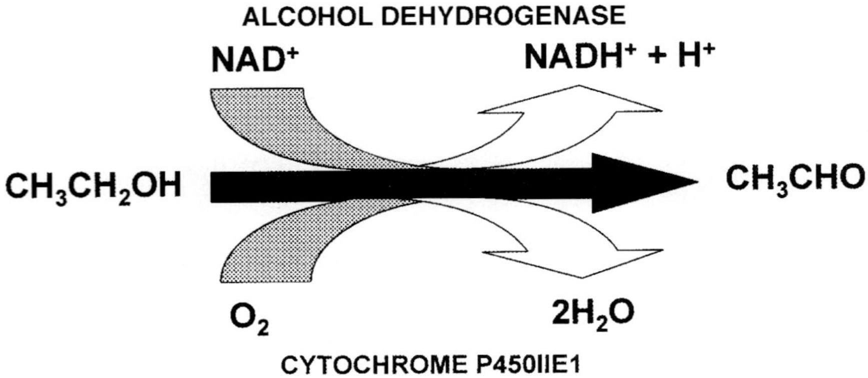

Figure 2 Ethanol (CH_3CH_2OH) is oxidized to acetaldehyde (CH_3CHO) primarily via two enzymatic pathways. The alcohol dehydrogenase pathway is the primary route of ethanol metabolism. This pathway, which results in conversion of NAD to $NADH^+$ and H^+, changes the redox state of the hepatocyte. The cytochrome P-450IIE1 pathway, a less important route, utilizes oxygen, and appears to be responsible for the generation of free radicals within the hepatocyte.

the lobule. Cytochrome P-450IIE1 utilizes oxygen directly (Fig. 2), whereas ADH produces $NADH^+$, requiring mitochondrial oxygen for regeneration of NAD. Splanchnic blood flow increases in a compensatory attempt to prevent hepatic hypoxia. However, this compensatory response is often inadequate. The resulting relative state of hypoxia renders the hepatocyte vulnerable to insults such as hypotension, hepatotoxins, or decreased inspired oxygen. In experimental animals, this hypermetabolic state can be prevented by administration of propylthiouracil.

Free Radical Formation. In addition to utilizing twice as much oxygen as ADH, cytochrome P-450IIE1 is active in forming reactive oxygen intermediates (superoxide radicals and peroxides). Formation of particularly toxic radicals appears to be facilitated by the availability of free iron, which can be mobilized either by hypoxia or by the altered redox state induced by alcohol metabolism. In addition, prolonged excessive alcohol intake reduces the enzymes and intrahepatic scavengers, such as glutathione and vitamin E, which protect the hepatocyte against oxidant injury. This imbalance is thought to result in the accumulation of a variety of toxic free radicals within the hepatocyte. Although the specific means by which these reactive intermediates adversely affect hepatocytes are not clear, a number of potential mechanisms have been proposed. These include the peroxidation of cellular lipids, damage to mitochondrial function and intrahepatic DNA, and changes in intrahepatic calcium homeostasis.

Acetaldehyde. Acetaldehyde is the primary oxidation product of ethanol metabolism. Its conversion to acetate in mitochondria is severely depressed in chronic alcoholics, resulting in accumulation of acetaldehyde within the hepatocyte. Acetaldehyde is electrophilic and binds to nucleophilic sites on proteins and enzymes, causing formation of acetaldehyde-protein "adducts," which result in functional impairment. One example of this is the binding of acetaldehyde to tubulin, a critical ingredient of the hepatic cytoskeleton. The adduct formation interferes with microtubule assembly and decreases movement of plasma proteins from the Golgi apparatus to the plasma membrane. The result is intrahepatic accumulation of lipids and proteins, which causes marked cell swelling, a classic feature of alcoholic hepatitis and cirrhosis. Adduct formation and lipid peroxidation induced by acetaldehyde can also cause derangement in a variety of other cellular functions, including depression of mitochondrial oxidative phosphorylation, enzyme inhibition, and impairment of cell-surface receptor recycling.

A great deal remains to be learned about the intracellular events that lead to hepatocellular necrosis from chronic alcohol abuse. However, a picture is emerging of a cell placed under unusual degrees of oxidative stress while at the same time having its normal defense mechanisms impaired by the by-products of ethanol metabolism (Fig. 3). The imbalance of these forces appears to be the first step in irreversible damage to the hepatocyte. However, the story does not end there. Emerging evidence suggests that these same intrahepatic events initiate a series of responses in adjacent cells that result in immunological injury to the hepatocyte as well as initiation of hepatic fibrosis.

Immunological Injury

Kupffer, endothelial, and stellate cells appear to play essential roles in facilitating toxic processes within the liver. Oxidant stress appears to trigger recruitment of these and other cells through the release of a variety of proinflammatory cytokines. For example, interleukin-8 (IL-8) stimulates release and activation of neutrophils and is thought to play an important role in stimulating the neutrophilia and hepatocellular neutrophilic infiltration characteristic of alcoholic hepatitis. Another prominent stimulus to cytokine release is endotoxin. Kupffer cells, which make up about 30% of the sinusoidal cells, clear particulate and foreign matter from the portal circulation and play a central role in the uptake and detoxification of endotoxins. These cells are activated by portal endotoxemia, which is common in patients with alcoholic liver disease, probably from alcohol-induced disruption

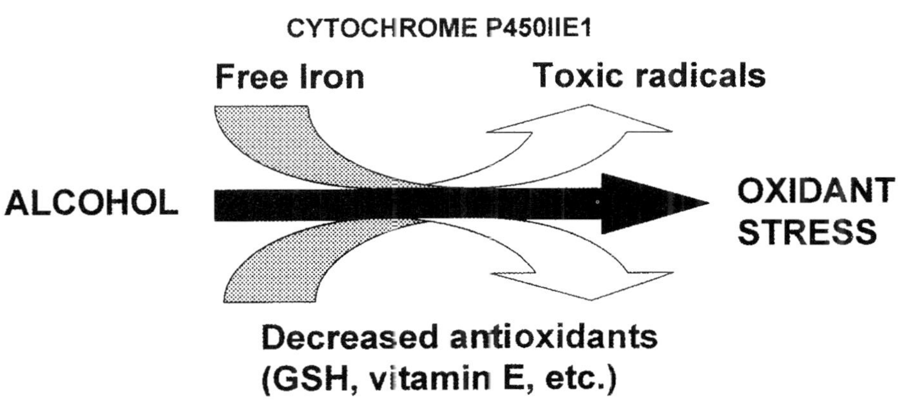

Figure 3 Ethanol metabolism, especially through the cytochrome P-450IIE1 pathway, appears to be responsible for the generation of free radicals within the hepatocyte. Production of the most toxic radicals is facilitated by the presence of free iron, which is promoted by hypoxia and the altered redox state of the hepatocyte. Alcohol abuse also reduces various antioxidants, including glutathione and vitamin E. This imbalance in the production of free radicals and diminution of antioxidant capacity leaves the hepatocyte vulnerable to oxidant stress.

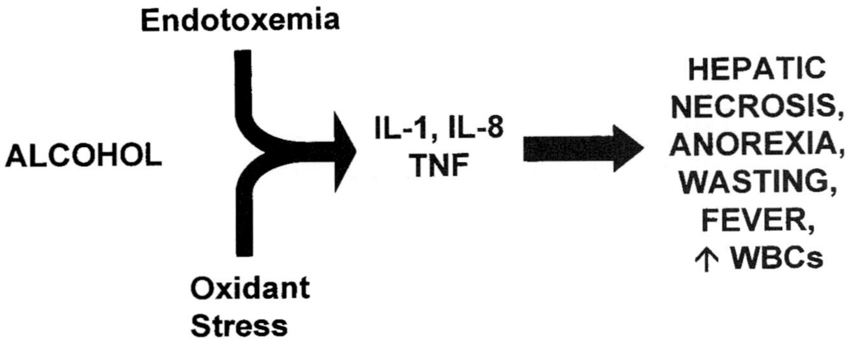

Figure 4 Oxidant stress and endotoxemia, each induced by chronic alcohol abuse, lead to release of a variety of proinflammation cytokines, including interleukin-1 (IL-1), IL-8, and tumor necrosis factor (TNF). The activity of these cytokines is thought to mediate many of the features of severe alcoholic liver disease, including hepatocellular necrosis, anorexia, and muscle wasting, fever, leukocytosis, and neutrophilic infiltration of the liver.

of the gut mucosal barrier. Kupffer cell activation increases production and release of IL-1, IL-8, and tumor necrosis factor alpha (TNF-α), each of which promotes hepatic damage, accounting for many of the clinical features of severe alcoholic liver disease such as fever, anorexia, and muscle wasting (Fig. 4).

Hepatic Fibrosis

Oxidant stress and Kupffer cell activation also appear to be major factors stimulating the development of hepatic fibrosis in patients with alcoholic liver disease. This is thought to occur through activation of hepatic stellate cells, which line the sinusoids. The stimulation of collagen synthesis appears to be mediated by TNF-α, which stimulates DNA synthesis of hepatic stellate cells, and by transforming growth factor beta (TGF-β), one of the most potent fibrogenic cytokines for stellate cells (Fig. 5).

Gender

The final factor to be considered in the pathogenesis of alcoholic liver disease is gender. Traditionally, women have drunk less than men, have been less likely to become alcoholic, and if they did, had a later onset of alcoholism than men. However, if they abuse alcohol, women develop alcoholic hepatitis and cirrhosis with a shorter duration and lower intake of ethanol than do men. This may be because women have higher blood ethanol concentrations for any amount of alcohol ingested.

The increased blood alcohol levels in women can be explained in part by their smaller body size. However, they also appear to have diminished gastric "first-pass" oxidation of ethanol. Gastric ADH is thought to facilitate oxidation of alcohol within the stomach prior to intestinal absorption and, as a result, to decrease blood ethanol levels. It has been speculated that this first-pass metabolism decreases the bioavailability of ethanol and represents a "protective barrier" against its systemic effects. Women have lower gastric ADH activity than men, perhaps in part explaining their greater susceptibility to alcohol-induced liver damage.

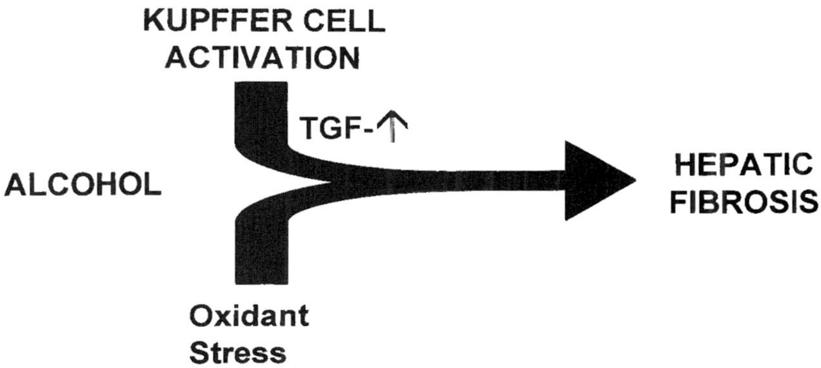

Figure 5 Oxidant stress and Kupffer cell activation appear to be major factors stimulating hepatic fibrosis in chronic alcoholics. Kupffer cell stimulation of hepatic stellate cell collagen production appears to be mediated by the cytokine transforming growth factor beta (TGF-β).

Summary

Clearly, we have a great deal yet to learn about the pathogenesis of alcoholic liver disease. However, recent advances in unraveling this complex process have enhanced our understanding of the clinical features of the various forms of alcoholic liver disease. These advances also have stimulated a number of innovative new approaches to treatment. Further understanding of the means by which chronic alcohol abuse can so severely damage the liver is essential to additional advances in our management of these patients.

CLINICAL SYNDROMES

Our understanding of the clinical features of alcoholic liver disease is due to elegant studies in the 1970s, in which the histological features of injury were carefully correlated with symptoms, physical findings, laboratory abnormalities, and the clinical course of disease. Although there is often considerable overlap, three major clinicopathological entities account for most patients with alcoholic liver disease. These include fatty liver, alcoholic hepatitis, and cirrhosis. Hepatic steatosis is the most common of these but is usually transient and benign. Alcoholic hepatitis and cirrhosis, serious conditions that can result in significant morbidity and mortality, require chronic abuse of large quantities of alcohol for years; even then, they develop in only the minority of chronic alcoholics.

Fatty Liver

Fatty liver can occur in association with a wide range of diseases, toxins, and drugs; however, the majority of cases are secondary to alcohol excess, diabetes, or obesity. Steatosis occurs in the majority of heavy drinkers. As little as 24 oz of 86-proof alcohol can result in fatty liver. Nonspecific fatigue, anorexia, abdominal discomfort, or pain in the right upper quadrant may be seen, although most patients are asymptomatic. Elevated liver enzymes and hepatomegaly are typically the only finding. The prognosis is usually benign and the hepatomegaly, abnormal liver function tests, and steatosis usually quickly resolve with abstinence. Deaths resulting directly from fatty liver are uncommon (see Chap. 26 for nonalcoholic fatty liver).

Alcoholic Hepatitis

Alcoholic hepatitis is associated with more significant morbidity and mortality. Patients with severe alcoholic hepatitis have a mortality rate approaching that seen in patients with fulminant hepatic failure. Alcoholic hepatitis is also a well-recognized precursor of cirrhosis. Alcoholic hepatitis generally follows consumption of large quantities of alcohol over an extended period, generally 15–20 years. Asymptomatic patients may be discovered when hepatomegaly is detected during routine examination or mild elevations in serum aminotransferase levels are noted on biochemical screening (see Chap. 1). However, many patients with symptomatic alcoholic hepatitis minimize or deny their symptoms.

Symptoms

Symptoms of more advanced disease, which are often vague and nonspecific, include abdominal pain, nausea, vomiting, weakness, diarrhea, weight loss, fatigue, and fever. There is usually a history of heavy alcohol intake, although some patients deny and many minimize the degree of alcohol intake. Many sicker patients discontinue alcohol a few days to weeks before hospitalization, often complaining of being "too sick" to drink. Severe alcoholic hepatitis is marked by fever, anorexia, weakness, jaundice, and bleeding. Frequently, patients will have had nothing to eat or drink for several days prior to presentation. Patients often complain of right-upper-quadrant pain; however, symptoms of end-stage liver disease—such as abdominal swelling, edema, and confusion—are infrequent.

Physical Findings

The most universal physical finding of alcoholic hepatitis is hepatomegaly, seen in about three-quarters of patients and ranging from mild to massive enlargement. This appears to result not from fatty infiltration but from the accumulation of intracellular proteins. Alcohol leads to both induction of microsomal enzymes as well as to diminished excretion of glycosylated proteins; the resulting intrahepatic accumulation of proteins leads to an osmotic flux of water, culminating in marked hepatocellular swelling. Many patients exhibit right-upper-quadrant tenderness to palpation and may have an audible hepatic bruit over the liver. Jaundice, spider angiomata, splenomegaly, ascites, and edema are common findings. In more severe cases, hepatic encephalopathy may be present. Fever, seen in many patients, is generally mild, but temperatures as high as 104–105°F have been seen. Fever may persist for weeks and often no source of infection can be found. Other common physical findings include testicular atrophy and peripheral neuropathy.

Laboratory Abnormalities

Patients with alcoholic hepatitis usually have only modest elevations in serum aminotransferase levels, even when the disease is severe. AST levels are usually less than 300–500 IU, with trivial elevations of ALT levels. An AST/ALT ratio greater than 3:1 is characteristically seen. Alkaline phosphatase values can range from normal to several thousand. Serum bilirubin levels can range from normal to 20–30 mg/dL, and serum albumin may be normal or depressed to levels as low as 1.0–1.5 g/dL. Plasma ferritin levels are often significantly elevated and may exceed 1000 μg/L. Most patients are anemic and have some degree of thrombocytopenia. The white blood cell count is usually normal but can be elevated to levels consistent with leukemoid states.

Histological Features

The symptoms, physical findings, and biochemical abnormalities in patients with alcoholic hepatitis often do not reflect the degree of hepatic injury. Classic histological features include ballooned degenerating hepatocytes concentrated in the pericentral areas, often containing alcoholic hyaline (Mallory bodies), with a surrounding infiltrate composed of polymorphonuclear leukocytes. Varying degrees of fatty infiltration may be seen, and some patients develop prominent perisinusoidal fibrosis, at times with partial or complete obliteration of the terminal hepatic venules (central hyaline sclerosis), which can lead to portal hypertension even in the absence of cirrhosis.

Cirrhosis

Cirrhosis is the final step in the spectrum of alcoholic liver disease. There is a strong dose-time relationship between alcohol consumption and risk of developing alcohol-related disease; however, only 20–50% of heavy drinkers develop cirrhosis. Alcoholic hepatitis is the most clearly defined histological precursor of cirrhosis. However, some patients with fatty liver appear to progress to cirrhosis without developing alcoholic hepatitis. Whether this represents an alternative pathway for the development of cirrhosis or whether, alternatively, intermittent episodes of alcoholic hepatitis were not recognized remains highly controversial (Fig. 6).

Clinical Features

The clinical features of alcoholic cirrhosis are similar to those seen in patients with alcoholic hepatitis. Parotid enlargement, palmar erythema, ascites, hepatic encephalopathy, spider angiomata, Dupuytren's contractures, and signs of portal hypertension are more common among patients with cirrhosis. However, reversible portal hypertension can be

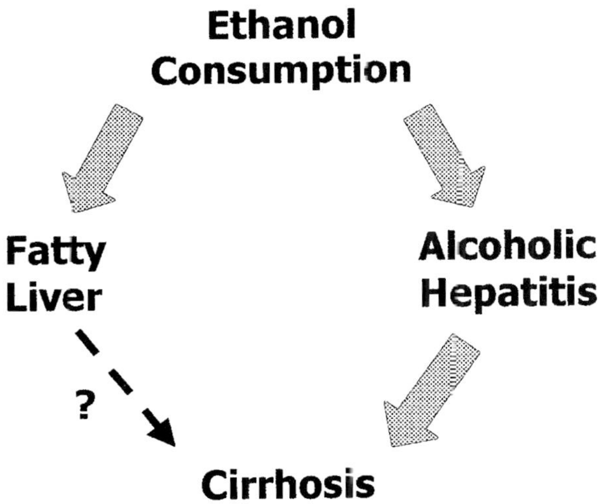

Figure 6 Alcohol consumption leads to a spectrum of disease, with cirrhosis marking the final step. Alcoholic hepatitis is the most clearly defined histological precursor of cirrhosis. It remains debated whether patients progress to cirrhosis from alcoholic fatty liver (steatosis).

seen in patients with alcoholic hepatitis, so the presence of ascites or esophageal varices does not reliably differentiate patients with alcoholic hepatitis from those with cirrhosis. As a result, liver biopsy is the only certain means of confirming the presence of alcoholic cirrhosis.

Histologic Features

The first evidence of fibrosis in alcoholics often is a lace-like pattern of perisinusoidal collagen deposition concentrated in the pericentral regions. This can progress to thin bands of fibrous tissue, which circumscribe small nodules of hepatocytes (micronodular cirrhosis). This often is accompanied by varying degrees of steatosis, centrilobular necrosis, alcoholic hyaline, and polymorphonuclear leukocytic inflammation, which help to establish the underlying etiology of the cirrhosis. With abstinence, these features often disappear. Fatty liver usually resolves within a month and the histological features of alcoholic hepatitis usually disappear within 2–3 months. Over time, parenchymal remodeling can occur and the micronodular cirrhosis is transformed to macronodular cirrhosis, indistinguishable from other causes of cirrhosis.

PROGNOSIS

The prognosis of patients with alcoholic liver disease varies greatly. Patients with uncomplicated fatty liver usually recover quickly with abstinence. Most patients with milder forms of alcoholic hepatitis recover, although this may take months to occur. Patients with severe alcoholic hepatitis have a very high short-term mortality, while patients with moderate disease are primarily at risk for developing alcoholic cirrhosis. The prognosis of patients with cirrhosis also varies considerably. Patients with well-compensated disease who can abstain have an excellent prognosis. In contrast, patients with decompensated disease, especially if they continue to drink, often die within 6–12 months.

Clinical Course of Severe Alcoholic Hepatitis

Patients with severe alcoholic hepatitis frequently deteriorate during the first 4–5 days of hospitalization, and biochemical measures of liver injury often increase for 2–4 weeks after admission. AST, ALT, serum bilirubin, creatinine, and prothrombin time values often worsen in the first few weeks after hospitalization. Patients who are alert on admission also may develop confusion and signs of hepatic encephalopathy within a few days. Clinical and laboratory features of alcoholic hepatitis such as fever, abnormal aminotransferase values, hyperbilirubinemia, and hypoalbuminemia often persist for months despite continued hospitalization and abstinence.

Acute Mortality

As many as 50% of patients with severe alcoholic hepatitis die within a month of initial hospitalization. Clinical features portending a poor prognosis include the presence of hepatic encephalopathy that persists despite adequate treatment, marked prolongation of prothrombin time values, elevation of serum bilirubin values above 20 mg/dL, depressed serum albumin values, serum creatinine greater than 2.0 mg/dL, and older age. A discriminant function calculated by the formula: $[(4.6 \times \text{prothrombin time}) + \text{serum bilirubin}]$ has

Table 1 Child–Pugh Grading of Severity of Liver Disease

Clinical and biochemical measurements	Points scored for increasing abnormality		
	1	2	3
Encephalopathy[a]	None	1 and 2	3 and 4
Ascites	Absent	Slight	Moderate
Bilirubin (mg/100 mL)	1–2	2–3	>3
Prothrombin time (seconds prolonged)	1–4	4–6	>6

[a]According to grading of Trey et al. (N Engl J Med 1966; 274:473.)

been shown to be the best predictor of mortality in patients with alcoholic hepatitis. Patients with values greater than 90 face the highest risk of short-term mortality.

Alcoholic Cirrhosis

The prognosis in alcoholic cirrhosis depends upon the number and degree of complications and the patient's ability to abstain from further alcohol intake. The Child-Pugh criteria give a good indication of prognosis (Table 1). Patients with scores of 5–6 have an excellent prognosis. In contrast, patients with Child-Pugh scores greater than 10 often succumb within 6–12 months, particularly if they continue to drink. Other ominous prognostic signs include intractable ascites, portal hypertension, esophageal variceal bleeding, hepatic encephalopathy, and the hepatorenal syndrome. The most common causes of death from alcoholic cirrhosis are hepatic failure (27–51%), gastrointestinal hemorrhage (9–47%), hepatocellular carcinoma (5–16%), infections (3–17%), and renal failure (1–8%).

COEXISTENT DISEASES

Patients with alcoholic liver disease often have coexistent diseases that can adversely affect their prognosis. Because of their altered metabolism of drugs, alcoholics are particularly vulnerable to drug-induced liver injury. Alcoholics are also frequently exposed to hepatitis infections, which can result in immediate mortality, enhanced progression of chronic liver injury, and increased risk for hepatocellular carcinoma.

Drug-Induced Liver Injury

The liver is central to the transformation and elimination of most drugs. Cytochrome P-450IIE1 is involved in the metabolism of acetaminophen, carbon tetrachloride, and a variety of other compounds. Following acute ingestion, alcohol competes for this enzyme, inhibiting drug metabolism. However, with chronic alcohol use, cytochrome P-450IIE1 activity can increase by 10- to 20-fold, particularly immediately after heavy drinking has been discontinued. This enzyme induction, in combination with depletion of protective scavengers such as glutathione and vitamin E, can lead to unopposed formation of toxic metabolites, which results in massive liver injury. Alcoholics can develop severe acetaminophen hepatotoxicity even after ingestion of only modest amounts of the drug (see Chaps.

24 and 25). These patients often present with AST and ALT values as high as 5,000–10,000 and can rapidly progress to decompensated liver disease, from which they often do not recover.

Viral Hepatitis

Viral hepatitis is quite common among alcoholics. In most serological surveys, 25–30% of alcoholics have antibodies to hepatitis B, C, or both. The typical serological pattern for hepatitis B includes anti-HBc and anti-HBs, indicating previous exposure to the virus. Few patients have active HBV infection. In contrast, chronic HCV infection with circulating HCV RNA is quite common among alcoholics. Active infection with either of these viruses appears to accelerate the progression of the liver disease and to enhance the risk of hepatocellular carcinoma.

Hepatitis A virus infection can also present a major risk, especially to patients with cirrhosis. Given their lack of hepatic reserve, these patients can develop severe, life-threatening disease, with reported mortality rates as high as 50%.

MANAGEMENT

Our current understanding of the pathogenesis of alcoholic liver injury leads to the inescapable conclusion that sustained abstinence is the most important step in the management of patients with alcoholic liver disease. Yet physicians often seem so unduly pessimistic about either the possibility or benefits of abstinence that they look instead for quick fixes and other forms of treatment. At the same time, they fail to educate patients about the remarkable benefits that can be obtained with complete, sustained cessation of alcohol intake. As a result, they often deny their patients the most effective treatment of this disease. The other crucial ingredient in the management of patients with prolonged alcoholism is the provision of a nutritious diet (see Chap. 16). In the management of patients with alcoholic liver disease, it is also important to see that they avoid hepatotoxic medications and hepatitis vaccinations. Corticosteroid therapy has been shown to provide transient though lifesaving benefits to a small group of patients with severe alcoholic hepatitis. Although many other forms of therapy have been tried for patients with alcoholic liver disease, none have proven to be useful. However, liver transplantation is extremely effective in selected patients with end-stage liver disease who are willing to make a lifetime commitment to abstinence.

Abstinence

Patients who have not yet reached end-stage alcoholic liver disease have a remarkable potential for recovery with abstinence. Even patients with profound jaundice, ascites, and synthetic dysfunction may become asymptomatic, develop normal liver function tests, and have a normal physical examination within 12–24 months of abstinence. The degree of recovery parallels that seen among patients with severe autoimmune hepatitis or Wilson's disease who are treated with corticosteroids or penicillamine. Patients with cirrhosis often show dramatic improvement in the clinical features of their disease. The only patients who have not been shown to respond to abstinence are those with severe portal hypertension.

Patients with compensated cirrhosis who abstain have almost a 90% chance of surviving at least 5 years (Fig. 7). Even among patients with decompensated cirrhosis,

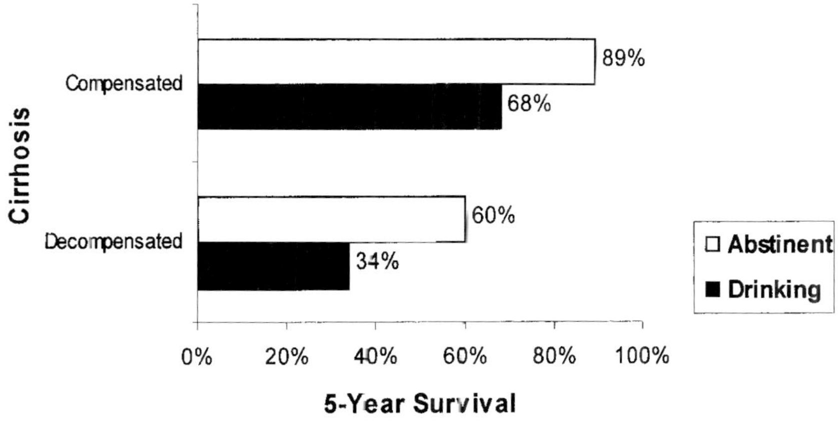

Figure 7 The 5-year survival rates in patients with alcoholic cirrhosis relative to drinking behavior and severity of liver disease. (From Powell, Am J Med 1968; 44:406.)

abstinence doubles the chance of survival for the subsequent 5–10 years. However, long-term survivors remain at risk for hepatocellular carcinoma even after years of abstinence.

Nutritional Support

Malnutrition is a major problem in patients with alcoholic liver disease (see Chap. 16). Protein-calorie malnutrition is seen in 75% of patients hospitalized with moderate to severe alcoholic hepatitis or cirrhosis. These patients are often profoundly anorectic and have increased muscle catabolism. Diverse vitamin and mineral deficiencies are seen, including depletion of zinc, magnesium, phosphorus, folic acid, thiamine, pyridoxine, and vitamins A, D, and B_{12}. Enhanced expression of cytokines such as TNF has been implicated in the pathogenesis of the anorexia, muscle wasting, and zinc deficiency of patients with alcoholic liver disease.

Provision of adequate nutritional support to patients with severe alcoholic liver disease can be quite challenging. Many patients suffer from severe anorexia and early satiety. Others require dietary sodium and protein restriction because of ascites and encephalopathy. Nevertheless, provision of adequate calories, vitamins, minerals, and protein is essential. An experienced dietitian can often do wonders for these patients. In selected patients with intractable ascites, a peritoneovenous or transjugular shunt may be extremely useful in overcoming early satiety, which can be such an obstacle to adequate nutritional intake.

Special amino acid preparations enriched with branched-chain amino acids have been extensively studied in patients with severe alcoholic liver disease. Neither enteral nor oral administration of these preparations has been conclusively proven to be beneficial. As a result, their high cost cannot be justified except under special circumstances.

Corticosteroids

Corticosteroids have been shown to dramatically improve the short-term survival of patients with severe alcoholic hepatitis (Fig. 8). Patients who have the best response to treatment are those with (1) spontaneous hepatic encephalopathy; (2) a discriminant func-

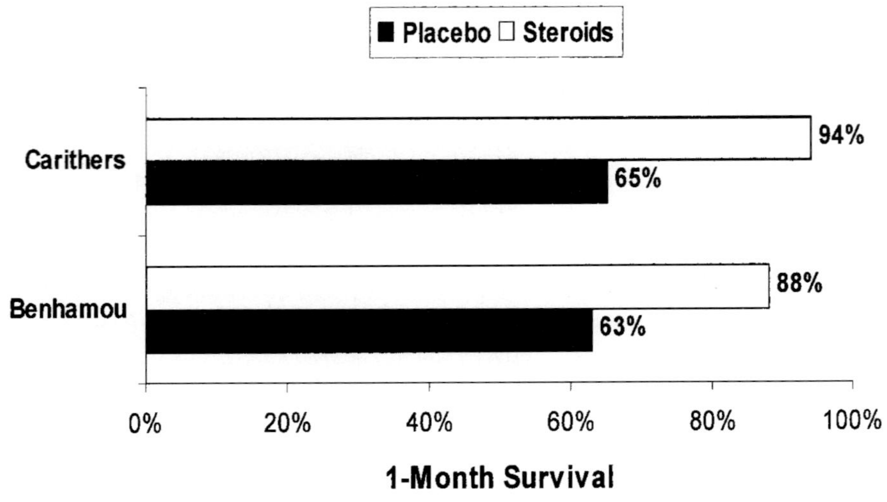

Figure 8 The 1-month survival rates in patients with alcoholic hepatitis receiving either corticosteroids or placebo. Both trials showed a statistically significant improvement in 1-month survival in patients receiving corticosteroids (Carithers, $p = 0.006$; Benhamou, $p = 0.001$.)

tion value above 90; and (3) no active bleeding, pancreatitis, or renal failure. It has been suggested that many of the benefits of corticosteroid therapy in these patients are achieved by blocking the formation and release of proinflammatory cytokines such as TNF.

Other Potential Modes of Therapy

Numerous other forms of treatment have been attempted in patients with alcoholic hepatitis and cirrhosis. These include propylthiouracil (PTU), glucagon/insulin infusions, anabolic steroids, and colchicine. Although each has a sound basis, none have been shown to be effective or safe enough for general clinical use.

Newer forms of treatment have been proposed which are based on current understanding of the pathogenesis of alcoholic liver disease. Most of these are directed at blocking the production and release of proinflammatory cytokines. These include specific antibodies against cytokines, such as TNF, which appear to be so integral to many of the clinical manifestations of severe alcoholic liver disease. However, until we clearly understand the relative role of these cytokines in producing inflammation, necrosis, and hepatic regeneration, such treatments must be confined to carefully controlled and monitored clinical trials.

Liver Transplantation

Liver transplantation has been shown to be very effective in selected patients with end-stage alcoholic liver disease. From 1988 to 1995, 23% of all liver transplants in the United States were performed for alcoholic liver disease. Another 25% of patients received transplants for end-stage liver disease secondary to chronic hepatitis C; many of them had a history of concomitant alcohol use. Both graft and patient survival in those with alcoholic liver disease compare favorably to that of patients transplanted for other condi-

Table 2 Crude Survival by Primary Liver Disease Among Adult Recipients of Liver Transplantation in the United States: 1988–1995[a]

	Cumulative percentage surviving							
	3 months		1 year		3 years		5 years	
Primary liver disease	Patient	Graft	Patient	Graft	Patient	Graft	Patient	Graft
ALD, no hepatitis C	87.3	83.3	81.6	77.1	73.9	69.2	59.6	55.1
ALD + hepatitis C	87.7	84.0	81.7	76.5	72.2	63.2	N/A	N/A
Hepatitis C, no ALD	88.2	83.0	80.7	74.4	71.7	65.4	57.3	50.3
Hepatitis B	88.2	83.9	74.8	69.2	60.5	54.4	49.3	43.6
Cryptogenic cirrhosis	85.5	80.3	79.0	72.6	72.3	65.8	60.4	52.9
PBC	90.1	84.9	85.7	79.9	81.6	75.8	75.9	69.2
PSC	91.6	85.3	86.3	77.9	79.9	71.5	70.1	61.3
Autoimmune	86.7	82.1	81.8	77.0	77.3	71.3	71.8	65.1
Metabolic	84.3	80.1	77.4	72.8	73.4	67.4	60.3	52.8
Malignancy	85.4	80.9	66.1	61.9	40.0	37.5	26.7	23.9
Miscellaneous	84.8	80.8	78.4	73.6	73.9	67.5	65.5	56.3

[a]Excludes recipients with acute liver failure.
Abbreviations: ALD, alcoholic liver disease; PBC primary biliary cirrhosis; PSC, primary sclerosing cholangitis; NA, not applicable.
Source: From Belle et al., Liver Transpl Surg 1997; 3:212.

tions (Table 2). The quality of life for most patients is excellent and recidivism rates are quite low following transplantation.

Nevertheless, fewer than 10% of the patients who die annually from alcoholic liver disease will ever be afforded the opportunity for transplantation. Most transplant programs require a fair but stringent preoperative evaluation, which includes intensive evaluation by experienced social workers, psychologists, or psychiatrists. In addition, most programs require patients to remain abstinent for at least 6 months before they can be seriously considered for transplantation.

SUMMARY

Alcoholic liver disease is one of the most important liver diseases in the United States and throughout the world. The exact mechanisms by which alcohol causes severe liver injury in selected patients remain obscure. However, improvements in our understanding of the basic biology of liver cell injury and fibrosis offer exciting promises for future advances in this area. As our knowledge of pathophysiology expands, new treatments will become available. Until then, abstinence, ongoing support by caring physicians, and liver transplantation for selected patients will remain the mainstays of management for patients with alcoholic liver disease.

REFERENCES

Akriviadis EA, Redeker AG. Fulminant hepatitis A in intravenous drug users with chronic liver disease. Ann Intern Med 1989; 110:838–839.

Belle SH, Beringer KC, Detre KM. Liver transplantation for alcoholic liver disease in the United States: 1988 to 1995. Liver Transpl Surg 1997; 3:212–219.

Carithers RL, Jr., Herlong HF, Diehl AM, Shaw EW, Combes B, Fallon HJ, Maddrey WC. Methylprednisolone therapy in patients with severe alcoholic hepatitis: a randomized multicenter trial. Ann Intern Med 1989; 110:685–690.

French SW, Nash J, Shitabet P, Kachi K, Hara C, Chedid A, Mendenhall CL. Pathology of alcoholic liver disease: VA cooperative study group 119. Semin Liver Dis 1993; 13:154–169.

Helman RA, Temko MH, Nye SW, Fallon HJ. Alcoholic hepatitis: natural history and evaluation of prednisolone therapy. Ann Intern Med 1971; 74:311–321.

Maddrey WC, Boitnott JK, Bedine MS, Weber FJ Jr., Mezey E, White RI Jr. Corticosteroid therapy of alcoholic hepatitis. Gastroenterology 1978; 75:193–199.

McClain CJ, Hill DB, Schmidt J, Diehl AM. Cytokines and alcoholic liver disease. Semin Liver Dis 1993; 13:170–182.

Munoz SJ. Nutritional therapies in liver disease. Semin Liver Dis 1991; 11:278–281.

Schiødt FV, Rochling FA, Casey DL, Lee WM. Acetaminophen toxicity in an urban county hospital. N Engl J Med 1997; 337:1112–1117.

Tsukamoto H, Kaplowitz N. Pathogenesis of alcoholic liver disease. In: Kaplowitz N, ed. Liver and Biliary Diseases. Baltimore: Williams & Wilkins, 1992:121–137.

16

Nutritional Support in Chronic Liver Disease

Michael Charlton
Mayo Clinic and Foundation, Rochester, Minnesota

BACKGROUND

The liver has the most diverse function of all the organs, including being central to the metabolism of fat, carbohydrates, and protein. A primary role of the liver is undoubtedly the regulation of the metabolism of amino acids and proteins.

The liver carries out four main functions in protein metabolism: formation of plasma proteins, amino acid interconversion, deamination of amino acids, and urea synthesis (for ammonia excretion). Hepatocytes manufacture a diverse set of proteins including many clotting factors, albumin (accounting for fully 40% hepatic protein synthesis), thyroid-binding globulin, VLDL apoB 100, and complement. Over 80% of the proteins synthesized by the liver are exported into the systemic circulation. These proteins are central to the maintenance of hemostasis, oncotic pressure, transport of hormones, lipid transport, and acute-phase reactions. Total hepatic plasma protein synthesis ranges from 30–60 g/day.

The liver's role in lipid metabolism has two principal components. First, the liver is the site of bile acid formation and is thereby essential to the efficient digestion and subsequent absorption of dietary fats. Second, the liver is the only site of synthesis of apolipoprotein B-100 and is responsible for the metabolism of other apolipoproteins and chylomicrons.

In carbohydrate metabolism, the liver is the primary site of the action of glucagon it is where glycogen stores are regulated for the maintenance of blood glucose levels between meals and during periods of physiological stress. In addition, there is evidence that the liver is important in the regulation of satiety.

Among the many other functions of the liver, it is responsible for the metabolism of many hormones that have discordant effects on protein, carbohydrate, and lipid metabolism, such as insulin, the sex hormones, and glucagon. It is thus not surprising that chronic liver disease should be associated with a high incidence of malnutrition and altered metabolism of proteins, carbohydrates, and lipids. An understanding of the changes in metabolism that take place in patients with chronic liver disease is essential to the development of rational guidelines for the nutritional support of these patients. This chapter provides an overview of the prevalence, consequences, pathophysiology, treatment, and future directions of malnutrition in chronic liver disease.

PREVALENCE OF MALNUTRITION IN CIRRHOSIS

Disordered metabolism may occur in patients without clinical consequence but is most frequently encountered in patients with liver disease who exhibit protein-calorie malnutrition (PCM), defined as a wasting condition resulting from a diet deficient in both calories and protein. Cirrhosis is a condition frequently associated with profound changes in body composition. The emaciated patient with PCM and a protuberant abdomen full of ascites is familiar to all who are involved in the care of patients with liver disease. Although the prevalence of PCM varies widely with both etiology and severity of the established liver injury, it is by any measure a common clinical manifestation of chronic liver disease.

Alcoholic liver disease is the form of liver disease most frequently associated with PCM. The reported prevalence of PCM (in studies in which detailed nutritional assessments were made) in patients with alcoholic liver disease varies between 29% in patients with compensated alcoholic liver disease in the community up to 100% in hospitalized patients with acute alcoholic hepatitis. For patients with compensated alcoholic liver disease, the prevalence of PCM has been reported to be between 10 and 42%. Reliable data, based on detailed nutritional assessment, of the prevalence of PCM in patients with nonalcoholic liver disease is scant compared to the relative wealth of data available for patients with alcoholic liver disease. In a study by Morgan et al., some 40% of patients with primary biliary cirrhosis were found to have evidence of PCM. In the same study, only 12% of patients with chronic hepatitis were found to be malnourished. Of interest is that the presence of malnutrition in this study was not on the basis of either inadequate caloric intake or steatorrhea.

In patients with end-stage liver disease, the existence of PCM is almost universal. In a detailed multivariate analysis by DiCecco et al., all of 74 patients being evaluated for orthotopic liver transplantation were found to have evidence of malnutrition. The great majority (78%) of these patients had loss of muscle mass, as determined by decreased midarm circumference. Similar results were obtained in a much smaller but equally detailed study of prospective transplant recipients.

Based on the aggregate of the data reported above, PCM might be considered to be the most common complication of cirrhosis.

PATHOGENESIS OF MALNUTRITION IN CIRRHOSIS

The pathogenesis of PCM in patients with cirrhosis is multifactorial and will differ from one patient to another, as the relative presence or absence of pathogenic factors varies between patients. The various contributing factors are best considered separately as those related to liver disease and those which are iatrogenic. An outline of the various contributing factors in PCM associated with liver disease is shown in Table 1.

Table 1 Pathogenesis of Protein Calorie Malnutrition in Patients with Cirrhosis[a]

Disease-related	Iatrogenic
Inability to maintain intake	Protein restriction
Anorexia	Acute
Encephalopathy	Persistent
Malabsorption/maldigestion	Diagnostic procedures
Portal enteropathy	Purgative associated nausea and vomiting
Decreased bile salt synthesis	
Metabolic derangement	Unpalatability of nutritional supplements
Lowered respiratory quotient	Drug-related, e.g., β-blocker-induced increase in amino acid oxidation
Attenuated protein synthesis	
Increased amino acid oxidation	
Increased resting energy expenditure	
Increased nutritional requirements during complications from liver disease	

[a]In most instances, disease-related factors will vary between patients according to etiology and severity of disease.

Iatrogenic Factors

While many of the pathogenic changes that lead to PCM in liver disease are related to changes in metabolism secondary to the presence of liver disease, nondisease-related changes in protein supply play a central role. Of all of the factors contributing to the development of PCM in liver disease, inadequate intake is the most readily identifiable and correctable. One of the most widely disseminated but fallacious "pearls" regarding nutrition in the setting of liver disease is the need to restrict protein to these patients. The restriction of protein intake to less than 1.0 g/kg/day greatly increases the risk of protein wasting and negative nitrogen balance in patients with stable cirrhosis. The risks of net nitrogen loss from protein restriction are amplified in patients with acute complications of liver disease, such as bacterial peritonitis, variceal hemorrhage, or acute alcoholic hepatitis, as the protein requirements increase in these settings. While the prevalence of inadequate nutrition has been demonstrated to be high in the outpatient setting, the prevalence *increases* during hospitalization. In a prospective study by Egan et al., patients admitted to hospital for the treatment of alcoholic hepatitis received a mean of 50% of their calculated caloric and 57% of their total calculated protein requirements. The poor protein intake in hospitalized patients with liver disease is partly attributable to the inherent difficulties in feeding patients with encephalopathy or the malaise associated with acute alcoholic hepatitis, but it is also in part iatrogenic. The prolonged periods of fasting imposed for the myriad investigations carried out during hospitalizations can greatly exacerbate the difficulties of maintaining intake in patients with liver disease and should be planned to minimize the time spent fasting. Furthermore, while protein restriction may have a role in the management of acute hepatic encephalopathy, there is no need for this practice in the medium- or long-term management of patients with liver disease. Indeed, medium- or long-term protein restriction should be avoided in this group of patients, as there is overwhelming evidence that the incidence of complications of liver disease increases with malnutrition. In the few patients who are intolerant of adequate protein intake in the diet secondary to chronic hepatic encephalopathy, consideration should be given to branded-chain amine acid (BCAA)-enriched formulas, additional vegetable protein, or casein supplements. There are no convincing data to support the use of BCAA-enriched formulas as initial therapy for the treatment of acute portosystemic encephalopathy.

Disease-Related Factors

Diminished Intake

There is considerable evidence that the liver plays an important role in the regulation of satiety. The mechanisms of hepatic control of appetite are thought to include hepatic vagal afferent monitoring of hepatic glycogen change. The reported incidence of anorexia in the setting of chronic liver disease is high. A review of the literature regarding nutrition in patients with alcoholic liver disease by Achord et al. reported the incidence of anorexia to be ~90% in patients with advanced alcoholic liver disease.

Increased Requirements

In the outpatient setting, the reported adequacy of micro- and macronutrient ingestion is varied. Some investigators have reported adequate intakes, while others have documented persistently low intakes. The requirements of cirrhotic patients are, however, often underestimated in the outpatient setting due to difficulties in assessing their nutritional requirements. There are also a number of factors that can contributed to increased nutritional requirements in cirrhosis. Maldigestion, secondary to diminished bile salt synthesis, with consequent impaired micelle formation, and malabsorption secondary to portal enteropathy and drugs, such as lactulose and neomycin, are all contributing factors in the increased nutritional requirements in cirrhosis. Steatorrhea has a prevalence of ~45% in patients with cirrhosis. In addition to the diminished delivery of bile acids to the intestinal lumen and the reduced absorption of long-chain fatty acids, pancreatic exocrine insufficiency is often quoted as a contributing factor to malabsorption in cirrhotics. This is unlikely, as it has been demonstrated that 5% of normal pancreatic exocrine function is adequate to prevent steatorrhea.

Although the pathogenesis is unknown, the prevalence of protein-losing enteropathy is high in patients with cirrhosis. Alfonso et al., who reported a prevalence of ~40% in cirrhotic patients, could not identify a correlation of protein-losing enteropathy with severity of underlying liver disease. There is some evidence that portal hypertension plays a role in the pathogenesis of excessive intestinal protein losses, including diminished losses following portocaval shunting, but the data are inconclusive.

Other factors contributing to increased nutritional requirements in patients with cirrhosis are the caloric cost of alcohol metabolism, complications of cirrhosis (e.g., spontaneous bacterial peritonitis, repeated large-volume paracentesis, and variceal hemorrhage), and altered utilization of substrates. The effect of ascites on resting energy expenditure was elegantly demonstrated by Dolz et al., who carried out indirect calorimetry before and after large volume paracentesis. Dolz et al. found that a mean weight reduction of 16.6 kg was associated with a 9.5% reduction in resting energy expenditure compared with levels recorded prior to paracentesis ($p < 0.005$). The presence of spontaneous bacterial peritonitis (which was absent in the study by Dolz et al.) would add to metabolic cost of ascites. Unusually, celiac sprue (in patients with primary biliary cirrhosis) or ulcerative colitis (in patients with primary sclerosing cholangitis) are contributing factors to the altered nutritional requirements in patients with cirrhosis.

There is some debate about whether the caloric needs of patients with cirrhosis are increased as compared with those of controls. Eight groups of investigators have addressed this issue by measuring the basal energy expenditure of patients with cirrhosis via indirect calorimetry. The results have been conflicting. Four groups found that the basal energy expenditure of patients with compensated cirrhosis was not significantly different from that of age-matched controls. In a study by Shanbhogue et al., the resting energy expenditure of cirrhotic patients was significantly higher than that of controls when expressed in terms of kilocalories per unit of lean body mass. The same conclusions were reached by four other groups of investigators. As energy expenditure is largely determined by the tissues that make up lean body mass, it is entirely appropriate to express energy expenditure in these units. Perhaps the best information can be gleaned from a large study by Muller et al., in which a heterogeneous group of 123 patients with varied stages and etiologies of liver disease were evaluated. Muller et al. reported that, when expressed per unit of lean body mass, 18% of patients with cirrhosis had increased resting energy expenditure, 51% had normal energy expenditure compared with that of controls, and 31% had a resting energy expenditure significantly lower than that of controls. The degree of increased energy requirements, in those patients who were hypermetabolic was seen to correlate with diminished body cell mass but not with the etiology or duration of liver disease. Biochemical parameters, such as bilirubin or albumin, were not predictive of hypermetabolism. Increased resting energy expenditure is thus not a universal finding in the setting of cirrhosis but is sufficiently common to require consideration when determining the nutritional requirements of these patients. Estimations of the caloric needs of patients with cirrhosis based on the Harris-Benedict equation are frequently inaccurate, tending to underestimate the caloric needs of patients with cirrhosis by 15–18% as compared with measurement using indirect calorimetry.

Altered Substrate Utilization

Clinically and physiologically, cirrhosis is a condition of accelerated starvation. There are several studies documenting a lowered respiratory quotient, as compared with controls, in patients with liver disease in the postabsorptive state (Table 2). The only two studies that

Table 2 Respiratory Quotients in Cirrhosis[a]

Study	Cirrhotics RQ (n)	Controls RQ (n)	$p < 0.05$ vs. controls
Mullen et al., 1986	0.75 ± 0.01 (6)	0.84 ± 0.03 (6)	Yes
Owen et al., 1983	0.74 ± 0.02 (8)	0.85 ± 0.02 (10)	Yes
Muller et al., 1992	0.73 ± 0.02 (123)	0.83 ± 0.01 (30)	Yes
McCullough et al., 1992	0.74 ± 0.01 (6)	0.83 ± 0.02 (6)	Yes
Schneeweiss et al., 1990	0.72 ± 0.01 (22)	0.84 ± 0.01 (20)	Yes
Merli et al., 1980	0.78 ± 0.04 (25)	0.87 ± 0.5 (10)	Yes
McCullough et al., 1992	0.77 ± 0.01 (7)	0.83 ± 0.1 (7)	Yes
Jhangiani et al., 1986	0.84 ± 0.00 (8)	0.83 ± 0.04 (7)	No
Petrides et al., 1991	0.82 ± 0.03 (8)	0.84 ± 0.01 (9)	No

[a]The figures given for the subjects with cirrhosis in the studies by Petrides et al. refer to the nonprotein portion respiratory quotient. The data for the subjects in the study by Jhangiani et al. were not corrected for urinary nitrogen excretion.

found the respiratory quotient of patients with cirrhosis to be lower, albeit not significantly so, are remarkable for the high respiratory quotient measured in the cirrhotic groups. The mean respiratory quotient of patients calculated from the combined means of these nine studies is 0.77 (n = 221) versus 0.85 (n = 105) for healthy controls. Lower respiratory quotients are indicative of increased utilization of alternative fuel substrates (i.e., protein and fat). Based on the results of these eight studies, following an overnight fast, patients with stable cirrhosis derive ~75% of their calories from fat. In healthy controls, the proportion of calories derived from fat is ~35%. This diminished respiratory quotient is secondary chiefly to the increased oxidation of lipids, with concomitantly attenuated glucose oxidation. The mechanism of the increased utilization of alternative fuels is unclear, although Petrides et al. have demonstrated marked insulin resistance in cirrhosis. Insulin resistance in liver disease is associated with reduced hepatic glycogen production and impaired muscle glycogen synthesis. Of note is that this early utilization of fat and protein can be ameliorated by frequent feeding. In a study by Swart et al., a late evening meal had a positive effect on nitrogen balance in patients with cirrhosis as compared with an equicaloric diet without a late evening meal.

Altered Protein and Amino Acid Metabolism

Changes in protein metabolism are the most important of the metabolic changes associated with chronic liver disease and are thus discussed in detail. When the liver fails, it is the loss of hepatic regulation of protein metabolism that results rapidly in death. The alterations in amino acid and protein metabolism associated with liver disease are characterized by low levels of circulating BCAA (leucine, isoleucine, and valine) and elevated levels of circulating aromatic amino acids (AAA) (phenylalanine and tyrosine, tryptophan, and methionine). It is widely believed that the changes in amino acid metabolism play a role in the pathogenesis of many of the complications of cirrhosis, such as portosystemic encephalopathy.

Despite the clinical associations of liver disease with emaciation, formal study of protein metabolism in the setting of liver disease has yielded conflicting results. A variety of methodologies have been utilized in the study of protein metabolism in liver disease, each with its own limitations. It is important to point out that the studies reviewed in this section comprise a heterogeneous mix of patients with liver disease. Although those studies that have best characterized their study populations are referred to, there is still remarkable diversity of:

Severity and characterization of liver disease
Degree of insulin resistance and/or deficiency in subjects with cirrhosis
Concomitant drug treatments
Biochemical and hormonal profiles
Age and gender matching of controls

As nitrogen is a major component of all protein molecules, the net whole-body balance of nitrogen has long been used as an index of protein balance. Even under optimal conditions, precise nitrogen balance studies involve an exacting process, with a multitude of associated pitfalls. Fecal nitrogen losses contribute substantially to total nitrogen excretion and are frequently altered in liver disease. Nitrogen losses from skin are presumed to be fixed and are derived from published estimations. Despite these limitations, there have been four major studies evaluating nitrogen balance in patients with liver disease. In a study by Gabuzda et al., patients with stable cirrhosis were given protein intake ranging from 0–100 g/day (approximately 0–1.4 g/kg/day). Gabuzda et al. reported that at a protein intake of 75 g/day (~1.1 g/kg/day), all of the study subjects with stable cirrhosis were in a positive nitrogen balance. Of 11 patients ingesting 50 g/day of protein, 2 were in positive nitrogen balance. These data have been confirmed by other authors. The sum of these studies suggests that the amount of protein required by patients with *stable* cirrhosis to maintain a positive nitrogen balance is similar to the requirements of subjects without liver disease. It is worth remembering, however, that nitrogen balance studies in patients with chronic liver disease have a bias to underestimate nitrogen losses.

The most recent and probably most informative data regarding protein metabolism in the setting of liver disease has incorporated the use of isotopes of leucine as tracers. Leucine is an essential amino acid and makes up from 6–8% of the constituent proteins of the body. Leucine contains six carbon atoms. The 1-carbon (carboxyl moiety) is not synthesized in mammals. Leucine is reversibly transaminated to its ketoacid, ketoisocaproic acid (KIC), in skeletal muscle and oxidized almost exclusively in the liver. The oxidation of KIC is irreversible and generates CO_2. If the 1-carbon of leucine is labeled (with ^{13}C or ^{14}C) and infused as a tracer, the label will appear in CO_2 breath samples (Fig. 1). Since it is possible to measure ^{13}C-KIC enrichment in plasma and KIC is the immediate precursor of oxidation, it is possible to directly quantify leucine oxidation. In the steady state, as the 1-carbon moiety is not synthesized in humans, dilution of labeled leucine occurs either by leucine appearing through protein breakdown (endogenous leucine flux) or through dietary leucine

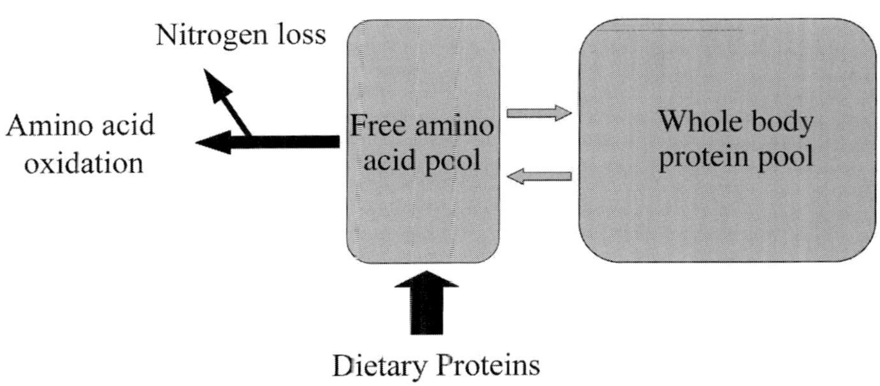

Figure 1 A simple model to study whole-body protein turnover in humans. In this model, the total protein content in the body is assigned to a single pool, the size of which is determined by the balance between protein breakdown and protein synthesis. The free amino acid pool (intra- and extracellular) is determined by the balance between the rate of appearance and disappearance of amino acids from this pool. The appearance of essential amino acids stems from protein breakdown and diet, although nonessential amino acids are synthesized in the body. The amino acids disappear from the system either by irreversible loss (oxidation) and eventual nitrogen loss or by incorporation into protein (protein synthesis). In the fasting state, essential amino acids such as leucine appear only from protein breakdown. A carboxyl moiety [e.g., L(1-^{13}C)] of leucine disappears only by its oxidation or synthesis. In a steady state leucine flux (estimated from the dilution of isotopic label) is the same as leucine appearance rate (protein breakdown) and leucine disappearance rate (synthesis and oxidation). By measuring flux and oxidation, synthesis rate (i.e., nonoxidative leucine flux) is calculated (i.e., flux minus oxidation).

Table 3 Leucine Tracer Studies of Postabsorptive (Fasting) Whole-Body Protein Turnover in Cirrhosis[a]

Author	Isotope	Cirrhotics (n)	Controls (n)	Protein breakdown	Leucine oxidation	Protein synthesis
Shanbhogue, 1987	L-(1-^{13}C)	32	7	↔	↓	N/A
Petrides et al., 1991	L-(1-^{14}C)	8	9	↔	↔	↔
Morrison, 1990	L-(1-^{13}C)	8	11	↔	↑	↓
Millikan et al., 1985	L-(^{15}N,1-^{13}C)	8	5	↔	↔	↔
McCullough et al., 1992	L-(1-^{13}C)	7	7	↑	↑	↑
Mullen et al., 1986	L-(1-^{13}C)	6	6	↔	N/A	↔
Tessari et al., 1994	^{13}C and ^{14}C	11	11	↑	N/A	N/A

[a]Upward arrows indicate a significant increase ($p < 0.05$), downward arrows indicate a significant decrease ($p < 0.05$) and horizontal arrows indicate no significant difference versus controls. The only study to normalize for body cell mass was by McCullough et al. The subjects in the study by Shanbhogue et al. had end-stage liver disease and were awaiting orthotopic liver transplantation.

absorption (exogenous leucine flux). Calculations of amino acid kinetics based on leucine metabolism are performed in the steady state based on a stochastic or reciprocal-pool model.

Table 3 summarizes the major studies of protein metabolism and liver disease incorporating leucine as a tracer. Examination of Table 3 reveals a diversity of results regarding whole-body protein metabolism in liver disease based on leucine tracer studies. The diversity of the results by the various authors of these studies can be explained on the basis of the disparate methods incorporated in each of the studies.

In the study by Shanbhogue et al., leucine kinetics were expressed as absolute values, without any normalization for body composition or weight. In the study of Mullen et al., total body water alone was measured as an index of fat-free body mass. Total body water will have included nonmetabolically active extracellular water, which is increased in patients with cirrhosis. The only study to calculate leucine kinetics normalized for the amount of metabolically active tissue (body cell mass) present was by McCullough et al. In this study, leucine oxidation was found to be higher in patients with cirrhosis as compared with controls when results were calculated using KIC as a precursor in a reciprocal-pool model but not when precursor calculations were made with leucine, using a reciprocal-pool model.

Protein and Amino Acid Metabolism in the Fed State

All of the isotope studies mentioned so far have studied protein kinetics in the postabsorptive state. Protein and amino acid kinetics may also be altered during or following a meal. The effect of cirrhosis on whole-body protein and amino acid metabolism during an amino acid load has been studied by several authors. Four of these studies compared fed leucine kinetics in patients with cirrhosis to those of controls (Table 4). Three of these studies found a similar inhibition of amino acid flux (protein breakdown) during amino acid ± insulin infusion in cirrhotic patients as compared with controls. Amino acid oxidation also increases in a similar fashion in response to a meal in patients with cirrhosis and controls. The effect of cirrhosis on amino acid and insulin stimulation of whole-body protein synthesis is

Table 4 Effect of Cirrhosis on Fed-State Amino Acid Kinetics Versus Controls[a]

Author	Isotope of leucine	Cirrhotics (*n*)	Controls (*n*)	Protein breakdown	Leucine oxidation	Protein synthesis
Tessari et al., 1994	(^{13}C) and ($^2H_3$)	11	11	↑	N/A	N/A
Petrides et al., 1991	L-(1-^{14}C)	8	9	↔	↔	↔
Tessari et al., 1996	(^{13}C) and ($^2H_3$)	11	11	↔	↔	↓
Millikan et al., 1985	L-(^{15}N,-1-^{13}C)	8	5	↔	↔	↔

[a]Upward arrows indicate a significant increase ($p < 0.05$), downward arrows indicate a significant decrease ($p < 0.05$) and horizontal arrows indicate no significant difference versus controls. The subjects in both of the studies by Tessari et al. had normal fasting plasma leucine levels, which are typically elevated in cirrhosis. These subjects may have had an early stage of disease. Histological evidence of cirrhosis was not available in all of the cirrhotic subjects in these studies. The study by Petrides et al. involved the infusion of much higher concentrations of aromatic amino acids than that of Tessari et al. The concentrations of amino acids administered in the study by Millikan et al. were not stated.

more controversial, however. In the most recently published work, by Tessari et al., there was a striking attenuation of aminogenesis-induced protein synthesis in patients with cirrhosis during a BCAA-enriched/AAA-deficient infusion (with concomitant insulin and glucose administration). Normal subjects underwent a 20% increase above baseline levels in protein synthesis (as measured by the nonoxidative portion of leucine flux) during the amino acid, insulin, and glucose infusions. The rate of protein synthesis failed to increase at all above baseline levels in the subjects with cirrhosis during similar infusions. This attenuation of aminogenesis- and insulin-induced increase in protein synthesis would contribute to an overall protein catabolic state in cirrhosis. Furthermore, the inability of patients with cirrhosis to mount the expected increase in protein synthesis during the infusion of BCAA and insulin may impair processes such as the maintenance of mucosal integrity, cellular immunity, and the production of acute-phase proteins. Secondarily, these changes may contribute to the failure of BCAA-based nutritional therapy to consistently improve outcomes in complications from chronic liver disease. The finding by Tessari et al. of an attenuation in the aminogenic increase in protein synthesis is in contrast to the results of an earlier study by Petrides et al. In that study, patients with stable cirrhosis and normals exhibited a similar increase in protein synthesis during the infusion of mixed amino acids and insulin. These apparently contradictory results might be explained on the basis of differences in the concentrations of amino acids and infusion rates during the two studies. Petrides et al. used a standard amino acid formula, richer in phenylalanine, than did Tessari et al. [(PHE) 232 mmol/L vs. (PHE) 6.1 mmol/L]. The ability of insulin to increase whole-body protein synthesis is dependent upon substrate (amino acid) availability. Furthermore, it was recently demonstrated that hyperglucagonemia is central in the disposal of amino acids during an amino acid load and that physiological hyperglucagonemia inhibits the aminogenic increase in protein synthesis. The relative lack of the aromatic amino acids in the infusate, together with hyperglucagonemia, may be responsible for an inability to increase protein synthesis during the amino acid, insulin, and glucose infusion by creating a relative unavailability of phenylalanine for incorporation into protein synthesis.

The pathogenesis of the changes in protein metabolism that occur in chronic liver disease is unclear. A number of changes in the levels of circulating hormones are associated with liver disease (Table 5), many of which are known to be important in the regulation of protein synthesis. It is likely that hyperglucagonemia, insulin resistance, diminished andro-

Table 5 Effect of Cirrhosis on Circulating Hormone Levels[a]

Hormone	Effect of cirrhosis	Hormone	Effect of cirrhosis
Growth hormone	↑	Testosterone	↓
Prolactin	↑	Cortisol	↓
Glucagon	↑	T_3, FT_3, FT_4	↓
VIP	↑	IGF-1 and IGF-2	↓
Insulin	↑		
Catecholamines	↑		
Estradiol	↑		

[a]Glucagon excess exerts a catabolic effect in the postabsorptive and the fed states. The insulin-like growth factors and testosterone, which are low in cirrhosis, have an anabolic effect in normal physiology. The physiological effects of hyperinsulinemia on protein metabolism are controversial. Growth hormone exerts much of its anabolic effects via the insulin-like growth factors, which are hepatically synthesized.

genic steroids, and insulin-like growth factors contribute to the overall protein-catabolic state of cirrhosis. The roles of the hormonal changes that occur concomitantly with cirrhosis have yet to be determined. Lowered levels of micronutrients and trace metals and elevated levels of cytokines, such as tumor necrosis factor alpha and the interleukins, may also play a role.

Summary of Altered Amino Acid and Protein Metabolism in Cirrhosis

Despite the constraints inherent to the methodologies incorporated in the studies discussed above, some features of altered amino acid and protein metabolism in the setting of cirrhosis seem likely:

Protein breakdown (as measured by endogenous leucine flux) and the use of amino acids as a fuel source (as measured by leucine oxidation) are increased in the postabsorptive state (when calculated using a reciprocal pool model and when normalized for body cell mass).

The whole-body protein synthesis response to a meal (an amino acid infusion) is diminished.

RECOMMENDATIONS FOR NUTRITIONAL SUPPORT OF PATIENTS WITH CHRONIC LIVER DISEASE

Based on the aggregate of the changes in metabolism associated with chronic liver disease that have been discussed in this chapter, it is possible to make some rational suggestions about the nutritional support of patients with chronic liver disease.

Assessment of Nutritional Status

Dr. Lee Schamroth is quoted as saying that "We only see what we look for and we only look for what we know." This is particularly pertinent to malnutrition in patients with chronic liver disease, which is often undiagnosed. Because of the high prevalence of malnutrition and micronutrient deficiencies, *all* patients with cirrhosis and patients with complications of alcoholic liver disease of any stage should be evaluated for the presence of malnutrition. Many tests that are used as part of a nutritional assessment are unreliable in the setting of liver disease, as they may be altered by liver disease in the absence of malnutrition. These include measurement of any of the hepatically synthesized plasma proteins (including albumin, prealbumin, pseudocholinesterase, and retinol-binding protein). Other tests are unreliable due to medications and complications of chronic liver disease (e.g., ascites). These tests include total-body potassium measurements, dual-photon densitometry, and total body electrical conductivity. Fortunately, some of the best measurements of nutritional status are also the cheapest and most widely available. Body cell mass measurement and neutron activation scanning are both highly accurate means of measuring body composition but are expensive, difficult to perform, and available at only a few centers. With these caveats in mind, the nutritional assessment should include the following:

Detailed history and physical examination incorporating the subjective global nutritional assessment. (Anthropometric measurements, such as skin-fold thickness, may be of use as an objective serial measurement)
Screening for common micronutrient deficiencies
Vitamins A, D, and E
Prothrombin time
Serum zinc level (serum zinc levels may be normal in the setting of depleted whole-body zinc stores but low serum zinc levels correspond to low whole-body zinc stores)

Supplemental doses of these micronutrients for patients with documented deficiencies are:

Vitamin D, 25,000–50,000 U thrice weekly
Vitamin E, 400 mg/day
Vitamin A, 25,000 U thrice weekly
Calcium, 500 mg PO tid
Zinc sulfate, 220 mg PO tid

Additional screening measures should include:

Calcium levels and bone mineral density in patients with cholestatic (primary biliary cirrhosis and primary sclerosing cholangitis) and autoimmune liver disease
Thiamine, B_{12}, and folate in patients with complications from alcoholic liver disease

NUTRITIONAL SUPPORT MEASURES FOR THE OUTPATIENT WITH COMPENSATED CHRONIC LIVER DISEASE

Frequent meals (including a bedtime snack)
Intake of 30 kcal/kg/day nonprotein calories (55% carbohydrate: 35% fat: 10% protein)
At least 1.1 g/kg/day protein

NUTRITIONAL SUPPORT MEASURES FOR THE OUTPATIENT WITH CHRONIC LIVER DISEASE AND ASCITES

As above plus:

- 2–4 g/day sodium (dietary education is extremely valuable in achieving this)
- Gentle fluid restriction (≥ 20 mL of liquids per kilogram of dry weight per day (Stringent fluid restrictions tend to result in prerenal azotemia.)
- Furosemide/spironolactone when the above fail (ascites increases basal energy expenditure and increases the risk of spontaneous bacterial peritonitis.)

NUTRITIONAL AND OTHER SUPPORT MEASURES FOR THE PATIENT WITH PORTOSYSTEMIC ENCEPHALOPATHY

Exclude precipitating cause:

- Poor compliance (diet or medications)
- GI bleeding
- Infection (e.g., spontaneous bacterial peritonitis)
- Drug effect (e.g., alcohol, benzodiazepines)
- Other metabolic causes of altered mental status (e.g., electrolyte disturbance)
- Subdural hematoma

When an evaluation for precipitating causes of PSE has been performed and, where possible, appropriate measures to correct contributing factors have been instigated, the following treatments should be administered:

- Lactulose (titrate to achieve two to four stools per day)
- Zinc sulfate 220 mg PO tid
- Metronidazole, 250–500 mg PO tid (only acutely in patients who have failed to respond to the administration of lactulose and zinc)
- Protein restriction (0.25 g/kg/day) until episode has resolved or for 5 days, whichever is shorter
- In patients who are refractory to or fail to tolerate standard therapies and in those who develop chronic PSE, consider branched chain amino acid (BCAA)-enriched/aromatic amino acid (AAA)-deficient supplements—e.g., NutriHep—to maintain protein intake at ≥ 1.0 g/kg/day. Other options in these rare patients include vegetable protein, casein, and alpha–keto acid diets. These alternative therapies are seldom required. (Alternative treatments of portosystemic encephalopathy are discussed in more detail in Chap. 36.)
- Long-term protein restriction is never indicated.

NUTRITIONAL SUPPORT MEASURES FOR THE HOSPITALIZED PATIENT WITH COMPLICATIONS OF CHRONIC LIVER DISEASE

- Initiate calorie counts.
- Obtain indirect calorimetry when possible (35 kcal/kg of ideal weight if indirect calorimetry unavailable).

Initiate nutritional supplements early (upon admission for alcoholic hepatitis; see Chap. 15) when intake is deficient—use the enteric route whenever possible.
Only restrict protein when absolutely necessary (i.e., in fulminant disease and PSE grades II–IV, and for as short a period as possible).

NUTRITIONAL SUPPORT MEASURES FOLLOWING ORTHOTOPIC LIVER TRANSPLANTATION

Presume that patients will need nutritional support
Give enteric supplementation day 1 postoperatively versus total parenteral nutrition (TPN)
Continue until calorie intake counts approach needs (needs based upon Harris-Benedict equation + 20%)
Add trace elements if TPN lasts longer than 7 days (trace element reserves are frequently depleted in transplant recipients).
Let the patient dictate diet; avoid rigid rules about introduction of liquids and regular diet
Low-bacteria diet when taking by mouth (continue for first month)
Avoid pharmacological treatment of constipation and diarrhea when possible

FUTURE DIRECTIONS

Clearly, the nutritional therapy of patients with chronic liver disease should be tailored to the individual patient. Ideally, nutritional therapy will be further directed at specific liver diseases. Alcoholic hepatitis has been the focus of recent investigation. In an animal model of this disease, saturated fatty acids (palm oil) were shown to ameliorate the histological and biochemical effects of acute alcoholic hepatitis. Human trials are currently under way. In a separate study, medium-chain triglycerides and vitamin E supplementation were shown to reduce the severity of established experimental alcoholic liver injury. Zinc supplementation has been shown to be efficacious in the treatment of portosystemic encephalopathy in four of five trials. The potential usefulness of omega-3 fatty acids and glutamine in the treatment of chronic liver diseases is also a matter of some speculation. While the failure of BCAA-enriched/AAA-depleted nutritional supplements to consistently improve outcomes in the management of portosystemic encephalopathy has been a source of frustration, recent work suggests a possible role for these preparations in the management of malnourished patients awaiting orthotopic liver transplantation. The potential appeal of safe and relatively inexpensive nutritional therapies for chronic liver diseases or their complications is obvious.

BIBLIOGRAPHY

Charlton MR. Protein metabolism and liver disease. Ballière's Clin Endocrinol Metab 1997; 10: 617–635.
DiCecco SR, Wieners EJ, Wiesner RH, Southorn PA, Plevak DJ, Krom RA. Assessment of nutritional status of patients with end-stage liver disease undergoing liver transplantation. Mayo Clinic Proc 1989; 64:95–102.
Dolz C, Raurich JM, Ibanez J, Obrador A, Marse P, Gaya J. Ascites increases the resting energy expenditure in liver cirrhosis. Gastroenterology 1991; 100:738–744.

Gabuzda GJ, Davidson CS. Protein metabolism in patients with hepatic cirrhosis of the liver. Ann NY Acad Sci 1954; 776–785.

Lockwood AH, Ginsberg MD, Rhoades HM, Gutierrez MT. Cerebral glucose metabolism after portacaval shunting in the rat: patterns of metabolism and implications for the pathogenesis of hepatic encephalopathy. J Clin Invest 1986; 78:86–95.

McCullough AJ, Mullen KD, Kalhan SC. Body cell mass and leucine metabolism in cirrhosis. Gastroenterology 1992; 102:1325–1333.

Mendenhall CL, Tosch T, Weesner RE, Garcia-Pont P, Goldberg SJ, Kiernan T, Seeff LB, Sorell M, Tamburro C, Zetterman R, et al. VA cooperative study on alcoholic hepatitis: II. Prognostic significance of protein-calorie malnutrition. Am J Clin Nutr 1986; 43:213–218.

Muller MJ, Lautz HU, Plogmann B, Burger M, Korber J, Schmidt FW. Energy expenditure and substrate oxidation in patients with cirrhosis: the impact of cause, clinical staging and nutritional state. Hepatology 1992; 15:782–794.

Petrides AS, Groop LC, Riely CA, DeFronzo RA. Effect of physiologic hyperinsulinemia on glucose and lipid metabolism in cirrhosis. J Clin Invest 1991; 88:561–570.

Swart GR, Zillikens MC, van Vuure JK, van den Berg JW. Effect of a late evening meal on nitrogen balance in patients with cirrhosis of the liver. Br Med J 1989; 299:1202–1203.

17
Management of Gallstones

Eneya Mulagha and Hans Fromm
The George Washington University Medical Center, Washington, D.C.

INTRODUCTION

This chapter focuses on the medical management of cholecystolithiasis. (See Chap. 18 for management of bile duct stones.) About 90% of gallstones are formed on the basis of a disturbance of cholesterol metabolism characterized by increased biliary secretion of cholesterol and consequent supersaturation of bile in cholesterol. The opportunities, as far as effective medical treatment of gallstones are concerned, are greatest in cholesterol stones, since, in selected cases, they can be dissolved with the bile acid ursodiol (ursodeoxycholic acid). A brief review of the pathogenesis of cholesterol gallstones appears useful because it provides the basis for an understanding of the mechanism of action of medical dissolution treatment with ursodiol.

PATHOGENESIS

The pathogenesis of cholesterol gallstones is characterized by several steps. The first and most important mechanism underlying gallstone formation consists of an increased biliary secretion of cholesterol. However, gallstones form only if cholesterol crystallizes, a process promoted by the action of nucleating proteins secreted in the presence of bile supersaturated in cholesterol. Stone growth is facilitated by incomplete emptying of the gallbladder. Animal studies suggest that this type of gallbladder dysfunction may be the result of the high concentrations of cholesterol in the bile.

Recently, two possibly important factors in the etiology and pathogenesis of gallstones have received attention. One is the role of a gallstone gene (*Lith* 1) in the high incidence of gallstones in inbred mice, which are characterized by a high biliary secretion of cholesterol. In this animal model, *Lith* 1 has been mapped to chromosome 2 by quantitative trait locus analysis. The gene for a sister-P-glycoprotein, which is a canalicular membrane bile acid transporter and also located in chromosome 2, is overexpressed in this mouse strain. It is not yet clear how the increase in bile acid secretion is linked to gallstone formation in this animal model. The second possibly important pathogenetic factor, which has recently come into focus, relates to the finding of bacterial DNA in the inner and outer layers of mixed cholesterol gallstones. It is of interest that, in a preliminary study, bacterial DNA was not detected in three out of three pure cholesterol gallstones. How bacteria influence gallstone formation is not clear. They may be involved in several mechanisms, including interaction with the bile duct epithelium via signal transduction and stimulation of the secretion of nucleating factors as well as by direct participation in the physical chemistry of gallstone growth.

Ursodiol ingestion and subsequent enrichment of bile fundamentally intervene in the chain of events leading to the formation of gallstones by decreasing the biliary secretion and saturation of cholesterol as well as by inhibiting the nucleation process in bile.

EPIDEMIOLOGY, NATURAL HISTORY, AND CLINICAL PRESENTATION

Gallstones are very common. They are present in about 10% of the population in the United States and Europe. Their prevalence increases with age. Approximately 90% of the gallstones are either cholesterol stones (> 50% cholesterol content) or mixed stones (20–50% cholesterol content). The remaining 10% are pigment stones.

Fortunately, 70–80% of the gallstones are asymptomatic. The risk for an asymptomatic gallstone carrier to develop biliary pain is 1–4% per year. Biliary pain is not "colicky." Typically, it is steady in character, localized to the epigastrium or right upper abdomen, has a crescendo-plateau-decrescendo course, and lasts at least 30 min. Most often, it occurs at night. Biliary pain is frequently accompanied by nausea, vomiting, and diaphoresis.

The annual risk of the development of a biliary complication, such as acute cholecystitis, acute pancreatitis, bile duct obstruction, or ascending cholangitis is much lower—i.e., about 0.1–0.4%. It is important to remember that a biliary complication is virtually always preceded by attacks, usually multiple attacks, of biliary pain. Exceptions to this rule occur in old age or such conditions as immunodeficiency, poorly controlled diabetes mellitus, and renal failure. In those conditions, complications may develop without preceding episodes of distinct biliary pain.

MANAGEMENT OF GALLSTONES

Asymptomatic ("Silent") Gallstones

Asymptomatic gallstones should be managed expectantly—i.e., nonoperatively—since the majority of gallstone carriers never develop significant symptoms or complications from their stones. Frequently, a cholecystectomy is performed for symptoms that are not caused by gallstones—i.e., nonspecific symptoms due to functional bowel disorders (irritable bowel syndrome, dyspepsia etc.)—or abdominal pain related to other conditions, such as peptic ulcer or inflammatory bowel disease.

In this context, it is also important not to overinterpret ultrasonographic findings. A thickened gallbladder wall or pericholecystic fluid collection, for example, is not a specific sign of acute cholecystitis. However, the ultrasonographic Murphy's sign (focal gallbladder tenderness under the ultrasound transducer), although somewhat operator-dependent, strongly points toward the presence of acute cholecystitis.

Symptomatic Gallstones

Symptomatic gallstones (i.e., stones that cause biliary pain or complications) are, in most cases, managed surgically. Cholecystectomy represents the treatment of choice for the majority of symptomatic gallstone patients. Laparoscopic cholecystectomy (LC) has become the main method for removing the gallbladder. Since LC has many advantages in comparison to open cholecystectomy—namely, faster postoperative recovery, less postoperative discomfort, and smaller incision scars—its introduction has lead to a markedly higher use of surgical treatment in the management of gallstones. Increases in the rate of cholecystectomy from 21–60% have been reported. Patients undergoing LC are younger and healthier than they were in the pre-LC era, indicating that the threshold for a cholecystectomy has been lowered. Although the safety of LC has been cited to be equal to that of open cholecystectomy when performed by surgeons experienced with this procedure, LC is associated with a "learning curve." Surgeons who are less experienced or who perform LC infrequently have an increased rate of complications. Overall, in comparison to open cholecystectomy, LC is associated with a higher rate and a greater severity of complications. Bile duct injuries are twice as common in LC (about 0.75%) than in open cholecystectomy (about 0.3%).

Careful consideration of the available medical treatment options, however, is critical for the management of those patients who either refuse surgery or present contraindications to operative treatment (see below). Once a decision is made that a patient is a candidate for surgery, the question that needs to be considered is whether the operation should be performed after the first episode of biliary pain or whether the patient may wait until the pain recurs.

An analysis addressing this question has indicated that there is virtually no difference in outcome—i.e., no difference in life expectancy—between these two management approaches. However, life expectancy would decrease if the patient waited until a complication occurred. While the cumulative risks for a 30-year-old gallstone patient dying from gallstone disease by the age of 50 would be 0.11 and 0.14%, respectively, with the first two treatment strategies, the figure is 0.46% if the patient waits until a complication occurs.

In terms of biliary pain recurrence, about 50% of the patients remain free of pain during the first year of follow-up and in about 30% of cases there is no recurrence of the pain in 10 years. In other words, approximately one-third of patients have no further symptoms after their first episode of biliary pain.

Therefore, the patient who experiences his or her first episode of biliary pain should be informed that, as far as life expectancy is concerned, waiting until the pain recurs has the same outcome as immediate surgery. The decision to wait until the biliary pain recurs rather than to operate after the first episode of pain is also influenced by the fact that biliary complications are, with the exceptions described above, virtually always preceded by repeated attacks of biliary pain.

Symptomatic patients who refuse surgery or present a significant surgical risk are eligible for medical management. The success of medical therapy is dependent upon the fulfillment of selection criteria specific for the different currently available treatment modalities. Unfortunately, only a minority of gallstone patients fulfill the selection criteria associated with a successful outcome.

Oral Dissolution Therapy with Ursodiol

Ursodiol is a naturally occurring dihydroxy bile acid that suppresses the secretion of cholesterol into bile to levels below saturation. As a result, cholesterol slowly leaches out of a gallstone, leading to its gradual dissolution. The recommended dose of ursodiol is 8–10 mg/kg/body weight/day divided into two doses, after breakfast and dinner, respectively. The treatment is successful (complete dissolution) in up to 90% of the cases with noncalcified stones not larger than 5 mm in diameter. Stones that are larger than 1 cm rarely dissolve. If dissolution takes place, it does so at a mean rate of approximately 1 mm per month. Gallstones recur after dissolution in about 30–50% of cases at an annual rate of about 10% during the first 3–5 years. The recurrence rate is lower in patients who had solitary stones as compared with those having multiple stones.

Bile acid dissolution treatment is effective only in patients with noncalcified cholesterol gallstones in a functioning (i.e., contractile) gallbladder. The presence of gallstone calcifications can be detected on either a plain x-ray film or by computed tomography (CT) of the abdomen. Although CT is about 30% more sensitive than conventional x-ray in the detection of calcifications, minor calcifications visualized only by CT do not preclude successful dissolution therapy. However, the success of ursodiol treatment is highest in gallstones showing no CT evidence of calcifications.

Fortunately, about 90% of symptomatic gallstone patients have a functioning gallbladder. The latter is almost invariably the case in patients who present without clinical or laboratory evidence of complications. Therefore, there is no need to document gallbladder function by an oral cholecystogram (visualization of the gallbladder) or an upper abdominal ultrasonogram (demonstration of contraction of the gallbladder after intravenous injection of cholecystokinin). In the National Cooperative Gallstone Study, no convincing relationship was documented between the success of dissolution therapy with chemodeoxycholic acid (the slightly hepatotoxic 7-alpha epimer of ursodiol) and visualization of the gallbladder by oral cholecystography.

A major advantage of ursodiol lies in its safety. It is not only virtually free of any side effects but also expresses hepatoprotective properties, which have led to the successful use of ursodiol in the treatment of primary biliary cirrhosis and of other cholestatic liver diseases.

As mentioned, gallstones recur in 30–50% of the cases after dissolution. The recurrence can be decreased by maintaining the patient on ursodiol—for example, generally 300 mg per day—which represents half the therapeutic dose. However, because of its cost, maintenance therapy is not recommended with the exception of cases that present a major surgical risk. In such cases, the full dose of ursodiol, generally 300 mg twice a day, should be considered to achieve optimal protection from recurrence.

Extracorporeal Shockwave Lithotripsy (ESWL)

ESWL is used in Europe and Japan, but despite an impressive body of data from the United States, Europe, and Japan proving its efficacy and safety, it has not been approved by the FDA for use in the United States. The lack of approval by this agency relates to its insistence on the performance of controlled clinical trials. Manufacturers of lithotriptors are reluctant to make the substantial investments necessary for controlled trials because profits are expected to be low owing to the wide use and popularity of LC.

ESWL has been extremely successful in properly selected patients with noncalcified gallstones. The successful outcome of ESWL is, to a large extent, determined by the degree of fragmentation of the gallstones. Gallbladder clearance of gallstones improves and stone recurrence decreases with decreasing fragment size. Fragments that are too small to be measurable by ultrasound ("pulverization" of gallstones) are associated with the highest success rate. As in the case of oral bile acid dissolution therapy, patient selection is an important determinant of the results of ESWL; radiolucency as well as the number and size of stones are critical factors. Emptying as well as residual and fasting volumes of the gallbladder also influence the outcome of ESWL.

The highest success rates, those above 80%, are seen with solitary stones that are not larger than 2 cm. Recent studies aiming at so-called pulverization of the stones by repeated ESWL sessions show success in up to 100% even with larger and multiple stones. High success rates with this pulverization method have also been reported with calcified stones. As mentioned, pulverization implies the fragmentation of the gallstones into very small, sand-like particles. It is of interest that high success rates were achieved without adjuvant therapy with ursodiol. The role of adjuvant bile acid therapy before and after ESWL of gallstones requires further study. However, it appears that patients with contractile gallbladders may not require ursodiol after ESWL.

The incidence of complications is very low after lithotripsy. Bile duct obstruction and gallstone pancreatitis caused by fragments lodged in the common bile duct occur in less than 1% of the cases. Consequently, ERCP and sphincterotomy are rarely needed in patients who have undergone ESWL. There is virtually no mortality with this procedure when properly performed.

Gallstone recurrence rates after lithotripsy vary from 11–26% for a 24-month period using actuarial analysis. In most studies, stones continued to recur as patients were followed after ESWL. However, the rate of recurrence usually declined with increasing length of follow-up and rarely exceeded a total of 50–60%. In patients with single gallstones, the recurrence seems lower than 50%. Furthermore, stone recurrence may be significantly reduced by application of the described "pulverization" method; it also appears to be lower in patients with unimpaired gallbladder emptying.

Topical Dissolution with Methyl Tert-Butyl Ether (MTBE)

This treatment method involves the perfusion of the gallbladder with a powerful organic solvent. The solvent is perfused through the gallbladder via a pigtail catheter, which is introduced either transhepatically or retrogradely using an endoscope. Special pumps designed to assure optimal perfusion of the solvent through the gallbladder are being studied, but there appear to be insufficient data to evaluate the efficacy and safety of such pump devices. Most published studies involve frequent manual injections of the solvent and aspiration of the solute over a period of several hours.

The gallstones can be dissolved within a few hours, but they must be noncalcified cholesterol stones. As noted, CT scan is the most sensitive and reliable method for excluding gallstone calcifications. The rarely used method of topical gallstone dissolution is reserved for properly selected patients who present a high surgical risk. The procedure is invasive and requires personnel who are familiar with the handling of MTBE, a volatile and potentially explosive solvent. In view of the hazardous aspects of this solvent, the procedure must be carried out in a well-ventilated room.

BIBLIOGRAPHY

Boscaini M, Piccini-Leopardi M, Andreotti F, Montori A. Gallstone pulverization strategy in patients treated with extracorporeal lithotripsy and follow-up results of maintenance treatment with ursodeoxycholic acid. Gut 1994; 35:117–121.

Friedman GD. Natural history of asymptomatic and symptomatic gallstones. Am J Surg 1993; 165: 399–404.

Fromm H, Malavolti M. Gallstone recurrence after medical therapy: viewpoints on digestive diseases. 1992; 24(1):1–7.

Lee DK, Tarr PI, Haigh SP, Lee SP. Detection and identification of bacterial gene sequences in mixed cholesterol gallstone by amplification of 16S rRNA genes. Gastroenterology 1997; 112:A513.

Leuschner U, Hellstern A, Schmid K, et al. Gallstone dissolution with methyl tert-butyl ether in 120 patients—efficacy and safety. Dig Dis Sci 1991; 36:193–197.

Legorreta AP, Silber JH, Costantino GW, Kobylinski RW, Zatz SL. Increased cholecystectomy rate after the introduction of laparoscopic cholecystectomy. JAMA 1993; 270:1429–1432.

Levenson DE, Fromm H. Medical management of gallbladder disease. In: Zakim D, Boyer TD, eds. Hepatology: A Textbook of Liver Disease. Philadelphia: Saunders, 1996:1877–1897.

Pauletzki J, Sailer C, Kluppelberg U, et al. Gallbladder emptying determines early gallstone clearance after shock wave lithotripsy. Gastroenterology 1994; 107:1496–1502.

Ransohoff DF, Gracie WA. Management of patients with symptomatic gallstones: a quantitative analysis. Am J Med 1990; 88:154–160.

Soehendra N, Nam V-C, Binmoeller KF, et al. Pulverization of calcified and non-calcified gallbladder stones: extracorporeal shock wave lithotripsy used alone. Gut 1994; 35:417–422.

Steiner CA, Bass EB, Talamini MA, et al. Surgical rates and mortality for open and laparoscopic cholecystectomy in Maryland. N Engl J Med 1994; 330:403–408.

Wang DQ, Paigen B, Carey MC. Phenotypic characterization of Lith genes that determine susceptibility of cholesterol cholelithiasis in inbred mice: physical chemistry of gallbladder bile. J Lipid Res 1997; 38:1395–1411.

18
Endoscopic Management of Gallstones

Ram Chuttani, Savant Mehta, and Gottumukkala Raju
Harvard Medical School and Beth Israel Hospital, Boston, Massachusetts

Up to the mid-1970s, the only management of common bile duct (CBD) stones was surgical. This has changed in the last two decades. Endoscopic retrograde cholangiopancreaticography (ERCP) in 1969 and sphincterotomy in 1974 have allowed endoscopic access to the bile duct. With the introduction of these techniques, the management of this problem has moved from the predominantly surgical domain to the arena of endoscopists. This chapter discusses the current endoscopic management of CBD stones, reviewing various diagnostic options, techniques of endoscopic access, and stone retrieval; principles of CBD stone management in various settings are discussed.

DETECTION OF BILE DUCT STONES

Clinical, Biochemical, and Noninvasive Imaging (Ultrasound and Computed Tomography)

Diagnosis of CBD stones starts with history, physical examination, and biochemical tests, followed by noninvasive imaging studies [ultrasound and computed tomography (CT) scan]. The published data suggest that there is no single clinical, biochemical, or noninvasive imaging study that can predict the presence of CBD stones with both high sensitivity and specificity.

Clinical syndromes suggestive of choledocholithiasis include cholangitis, pancreatitis, combined cholangitis and pancreatitis, and biliary pain with abnormal liver tests. The diagnostic yield of choledocholithiasis is dependent on the clinical presentation. Choledocholithiasis is found in 36% of patients with biliary pancreatitis, 72% of patients with biliary pain and abnormal liver tests, 87% of patients with cholangitis, and nearly 100% of patients with combined cholangitis and pancreatitis.

Serial rather than a single determination of liver test abnormalities (total bilirubin, alkaline phosphatase, AST and ALT) are helpful for better stratification of patients more likely to be harboring CBD stones. In a prospective study of the value of serial determinations of liver tests abnormalities in the diagnosis of CBD stones, four patterns of liver enzyme abnormalities were observed. In patients with normalized liver tests, the diagnostic yield of CBD stones at ERCP was 13%. In those with a rapid decrease in value (> 50% as compared to the initial elevated levels), 50% had CBD stones at ERCP. In those with slowly falling values, 67% had CBD stones; while in patients with increasing abnormalities, 94% harbored CBD stones. A number of factors have been investigated to predict the presence of CBD stones. Age greater than 55, a total bilirubin level over 1.7 mg/100 mL, a dilated CBD (> 6 mm) on ultrasonography, and suspected or detected bile duct stone on ultrasonography are four independent predictors of CBD stones. The probability of finding a stone based on this four-predictor model ranged from 18% if none of them was present to 94% if all were present. Increased CBD diameter or the presence of common duct stones on ultrasonography had the highest predictive value for detecting a CBD stone (64 and 78% respectively).

Ultrasound has good sensitivity for detecting ductal dilatation. However, its sensitivity for detecting CBD stones is poor (10–50%). In fully one-third of patients with CBD stones, there may not be ductal dilatation. CT scan is superior, reaching a 70–88% sensitivity if careful thin-slice sections are studied in the pancreaticobiliary region (Fig. 1).

Newer Imaging Techniques

Endoscopic ultrasonography (EUS), spiral CT cholangiography, and magnetic resonance imaging (MRI) cholangiopancreaticography (MRCP) are recent additions for noninvasive

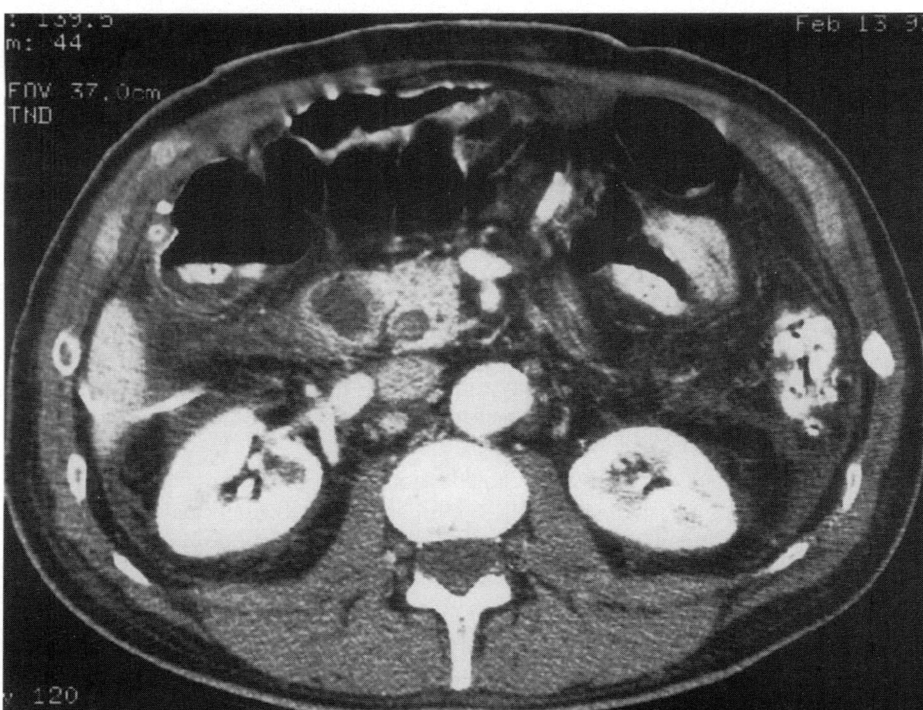

Figure 1 Helical CT scan showing a stone at the lower end of the CBD.

methods of diagnosing gallstones. All these imaging modalities, especially MRCP, have extremely high sensitivity in diagnosing CBD stones and approach that of ERCP. Their precise role in the imaging algorithm of patients suspected of having CBD stones has yet to be determined.

Biliary Endoscopic Ultrasonography (EUS)

Biliary EUS is a new, minimally invasive procedure that is highly accurate in the diagnosis of pancreatic diseases and extrahepatic cholestasis. Several centers have evaluated the diagnostic potential of EUS in patients with choledocholithiasis. Sensitivity of EUS approaches 100% for the diagnosis of CBD stones. EUS was shown to be more sensitive in the diagnosis of CBD stones than either conventional ultrasound (25%) or CT (75%). The specificity and positive predictive value were not significantly different. The negative predictive value of EUS (97%) was significantly better than that of conventional ultrasound (56%) and CT (78%). In a recent study, EUS was compared with ERCP in the evaluation of patients with CBD stones prior to surgery. Comparison of EUS with surgical exploration in 185 patients showed a sensitivity of 95%, a specificity of 96%, a negative predictive value of 96%, a positive predictive value of 95%, and an accuracy of 96%. The high negative predictive value of EUS makes it a valuable tool of great potential in avoiding an ERCP. In pregnant patients with clinical features suggestive of CBD stones, where the use of fluoroscopy is relatively contraindicated, a negative EUS study for CBD stones is very helpful. The value of high positive predictive value of EUS in the diagnosis of CBD stones is of limited clinical significance, however, as all these patients need an ERCP which can provide not only the diagnosis but also provide therapy. Other limitations of EUS in the diagnosis of CBD stones include the inability to insert the thick EUS scope with a relatively rigid distal segment into the duodenum and examine the CBD when there has been gastric surgery, especially with a Billroth II type anastamosis, the presence of pancreatic calcification or severe acute pancreatitis which interferes with visualization of distal portion of the CBD, and the presence of air in the biliary tract following endoscopic sphincterotomy or choledochal bypass. Finally, the technical skills required for both performance of the procedure and interpretation of the images prevent EUS from becoming widely available outside of referral centers.

MRCP

MRCP (Fig. 2) is an important addition to more conventional MR imaging of the pancreaticobiliary system. It visualizes static fluid-filled structures using heavily T2-weighted images with fat suppression. It is completely noninvasive, easy to perform, and does not require the use of any contrast agents or intravenous sedation. Blood clot, air, or sludge in the bile duct may result in a false-positive finding. Motion creates artifacts that limit the resolution of the image, and the patient must therefore be capable of breath-holding for short periods. This may not be necessary with the introduction of newer MRI protocols, which complete the scan within periods as short as a few seconds. It is too early to predict whether MRCP will be able to substitute routinely for diagnostic ERCP; however, it can clearly provide valuable information in patients for whom ERCP is unsuccessful or inadequate. There has been considerable improvement in technique which has increased the sensitivity and specificity of MRCP in the diagnosis of choledocholithiasis. In 1995 Guibaud et al. reported a sensitivity of 81% and a specificity of 98% in 126 patients using a

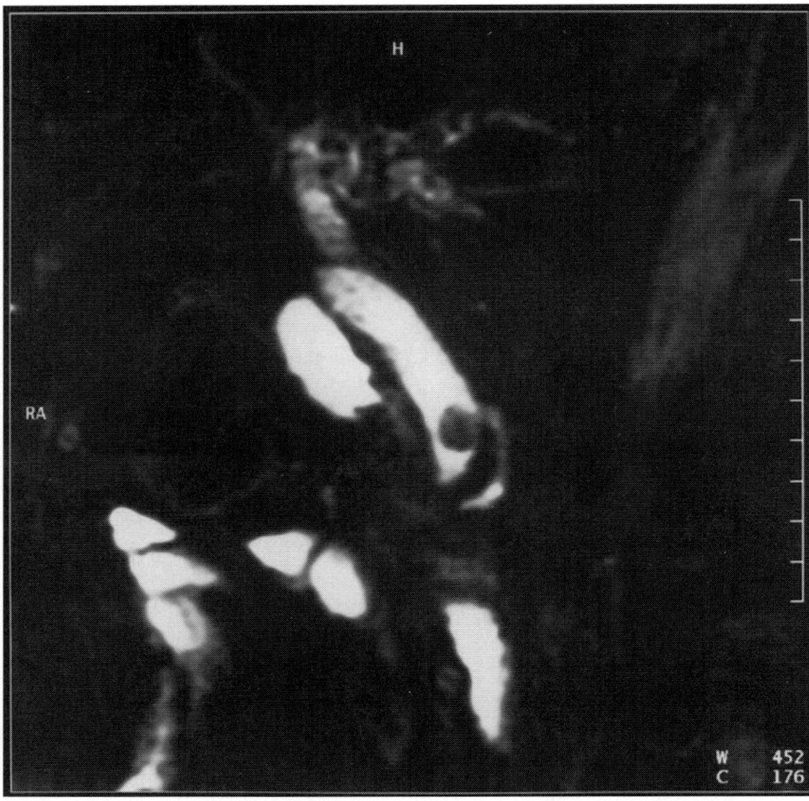

Figure 2 MRCP demonstrating a signal void in the distal CBD consistent with a stone.

body coil with lower-resolution imaging parameters. In a study by Reinhold et al. using phased-array multicoil in 110 patients scheduled for ERCP, of whom 27 proved to have CBD stones, a sensitivity of 90% and a specificity of 99% were attained. These figures have been reproduced in several recent studies. Hence it is clear that MRCP has a very high sensitivity and nearly 100% specificity and can be very useful in diagnosing choledocholithiasis.

CT Cholangiography

Recent studies have shown that CT cholangiography using high-speed helical scanners is better at illustrating the biliary system than conventional CT scanning, but the resolution of CT does not approach that of ERCP. In a recent study by Raptopoulos et al. using projectional computed tomographic cholangiopancreatography (CTCP) in 61 patients, of whom 35 had ERCP, there was no statistically significant difference between the number of biliary and pancreatic duct segments missed with ERCP compared with those missed with CTCP. CTCP provided additional information in 11 patients, less information in 7 patients, and equal information in 24 patients.

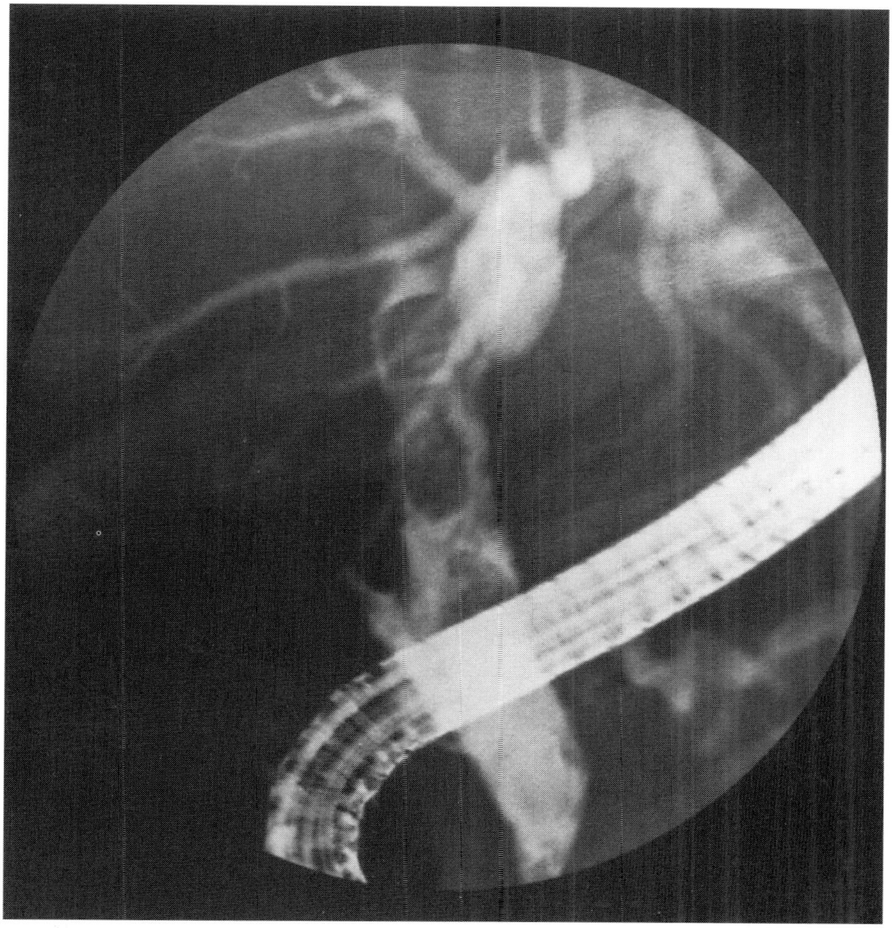

Figure 3 ERCP demonstrating three large intraductal faceted calculi.

ERCP

The diagnosis of a CBD stone is made by findings of a mobile and/or persistent filling defect on injection of iodinated contrast into the CBD. ERCP (Fig. 3) is currently regarded by most clinicians as the "gold standard" for diagnosing CBD stones, with sensitivity close to 100%.

ENDOSCOPIC MANAGEMENT OF COMMON BILE DUCT STONES

CBD stone diagnosis and removal involve several steps of highly skilled endoscopic maneuvering:

1. Successful cannulation of the CBD
2. Free access into the CBD

3. Biliary sphincterotomy or sphincteroplasty
4. Stone extraction

Cannulation of the Bile Duct

Gaining endoscopic access to the CBD is the most crucial step before stones can be removed. Operator experience determines the outcome of endoscopic management of CBD stones. Unlike other endoscopic procedures, the learning curve for ERCP is quite steep. Physicians who had performed more than 200 procedures were able to obtain diagnostic information in 85%, whereas the inexperienced endoscopists were successful only one-third of the time. With additional experience, better instruments, and special techniques, biliary experts now approach nearly 100% success in diagnostic and therapeutic ERCP. In this procedure, one looks for small mobile stones during slow injection of contrast into the CBD. One should take extra precaution to avoid the accidental injection of air into the CBD, as the air bubbles may mimic stones.

Free Access into the Bile Duct

Free cannulation of the CBD is essential to removing stones. Endoscopists may need to use hydrophilic guide wires and/or sphincterotomes to achieve deep cannulation of the bile duct. Rarely, there may be a need to "precut" the major papilla. This technique has higher risks but has proven to be safe in experienced hands. It may be cost-effective to start the procedure with a sphincterotome in patients with a high of suspicion for CBD stones.

Biliary Sphincterotomy

Endoscopic sphincterotomy allows access into the CBD for removal of stones. Sphincterotomy is performed by orienting and bowing the sphincterotome toward the roof of the papilla and cutting the sphincter using electrocautery. The cut is always made in the 11 o'clock–1 o'clock direction to minimize the risks of bleeding and perforation. In addition, safe sphincterotomies are done using short sequential bursts of current. The size of the opening created by sphincterotomy is greatly dependent on the length of the intramural segment of the CBD (Figs. 4 and 5).

The procedure carries a small risk of acute complications such as pancreatitis, bleeding, and duodenal perforation, with a fatal outcome in a very small minority of patients. There are also some concerns regarding the long-term effects of sphincterotomy, particularly in young adults. In a prospective multicenter study reported by Freeman et al. using standard definitions and grading of severity of complications, the complication rates and risk factors were calculated from 2347 sphincterotomies performed in 11 university centers and 6 community hospitals. The overall complication rate was about 10%. Pancreatitis occurred in 5.4% and hemorrhage in 2.0%. Death from all causes occurred in 2.3% within 30 days. However, death was thought to be directly or indirectly due to ERCP in 10 of 2347 patients (0.4%). Five significant risk factors for complications were identified in a multivariate analysis: suspected dysfunction of the sphincter of Oddi as an indication for the procedure, cirrhosis as a comorbid condition, difficult cannulation of the bile duct, "precut" sphincterotomy to achieve access to the bile duct, and combined percutaneous-endoscopic procedure to achieve access of the bile duct. The overall risk of complications was not related to patient age, the number of coexisting illnesses, or the diameter of the bile

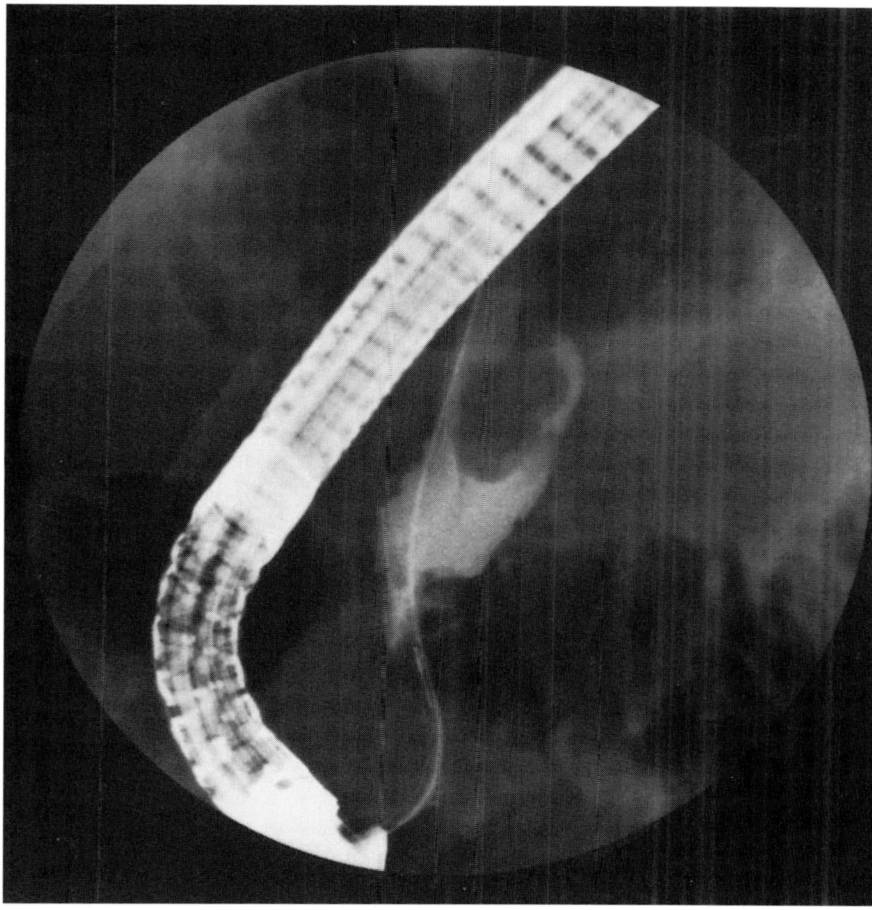

Figure 4 Sphincterotome being inserted into the CBD over a guide wire. There is one large stone seen in the CBD along with some sludge near the lower end.

duct. The rate of complications was highest when the indication for the procedure was a suspected sphincter of Oddi dysfunction (21.7%) and lowest when the indication was removal of CBD stones within 30 days of laparoscopic cholecystectomy (4.9%). As compared with those who performed fewer procedures, endoscopists who performed more than one sphincterotomy per week had lower complications (8.4 versus 11.1%, $p = 0.03$).

The protease inhibitor gabexate has been shown to have a beneficial effect in preventing pancreatitis. In a study by Cavallini et al., acute pancreatitis developed in 16 of 210 patients in the placebo group and 5 of 208 patients in the gabexate group (1 g dissolved in 500 mL of 0.9% saline solution or 5% glucose solution and administered by continuous intravenous infusion beginning 30 to 90 min before the endoscopy session and continuing for 12 h afterward). Direct cost analysis of this approach is needed.

Long-term complications of sphincterotomy is the subject of a recent study, since endoscopic sphincterotomy permanently destroys the biliary sphincter. This has been of concern, especially in younger patients who may be exposed to biliary complications

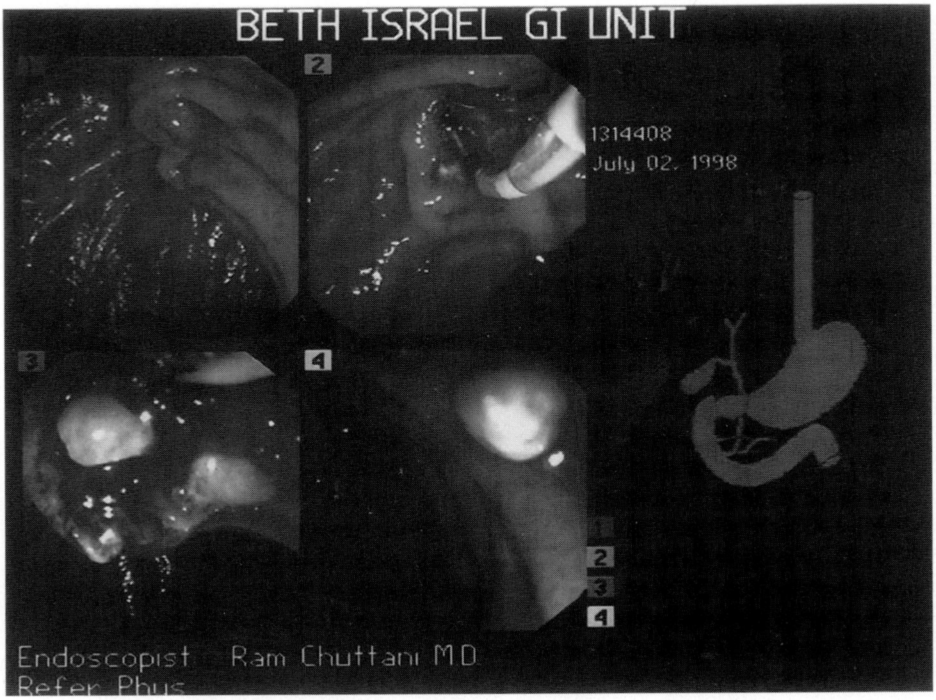

Figure 5 Serial steps (1–4) in a patient with CBD stones showing a bulging papilla, sphincterotomy, balloon extraction of the stones, and stones successfully removed and lying in the duodenum.

secondary to duodenobiliary reflux, bacterial contamination, and chronic inflammation of the biliary system. An Amsterdam group followed a cohort of 100 patients (without gallbladders) who had undergone sphincterotomy for stones more than 10 years previously, at a time when they were all less than 60 years old. Twenty-two patients developed a total of 36 late complications. Stone recurrence was the most important problem. Twenty-one patients developed symptoms of recurrent bile duct stones and one patient developed biliary pancreatitis. Other late complications, such as recurrent ascending cholangitis and malignant degeneration, were not observed. ERCP was performed in 20 of the 22 patients with late complications and demonstrated bile duct stones in 13, combined with stenosis in 9 patients. These late complications were, however, easily managed endoscopically.

Balloon Sphincteroplasty

Endoscopic balloon dilation (EBD) is an alternative for removal of CBD stones. In this procedure the opening of the CBD is enlarged by inflation of a balloon. In contrast to sphincterotomy, which destroys the sphincter permanently, the function of the sphincter of Oddi is preserved after balloon dilatation. This may be an attractive option to manage CBD stones in younger patients. The size of the lumen created safely by balloon dilation is 8–10 mm. The small orifice obtained with balloon dilatation limits the size of stone that can be removed from the CBD without resorting to lithotripsy. Blackstone et al. reported a randomized controlled trial comparing balloon dilatation with sphincterotomy for the removal of CBD stones. There was an equally high bile duct clearance with both techniques (90%), but mechanical lithotripsy was required more often in the balloon dilatation group than the sphincterotomy group. There was no difference in the early complication rate between the two groups. Preliminary data from a recent large study suggest a higher complication rate using balloon sphincteroplasty, but long-term effects of balloon sphincteroplasty have yet to be determined.

Removal of Bile Duct Stones (Small Versus Large Stones)

Successful stone retrieval from the CBD depends upon the size of the stone and the shape of the duct. Stones of less than 1 cm can usually be retrieved from the CBD with an inflatable soft retrieval balloon or a basket under fluoroscopic guidance (Figs. 6 and 7). It is generally easier to extract a larger stone with a basket and a smaller one with a balloon. When

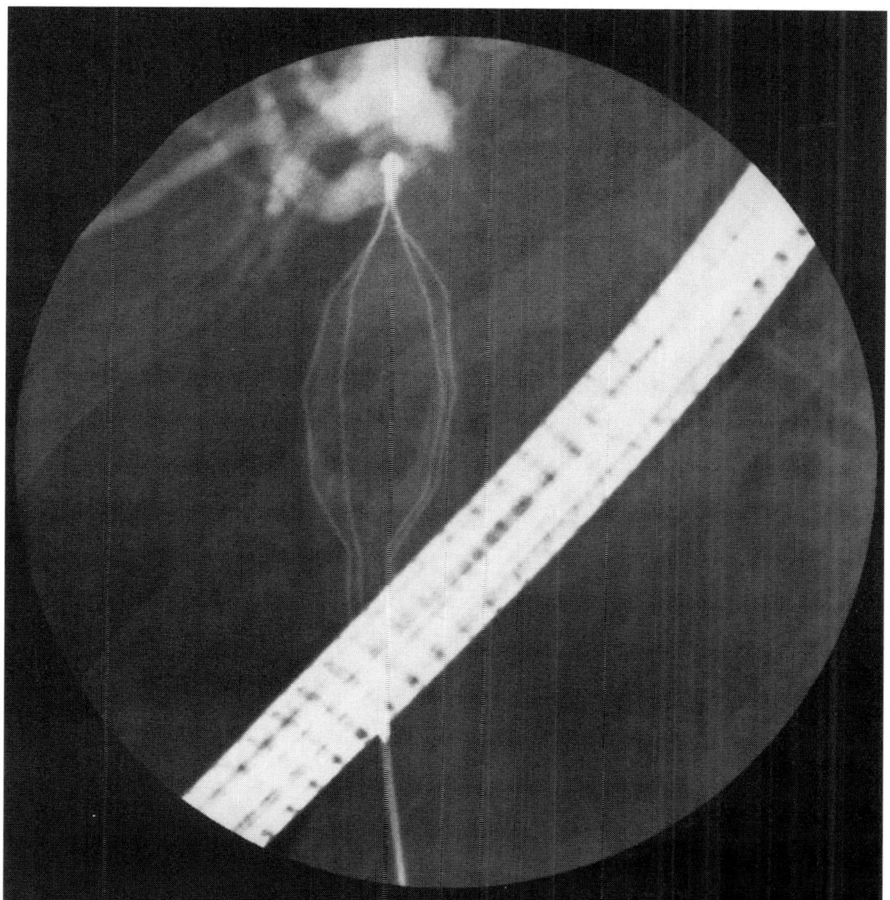

Figure 6 Stone trapped in a dormia basket in the CBD.

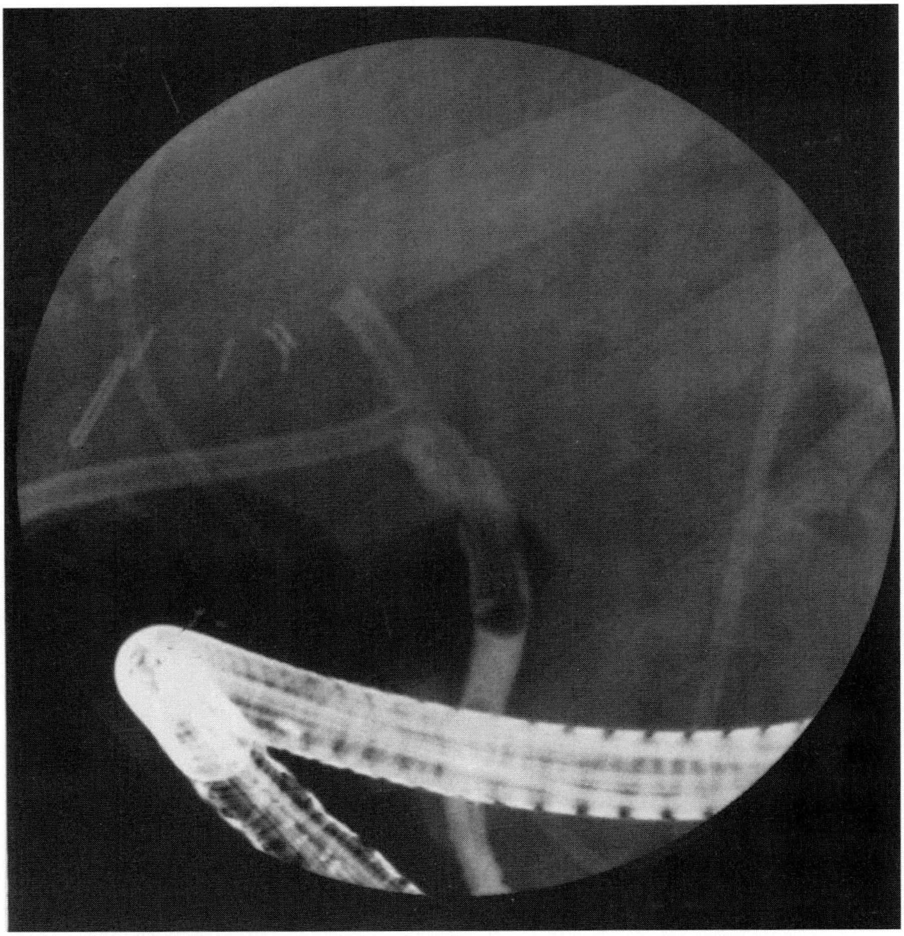

Figure 7 A retained CBD stone in a patient following cholecystectomy. The T-tube is being extracted with a balloon.

additional manipulation is required, the use of guide wire to maintain bile duct access is essential to prevent additional trauma of the papilla. Results from a prospective study of endoscopic therapy of choledocholithiasis conducted in Poland give a bird's eye view of the various techniques required to clear CBD stones. Endoscopic sphincterotomy alone was sufficient to clear the CBD of small stones by spontaneous expulsion in 23% of patients; balloon or basket retrieval was required in 64%; and lithotripsy techniques (mechanical lithotripsy, 9%; electrohydraulic lithotripsy, 3%; extracorporeal shock-wave lithotripsy, 1%) are needed to clear large stones in the CBD.

Lithotripsy

Stones larger than 1 cm may impact the orifice or be difficult to entrap. Removal of such stones is facilitated after fragmentation into smaller pieces. A number of different lithotripters are available to fragment the CBD stones. Stones that are located above a stricture, such as those seen in primary sclerosing cholangitis (see Chap. 13), with a surgical anastomosis or recurrent pyogenic cholangitis are difficult to remove. These cases are best managed in centers where expertise in stricture, dilatation, stone fragmentation, and direct choledochoscopy are available.

Lithotripsy may be performed using mechanical, electrohydraulic, and laser technology. In mechanical lithotripsy, stone fragmentation is accomplished by trapping the stone in a basket of tensile steel wires capable of withstanding traction of > 100 kg and crushing the stone into smaller pieces. The mechanical lithotripters may be "through the scope" lithotripters or may need withdrawal of the endoscope prior to lithotripsy. The success rate of mechanical lithotripsy and CBD stone clearance has been reported in the range of 85–95%. Failure of mechanical lithotripsy is due to inability to trap the stone within the lithotripter basket or improper basket deployment within a tight space. Electrohydraulic lithotripsy (EHL) fragments stones by emitting an electrical spark at the tip of a bipolar coaxial probe in a fluid medium (bile). Although this technique was originally used in combination with a stone-trapping basket under fluoroscopic guidance, it is now applied mostly under direct vision with a "mother-baby" endoscopy system to reduce the chance of bile duct injury. With this new technique, complications such as perforation and hemorrhage are decreased substantially. This system is highly successful for stones located within the larger bile ducts. Difficulty in maneuvering the "baby scope" into the intrahepatic ducts significantly reduces its success for intrahepatic stones (see below). Laser lithotripsy is also applied using a mother-baby system. It utilizes a pulsed dye laser to fragment stones in a similar fashion as EHL. Stone-recognition technology in laser lithotripsy may avoid the need for this system.

Infusion of stone-dissolving medications like monooctanoin, methyl tert-butyl-ether (MTBE), and EDTA have been used to dissolve difficult CBD stones, using placement of a nasobiliary catheter. However, success rate is poor.

Large Irretrievable Bile Duct Stones

Endoscopic sphincterotomy and stone extraction can clear the CBD in 90–95% of patients. In case endoscopic stone extraction fails, insertion of a biliary endoprosthesis is an alternative. Short-term stenting is a simple and useful procedure to establish biliary drainage when stones cannot be extracted endoscopically. The situation should then be assessed carefully and the patient advised about further treatment options, including surgical management. Endoscopy may be repeated after a few months of oral ursodeoxycholic acid (see Chap. 17), since stones may pass or prove easier to remove on the second attempt. A Milwaukee group demonstrated that 9 of 10 patients treated with ursodeoxycholic acid had complete stone clearance, and 41 of 42 stones were removed during a follow-up of 9 ± 2 months; in contrast, none of the 12 patients in the control group had complete clearance and only 6 of 40 stones were removed after a follow-up period of 31 ± 6 months.

Permanent stenting after sphincterotomy is an alternative in high-surgical-risk patients. However the Amsterdam study highlights the risk of long-term complications. During a follow-up of up to 10 years (median 3 years), 44 of the 58 patients died, 9 with cholangitis (despite active intervention in 4). No fewer than 23 (40%) developed a total of 34 complications. The overall complication rate was 16% at 1 year but had risen to 50% at 4 years. The investigators concluded that permanent stenting should be used only in patients with severe comorbid conditions and a short life expectancy. Some of the technical aspects of stenting need further evaluation. The Amsterdam group used "straight" stents and had two early duodenal perforations due to stent migration. Unanswered questions include the use of pigtail stents, Teflon stents, or metal stents in this situation.

Endoscopic Management of Biliary Pancreatitis

Untreated, 40% of gallstone pancreatitis will recur within 6 months of presentation, and definitive treatment is generally required to prevent potentially serious attacks. The classic textbook approach in the management of gallstone pancreatitis is to perform cholecystectomy, and it is best performed as soon as the pancreatitis has subsided. With the widespread availability of ERCP and the routine use of laparoscopic cholecystectomy, endoscopists are playing an important role in the management of biliary pancreatitis. A number of clinical studies conducted in the last 15 years have clarified the role of ERCP in the management of patients with biliary pancreatitis:

1. Patients who have cholangitis or progressive jaundice benefit from early ERCP (within 24–72 h after the onset of symptoms).
2. Patients with severe or worsening pancreatitis but without biliary obstruction may not benefit from emergent ERCP.
3. Patients with no evidence of biliary obstruction and stable (mild) or improving biliary pancreatitis do not benefit from emergent ERCP.

In a randomized trial at one center reported by Neoptolemos et al. in 1986, 121 patients with acute biliary pancreatitis were assigned to either ERCP (and papillotomy if bile duct stones were found) or conventional treatment, within 72 h after admission to the hospital. Patients with mild pancreatitis had similar outcomes regardless of the treatment. Among patients with severe pancreatitis, the morbidity but not the mortality was significantly lower for those who underwent early ERCP.

In a study from Hong Kong reported by Fan et al., 195 patients with acute pancreatitis from various causes were randomly assigned to either ERCP with papillotomy or conservative treatment within 24 h after admission. The rates of mortality and local and systemic complications were similar in the two groups; the incidence of biliary sepsis was significantly lower with early ERCP and papillotomy.

Folsch et al. reported the results of a multicenter prospective trial in Germany in which patients with biliary pancreatitis but without obstructive jaundice were randomly assigned to invasive treatment with ERCP and biliary decompression (if indicated) within 72 h of the onset of symptoms or to conservative treatment. They demonstrated that patients with acute biliary pancreatitis without biliary obstruction or biliary sepsis did not benefit from ERCP. The overall rate of complications with similar in the two groups, but patients in the invasive-treatment group had more severe complications. Therefore, emergent ERCP is generally indicated in severe or worsening acute pancreatitis with evidence of persistent biliary obstruction.

Endoscopists are frequently consulted to "clear" the bile duct in patients with resolved pancreatitis or cholangitis prior to laparoscopic cholecystectomy. There are scant data to recommend this approach in the absence of liver test abnormalities. In a classic study by Acosta et al. reported in 1974, 90% of patients with acute pancreatitis were found to have gallstones in the stools during the 72 h after presentation. This suggests that the vast majority of patients with gallstone pancreatitis will pass the stone(s) spontaneously.

Endoscopic Management of Cholangitis with CBD Stones

Until the 1980s, the management of cholangitis included parenteral antibiotics and emergent surgery. Endoscopic biliary drainage decreases both morbidity (34 versus 66%) and mortality (10 versus 32%) of severe cholangitis as compared to surgical biliary decompression, as demonstrated by Lai et al. A more recent report by Seigel et al. showed no procedure-related mortality in 898 patients with severe cholangitis. There are several issues that need special comment, however. Care must be taken to avoid excessive manipulation or injection of contrast during an acute infection, as this has been known to disseminate the bacterial infection. Bile fluid should be aspirated at ERCP for Gram stain and culture, as culture positivity occurs in 97% of cases. In the acute setting, in patients with large stones, numerous stones or stones above a stricture, the aim should be to provide immediate adequate biliary decompression. This may either be done using a nasobiliary drain for thick purulent bile or a bile duct stent for thin infected bile. Most of these patients will require a definitive ERCP or surgical biliary decompression after the acute infection has cleared. In patients where the biliary infection is under control, the bile ducts can be cleared of the stones in the same setting.

Endoscopic Management of Bile Duct Stones with Gallbladder In Situ Versus Postcholecystectomy

The role of cholecystectomy after the endoscopic removal of CBD stones for patients still harboring gallstones is controversial. In elderly patients with significant comorbid conditions that increase the risk of cholecystectomy, leaving the gallbladder in situ as an acceptable alternative. In a study from Sweden that compared endoscopic stone removal and leaving the gallbladder in situ versus cholecystectomy in middle-aged and elderly patients (median age, 75 years), the two therapies were equally effective. In a study from a Dutch group in 71 patients, all younger than 80 years of age, of the 26 patients in whom the "wait and watch" policy was adopted, 6 developed symptoms over a median follow-up of 12 months. In these patients, the outcome of surgery was no worse than that in the surgical group, challenging the conventional wisdom that all patients should have their gallbladders removed after endoscopic stone removal. In a retrospective study of 1272 patients reported by Siegel et al. in whom ES was performed and who had not undergone cholecystectomy previously, only 8.5% required cholecystectomy within 3 years of ES for recurrent symptoms referable to the biliary tract.

Usually most gallstone-related complications occur during the year after ES; the range for acute cholecystitis is 0–3%. After 2 years, the incidence of gallstone-related complications is comparable to that with asymptomatic gallstones, with the annual incidence of acute cholecystitis in the range of 1–2%. However, patients with a nonfilling gallbladder at the time of ERCP may have a higher incidence of cholecystitis and hence should be offered cholecystectomy. The issue is further open to debate with the ever-improving technique of laparoscopic cholecystectomy, as most of the published trials did not compare this with expectant treatment after endoscopic stone removal. At this time it seems prudent to recommend laparoscopic cholecystectomy in younger patients with gallbladder stones after endoscopic stone removal. In older or high-risk patients, provided the cystic duct is patent and the patient has had no prior episodes suggesting chronic cholecystitis, advocating no further therapy may be reasonable.

Management of Intrahepatic Stones

Intrahepatic stones are infrequent in western countries but are endemic in East Asia. Primary intrahepatic stones, which are formed in the proximal bile ducts, are typically brown or orange in color and contain less than 20% cholesterol. They are mainly calcium bilirubinate stones and are often associated with biliary strictures and recurrent cholangitis, secondary biliary cirrhosis, and portal hypertension. These are best managed by a combined surgical and percutaneous choledochoscopic approach. If limited to the left lobe and associated with recurrent cholangitis, resection of the left lobe can be curative. In other situations, or in patients at high risk for surgery, a surgical drainage procedure with percutaneous stone extraction with or without lithotripsy is associated with good success rates. In these patients the role of ERCP is limited and must be undertaken after careful review for the fear of precipitating acute cholangitis. These patients have a significantly increased risk of developing cholangiocarcinoma.

Secondary intrahepatic stones, which are often associated with CBD stones or intrahepatic strictures, are far less common. ERCP still remains the mainstay of treatment for secondary intrahepatic stones.

REFERENCES

1. Roston AD, Jacobson IM. Evaluation of the pattern of liver tests and yield of cholangiography in symptomatic choledocholithiasis: a prospective study. Gastrointest Endosc 1997; 45:394–399.
2. Sugiyama M, Atomi Y. Endoscopic ultrasonography for diagnosing choledocholithiasis: a prospective comparative study with ultrasound and computed tomography. Gastrointest Endosc 1997; 45:143–146.
3. Aubertin JM, Levoir D, Bouillot JL, et al. Endoscopic ultrasonography immediately prior to laparoscopic cholecystectomy: a prospective evaluation. Endoscopy 1996; 28:667–673.
4. Regan F, Fraden J, Khazan R, Bohlman M, Magnuson T. Choledocholithiasis: evaluation with MR cholangiography. AJR 1996; 167:1441–1445.
5. Raptopoulos V, Prassopoulos P, Chuttani R, McNicholas MMJ, McKee JD, Kressel HY. Multiplanar CT pancreatography and distal cholangiography with minimum intensity projections. Radiology 1998; 207:317–324.
6. Freeman ML, Nelson DB, Sherman S, et al. Complications of endoscopic sphincterotomy. N Engl J Med 1996; 335:909–918.
7. Cavallino G, Titibello A, Frulloni C, et al. Gabexate for the prevention of pancreatic damage related to ERCP. Gabexate in digestive endoscopy—Italian group. N Engl J Med 1996; 335: 919–923.
8. Bergman JJGHM, Van der Mey S, Rauws IEAJ, et al. Long-term follow-up after endoscopic sphincterotomy for bile duct stones in patients younger than 60 years of age. Gastrointest Endosc 1996; 44:643–649.
9. MacMathuna P, Siegenberg D, Gibbons D, et al. The acute and long term effects of balloon sphincteroplasty on papillary structure in pigs. Gastrointest Endosc 1996; 44:650–655.
10. Folsch UR, Niesche R, Ludtke R, Hilgers RA, Creutfeldt W. Early ERCP and papillotomy compared with conservative treatment for acute biliary pancreatitis: The German study on acute biliary pancreatitis. N Engl J Med 1997; 336:237–242.
11. Keulemans YCA, Rauws EAJ, Huibregtse K, Gouma DJ. Current management of the gallbladder after endoscopic sphincterotomy for common bile duct stones. Gastrointest Endosc 1997; 46:514–519.
12. Targarona EM, Ayuso RMP, Bordas JM, et al. Randomised trial of endoscopic sphincterotomy with gallbladder left in situ versus open surgery for common bile duct calculi in high-risk patients. Lancet 1996; 347:926–929.

19
Management of Liver Abscess

Christopher J. Grace, W. Kemper Alston, and Mary Beth Ramundo
University of Vermont College of Medicine, Burlington, Vermont

INTRODUCTION

This chapter reviews the problem of pyogenic liver abscess (PLA), as defined by one or more focal, purulent infections of the liver due to bacteria or fungi. Parasitic infections are addressed in the following chapter. Although infrequent (approximately one case per 10,000 hospital admissions), PLA is life-threatening and presents substantial diagnostic and therapeutic challenges. During this century all aspects of the treatment of this disease have evolved, including the identification of host factors and predisposing conditions, diagnostic imaging, microbiological methods, surgical techniques, and antimicrobial agents. These advances have achieved a significant decline in attributable mortality, from 80–10% in some series. Unfortunately the presentation of PLA remains nonspecific, and the wide array of diagnostic and therapeutic modalities available leaves the physician with complex, controversial decisions to be made.

EPIDEMIOLOGY

Although rare in children, PLA may be encountered in all age groups. During the antibiotic era, as in the case of many other infectious diseases, these patients are now more likely to be older and to have more comorbid conditions. Young adults with appendicitis are no longer typical; older patients with biliary disease, often malignant, are now the norm. Diabetes, cirrhosis, cancer, trauma, sepsis, inflammatory bowel disease, and malnutrition are host risk factors at all ages, while chronic granulomatous disease and sickle cell anemia are frequent in children with liver abscess. Iatrogenic factors include use of corticosteroids, organ transplantation, central venous catheters, hepatobiliary procedures, and cytotoxic chemotherapy. The sexes are equally affected.

PATHOGENESIS

The liver is very resistant to bacterial infection. While portal vein bacteremia is probably a common event, hepatic abscess formation is relatively rare. Presumably, the reticuloendothelial system provides excellent local immunological defense. For infection to occur, there must be a portal of entry as well as a breakdown in resistance, either within the liver itself or the host in general. Table 1 lists the general routes for intrahepatic infection.

The most common (approximately 30%) is now biliary disease, where stasis due to calculus, stricture, or malignancy results in ascending cholangitis and hepatic abscess. As pancreatic and biliary neoplasms are treated more aggressively, this group may continue to increase in frequency.

Cryptogenic liver abscess indicates that no cause of infection can be determined. This accounts for an estimated 25% of cases and is frequently solitary. It is unclear if these cases result from occult or previously treated portal infection, occult bacteremia seeding the liver, or secondary infection of devitalized hepatic tissue. Some authors have suggested a dental source in cases of cryptogenic liver abscess.

Any intraabdominal infection drained by the portal vein may predispose to liver abscess. Conditions such as appendicitis, diverticulitis, intestinal perforation, or inflammatory bowel disease, which cause portal "pylephlebitis," may set the stage for PLA. These are often solitary lesions, more often in the right lobe than the left, reflecting the distribution of hepatic blood flow. Occult colorectal inflammation may result in cryptogenic abscesses.

Systemic, disseminated infections may involve the liver via the hepatic artery. Umbilical vein infections in newborns are rarely complicated by liver abscess.

A special circumstance is hepatosplenic candidiasis, also termed chronic systemic candidiasis. This infection is most often a complication of prolonged, severe neutropenia, as occurs during therapy of acute leukemia. Numerous poorly defined microabscesses result in fever despite broad-spectrum antibiotics. With recovery of neutrophil counts, the lesions become pyogenic and organized and are then recognized radiologically. Impaired mucocutaneous defense with catheters and chemotherapy, corticosteroids, and fungal overgrowth encouraged by antibiotics are all important factors. This infection is becoming more common as patients with acute leukemia receive more aggressive therapy and better supportive care, so that they survive longer. Antemortem diagnosis depends on a high index of suspicion.

Pyogenic liver abscess may also occur via direct inoculation or extension from a contiguous focus of infection. Penetrating trauma, especially involving foreign bodies, or blunt trauma complicated by infarction and stasis of blood or bile, may allow abscess formation. Sepsis involving a perforated gallbladder, subhepatic abscess, or subphrenic abscess may extend to involve the liver. Finally, liver biopsy, percutaneous biliary drainage, and local treatment of hepatic malignancy rarely predispose to liver abscess. Liver trans-

Table 1 Pathogenesis of Pyogenic Liver Abscess

1. Biliary tract: obstruction or manipulation
2. Cryptogenic: no source identified
3. Portal vein: primary intraabdominal infection
4. Hepatic artery: hematogenous spread
5. Direct extension: penetrating trauma, surgical site infection, biliary infection

plantation may be complicated by abscess. usually recognized in the month following surgery during which technical problems were encountered.

CLINICAL FEATURES

The clinical presentation of PLA is nonspecific and may vary with underlying etiology, host factors, and causative organisms. The most common symptoms are fever and malaise. Abdominal pain is often present but is not always localized to the right upper quadrant. Other complaints include chills, nausea, vomiting, and weight loss. Most patients have symptoms for more than 2 weeks prior to the diagnosis.

The most common findings on physical examination are right-upper-quadrant tenderness and hepatomegaly. Jaundice can occur but is more likely to be present in patients with a biliary source for their hepatic abscess. Abnormal findings on examination of the right lung base are present in approximately 25% of patients.

Leukocytosis is the most common laboratory abnormality observed in patients with PLA. Elevation of alkaline phosphatase is the most significant finding on liver function studies, although mild elevations of the transaminases are not unusual. Decreased albumin and anemia of chronic disease can also be seen. Bilirubin is elevated in approximately one-third of patients. Chest x-ray findings such as right-sided pleural effusion and right-lower-lobe atelectasis are observed in half of the patients.

The differential diagnosis for the above constellation of signs and symptoms, in addition to liver abscess, would include cholecystitis, cholangitis, subphrenic or subhepatic abscess, malignancy, acute alcoholic hepatitis, pancreatitis, and pneumonia. Radiological studies may then demonstrate a defect consistent with a liver abscess (Fig. 1). Necrotic tumor, hydatid cyst, and amebic abscess would also be in the differential diagnosis of a hypodense lesion in the liver. The diagnosis of amebic liver abscess can be made with the appropriate exposure history and a positive serology for *Entamoeba*.

Blood cultures are positive in approximately 50% of patients with PLA. There is a greater yield on culture of material aspirated from the abscess, often growing additional organisms not isolated from the blood. Therefore, although blood cultures are useful, material should be obtained from the abscess and sent for aerobic and anaerobic culture. Fungal cultures should be considered in immunocompromised individuals such as transplant recipients and patients with hematological malignancies. Aerobic gram-negative bacilli such as *Escherichia coli*, anaerobic gram-negative bacilli, and streptococci have been the most commonly isolated organisms. This is not surprising, as these organisms are normal flora in the gastrointestinal tract and the majority of pyogenic liver abscesses are related to an intraabdominal source of infection. Negative cultures have been associated with fastidious or anaerobic organisms as well as with previous antimicrobial therapy.

Both increasing numbers of immunocompromised hosts and the development of new invasive procedures have contributed to the increasing variety of organisms reported to be present in liver abscesses (Table 2). There are associations between certain pathogens and specific underlying diseases. *Yersinia* hepatic abscess has been associated with hemachromatosis. *Candida* hepatic abscesses are seen in patients with hematological malignancies who have experienced prolonged neutropenia. *Staphylococcus aureus* hepatic abscess is associated with chronic granulomatous disease. An organism such as *Staphylococcus hominis*, which is felt to be a nonpathogen, can cause a liver abscess in an individual who is

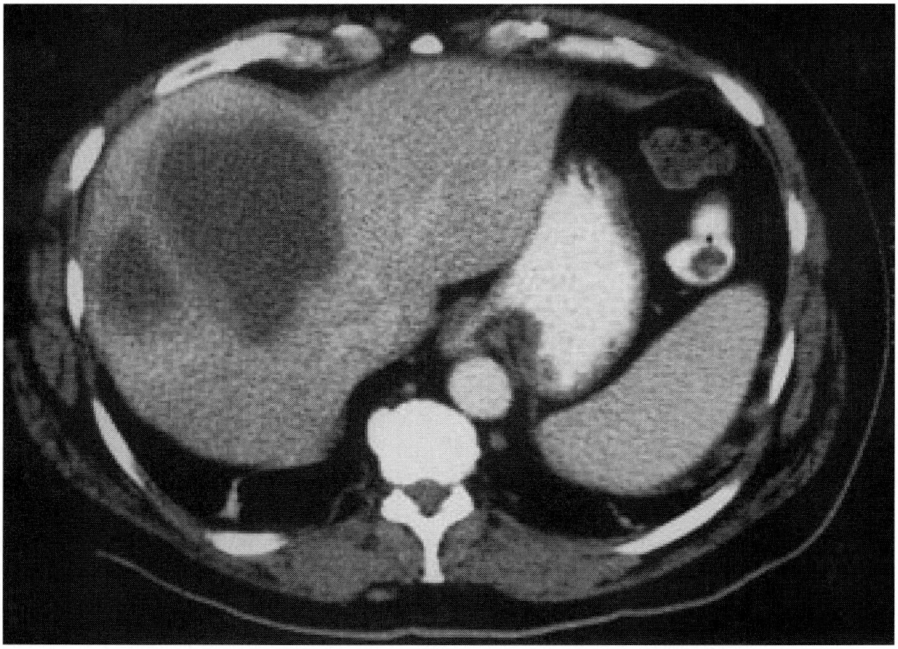

Figure 1 Computed tomography of the liver showing multiple hypodense lesions with thickened rims, consistent with pyogenic liver abscesses. The largest abscess is 10 cm in diameter. Some 200 mL of pus was aspirated from the largest collection.

immunocompromised as a result of liver transplantation. Antimicrobial therapy should be directed by the results of culture of the material obtained from the abscess and blood.

Factors associated with increased mortality have not been clearly identified. Some studies suggest that increased mortality is associated with multiple abscesses, hypoalbuminemia, underlying malignancy, or PLA caused by fungi or gas-forming organisms.

Table 2 Microbiology of Pyogenic Liver Abscess

Gram-negative bacilli	Gram-positive cocci
Escherichia coli	*Enterococcus*
Klebsiella	*Streptococcus*
Enterobacter	*Staphylococcus*
Proteus	Gram-positive bacilli
Pseudomonas	*Listeria monocytogenes*
Citrobacter	*Corynebacterium jeikeium*
Serratia	Anaerobes
Morganella	*Actinomyces*
Salmonella	*Bacteroides*
Yersinia	*Fusobacterium*
Eikenella	*Clostridium*
Aeromonas	Fungi
Haemophilus	*Candida*
Campylobacter	*Aspergillus*

Sepsis is a potential complication of PLA, which has consistently been associated with increased risk of death. Rupture of the abscess can result in peritonitis or empyema. Septic pulmonary emboli have also been observed as a complication of PLA.

Early diagnosis and treatment have been associated with decreased mortality. However as symptoms are nonspecific, diagnosis is frequently delayed. Therefore, PLA, although uncommon, always needs to be considered in the differential diagnosis of patients with the constellation of signs and symptoms presented above.

DIAGNOSIS

The diagnosis of a PLA begins with a strong index of suspicion based on history, physical exam, and initial laboratory data (Fig. 2). The initial suspicion is then supported with hepatic imaging and confirmed by drainage of purulent material from the abscess.

Once PLA is suspected, the liver should be imaged. Techniques include radionuclide scans, ultrasonography (US), computed tomography (CT), and magnetic resonance imaging (MRI). Radionuclide scans include technetium-99 sulfur colloid–, gallium-67–, and indium-tagged white blood cell scans. These nuclear scans have sensitivities of 80–85% but are nonspecific and are no longer first-line imaging techniques. Abnormalities are usually pursued with US or CT.

MRI is a relatively new technique; published reports describing its use with PLA are limited. PLA have low signal intensity on T1-weighted spin-echo images and very high signal intensity on T2 images. Gadolinium may demonstrate enhancement of the abscess rim. Studies by Mendez et al. with small numbers of patients suggest that MRI may be more sensitive than CT or US for imaging small abscesses, although these scans are also nonspecific. MRI may be considered when intravenous contrast, which is used with CT imaging, is contraindicated. The role of MRI in the diagnosis and management of PLA has yet to be fully determined.

The introduction of US and CT over the last two decades has revolutionized the management of PLA, and they have become the imaging techniques of choice. Both have proven to be very effective in the diagnosis and treatment of PLA. The choice of starting with one or the other modality will depend on the expertise and experience of the radiologist.

By continuous real-time ultrasonography, hepatic abscesses appear as round or ovoid lesions. Ultrasound has an overall sensitivity of 79–87%, being somewhat more sensitive for detecting multiple lesions than single abscesses. Advantages of US include differentiation of cystic from solid hepatic lesions and delineation of biliary tract abnormalities such as stones and intra- and extrahepatic obstruction. These abnormalities are important to recognize, since they may alter the approach to abscess drainage of necessitate other procedures such as, in the case of extrahepatic biliary obstruction, endoscopic retrograde cholangiopancreatography (ERCP). Ultrasound is less sensitive in patients with fatty liver or cirrhosis, in which the liver parenchyma may have variable echogenicity. Other reasons for false-negative US include a single right-sided abscess near the diaphragm and hepatic candidiasis. Patients suspected of having a PLA but with a negative US should have further imaging with CT.

CT is the most sensitive of the imaging techniques. Intravenous contrast enhancement is given unless contraindicated. Overall sensitivity is 94–97%, being slightly better for multiple lesions than for single abscesses. Some 7–21% of lesions reveal gas within the abscess cavity. CT scanning has the additional advantage of identifying other nonhepato-

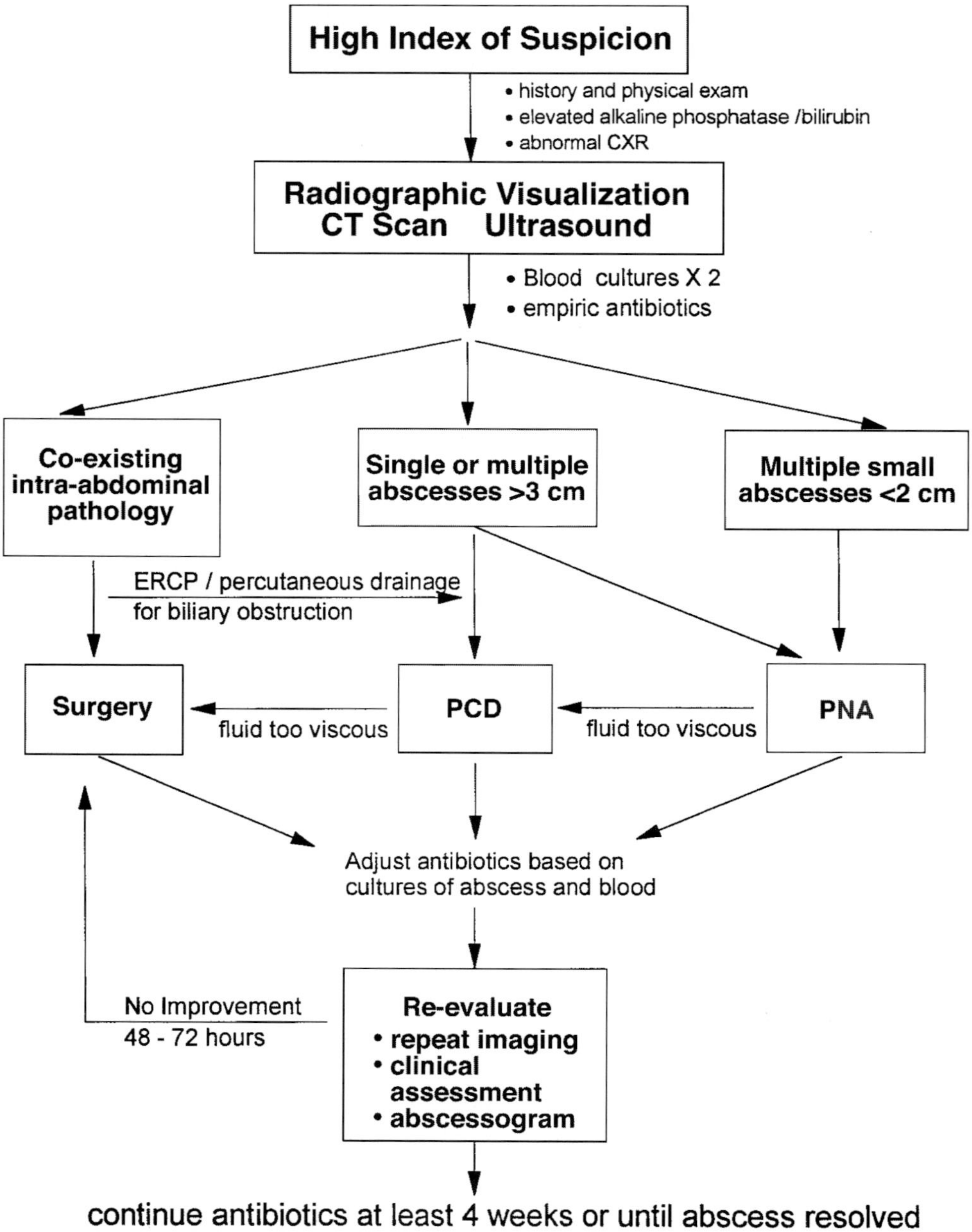

Figure 2 Diagnosis and treatment of liver abscess.

biliary lesions such as diverticular or appendiceal abscesses, malignancies, or free air. These findings may affect the choice of drainage approach to PLA.

The majority of PLAs are single (60–75%) and right sided (60–80%), as demonstrated by CT or US. Multiple abscesses (25–40%) can involve one or both lobes. It is important to recognize that multiple abscesses may actually connect. Abscesses may also fistulize to or from the intra- or extrahepatic biliary tree.

Once a PLA has been identified radiographically, antimicrobial therapy should be started and approaches to drainage assessed. The key to appropriate antimicrobial therapy is identification of the offending pathogens. Two sets of blood cultures should be drawn prior to initiating antibiotic therapy. Blood culture results need to be interpreted in conjunction with cultures of the aspirated pus.

TREATMENT

Successful treatment involves drainage of the abscess(es), appropriate antibiotic therapy, and management of the underlying cause of the PLA. Although the rare patient has been cured with antibiotics or drainage alone, the vast majority of patients benefit from both interventions.

Drainage may be accomplished surgically or percutaneously. Despite the fact that McFadzean performed the first successful percutaneous drainage of a PLA in 1953, open surgical drainage remained the standard of care until the advent of US and CT imaging.

Percutaneous drainage has been shown to be at least as effective as surgical drainage, but it avoids general anesthesia, open laparotomy, and prolonged postoperative recovery. Overall cure rates with percutaneous drainage range from 77–90%. This is true for patients with both solitary and multiple PLAs, although success rates have been higher with the former. CT- or US-directed percutaneous drainage is the preferred approach for the great majority of patients. The percutaneous approach can be accomplished by catheter drainage (PCD) or needle aspiration (PNA).

PCD involves CT- or US-guided placement of an 8- to 14-Fr pigtail catheter into the abscess cavity and leaving the catheter in place for continued drainage. The catheters are placed under local anesthesia and may remain in place on average for 3–20 days or until drainage stops. Daily irrigation of the catheter with sterile saline is needed to maintain patency. Infusion of antibiotics or mucolytic agents into the abscess cavity is not proven or recommended. The presence of multiple abscesses generally does not require multiple catheter placements, since many of the abscesses communicate and can be drained with a single catheter. If follow-up scans demonstrate incomplete drainage, additional catheters can be placed. CT-directed PCD has been successful in 75–83% of patients.

The review by Dondelinger et al. of 14 reports with 252 patients revealed an overall mortality of 6.2% and a catheter-related mortality of 1.5%. Complications, in less than 5% of the patients, included puncture of the pleura or peritoneum, sepsis after catheter placement, hemorrhage, and catheter displacement. In the review by Seeto, 7% of patients had recurrence and 10% ultimately needed surgical intervention. This failure of PCD was due to viscous pus that could not be drained, catheter displacement, presence of extrahepatic abscess, biliary obstruction, and malignancy.

Contrast injection into the catheter ("abscessogram") can be useful to determine the placement of the catheter, further delineate the size of the residual abscess cavity, and—most importantly—determine the presence of fistulas. An abscessogram should be considered several days after the initial drainage, particularly in those patients suspected of having a biliary source. The contrast should be injected slowly under low pressure. Abscessograms may reveal fistulas that communicate with the intra- or extrahepatic biliary tree. Fistulas to the extrahepatic biliary tree often necessitate biliary diversion (ERCP, percutaneous biliary drainage, or surgery) for cure, while intrahepatic fistula will often heal with abscess drainage alone. Patients with biliary fistulas will require longer periods of catheter drainage.

Percutaneous needle aspiration involves the insertion of a needle into the abscess cavity, aspiration of as much of the pus as possible, and then removal of the needle. Like PCD, it is performed under local anesthesia. This approach has been successful in treating patients with both single and multiple abscesses. Of the patients treated by Baek et al., 72% required a single aspiration. Only 3 of these 25 patients needed three or four aspirations. The size of the abscess did not correlate with the number of needle aspirations required, though multiloculated abscesses required multiple aspirations in 33% of patients. Repeat aspiration may be needed in 3–7 days if there is no decrease in the size of the abscess. The overall success rate of CT-guided PNA has been reported to be as high as 80–87%. Of the small number of patients treated by PNA who were reviewed by Seeto et al., 12% relapsed. This technique may be indicated if a transpleural route is necessary and catheter placement contraindicated.

Surgical intervention is now rarely needed. Indications include viscous pus too thick to drain percutaneously, a bleeding diathesis that cannot be easily corrected, need for surgical repair of a primary intraabdominal lesion, lesions that are inaccessible to percutaneous drainage, failure of percutaneous drainage, or the need to rule out intraabdominal malignancy. Patients presenting with biliary tract obstruction will need either surgical-, ERCP-, or percutaneous-directed decompression.

The approach taken with a particular patient must be individualized. There are strong advocates for CT and US as well as the two percutaneous drainage techniques. Prospective studies are needed comparing CT with US and PCD with PNA. For the young, clinically stable patient with a single large (> 3.0 cm) abscess or multiple smaller abscesses without a biliary fistula, PNA may be adequate. For the patient with multiple large abscesses, especially if there is concern of a biliary fistula, PCD would be the preferred approach. A collaborative approach with the radiologist and surgeon is needed. Whatever percutaneous drainage approach is taken, there should be clinical improvement within 48–72 h, characterized by decrease in temperature and white blood cell count and improvement in the general well-being of the patient. The average time to complete defervescence has ranged from 1–6 days. The three drainage approaches and potential patient candidates are summarized in Table 3.

Antimicrobial therapy should be started as soon as the diagnosis of PLA is made. It is suggested that empirical antibiotics be started after two sets of blood cultures are drawn but prior to any drainage procedure in order to treat possible bacteremia and sepsis that may accompany the manipulation of the abscess.

Since many PLAs are polymicrobic, initial empirical antibiotics need to have activity against aerobic gram-negative bacilli and anaerobes (predominantly *Bacteroides fragilis*). Empiric coverage for enterococcal species is not always needed for community-acquired infections. For patients with nosocomial infections or those who are critically ill, the use of agents with activity against *Pseudomonas aeruginosa* and *Enterococcus* is warranted. Table 4 outlines the most commonly used agents and their spectrum. There is no one correct or best regimen, although it is important to include antibiotics that have activity against the major suspected pathogens. Whenever *P. aeruginosa* is suspected, beta-lactam antibiotics with antipseudomonal activity (piperacillin, piperacillin-tazobactam, imipenem-cilastatin, aztreonam) should be used in combination with an aminoglycoside.

Two or three narrow-spectrum agents can be used in combination. Such regimens can include an aminoglycoside or ceftriaxone plus clindamycin or metronidazole. Ampicillin or vancomycin can be added to either regimen to add enterococcal coverage. Agents that have a broad spectrum of coverage—such as cefotetan, imipenem-cilastatin, or piperacillin-tazobactam—can be used alone.

Table 3 Drainage Techniques and Potential Patient Candidates

Percutaneous needle aspiration (PNA):
- Age $<$ 40 years
- No significant comorbidities
- Not critically ill
- No fistula formation
- Single large abscess
- Multiple small ($<$ 2 cm) abscesses
- Transpleural approach required

Percutaneous catheter drainage (PCD):
- Elderly
- Large abscess
- Biliary obstruction
- Biliary fistula

Surgery
- Bleeding diathesis
- Viscous pus
- Lesion not accessible by percutaneous route
- Other intraabdominal lesoins requiring surgery
- Failure of percutaneous drainage

Reasonable empirical coverage for a patient with a community-acquired PLA who is not critically ill could include the combination of an aminoglycoside and clindamycin or monotherapy with cefotetan. For critically ill patients or those with nosocomial infections, piperacillin/aminoglycoside, piperacillin-tazobactam/aminoglycoside, or imipenem-cilastatin/aminoglycoside combinations would be appropriate. For patients suspected of

Table 4 Antibiotics with Activity Against Common Bacteria Causing Pyogenic Liver Abscess

	Aerobic GNR	Anaerobic GNR	*P. aeruginosa*	Enterococcus
Aminoglycoside	++−+	−	+++	−
Ampicillin	+	−	−	+++
Aztreonam	++++	−	++	−
Cefotetan	++	++	−	−
Ceftriaxone	+++	−	−	−
Ciprofloxacin	++++	−	++	−
Clindamycin	−	+++	−	−
Co-Trimoxazole	+++	−	−	−
Imipenem-cilastatin	++++	++	+	++
Metronidazole	−	++++	−	−
Piperacillin	++	++	+	+++
Piperacillin-tazobactam	++++	+++	+	+++
Vancomycin	−	−	−	+++
Amoxacillin-clavulanate	++	++	−	+++

Key: ++++, strongest activity; +++, relatively strong; ++, relatively weak; +, weak activity; −, no activity; GNR = gram-negative rod.

having a PLA secondary to bacteremia, agents such as nafcillin, cefazolin or vancomycin, which have activity against *Staphylococcus aureus* and streptococci should be added. Hepatosplenic candidiasis can be treated with amphotericin B or fluconazole.

Once results from the blood and abscess cultures are available, antibiotic coverage can be reassessed and tailored appropriately. There is no defined duration of antimicrobial therapy, though most patients will need treatment for at least 1 month. Multiple abscesses may need a longer duration of therapy than single lesions. Once the patient has stabilized and abscesses have been demonstrated to be shrinking, the patient may be switched to an oral regimen that covers the suspected or isolated organisms. Prior to discontinuing antibiotics, the patient should be clinically improved and the abscess completely or almost completely resolved on follow-up radiological studies.

SUMMARY

Pyogenic liver abscess remains an unusual but life-threatening infection. As invasive procedures and immunocompromised hosts become more common, more unusual presentations and organisms can be expected. Advances in early diagnosis and nonsurgical therapy have led to a significant reduction in mortality. Ultrasound and CT scan have led to the prompt recognition of intrahepatic pus in patients presenting with fever and abdominal pain. Percutaneous catheter drainage and percutaneous needle aspiration allow the prompt recovery of abscess fluid for culture as well as relatively noninvasive drainage. Potent antimicrobial agents guided by blood and abscess cultures act in synergy with adequate drainage. The challenge for clinicians remains to have a high index of suspicion and then to collaborate effectively with radiological and surgical colleagues to prevent the complications associated with unrecognized infection.

BIBLIOGRAPHY

Baek SY, Lee M, Cho KS, Lee SC, Sung K, Auh YH. Therapeutic percutaneous aspiration of hepatic abscesses: effectiveness in 25 patients. AJR 1993; 160:799–802.

Dondelinger RF, Kurdziel J, Gathy C. Percutaneous treatment of pyogenic liver abscess: a critical analysis of results. Cardiovasc Intervent Radiology 1990; 13:174–182.

Kandel G, Marcon NE. Pyogenic liver abscess: new concepts of an old disease. Am J Gastroenterol 1984; 79:65–71.

Huang C, Pitt HA, Lipsett PA, Osterman FA, Lillemoe KD, Cameron JL, Zuidema GD. Pyogenic hepatic abscess: changing trends over 42 years. Ann Surg 1996; 223:600–609.

McDonald MI, Corey GR, Gallis HA, Durack DT. Single and multiple pyogenic liver abscesses: natural history, diagnosis and treatment, with emphasis on percutaneous drainage. Medicine 1984; 63:291–302.

Mendez RJ, Schiebler ML, Outwater EK, Kressel HY. Hepatic abscesses: MR imaging findings. Radiology 1994; 190:431–436.

Seeto RK, Rockey DC. Pyogenic liver abscess: changes in etiology, management, and outcome. Medicine 1996; 75:99–113.

20
Management of Parasitic Liver Diseases

Raymundo Paraná and Luiz Guilherme Costa Lyra
University Hospital of Bahia, Salvador, Brazil

Ana Lúcia Coutinho Domingos and Victorino Spinelli Barreto
University Hospital of Pernambuco, Recife, Brazil

INTRODUCTION

Hepatic involvement in parasitic diseases is a significant worldwide public health problem. In this chapter we address the clinical picture and therapeutic approach to parasitic diseases, emphasizing those that primarily involve the liver.

LIVER DISEASE IN SCHISTOSOMIASIS

It is estimated that 200 million people are afflicted by schistosomiasis, a disease caused by schistosomes, trematode worms that, unlike other human parasites, have as their habitat the bloodstream instead of the intestinal lumen. Five species are involved in human pathology: *Schistosoma mansoni*, *S. japonica*, *S. haematobium*, *S. intercalatum*, and *S. mekongi*. Only *S. mansoni*—which is highly prevalent in northeastern Brazil, parts of the Middle East, and the Caribbean—is discussed here. The life cycle of *S. mansoni* includes a snail as an intermediate host, where its larvae mature to become cercariae, which penetrate the healthy human skin of individuals bathing in rivers or other infected waters. Facilitated by a proteolytic enzyme secreted by the cercariae, this process of penetration is associated with a generalized pruritus known as *swimmer's itch* and irritation of exposed skin, known as *cercarial dermatitis*.

The proteolytic enzyme and other worm antigens lead to both T- and B-cell immune responses that ultimately lead to an immune-mediated process blocking the penetration of new cercariae and thus limiting the "infecting worm burden." From the skin, larvae travel to the lungs and then to their final habitat in the mesenteric veins, where they mature, mate, and produce eggs. Each female is able to produce about 300 eggs a day. To complete the life

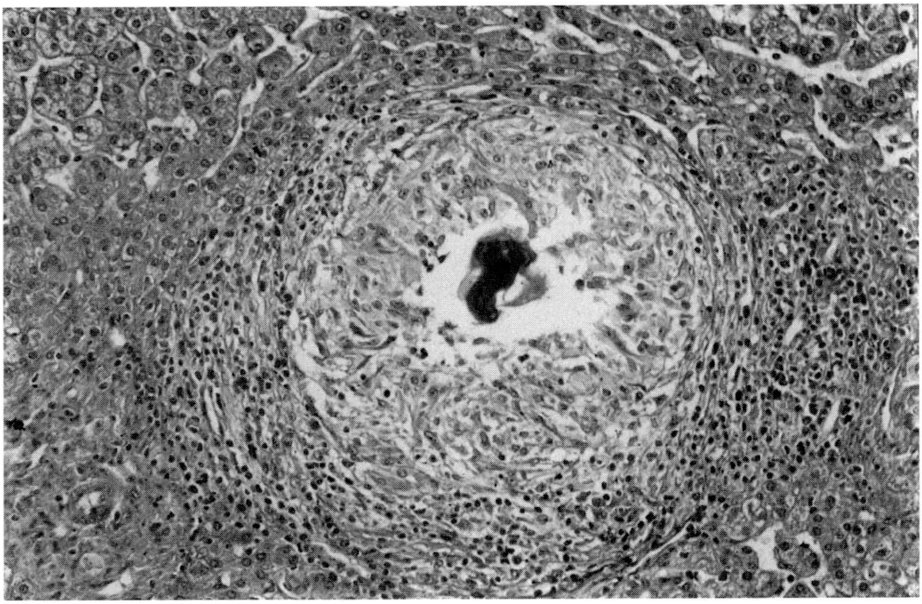

Figure 1 Granuloma around a schistosomal egg.

cycle, the eggs must find their way through the intestinal mucosa in order to be eliminated in the feces. Some eggs do not succeed in crossing the mucosa and remain in the gut wall, while others are carried away by the bloodstream through the mesenteric and portal veins into the liver. "Trapped" eggs expose larval antigens, leading to an inflammatory and granulomatous reaction with fibrosis, the basic pathological features of the disease (Fig. 1).

Clinical Classification

Schistosomiasis has a diversity of clinical presentation, which depends on a complex interaction of parasite and host factors. This variability has been classified by Coutinho as shown in Table 1.

As an in-depth discussion of each one of these clinical forms is beyond the scope of this chapter, we shall restrict our discussion to the hepatosplenic form, emphasizing the particular aspects of the liver disease that are important for clinical management.

HEPATOSPLENIC SCHISTOSOMIASIS

This severe form of the disease represents 5–7% of the infected population and is thought to be associated with larger worm burdens as well as a yet undefined genetic predisposition.

Pathology

The liver has a characteristic macroscopic appearance (Figs. 2 and 3), which resembles a turtle shell and, on the cut surface, exhibits a coarse portal fibrosis but no nodule formation except in the immediate subcapsular region, where one can see some small nodules of

Table 1 Coutinho's Clinical Classification of Schistosomiasis

Form	Major symptoms
Asymptomatic	"Healthy carrier"
Intestinal	Periodic diarrhea
Hepatointestinal	Periodic diarrhea, mild liver fibrosis, no portal hypertension
Hepatosplenic	Left love hepatomegaly, splenomegaly; portal fibrosis Portal hypertension
Cardiopulmonary	Features of the hepatosplenic form and pulmonary hypertension
Hypertensive	
Cyanotic	Cyanosis
Ectopic	Granulomatous lesions in extrahepatic tissues (e.g., central nervous system)
Pseudoneoplastic	Localized masses in several tissues caused by accumulation of eggs and augmented fibrosis
Glomerulonephritic	Immune complex–mediated disease caused by schistosomal antigens
Acute	Severe systemic febrile illness occurring about 45 days after initial exposure thought to be caused by an immune reaction to the massive exposure of antigens released by the first shedding of eggs in tissues.

uncertain significance. The gross appearance is also modified by marked hypertrophy of the left lobe and a corresponding atrophy of the right lobe, thought to be a result of hemodynamic changes in the portal circulation (see below).

Another striking gross pathological finding is massive splenomegaly, much out of proportion to what one sees in patients with cirrhosis with comparable degrees of portal

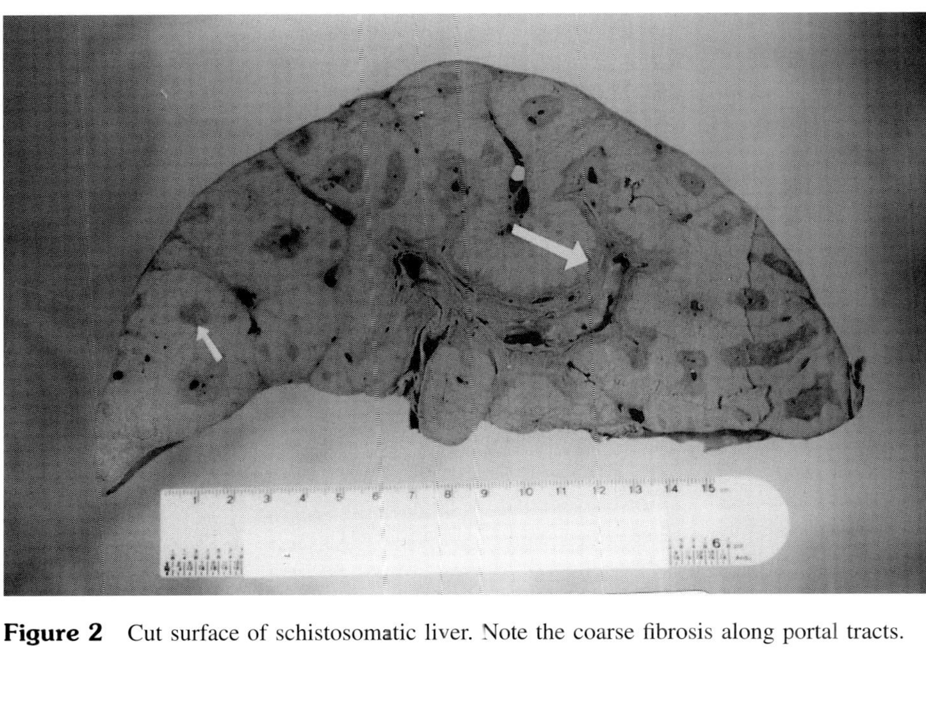

Figure 2 Cut surface of schistosomatic liver. Note the coarse fibrosis along portal tracts.

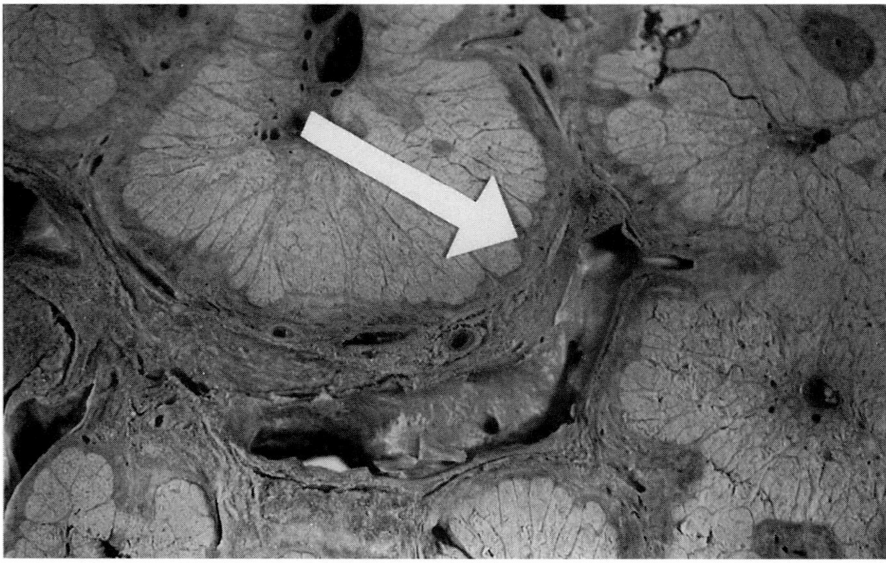

Figure 3 Detail of portal tract showing the typical "clay-pipestem" fibrosis.

hypertension. This is due to marked splenic hyperplasia, which results from long-lasting immunostimulation by worm antigens, in addition to the congestive changes of portal hypertension. Sometimes the spleen may be so large as to fill the entire left abdomen and reach the right lower quadrant, leading to a differential diagnosis of lymphosarcoma.

Histologically (Fig. 4), the hallmark of hepatic schistosomasis (also known as Symmer's fibrosis) is a coarse fibrotic enlargement of portal triads associated with septal fibrosis. Typically also, enlarged triads are filled with newly formed veins giving an angiomatoid appearance, which is a result of an extensive collateral circulation to the obstructed portal vein branch caused by the embolic schistosomal eggs. Bile duct lesions can also be observed, as well as an inflammatory infiltrate rich in lymphocytes, macrophages, and eosinophils. Epithelioid-cell granulomas around the eggs or, rarely, around dead adult worms may also be seen. As a striking differential feature from cirrhosis, the liver lobules are well preserved, with normal, single cell plates, central veins, and a reticulin framework.

Clinical Picture: Compensated Patient

Patients with hepatosplenic schistosomiasis are, for the most part, asymptomatic and are recognized at the time of physical or ultrasound examination. Some seek medical attention for evaluation of nonspecific symptoms; a significant proportion will present for the first time with an episode of variceal hemorrhage. Unlike the case with cirrhosis, however, mortality from this first bleeding episode is low, approaching zero with sound medical care. Indeed, bleeding tends to cease spontaneously in about 90% of patients. This is related to well-preserved hepatocellular function despite severe portal hypertension. This preservation of liver function reflects the essentially normal histology of the functional unit (liver lobule) as described above.

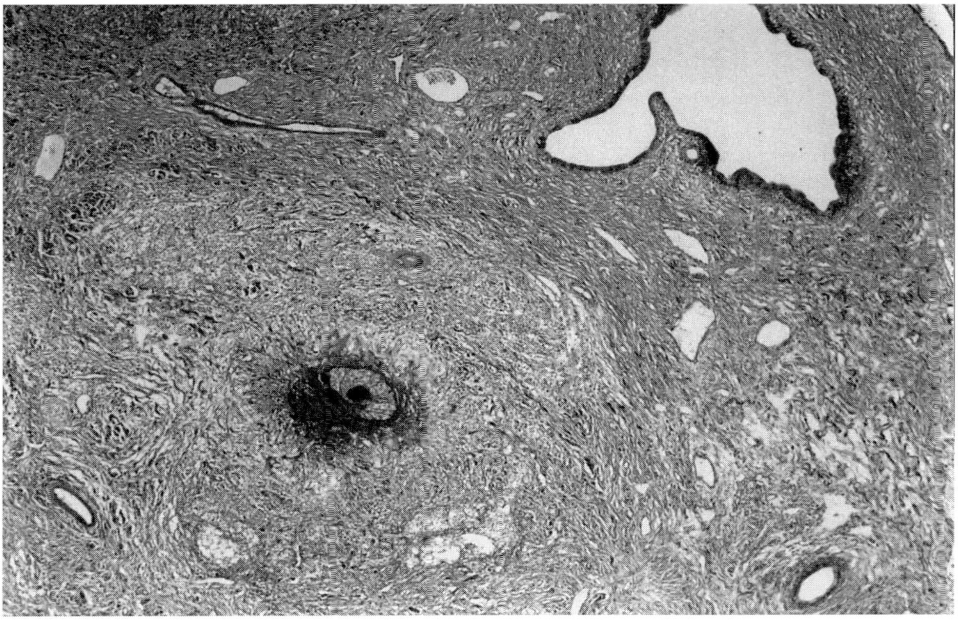

Figure 4 High-power view of a fibrotic portal triad. Note large granuloma around dead worm (transverse cut) and multiple collateral veins (angiomatoid).

On physical examination the patient usually appears well, with no wasting, jaundice, or stigmata of chronic liver diseases except when associated with other conditions (such as chronic viral hepatitis). These account for over 90% of the so-called decompensated patients who have a form of the disease that is almost indistinguishable from other types of cirrhosis. In contrast with the apparently benign clinical picture, however, gross collateral circulation may be observed in the abdominal and thoracic wall, reflecting the severe underlying portal hypertension (Fig. 5). The liver is hard, with a characteristic enlargement of the left lobe contrasting with a small, atrophic right lobe, barely palpable or not palpable at the costal margin. The other typical finding is that of pronounced splenomegaly (Fig. 6). Ascites and peripheral edema are never present until after an episode of upper GI bleeding when they occur transiently. Asterixis or other signs of hepatic encephalopathy are also conspicuously absent.

Portal Hypertension

Portal hypertension is the hallmark of hepatosplenic schistosomiasis and has a unique pathogenesis, leading to some striking differences from cirrhosis and to a different approach to therapy. First, since there is preservation of the liver's lobular architecture, there is no distortion of the sinusoidal network (a key pathological change in cirrhosis) and therefore no outflow block. Thus, sinusoidal pressure is kept under normal limits, as demonstrated by Coutinho in his pioneer work in 1960. Portal pressure builds up in schistosomiasis as a result of an increase in portal inflow resistance due to obstruction of many of the liver's small branches (Fig. 7) and a parallel increase in portal venous flow as a result of the increased splenic outflow due to the increased splenic mass, requiring a greater blood

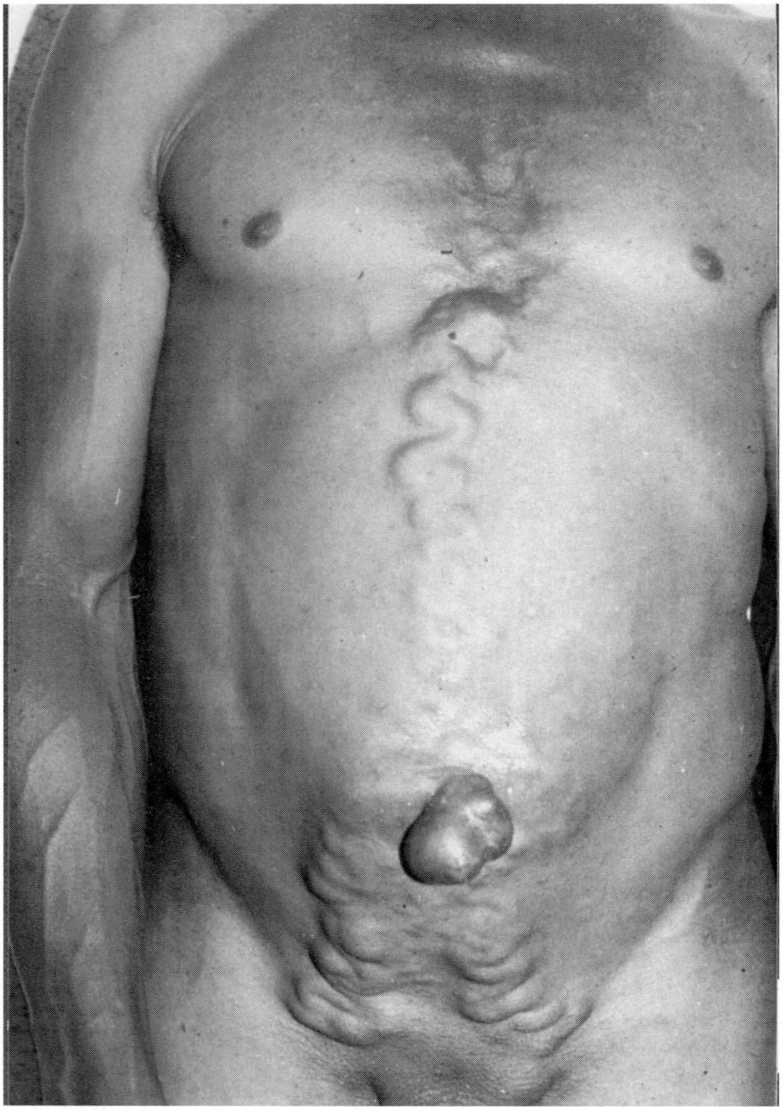

Figure 5 Dilated collateral veins in thoracic and abdominal wall in hepatosplenic schistosomiasis.

volume. This is in contrast to the portal hypertension of cirrhosis, where portal pressure is directly related to increased hepatic resistance.

Diagnosis and Management

The diagnosis of schistosomiasis is twofold: (1) identifying the infection with *S. mansoni* and (2) diagnosing and staging the liver disease. The former is usually accomplished by the identification of the typical side-spiked egg on a routine stool examination (Fig. 8) by the method of Hoffmann or by the quantitative method of Kato-Katz, which also permits an evaluation of the worm burden. Ultrasound is currently the most important imaging

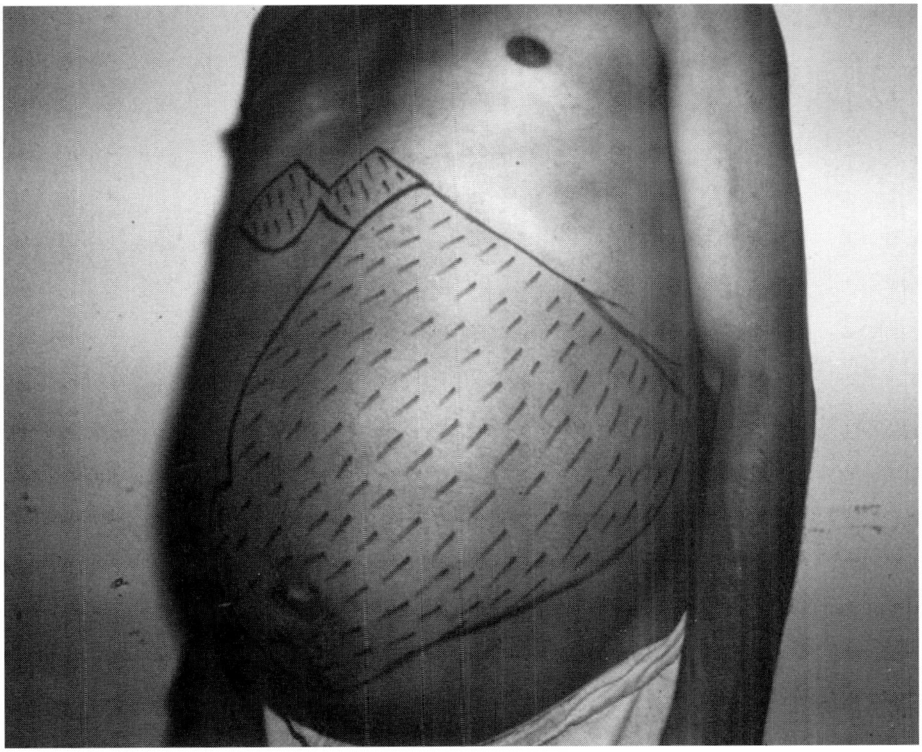

Figure 6 Massive splenomegaly in a patient with hepatosplenic schistosomiasis.

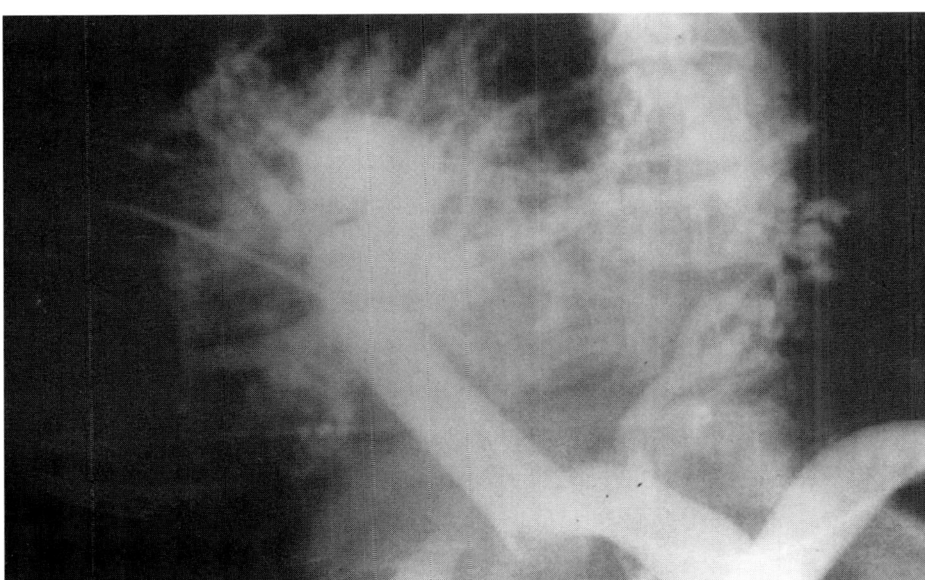

Figure 7 Transhepatic portography. Note the block of many portal vein branches and a rich collateral circulation around obstructed branches.

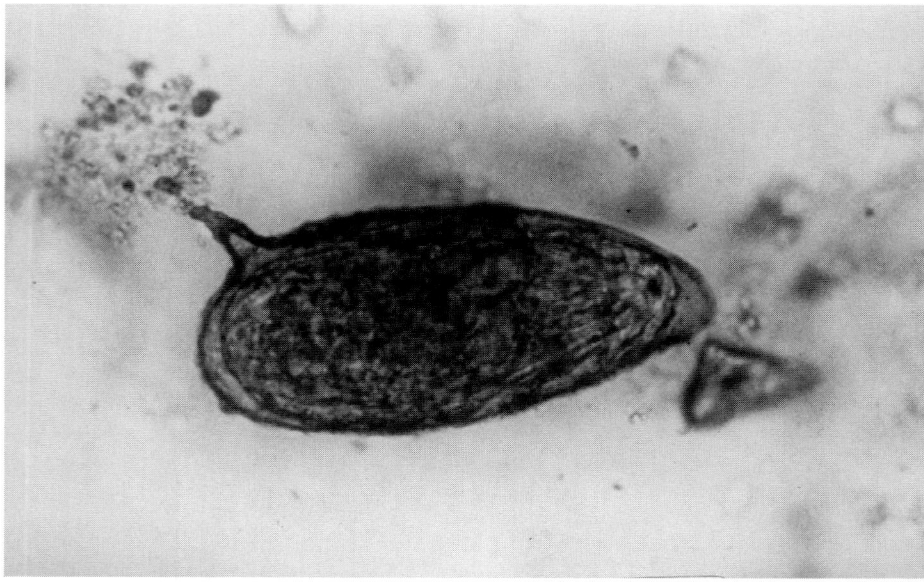

Figure 8 *Schistosoma mansoni* egg on a stool smear by the Hoffman method.

procedure in this regard, identifying the fibrosis and preserved liver parenchyma characterizing Symmers' disease. It also permits grading of the disease, based on the degree of fibrosis, measurements of right and left lobe, size of the spleen (Fig. 9), and a thorough evaluation of the portal hypertension, yielding important information for therapeutic decisions.

Some interesting observations were recently made in our department by Arruda, using a duplex-Doppler technique in a group of 24 patients with hepatosplenic schistosomiasis, with calculation of the "congestion index" (CI) developed by Moriyasu et al. Using the same equation as applied by Moriyasu to patients with cirrhosis (CI = cross-sectional area of portal veins in square centimeters divided by blood-flow velocity of the portal veins in centimeters per second), he found that the CI varies inversely with the portal pressure (Table 2). This reflects the different pathogenesis of portal hypertension, as mentioned above.

Thus, this simple, noninvasive, and easily performed exam not only helps to identify the patient more likely to bleed but provides important information as to the underlying physiopathology of the portal hypertension and information helpful in making sound therapeutic decisions.

Therapy

Treatment of schistosomiasis may be divided into (1) treatment of infection with *S. mansoni* and (2) treatment of liver disease, particularly the portal hypertension and its complications.

Antiparasitic Therapy

Antiparasitic treatment in schistosomiasis is always indicated if there is evidence of active disease, as demonstrated by a positive stool examination or the finding of viable eggs on a rectal biopsy. Although there might be some question as to the renal benefit of such therapy

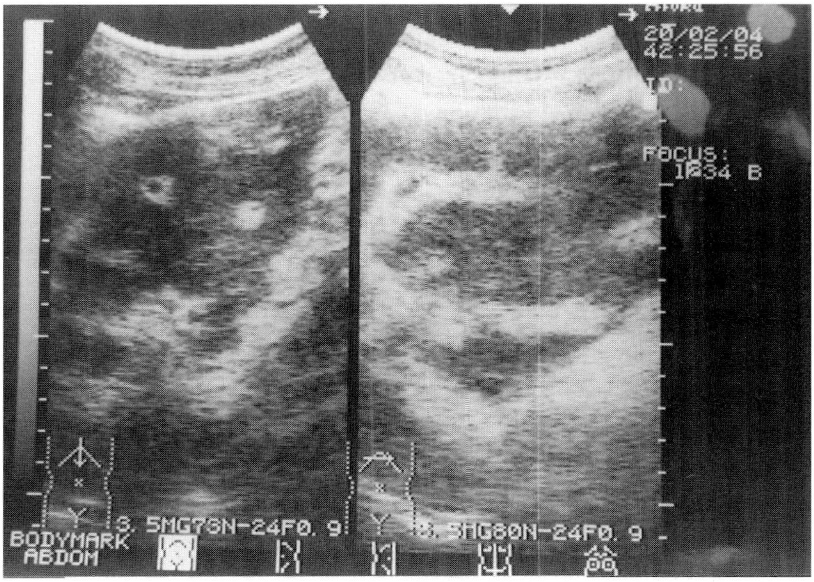

Figure 9 Hepatosplenic schistosomiasis with grade II portal fibrosis as demonstrated by ultrasound.

for an already fibrotic liver and to its harmful and potentially lethal effect (because of the massive embolization by dead worms carried by the portal circulation into the liver). However, the 40-year experience of our group in managing these patients has always pointed to beneficial effects of therapy, both subjectively, with improvement of symptoms and general sense of well-being, and objectively, by normalization of liver function tests and reduction of liver and spleen size in more than half the cases, with the spleen becoming nonpalpable in 15%. Moreover, reduction of hepatic fibrosis has also been demonstrated by follow-up ultrasonographic evaluation of treated patients. Experimental evidence in mice also indicates prevention of liver fibrosis by treatment before egg deposition, regression of hepatosplenomegaly, involution of granulomas, and regression of hepatic fibrosis and vascular changes in the liver.

Over the last 50 years, several drugs have been used for treating schistosomiasis but have been abandoned because of side effects. Currently, oxamniquine (OX) and prazi-

Table 2 Congestion Index in Portal Hypertension in Hepatosplenic Schistosomiasis[a]

Cirrhotics	0.171
Normal subjects	0.070
Patients without bleeding	0.073
Patients with bleeding	0.057

[a]Median (values combined from the data of Moriyasu and Arruda).

quantel (PZQ) are the drugs of choice for their efficacy (around 80%) and excellent tolerance.

OX (6-hydroxymethyl-2-isopropylaminomethyl-7-nitro 1, 2, 3, 4, tetrahydroquinoline) is the most widely used drug. Dosage is 15 mg/kg for adults and 20 mg/kg for children weighing less than 30 kg. Side effects are usually absent or mild and transient and consist of dizziness, somnolence, and headache rarely requiring medication. Infrequently, restlessness, hallucinations, and seizures have been reported, probably in predisposed patients. We tend to give this drug in a single nightly dose, but it may also be administered in two divided doses 4 h apart. With this dose we have observed cure rates of 80–85% in adults and 75% in children with a single course of therapy and an 80% reduction of egg counts in patients who have not been cured.

PZQ (2-cyclo-hexacarbonyl, 1,2,4,6,7,11, b-hexahydropyrazino-2,1-isoquinoline-1-4 one) is gaining popularity as an antischistosomal drug in many parts of the world. In Brazil it is used as an alternative drug because of the clinical success and the lower cost of OX. It is used as a single dose of 40–60 mg/kg for adults and 60–80 mg/kg for children. Its main side effects are abdominal pain and diarrhea, which are usually mild and transient. The cure rate with a single course is 80–90% and, as with OX, the reduction of egg counts is on the order of 80%.

Patients who fail to achieve a cure with either drug are better managed by retreatment with the same drug rather than with the other, since no cross-resistance has been observed.

Treatment of the Liver Disease

The treatment of liver disease of schistosomiasis essentially involves managing portal hypertension and its complications. The therapeutic "tools" are pretty much the same, namely, drugs aiming at lowering portal pressure (beta blockers, vasodilators, etc.), endoscopic injection sclerotherapy, and surgery. The estimated probability of upper gastrointestinal bleeding in prospectively followed patients has been reported to be 8–28%. Domingues and Coutinho, following 42 patients for 5 years, observed a bleeding rate of 43% among those who had previously bled versus 12% for those who had never bled.

Prophylaxis of bleeding is as yet an unresolved issue. Clearly, sclerotherapy or surgical intervention is not beneficial and may be harmful. There may be a place for drug therapy, but its efficacy is yet to be proved. Lack of a simple, noninvasive, reproducible method of monitoring portal pressure is a major obstacle to evaluating and guiding this form of therapy. One additional problem is that in schistosomiasis, probably due to different drug pharmacokinetics, the required dose of propranolol to achieve effective beta blockade (25% reduction of heart rate) is much higher than in cirrhosis. This "resistance" to propranolol in schistosomiasis was clearly demonstrated in human studies done by Braghirolli, with the effect on portal hemodynamics evaluated by monitoring azygous vein flow. The average effective dose was found to be 420 mg. In summary, although it remains an open issue, and keeping these difficulties in mind, pharmacological therapy with propranolol, nadolol, or isosorbide mononitrate is recommended in selected patients with a high probability of bleeding based on the usual indicators.

Management of acute variceal or portal hypertensive gastropathy bleeding follows the same general principles as in the cirrhotic patient, with three major considerations: (1) mortality is minimal, (2) spontaneous cessation of bleeding is the rule (around 90%), and (3) any shunting procedure must be avoided. Standard supportive care is usually sufficient. Endoscopy must be done as soon as possible and, if a ruptured varix is identified, sclerotherapy should be performed immediately. If the site of bleeding appears to be in the stomach, a vasoactive drug like somatostatin is our first choice and has virtually always been effective. Transfusion of blood or blood products must be kept to a minimum, particularly in areas where transfusion-transmitted virus control is not good, so as to avoid the transmission of hepatitis B or C to a patient with hepatosplenic schistosomiasis. This may be a disaster, adding a hepatocellular disease in someone already suffering from severe portal hypertension and leading to so-called decompensated hepatosplenic schistosomiasis. Since hepatocellular function is preserved, transfusion of blood clotting factors is usually not necessary and the transfusion of "volume" and red cell mass should be restricted to those who really need them—i.e., those with hemodynamic instability and significantly low blood oxygen content.

Despite the good tolerance to the initial bleeding episode, prevention of additional episodes of hemorrhage is clearly indicated. First of all, as pointed out above, the probability of rebleeding is four times as great as the initial bleeding episode. Second, each episode of bleeding exposes the patient to the hazards of the hospital setting through blood transfusions and iatrogenic diseases in addition to the hepatic ischemia resulting from the hemodynamic changes of the hemorrhagic episode itself.

Before the advent of sclerotherapy, surgery was the only modality of treatment for this condition. Splenectomy, advocated by Kelner and his group at the Federal University of Pernambuco, was the mainstay of therapy. For the reasons discussed above, splenectomy has a major impact on portal pressure in schistosomiasis, lowering it by as much as 30%. Evaluation of this procedure associated with intraesophageal ligation of varices in a follow-up of 358 patients for 1–25 years showed a rebleeding rate of 13% at 10 years and a 90% survival rate. Shunting procedures have been abandoned by our group for over 30 years because of its high incidence of encephalopathy and deterioration of liver disease. Raia et al., comparing proximal splenorenal shunt, distal splenorenal shunt, and splenectomy with esophagogastric devascularization, concluded the last was superior because it did not result in encephalopathy and had a lower mortality rate and higher efficacy. In 1991, Lacerda, using angiography, noted a progressive decrease in portal vein diameter with a corresponding increase in the hepatic artery, leading to "arterialization" of hepatic blood flow and less portal (containing trophic factors) blood, with deleterious effects on the liver in the long run. He attributed this to a "steal" of mesenteric/portal blood through a dilated left gastric vein. These observations led to ligation of this vein during splenectomy, as a standard procedure (Fig. 10). This practice has also been adopted by our department of surgery after being prospectively evaluated in randomized fashion by Ferraz et al.

Although very effective for control of the acute variceal bleeding, sclerotherapy, as a single modality of treatment for the eradication of varices and prevention of rebleeding, has some limitations in schistosomiasis. El-Zayadi et al. in 1988 and Cordeiro in 1990, both in controlled trials, found a significant decrease in mortality and a trend toward a decreased rebleeding rate. Sakai et al. in 1988, treated a group of 78 patients by sclerotherapy; after follow-up for 2 years, they reported a recurrence rate of 13%, with only one death. In a group of cirrhotics followed in parallel the results were as follows: Child A, 24% recurrence with 4% mortality; child B, 38% recurrence and 50% mortality; and child C, 73% recurrence and 100% mortality. Two years later, Sakai et al., analyzing a larger group of 97 patients, noticed that previous surgery, particularly splenectomy, had a significant impact on the results of sclerotherapy. For the 75 patients who had undergone previous surgery, control of rebleeding was achieved in 97%, while for the 22 who did not, control of rebleeding was only 73%, a statistically significant difference at p value < 0.05. Moreover, in a randomized trial conducted at the University Hospital of Pernambuco to prospectively

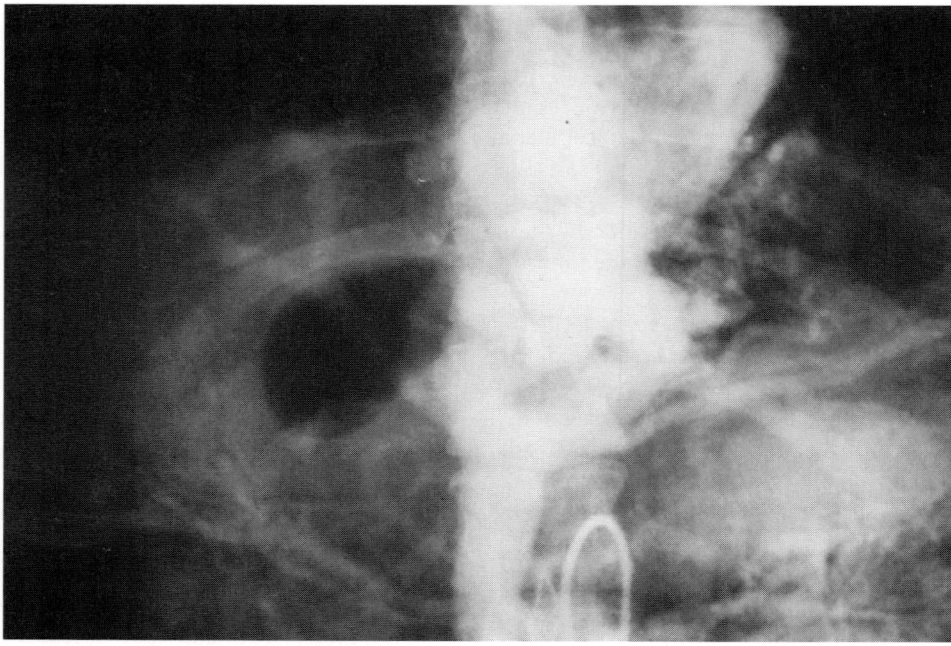

Figure 10 Hepatosplenic schistosomiasis patient after splenectomy. Note a very dilated left gastric vein and an extremely reduced portal vein.

evaluate three modalities of treatment for prophylaxis of rebleeding in patients with no previous therapy, the first evaluation of results at 3 years of follow-up, with roughly 19 patients assigned to each group, has shown a recurrence of bleeding of 37% with sclerotherapy alone, 10% in group with splenectomy plus sclerotherapy, and 6% with splenectomy plus surgical ligation of varices. Limiting surgery to splenectomy also had the advantage of reducing operative time by as much as 80% (204 min versus 135 min). We conclude that splenectomy combined with sclerotherapy is probably the best approach to these patients. Higher levels of portal pressure are likely to be the underlying cause of poor results: sclerotherapy and splenectomy appears to be the best means to lower portal pressure in this condition, as discussed above. In a group of 38 patients undergoing sclerotherapy in our department, 18 achieved good results with eradication of varices and 20 did not, of which 13 rebled during the follow-up period. Although the numbers are small, the presence of large varices with red spots, gastric fundic varices, and identifiable collaterals on ultrasound (all possible indicators of higher portal pressure) were all predictive of nonresponse to sclerotherapy. Thus, sclerotherapy in schistosomiasis is useful in the acute episode of variceal hemorrhage as an alternative for the patient who cannot undergo surgery or as adjunctive therapy with splenectomy. Addition of beta blockade to sclerotherapy until varices are eradicated has been considered but is still an open issue.

In summary, one can state that, in dealing with portal hypertension in schistosomiasis, (1) mortality at the first bleeding episode is very low and good supportive care, including the use of vasoactive drugs such as somatostatin and/or emergency sclerotherapy, are helpful in management; (2) splenectomy supplemented by sclerotherapy appears to be the best way to prevent rebleeding; (3) the role of beta blockers is still undefined; (4) surgical ligation of the left gastric vein to prevent posterior "steal" of mesenteric-portal blood from the liver, with progressive deterioration of liver function, seems warranted; and (5) esophageal ligation of varices is still under evaluation. (In our experience with 30 cases, we have had less side effects and results as good as those obtained with sclerosis.)

Liver Transplantation

Owing to the preservation of liver function, transplantation is rarely needed for hepatosplenic schistosomiasis except in the decompensated state. Indications follow the same rules as for other causes of end-stage liver disease. Moreover, because of the good results obtained with the surgical treatment of portal hypertension, as outlined above, one rarely needs to consider transplantation to control recurrent bleeding.

Schistosomiasis and Hepatotropic Viruses

Studies that have focused on the decompensated form of hepatosplenic schistosomiasis have revealed an important association with hepatitis B superinfection. More recently, hepatitis C infection was also found to be more frequent in decompensated schistosomiasis.

The association of hepatotropic viruses with schistosomiasis can be explained by transfusion and/or nosocomial transmission, since these patients present with gastrointestinal bleeding requiring hospitalization. On the other hand, epidemiological studies in endemic areas do not confirm the association of hepatotropic viruses with hepatosplenic schistosomiasis. Probably, patients who come to referral centers have more severe disease, selecting a subgroup where hepatitis B and C infection are more frequent. There are no controlled studies regarding antiviral treatment in patients with chronic viral hepatitis and schistosomiasis. As these patients have severe disease, interferon probably has a limited role.

DISEASES CAUSED BY PROTOZOANS

Visceral Leishmaniasis (Kala Azar)

Visceral leishmaniasis is the result of the infestation of cells of the reticulo-endothelial system (macrophages) by a parasite from the suborder Trypanosomatina, of the genus *Leishmania* and the species *donovani*. *L. donovani* is transmitted to humans by insects of the genuses *Lutzomya* and *Phlebotomus*, causing a disease whose clinical spectrum is extremely variable. During the process of ingesting blood, the insects also ingest the parasite, which generates a series of transformations in its digestive tract until it is ready to be introduced into another host during subsequent ingestion.

While endemic worldwide, visceral leishmaniasis is especially common in tropical and subtropical countries. It is estimated that 500,000 new cases of kala azar (the classic form, also known as black fever) are diagnosed annually worldwide, demonstrating that the disease is far from being conquered. The incidence is increasing in southwestern Europe and in Mediterranean countries; it has reached epidemic proportions in some countries, including Ethiopia and Sudan.

Pathogenesis

The parasite reproduces in the cytoplasm of the macrophages until the cell ruptures, releasing the parasite into the circulatory system and infecting new macrophages. As intracellular parasites, leishmania, once established in the cytoplasm of antigen-presenting cells, disrupt their principal functions. Many cell-mediated functions are disturbed by leishmania. There is also a polyclonal activation of B lymphocytes, generating hyperglobulinemia and resulting in excessive IgG and IgM production. In the acute phase of the disease, considerable elevation of tumor necrosis factor is observed, partly explaining the loss of muscle mass seen in infected patients.

Clinical Findings

The classic (polar) form of kala azar is characterized by prolonged fever accompanied by weight loss, malnutrition, and hepatosplenomegaly. The hepatic appearance is characterized by a significant increase in the size of the organ, which can grow to occupy a large part of the peritoneal cavity (Fig. 11).

The hepatic histopathology demonstrates hyperplasia and hypertrophy of the Kupffer cells, in whose cytoplasm the parasite can be found. Lymphoplasmacytic infiltration can also be observed in the lobular and portal areas. Necrosis of isolated cells and balloon degeneration of hepatocytes also occurs, and steatosis is a relatively frequent finding. The infiltrate may have aggregates of T and B lymphocytes. In some cases fibrosis occurs, generally demonstrating collagen deposits in the sinusoids. More rarely, there can be a pattern of portal and septal fibrosis without concomitant regenerative nodules. Patients who show marked sinusoidal and portal fibrosis, can develop portal hypertension and hepatic insufficiency, which are probably related to the difficulty of exporting the hepatic proteins to the sinusoids, thus causing a functional hepatic insufficiency. This array of symptoms can be called Roger's cirrhosis, although the patient does not show the histopathological criteria (regenerating nodules) necessary to diagnose classic hepatic cirrhosis.

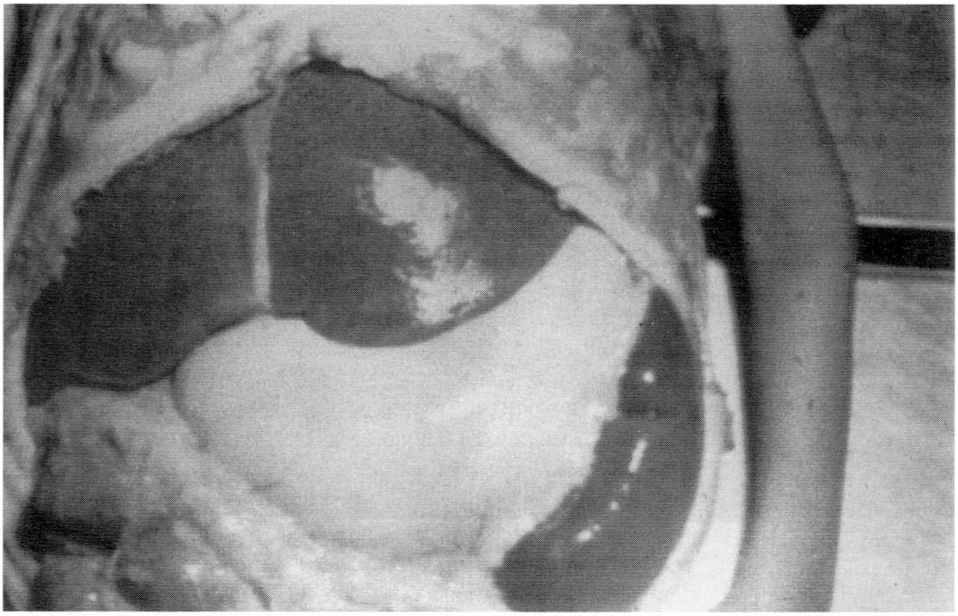

Figure 11 Liver enlargement in visceral leishmaniasis seen at autopsy in a young boy.

Laboratory Diagnosis

Kala azar is characterized by the presence of anemia, leukopenia, thrombocytopenia, and hypergammaglobulinemia. Hepatic involvement is indicated by elevations in serum aminotransferase, although the values observed are rarely higher than three times the upper limit of normal.

When the disease has been present over long periods of time, hypoalbuminemia can be observed, caused not only by the malnourished state but also by the difficulty of hepatic export of albumin. Serum protein electrophoresis demonstrates a polyclonal pattern of hypergammaglobulinemia.

As indirect, nonspecific, diagnostic tests, the protein precipitation reactions such as formol gel, Bramachari reaction, and Rey reaction are strongly positive. Currently, the direct hemagglutinin test and enzyme-linked immunosorbent assay (ELISA) are preferable for serological diagnosis, given their sensitivity and specificity. The presence of the parasite in the peripheral blood (amastigote forms) as well as in tissues, can be demonstrated in 30% of patients, especially on liver biopsy or fine needle aspirates from the spleen. Amastigotes may also be found in aspirates from lymph nodes and bone marrow. A field test for the rapid diagnosis of active visceral leishmaniasis, based on circulating IgG directed against the leishmanial antigen K39, has been utilized in India.

Treatment

The key to the treatment of visceral leishmaniasis lies in the use of pentavalent antimonials, which have been widely utilized for more than eight decades but whose mechanism is still largely unknown. Apparently, they affect the amastigote forms, inhibiting some oxidative processes vital to metabolism. The two forms of the drug available on the market are glucantine and Pentostam. Over the first 3 h after intravenous or intramuscular injection, plasma concentrations become markedly elevated, reaching levels as high as 10–15 μg/mL, and then progressively decrease over the subsequent 12 h. One part of the medication becomes concentrated in the tissues, creating a reservoir, while another part is excreted in the urine. After 10–15 days, the drug reaches a maximum concentration in the tissues, at which point its principal adverse effects may appear, most commonly those related to disturbances of the cardiovascular system and nephrotoxicity.

The doses and the duration of treatment with pentavalent antimonials are extremely variable. Generally, doses should vary between 15–20 mg/kg/day, over a period of not less than 15 days. Some groups prefer 20 mg/kg/day in a single dose for a minimum of 20 days, attempting to avoid recurrence of disease and/or the appearance of resistance. Some authors suggest utilization of smaller doses, such as 10 mg/kg twice a day for a period of 30 days, or even 10 mg/kg three times a day for 10 consecutive days. This has proven to have therapeutic effects. More recently, doses of 10 mg/kg three times a day for 10 days has been the most generally recommended because this regimen is simple and of short duration.

The resistance of leishmaniasis to pentavalent antimonials has frequently been described in the literature. Probably this phenomenon is related to the use of insufficient doses of the medication, disruptions in treatment, or even genetic mutations of the parasite, which increase the parasite's intrinsic resistance to the drug. Thus, therapeutic strategies and modeling become key points in the conduct of patients suffering from visceral leishmaniasis.

The therapeutic schemes most commonly used in Brazil focus on the parasite and on the clinical findings. This being the case, parasitism of less than 10 parasites per area aspirated in the spleen or bone marrow has a recommended dose of 20 mg/kg/day by intramuscular injection, with ambulatory treatment if the clinical condition of the patient permits. In the event that the patient should need to be hospitalized, a dose of 10 mg/kg every 12 h for 15 consecutive days will have a similar effect.

For refractory patients—that is, patients who do not respond to the protocol described above or those who develop more serious disease, with greater infestation—the recommended practice is 10 mg/kg every 8 h by intravenous injection for 10 consecutive days, afterwards shifting to an intramuscular dose of 20 mg/kg/day for a period of 10 to 15 days. Alternatively, 20 mg/kg/day can be used in a single dose for 40 consecutive days, preferably intravenously for the first 10 days and subsequently intramuscularly.

Patients with AIDS are resistant to treatment and frequently need to receive prophylaxis with 15-day doses of 20 mg/kg intramuscularly for an indeterminate period. Special care should be taken with patients who have cardiac arrhythmias. Because pentavalent antimonials accumulate in tissues, adverse effects appear during the course of treatment, especially after the fifteenth day. The most common clinical manifestations during treatment are myalgia, arthralgia, cephalia, anorexia, and gastric disturbances, necessitating treatment with antiemetics. Evidence of hepatocellular effects may be observed, as shown by transitory elevated aminotransferase levels.

An alternative treatment involves the use of capsulated amphotericin B, which produces elevated plasma levels with a shorter half-life, since it is rapidly sequestered by Kupffer cells. A dose of 10 mg/kg/day has proven to be advantageous in that it diminishes nephrotoxicity as well as other side effects.

An aromatic diamine (pentamidine) is also being utilized as an alternative treatment for kala azar. While the specific mechanism of its action is unknown, it is recognized that the drug interferes in the mitochondrial processes of the parasite. Initial dosages can be administered at longer intervals, since its half-life is much longer than that of amphotericin B. Its toxicity is related to hypertension, hyperglycemia, the onset of diabetes, nephrotoxicity, and immunosuppression.

More recently, ketoconazole has been suggested as alternative therapy for leishmaniasis, but its efficacy is still under evaluation. Interferon gamma, in conjunction with pentavalent antimonials, may be of benefit in cases resistant to the antimonials used as monotherapy.

Hepatic Amebiasis

Amebiasis is a disease caused by *Entamoeba histolytica*, a protozoan that moves by means of pseudopods. It resides in the human large intestine in the form of trophozoites and cysts. Human infection generally occurs through ingestion of cysts, which, when they reach the large and small intestine and under ideal conditions, undergo a process of decystation, generating trophozoites.

Epidemiology

Amebiasis occurs throughout the world, although it tends to be more prevalent in countries with hot, humid climates, especially in areas where the socioeconomic conditions are poor.

Pathogenesis

The majority of individuals with amebiasis show no clinical symptoms, and the parasites behave like commensals. However, pathogenic species do exist. These present a wide spectrum of disease, varying from subclinical forms to more serious forms. It is believed that only 10% of individuals with amebiasis develop problems related to the parasite's invasion of the intestinal wall. Although *E. hystolytica* generates antibody and cellular immune responses, its treatment does not prevent the recurrence of the disease.

The distinction between the pathogenic and nonpathogenic forms is an important factor in defining whether patients who are carriers of the cysts should be treated. It is possible to differentiate between amebic forms that are pathogenic and nonpathogenic by characterizing immunoenzymatic patterns. Nonpathogenic forms may undergo genomic mutation, thereby becoming pathogenic forms.

Determination of adhesions, molecules that promote the organisms' adherence to the surface of the colon, is another way of distinguishing pathogenic species from those that are nonpathogenic. The molecule GIAP (galactose inhibitable adherence protein) measured by solid-phase ELISA is positive in 99% of patients with hepatic amebic abscesses. Finally, molecular biological testing with analysis of amebic genomes can be utilized in distinguishing pathogenic from nonpathogenic forms, although it presents certain difficulties in routine laboratory utilization.

Clinical Findings

The principal clinical manifestation of amebiasis is dysentery—that is, bloody diarrhea caused by colitis. Patients generally present with a predictable array of symptoms characterized by mild or severe forms of diarrhea and the presence of mucus and blood in the feces. Proctosigmoidoscopic or colonoscopic findings may include an altered vascular pattern, friability, hemorrhage, and ulcerations. The liver is the most common site for extraintestinal manifestations of amebiasis. Organisms reach the liver through the mesenteric and portal veins. It should be noted, however, that only 50% of patients with amebic abscesses have a previous history of intestinal disease, indicating the possibility of parasitic penetration even in subclinical forms of the disease. Generally, there is only one hepatic lesions, which is usually found in the right lobe; however, multiple lesions can occur. If the lesions go untreated, there is a tendency toward dispersion, with the eventual possibility of rupture into the abdominal cavity, which can result in shock. The most common clinical manifestations are fever, weight loss, and abdominal pain, which are more intense in the acute processes. On the other hand, entirely asymptomatic cases have been noted and incidental diagnosis is made at the time of imaging studies. The liver, when palpated below the right ribs, may be tender and have a hardened consistency.

Some patients show clinical symptoms corresponding to sepsis, with fever, chills, nocturnal sweating, anorexia, and malaise. Jaundice may be present in rare cases, and invasion of the abscess into the biliary ducts or biliary compression through the inflammatory process may cause biliary obstruction. Respiratory discomfort, shortness of breath, and a productive cough can indicate dispersion into the pleural region or even into the lungs.

Laboratory Diagnosis

Leukocytosis with neutrophilia and accelerated erythrocyte sedimentation rates are nonspecific findings. Mild hyperbilirubinemia can occur, with elevations of serum alkaline phosphatase, gamma glutamyl transpeptidase, and sometimes aminotransferases. Long-term chronic abscesses can be accompanied by hyperglobulinemia. Hypoalbuminemia can be caused by a patient's advanced catabolic state or even by the loss of hepatic function due to the size of the hepatic cavitation.

Specific serological diagnosis is important when amebic abscess is suspected because parasites are observed in the feces only in 2–30% of the patients with liver abscess. On the other hand, searching for parasites by fine-needle aspiration of abscesses has been disappointing, with organisms being encountered in less than 50% of the cases. This low sensitivity points to the fact that parasites are not found in the large central necrotic area but are more often located in peripheral areas of abscesses. It may be necessary to obtain tissue from the periphery of the abscess under ultrasonic guidance in order to increase the chances of finding trophozoites.

Despite the low positivity of identification of organisms after aspiration of amebic abscesses, it still is useful to *culture this material* to rule out the possibility of pyogenic abscess (see Chap. 19) or secondary infection of the amebic abscess.

Serological tests are based on the detection of serum antibodies against amebic antigens. In the invasive form of the disease, antibody levels are high enough to be detected through these tests. Many serological tests have been utilized, the most extensive being those that measure through indirect hemagglutination, latex agglutination, double diffusion, ELISA, and electrophoresis, whose sensitivity in the amebic abscess is 95–99%. With the purification of GIAP, the possibility of better characterization of antibodies and of the pathogenic potential of the infectious forms has opened up considerably. More recently, the presence of an IgM fraction has been demonstrated, indicating acute illness. The loss of the IgM fraction accompanied by elevation of the IgG fraction indicates chronic illness.

Imaging

Ultrasonography is the key to the diagnosis of amebic abscesses. Computed tomography serves to complement ultrasonography. These two imaging techniques permit a precise measurement of the diameter of the cavity and the reduction in its size that occurs after chemotherapy or aspiration and/or external drainage.

Treatment

Sine qua non conditions for the treatment of amebic abscesses are the utilization of amebicides that reach adequate tissue concentrations and are capable of eliminating the parasite from the intestinal lumen. The most frequently utilized medication for invasive amebiasis is metronizadole, which blocks the synthesis of the parasite's components and is rapidly absorbed. Intraluminal concentrations, however, are insufficient to eliminate intestinal parasites. If the patient is otherwise in good health and eating normally, doses of 500–750 mg three times a day can be utilized over a period of 10 days, with good therapeutic effects. In more severe cases, in which the patient is unable to use the oral medicines, the recommended intravenous dose is 500 mg every 8 h. For children weighing less than 40 kg, doses of 35–50 mg can be administered orally three times a day for 10 days.

After the treatment of invasive amebiasis, the intestinal parasite should be eliminated by the utilization of an intraluminal amebicide. Of these, epophimyde can be used in doses of 200 mg three times a day for 5 days. Other options, such as teclozan, in doses of 100 mg three times a day for 5 days, have had similar results. These are the medications used most frequently in Brazil. In other countries preference is given to other medications, with treatment varying between 7 and 20 days. In the Brazilian experience, the use of metronizadole associated with luminal agents resolves most cases. Resistance to this therapeutic scheme is exceptional; however, in the literature, some authors have cited cases that impose therapeutic difficulties.

It is important to remember the collateral effects of metronizadole, among them the induction of nausea and vomiting, and, in some patients, the appearance of peripheral neuropathy, rarely occurring before 10 continuous days of treatment. Alcohol needs to be proscribed for the duration of metronidazole treatment.

Therapeutic alternatives utilized in exceptional cases include the use of emetine and of its less toxic derivative, dehydroemetine. The cardiovascular toxicity of these drugs places them in a secondary position in the treatment of amebic abscesses. They should be used only in exceptional cases. Chloroquine phosphate can also be used to obtain adequate tissue concentration; however, this requires a longer period of treatment, varying from 2–3 weeks. The principal side effects are irritability of the gastrointestinal tract, sometimes provoking vomiting and diarrhea, dizziness, and visual disturbances. These therapeutic schemes have not been demonstrated to be superior to the use of metronizadole. Their use should be confined to cases when the use of imidazole derivatives is impossible due to hypersensitivity or, more rarely, in cases of resistance.

Close to 10% of untreated amebic abscesses can develop secondary bacterial or anaerobic microbial infections. Because of this, as noted above, the cultivation of aspirated material or isolation of the infectious form is fundamental in defining therapeutic strategies with adequate antibiotic therapy. Bacterial superinfection in amebic abscesses should be suspected when persistent fever occurs after metronizadole has been introduced, with persistent leukocytosis, and when multiple abscesses are present.

DISEASES CAUSED BY HELMINTHS AND CESTODES

Toxocariasis

Toxocariasis is a prevalent disease in the tropics and is responsible in part for tropical eosinophilia. The etiologic agents are *Toxocara canis* and, less commonly, *Toxocara catis*. It is transmitted through close contact with domestic dogs and cats. The toxocara larvae penetrate the human intestinal mucosa, entering the circulatory system; however, they are unable to complete the cycle, since humans are inadequate hosts. They therefore migrate erratically through the intestines and generate a spectrum of diseases from least serious and most common to more severe forms. Children are the principal victims of the disease; up to the age of 15, milder forms prevail and are without important clinical manifestations.

Pathogenesis

Human infection occurs through ingestion of eggs, the life cycle of the parasite being similar to that of *Ascaris lumbricoides* (see below). Larvae are liberated in the small intestine and then penetrate the ileum and the colon, entering the circulatory system through the mesenteric vein and lymphatic ducts, arriving in the liver through the portal circulation, passing through the sinusoids, reaching the pulmonary capillaries, and arriving in the left heart, where they are dispersed through hematogenous pathways. The larvae can secrete substances affecting capillaries, thus facilitating their capillary transposition.

During the migratory process, the larvae liberate antigenic substances that stimulate the immune system, causing local inflammatory reactions and hypereosinophilia. In the immunocompetent host, the larvae are contained by the immune response, generating a local inflammatory reaction with granuloma formation and preventing continuation of migration. For reasons still not well understood, in some individuals the process of migration is not halted by the immunological reaction of the host, thereby permitting dissemination of disease. It is probable that larvae change their integument successively when there is an antibody response directed against their proteins.

Epidemiology

In seroepidemiological studies, antitoxocara antibodies have been found to be present in humans from many continents, demonstrating the endemic nature of the infection. Cohabitation with animals, such as dogs and cats, predisposes people to infection and is increasingly common in modern western societies.

Clinical Findings

The disease is, in general, benign. During the period of larval migration, the patient presents with nonspecific clinical manifestations such as nausea, vomiting, fever, and itching. In most cases the immune system will be able to deter larval migration by forming granulomas around the larvae in the affected tissue, which results in resolution.

The liver and spleen are commonly affected organs, which may result in hepatosplenomegaly. In the initial phase of the process, the patient may have a cough, fever, allergic manifestations such as itching and bronchial spasm, hepatosplenomegaly, and eosinophilia.

The spectrum of clinical laboratory findings is dependent on the parasitic load as well as on the capacity of the host immune response. Thus, infection by small numbers of larvae generally brings on only eosinophilia. The most severe form, visceral larva migrans, affects children and presents a wide clinical range of signs and symptoms, including hepatosplenomegaly, eosinophilia, hypergammaglobulinemia, irritability, nausea, and vomiting. Eventually the erratic migration of the larvae can reach the brain or even the eyes, bringing on clinical manifestations peculiar to those two organs.

Laboratory Diagnosis

One of the most dramatic effects of infection by toxocara is hypereosinophilia, which can reach levels of 100,000 cells per cubic millimeter. Depending on the seriousness of the disease, hyperglobulinemia may also be observed, reflecting a high level of IgE.

Currently the diagnosis of toxocariases can easily be made by detecting the presence of antibodies through an ELISA technique, whose sensitivity and specificity are satisfactory, especially in the presence of liver and spleen involvement.

Liver biopsy has limited value. The detection of larvae in the liver tissue is difficult in cores obtained by needle biopsy, requiring multiple samples, and it has the limitation of sampling error.

Treatment

Many antihelminthics have been used in the treatment of toxocariasis, especially diethylcarbamazine, ivermectine, tiabendazole, and albendazole. Because it is well tolerated and has been used extensively worldwide, albendazole treatment is felt to be the best therapeutic option, the usual dose being around 10 mg/kg/day for 5 to 15 days.

In more severe forms, where bronchial spasm and ocular involvement occur, patients can theoretically benefit from corticosteroids; however, it must be noted that there are possible undesirable side effects from the corticosteroids, which diminish immunological activity, thereby permitting greater larval migration.

Ascariasis

Ascariasis is a helminthic infection known since antiquity and caused by *Ascaris lumbricoides*. Despite the fact that this condition is clinically benign in most cases and is easily treatable, it is estimated that mortality due to ascariasis reaches 20,000 per year. It is generally more prevalent in underdeveloped countries and in populations of lower socioeconomic levels. It is the most common of human parasitoses, with the greatest prevalence occurring in countries with tropical and temperate climates.

Pathogenesis

Ascarids normally live in the lumen of the small intestine, although in severe parasitosis they can be found in the stomach and the colon as well. Human infestation occurs through ingestion of viable eggs. The eggs are digested in the stomach, thereby freeing larvae to migrate to the duodenum and the jejunum. The larvae then migrate to the ileum and the cecum, which they penetrate, reaching the portal vein through the mesenteric vein, then passing through the hepatic sinusoids, and reaching the lungs and the right heart. At the level of pulmonary capillaries, the secretion of enzymes facilitates transposition to the bronchial tree, causing coughing and dislocating the larvae to the larynx and pharynx, where they are swallowed. Ultimately they arrive in the intestine, where they achieve sexual maturity. The larval migration is asymptomatic and lacking in laboratory manifestations except eosinophilia. In instances of repeated infection there can be hypersensitivity, itching, bronchial spasm, and, in rare cases, pulmonary infiltration. During the process of hepatic migration, some of the larvae may be trapped in the hepatic sinusoids, generating a local inflammatory response that gives rise to the formation of hepatic granulomas, which may later be detected by imaging examinations. Rarely, the larval migration can be erratic, arriving at the biliary tree and/or the pancreatic duct as well as other abdominal organs. The adult parasite lodges in the digestive tract, where it completes its life cycle within the intestinal lumen.

Clinical Findings

Infection by *Ascaris lumbricoides* tends to be asymptomatic. In the larval migration phase, there may be pulmonary manifestations as described above. Loeffler's syndrome is occasionally observed. With hyperinfestation, there can be signs of intestinal occlusion which may require surgical resolution. The hepatic involvement occurs through erratic migration of adult parasites through duodenal papilla, causing biliary obstruction and consequently acute suppurative cholangitis and hepatic abscess formation (Fig. 12). Cases of pancreatitis are also described. This type of migration is commonly associated when inadequate doses of antihelminthics are prescribed in hyperinfected patients.

Laboratory Diagnosis

Examination of feces is the best method for establishing the diagnosis. The Lutz or Hoffman techniques have been generally preferred, but the Faust method is more sensitive for the detection of viable eggs.

Eosinophilia and hypergammaglobulinemia are self-limited and generally found only in the phase of larval migration; however, adult worms in the intestinal lumen can stimulate the production of eosinophils and maintain the eosinophilia.

In the presence of biliary obstruction with clinical symptoms including pain, fever and jaundice, the principal laboratory alterations are elevations of serum aminotransferases, alkaline phosphatase and gammaglutamyl transpeptidase. Patients may also develop suppurative cholangitis with a classical Charcot's triad.

In cases where the worms manage to pass beyond the common duct and reach smaller ducts, local infection may occur, with the formation of hepatic abscesses. In this situation, abdominal ultrasonography may reveal dilation of the intrahepatic biliary tree and evidence of intrahepatic abscess. When worms are impacted in the biliary tree, endoscopic retrograde cholangiography may be useful in diagnosis as well as in treatment (Fig. 13).

Treatment

Many antihelminthics are active against ascaris. Currently, albendazole is preferred owing to its ovocidal, larvicidal, and vermicidal action. It is prescribed in doses of not less than

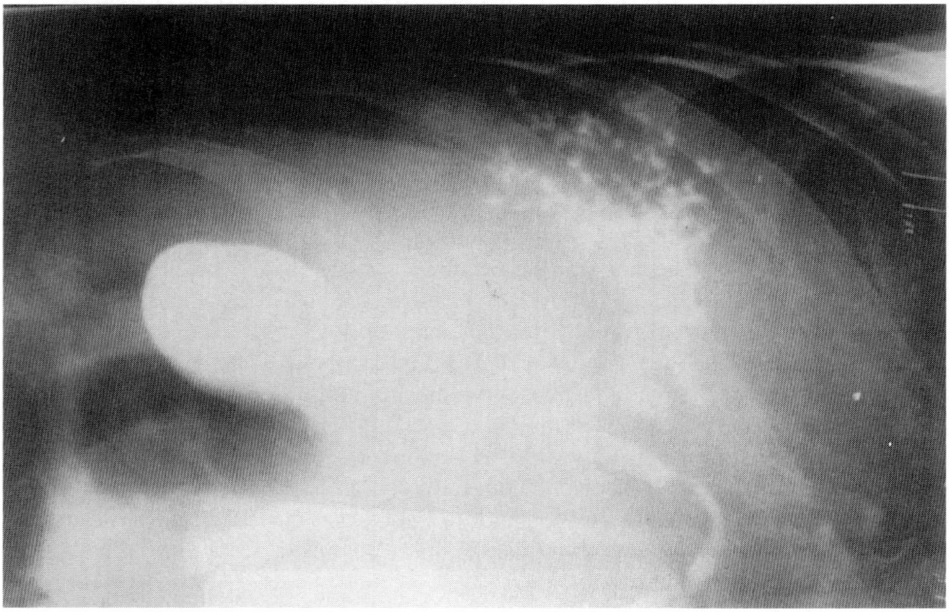

Figure 12 Liver abscess in ascariasis demonstrated by cholangiography.

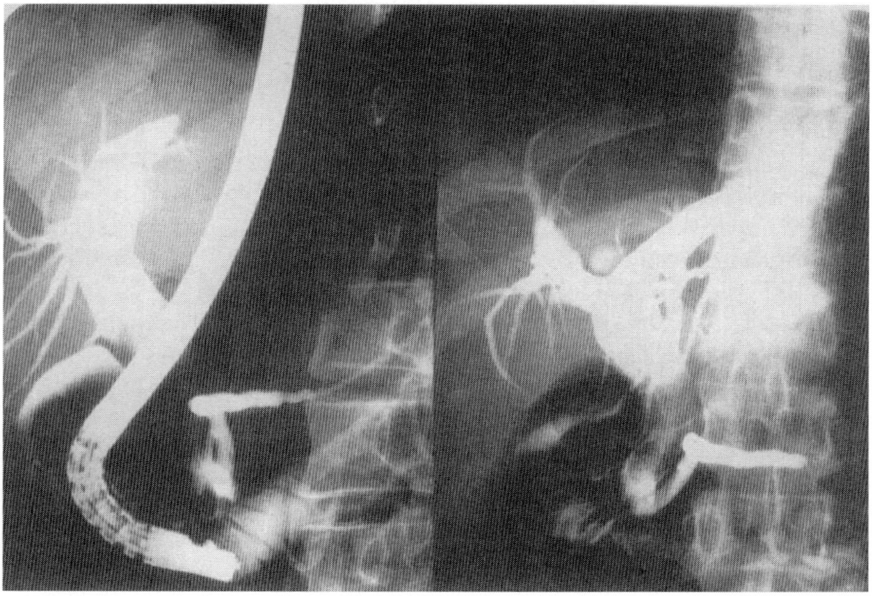

Figure 13 Biliary ascariasis causing common duct dilation demonstrated by endoscopic retrograde cholangiography.

400 mg for adults or 10 mg/kg for children. In cases of hyperinfestation, with the risk of intestinal obstruction, piperazine may be used, accompanied by mineral oil. Levamiscle, mebendazole, and pamoate or pirantel are drugs also recommended in the treatment of ascariasis.

In the case of biliary obstruction, extraction of worms may be accomplished at the time of endoscopic retrograde cholangiography, thereby resolving the obstructive process. Antibiotics are necessary as well, since bacterial infection generally accompanies helminthic invasion of the biliary tract. Administration of albendazole into the common duct at the time of cholangiography has recently been performed in patients with a heavy infestation. Patients with hepatic abscesses should be subjected to antibiotic treatment; in cases with large abscesses, percutaneous drainage or even surgery may be indicated.

Abdominal Angiostrongyliasis

Abdominal angiostrongyliasis is caused by the Costa Rican *Angiostrongylus morena*. In humans, the adult worms are found in the ileocecal area, where they generate inflammatory vascular reactions, sometimes presenting as a pseudotumor, and can mimic Crohn's disease (see Fig. 14). Rarely, other organs are affected, the liver among them.

Human abdominal angiostrongyliasis is accidental. The rodents are the preferred hosts and molluscs intermediate hosts. The clinical manifestations in humans are extremely variable, ranging from asymptomatic to the serious form of pseudotumors. The mesenteric location directs clinical symptoms toward the left and right lower quadrants of the abdomen, characterized as recurring abdominal pain accompanied by hypereosinophilia and

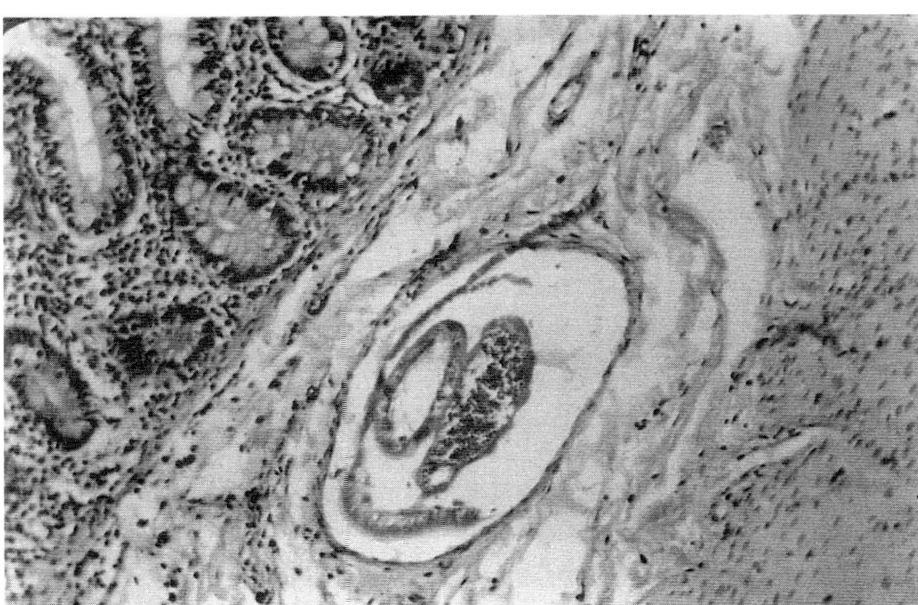

Figure 14 Larvae of *Angiostrongylus* in the small intestinal wall.

fever. More serious cases have been described, which resulted in destruction of ileocecal vessels, microhemorrhage, and intense local reaction, often requiring surgical correction.

Liver involvement is less common but is characterized by episodes of abdominal pain and hepatomegaly. In this situation it is common to observe eosinophilia and elevated circulating enzymes. The histopathological picture is nonspecific, with hepatic eosinophilic infiltration and, very rarely, the presence of larvae in the parenchyma. However, larvae can frequently be found in the intestinal submucosa.

The ideal treatment is still unknown. The use of antihelminthics in experimental models has demonstrated erratic migration of the larvae with death of the animals. Surgical treatment can be useful, but it does not guarantee eradication of the worms. It is recommended that, in hyperendemic areas, the mollusc population be controlled, as these are the intermediate hosts. It is also recommended that food and water should be boiled.

Strongyloidiasis

Strongyloidiasis is caused by *Strongyloides stercoralis*, as well as by *S. fülleborni*. Strongyloidiasis predominates in countries with hot, humid climates. In these types of environments, the larvae are able to survive on the ground. Human infection occurs when the larvae come into contact with the skin, which they then penetrate. The principal clinical characteristics include abdominal pain and diarrhea.

A clinical peculiarity of this disease is its capacity to invade organs, which is facilitated in immunosuppressed conditions such as corticosteroid therapy and HIV infection. Corticosteroid therapy has been known to bring on serious forms of the disease, with worms penetrating the mucous membranes of the walls of the small intestine and of the colon, reaching the circulatory system and bringing on a range of systemic inflammatory responses and even of sepsis.

Curiously, despite being the locus of the parasite's migration, the liver gives rise to few clinical, laboratory, or histological manifestations. This is probably related to the immunodepressed state of the patients, who are unable to generate satisfactory inflammatory responses to the parasite. Hepatic autopsy findings indicate nonspecific conditions such as steatosis, which can be related to the patient's underlying disease, the use of corticosteroids, or even metabolic perturbation generated by the systemic inflammatory response.

Strongyloidiasis can be treated using *thiabendazole* or *cambendazole*. More recently, some authors have suggested the use of higher doses of albendazole, although the place of this medication is still undetermined.

Hepatic Fascioliasis

Hepatic fascioliasis is a disease caused by *Fasciola hepatica*, a fluke that attacks humans accidentally. Its preferred hosts are bovine and ovine. Snails are intermediate hosts; the larvae capable of infecting mammals (cercarias) are released from them. Adult worms situate themselves in the biliary tree of the host. Human infection occurs through the ingestion of contaminated vegetables, water, fish, or the inadequately cooked liver of sheep or beef. In Brazil, hepatic fascioliasis is found in the cattle- and sheep-producing regions of the southern part of the country; few cases are reported, however, indicating that in most cases a definitive diagnosis is not made.

Clinical Findings

After ingestion of the cercariae, there is an acute phase of infection lasting for up to 30 days and characterized by the migration of the larvae through the liver, trying to reach the biliary tree. During this phase, fever, abdominal pain, and intense eosinophilia—in addition to less specific gastrointestinal disturbances such as nausea, vomiting, and diarrhea—occur. In the case of intense migration, there can be hepatocellular necrosis with jaundice and elevated levels of circulating cholestatic enzymes and aminotransferases.

After the parasites reach the biliary tree, there is a latent phase without specific symptoms that can last for years. After a long period of parasitism, the parasites lodge themselves in the biliary tree, causing inflammation and destruction of the ducts. The presence of the parasite in the lumens of the biliary ducts stimulates the secretion of proteins deriving from the parasite, which stimulate an inflammatory reaction. The proline secreted by the parasite stimulates a fibrotic reaction around the biliary ducts.

During infection, many hosts may show no symptoms for extended periods of time, making diagnosis extremely difficult. There may be intermittent signs of suppurative cholangitis, cholecystitis, or intermittent right- upper-quadrant abdominal pain. Diagnosis should be considered in patients in an endemic region showing biliary symptomatology, especially in an individual who works in an area where cattle and/or sheep are raised and/or is regularly exposed to contact with these animals.

Laboratory Diagnosis

In the phase of larval migration, eosinophilia with nonspecific symptoms such as fever and lethargy occurs. Elevated levels of hepatic enzymes may also be present. The detection of parasite eggs in the feces can be a diagnostic tool, but in humans the development of the parasite is often incomplete and eggs are frequently not produced. An ELISA detects antibodies produced against the worm. It is a sensitive method, and the presence of the IgM antibody marker is characteristic of the acute phase of the disease. Immunoprecipitation reactions have satisfactory specificity, although they lack sensitivity. A complement fixation reaction higher than 1/1000 is extremely suggestive.

Imaging and Cholangiography

Ultrasonographic findings are nonspecific, especially when the examiner is not specifically on the lookout for the disease. The presence of microhepatic abscesses has been reported in isolated cases. Computed tomography may reveal the presence of hyperdense areas in the liver, which can be found as a consequence of the larval migration phase. Previous infections manifest themselves as calcified areas.

Endoscopic retrograde cholangiographic findings may be similar to those observed in primary sclerosing cholangitis, as parasites in the biliary tree can mimic stenosis.

Treatment

Biphional in doses of 30–60 mg/kg on alternate days for 15 days is the treatment of choice. Principal collateral effects are those related to irritability of the digestive system, including pain, colic, nausea, vomiting, and diarrhea. Triclabenzole is an alternate treatment, used even in veterinary medicine. Praziquantel, used in oral doses of 25 mg/kg three times per day, can be effective, although for unknown reasons it is totally ineffective in some cases. Finally, surgery may be indicated in special cases in order to remove biliary obstruction, especially when the biliary tree shows signs of infection.

After treatment there is a decline in antifasciola antibodies, detected by ELISA. This test should be applied in order to evaluate resolution of the process.

Hydatid Cysts

Hydatid cysts result from infestation by the larval stage of cestodes, which belong to the genus *Echinococcus*. The preferred hosts of the adult parasites are wild and domestic carnivores. At least four species of *Echinococcus* can eventually parasitize humans: *E. granulosus*, *E. multiloculares*, *E. vogeli*, and *E. eligartros*. The most important of these is *E. granulosus*. The definitive hosts acquire the infection through ingesting animal viscera that contain cysts, which are freed once they enter the host's small intestine; there they develop and eventually reach the adult phase.

The adult parasite is a 3- to 6-mm tapeworm whose natural habitat is the intestines of canines and felines. The eggs are eliminated by the primary hosts and later ingested by intermediate hosts, including humans. They then appear in the duodenum, liberating the oncoferas—larvae that pass through the abdominal wall and enter the mesenteric vascular system, and they are disseminated more commonly through the liver and lungs.

In these organs, the larvae develop slowly, forming differentiated cysts with walls whose interior is occupied by the developing larvae. Generally, there is only one cyst with *E. granulosus*; other *Echinococcus* species produce multicystic lesions of the liver.

Epidemiology

Echinococcus granulosus is found on practically every continent. In the Americas, the infection is found most commonly in sheep-raising regions, such as the south of Brazil, Argentina, and Uruguay. In Europe and Asia, *Echinococcus* is present in virtually all countries where sheep are raised.

Most carriers of hydatid cysts are asymptomatic. Today, diagnosis is generally made incidentally through modern imaging methods such as ultrasound. On the other hand, depending on the size and location of the cyst, symptoms may occur because of compression of adjacent structures. The hydatid cyst can compress biliary ducts, generating obstruction, or hepatic vessels, possibly giving rise to thrombosis of the suprahepatic veins. If the cyst exerts pressure on the biliary tree, the patient may present with a classic array of cholestatic signs and symptoms, although this occurs only rarely. Eventually the hepatic cyst can break open into the abdominal cavity, generating hypersensitivity reactions or even a form of hydatidosis called secondary hydatidosis.

Imaging

Ultrasound and computed tomography are extremely useful methods in diagnosis. It should be noted that in some patients with long-term cysts, a simple abdominal x-ray can show hepatomegaly and calcifications in the region of the cyst. Ultrasonographic characteristics include the presence of fine or somewhat thickened walls, multiloculation, and small vesicles in the interior of the cyst. When multiple cysts are present, diagnosis is more difficult. The principal differential diagnosis is polycystic disease with hepatic involvement and congenital liver cysts, although ultrasonography and computed tomography give a relative degree of certainty to the diagnosis.

Laboratory Diagnosis

The serological techniques most frequently used are indirect hemagglutination or agglutination with latex particles, whose specificity is low but whose sensitivity is satisfactory.

More recently various ELISA techniques have been introduced, which have proved sensitive and specific in detecting antibodies against hydatid cysts.

Therapy

In general, the treatment of hydatid cysts is surgical, and only experienced surgeons should remove them. The surgical process carries some risks, such as the possibility of the cyst rupture into the abdominal cavity, thereby generating an anaphylactic reaction as well as the dissemination of scolices. Thus, it is important to isolate the surgical area when performing cystectomies, to empty the cyst before removing it, and to treat the surgical area with a 20% saline solution or 0.1% cetrimonium bromide. The injection of these substances into the empty cyst has the advantage of treating the viable parts of the parasite, thus avoiding their possible dissemination and reappearance—the latter occurring in 10% of the surgical cases.

The benzimidazoles—mebendazole and albendazole—have scolicidal activity. Elevated and prolonged doses of mebendazole (50/100 mg/kg/day) for a period of not less than 3 months and not longer than 6 months have been utilized, although with conflicting results. More recently, albendazole, also in elevated doses (10–15 mg/kg/day over a period of 3 months), has proved to be as effective as mebendazole, with less possibility of toxicity. The utilization of these drugs can postpone or even eliminate the need for surgery. Ultrasound after treatment can reveal diminution or even disappearance of the cysts in the case of successful treatment. As with all imidazole derivatives, reactions of hypersensitivity, hepatotoxicity, neutropenia, and peripheral neuropathy are possible. These generally disappear when the drug is discontinued.

Percutaneous drainage of cysts with ultrasonic guidance after albendazole treatment, with subsequent injection of 20% saline and irrigation, has been proposed as an alternative method for the treatment of uncomplicated cysts. This method requires caution in order to avoid the dissemination of the cyst contents in the peritoneal cavity and consequent anaphylactic reactions.

CYSTICERCOSIS

Hepatic cysticercosis results from infestation by *Taenia solium* larvae. Humans are the definitive hosts of *T. solium*, while swine are the intermediate hosts. Human ingestion of the ova results in the development of the intermediate stage of the disease—that is, larval migration through the organs and the formation of small cysts, within which the larvae develop. When humans ingest contaminated pork, the larvae begin to develop; they reach maturity in the human intestines. The organs most commonly reached are the brain, liver, spleen, striated muscles, lungs, and heart. The disease is generally asymptomatic, with the diagnosis made incidentally at the time of ultrasonography.

Treatment of hepatic cysticercosis is considered unnecessary if there are no symptoms. Since the organ most commonly affected is the central nervous system, there may be an array of neurological manifestations. Patients who are suspected of having liver involvement should be investigated for possible cerebral involvement. In those cases, the disease can be treated with cysticides such as praziquantel at a dose of 50 mg/kg/day for 15 consecutive days. More recently, albendazole has been utilized in doses of 15 mg/kg/day for 30 days, with good tolerability and satisfactory results.

BIBLIOGRAPHY

Arruda SMB. Dopplerfluxometria em esquistossomóticos com e sem hemorragia digestiva: tese mestrado. UFPE, 1996.

Coutinho A, Domingues ALC. Esguitossomose mansonica. In: Dani R, Castro LP, eds. Gastroenterologia Clínca, 3d ed. Rio de Janeiro: Guanabara, 1993:1697–1728.

Domingues ALC, Coutinho AD. Reduction of morbidity in hepatosplenic schistosomiasis mansoni after treatment with praziquantel: a long term study. Rev Soc Bras Med Trop 1990; 23:101–107.

Domingues ALC, Dias HS, Lima ARF, Cordeiro F, Coutinho AD. Analysis of possible predictive factors of no success of sclerotherapy of esophageal varices in schistosomotic patients. Annals of the Fifth International Symposiumon Schistosomiasis in Salvador-BA, 1995.

Domingues ALC, Dias HS, Pessoa AL, Cordeiro F, Barreto VST, Ferraz EM. Prospective evaluation of three modalities of treatment in Schistosomiasis mansoni—Annals of the Fifth International Symposium on Schistosomiasis in Salvador-BA, 1995.

Fallon PG, Doenhoff MJ. Drug resistant schistosomiasis: resistance to praziquantel and oxamiquinine induced in Schistosoma mansoni in mice is drug specific. Am J Trop Med Hyg 1994; 51(1): 83–88.

Golematis BC, Pevertetos PJ. Hepatic hydatid disease: current surgical treatment. Mt Sinai J Med 1995; 62:71–76.

Katz N et al. Clinical trials with oxamniquine, by oral route, in schistosomiasis mansoni. Rev Inst Med Trop São Paulo 1976; 13:57–70.

Khuroo MS. Ascariasis. Gastroenterol Clin North Am 1996; 2:553–577.

Khuroo MS, Wani NA, Javid G, Khan BA, et al. Percutaneous drainage compared with surgery for hepatic hydatid cysts. N Engl J Med 1997; 337:881–887.

Liu LX, Harinasuta KT. Liver and intestinal flukes. Gastroenterol Clin North Am 1996; 25:627–635.

Mohamed-Ali Q, et al. Ultrasonographical investigation of periportal fibrosis in children with Schistosoma mansoni infection: reversibility of morbidity seven months after treatment with praziquantel. Am J Trop Med Hyg 1991; 44:441–451.

Pedretti L Jr, Badogue E, Morales JS, Brutto OH. Cisticercose. In: Veronesi R, Foccacia R, eds. Tratado de Infectologia. São Paulo: Atheneu 1996:1332–1338.

Pal S, Sengupta K, Mann B, Sarkar S, Bhattachaya S, Das P. Comparative evaluation of somatic and excretory-secretory antigens of E. histolytica in serodiagnosis of human amoebiasis by ELISA. Indian J Med Res 1996; 104:152–156.

Punda-Políc V, Sardelíc S, Bradaríc N. Visceral leishmaniasis in southern Croatia. Lancet 1998; 351:188.

Raia S, Silva LC, Gayotto LCC, Forster SC, Fukushima J, Strauss E. Portal hypertension in schistosomiasis: A long-term follow-up of a randomized trial comparing three types of surgery. Hepatology 1994; 20:398–403.

Rashid JR, Wasunn KM, Gachihi GS, Nyakundi PM, et al. The efficacy and safety of ketoconozole visceral leishmaniasis. East Afr Med J 1994; 71:392–395.

Ravdin. Amebiasis. Clin Infect Dis 1995; 20:1453–1463.

Restrepo MI, Restrepo Z, Elsa-Villareal CL, Aguirre A, Restrepo M. Diagnostic tests for amoebic liver abscess. Rev Soc Bras Med Trop 1996; 29:27–32.

Sturchler D, Schubarth P, Gualzata M, et al. Thiabendazole vs albendazole in treatment of toxocariasis: a clinical trial. Am Trop Med Pas 1989; 83:473–478.

Stokvis H, et al. Seizures associated with oxamniquine therapy. Am J Trop Med Hyg 1986; 35: 330–331.

Sundar S, Reed SG, Singh VP, Kumar PCK, Murray HW. Rapid accurate field diagnosis of Indian visceral leishmaniasis. Lancet 1998; 351:563–565.

Van den Bogaerde JB, Jordaan M. Intraductal administration of albendazole for biliary ascariasis. Am J Gastroenterol 1997; 92:1531–1533.

Wynants H, Van den Ende J, Randria J, Van Gompel A, et al. Diagnosis of amoebic infection of the liver: report of 36 cases. Ann Soc Belg Med Trop 1995; 75:297–303.

21
Management of HIV-Related Hepatobiliary Disease

Michael A. Poles
University of California School of Medicine, Los Angeles, California

Douglas T. Dieterich
New York University School of Medicine, New York, New York

INTRODUCTION AND OVERVIEW

By the year 2000, it is likely that 15 to 20 million people will be infected with the human immunodeficiency virus (HIV). AIDS has become the third leading cause of death among American women 25–44 years of age, and is already the leading cause of death in male Caucasians of the same age group. The availability of potent antiretroviral agents combined with the ability to directly assess their effect on viral burden is expected to result in a dramatic prolongation of life of HIV-seropositive patients. Thus, greater attention needs to be focused on concurrent illnesses that may increase mid- to long-range morbidity and mortality in patients with HIV infection. After infection with HIV, patients are susceptible to a variety of hepatic processes that may contribute to morbidity and mortality. Hepatic disease is quite common in this population; intrahepatic opportunistic infections and malignancies are found in 30–80% of patients with AIDS at autopsy.

Liver disease in patients with AIDS presents in a myriad of ways including fever, right-upper-quadrant pain, hepatomegaly, but—most commonly—with isolated laboratory abnormalities. Up to 90% of patients with AIDS have abnormalities of their liver-associated enzymes, usually when CD4 cell counts are $<200/mm^3$. An enlarged liver can be detected on physical exam in 60–73% of these patients, but when their livers are examined histologically, abnormalities are almost uniformly seen. Every physician caring for patients with AIDS requires a systematic method of evaluating and treating patients with hepatobiliary disease to ensure that morbidity and mortality are minimized and quality of life and medical care costs are optimized.

The etiology of hepatic disease in these patients may be divided into categories to facilitate discussion (see Table 1). While this chapter has been partitioned into hepatitis, granulomatous disease, mass lesions, vascular lesions, hepatotoxic drugs, and nonspecific findings, inspection will reveal that this classification scheme is somewhat arbitrary, as many of the infections and neoplasms discussed have varied presentations.

Table 1 Etiologies of Hepatic Disease in HIV Infection

Hepatitis	Granulomatous inflammation	Mass lesions
Hepatitis B, C, D	Mycobacterial	Kaposi's sarcoma
Cytomegalovirus	*Mycobacterium avium* complex	Non-Hodgkin's lymphoma
Epstein-Barr virus	*Mycobacterium tuberculosis*	Other neoplasms
Herpes simplex virus	Other atypical mycobacteria	Vascular lesions
Adenovirus	Fungal	Peliosis hepatis
Varicella zoster virus	*Histoplasma capsulatum*	Kaposi's sarcoma
HIV	*Cryptococcus neoformans*	Nonspecific findings
Hepatotoxic drugs	*Coccidioides immitis*	
Ethanol	*Candida albicans*	
	Protozoa	
	Pneumocystis carinii	
	Toxoplasma gondii	
	Microsporidian species	
	Schistosoma sp.	
	Cryptosporidium parvum	
	Hepatotoxic drugs	

Hepatitis

Hepatocellular necrosis is not an uncommon finding in patients with AIDS. It is usually due to infection by viral pathogens or use of hepatotoxic drugs. The most common viral cause of hepatitis is the hepatitis B virus (HBV). Given the shared epidemiological risks of sexual contact, intravenous drug use, and—in the past—use of blood products, it is not surprising that up to 95% of patients with AIDS have serological markers of past HBV infection (anti-HBs or anti-HBc positive) and 10–15% are chronic carriers HBsAg-positive). Immunological dysfunction induced by HIV may modify the course of HBV infection. The likelihood of chronic HBsAg carriage is increased in HIV-seropositive patients if infection by HIV precedes that of HBV, but it is unchanged if HBV infection precedes that of HIV. It appears that lower CD4 cell counts are associated with an increased risk of developing chronic HBV infection. After resolution of acute hepatitis, patients with HIV may suffer reactivation of quiescent HBV, a rare occurrence in the immunocompetent patient. Interestingly, HIV patients infected with HBV, exhibit greater HBV replication, with higher levels of DNA polymerase and increased hepatocyte HBsAg titers. While these characteristics predict poor survival in immunocompetent patients, there are lower transaminase levels as well as less histological damage in this immunocompromised population, which may be correlated with the degree of immunosuppression. The presumed pathogenesis of HBV offers an explanation of this phenomenon. CD4 lymphocytes are thought to play an essential role in the host's immune response to hepatocytes infected with HBV; CD4 infiltration of the liver triggers cytotoxic CD8 cell activity, resulting in hepatocellular necrosis. Thus, HIV-induced cell-mediated immunosuppression diminishes immunological damage to infected hepatocytes and allows for augmented HBV replication. Since hepatic inflammation is minimized, progression to cirrhosis is unusual.

It is unclear whether HBV infection alters the clinical course of HIV infection. HIV and HBV do appear to interact at the molecular level. The HBV transactivation protein X, through production of NF-κB, a nuclear factor, appears capable of increasing the replication of HIV in vitro and in vivo. This suggests that coinfection by HBV and HIV might result in stimulation of HIV acting as a cofactor in disease progression. Elevated levels of cytokines, such as tumor necrosis factor, and depressed levels of interferon, due to infection with HBV, may also enhance HIV replication. Small studies have suggested an association between HBV infection and HIV progression, but larger epidemiological studies have refuted this, showing that progression to AIDS, CD4 cells titers, and survival are not affected by HIV-HBV coinfection.

Hepatitis delta virus (HDV), the defective RNA virus that requires concurrent infection with HBV (coinfection) or chronic HBV carriage (superinfection), causes severe liver disease with progression to cirrhosis in 70–80% of immunocompetent patients. The incidence of this virus is low in homosexual populations, but up to 70% of parenteral drug users carry HDV, many of whom are also HIV-positive. HDV is cytopathic to hepatocytes, and disease appears to be worse in patients who are immunosuppressed, perhaps due to increased viral replication. Some studies have failed to show an influence of HIV on the clinical course of HDV infection. HIV-seropositive patients have a decreased antibody response to HDV and are more prone to reactivation of HDV disease.

HCV, which is responsible for 70–80% of cases of non-A, non-B hepatitis, can cause acute hepatitis but more commonly does not give rise to symptoms. More than half of all HCV-infected patients progress to chronic hepatitis (Fig. 1), and about 20% of these patients will go on to develop cirrhosis after 10–20 years. HCV commonly coinfects patients with HIV; the greatest incidence is in intravenous drug users (IVDUs), though

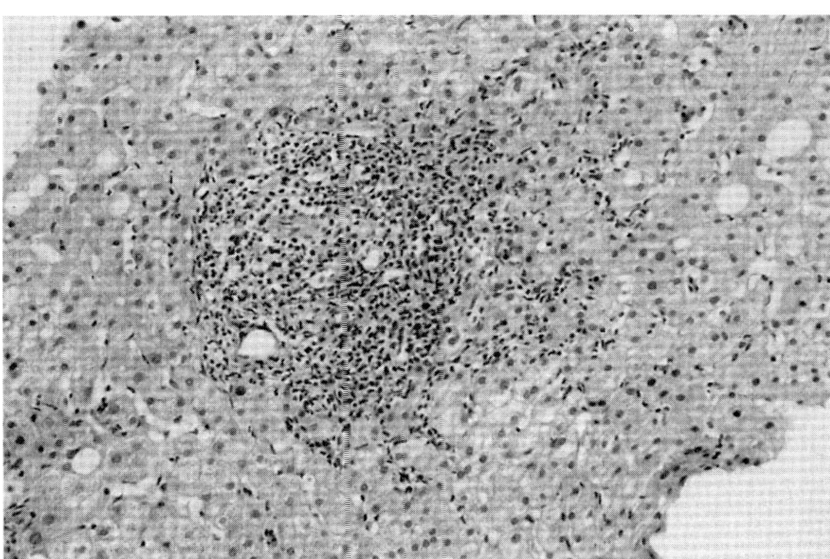

Figure 1 Medium-power photomicrograph of a needle core biopsy of liver showing portal, predominantly mononuclear inflammatory infiltrate that extends across the limiting plate, consistent with chronic hepatitis. Serological studies were positive for hepatitis C antibody. (H&E stain; original magnification ×200.)

recipients of blood transfusions and hemophiliacs are also at risk. The incidence among homosexual men is approximately 8–15%. Cell-mediated immunity appears to be important in the control of HCV, and HIV-induced immunosuppression may influence the transmission and clinical course of HCV disease.

The risk of sexual transmission of HCV is small, but male-to-female sexual transmission is five times more efficient when HIV infection is present. HIV-induced immunosuppression may enable increased HCV replication, higher HCV RNA levels, and increased progression to chronic HCV. In contrast to HBV, this appears to augment the virulence of HCV. One study demonstrated that over 5–12 or more years, the mean HCV RNA levels increased eightfold faster in HIV-seropositive as compared with HIV-seronegative hemophiliacs. Another study found that the level of HCV RNA was 10-fold higher in patients coinfected with HIV. Studies conflict regarding the correlation of depressed CD4 levels and the degree of HCV replication. Increased HCV replication appears to boost the risk of liver failure. In a study of 223 patients with hemophilia, 9% of HIV-HCV coinfected patients developed liver failure over a 10–20 year period in comparison to none of the patients with chronic HCV alone. Another study reported that the relative risk of developing liver failure was 21 in HCV/HIV coinfected hemophiliacs as compared with hemophiliacs who had HCV alone. The majority of patients who developed liver failure had CD4 cell counts < 100. A handful of studies, however, have concluded that HIV coinfection does not influence the course of HCV disease.

While it appears that HIV alters the course of HCV disease, the effect of HCV infection on the course of HIV disease is less obvious. HCV RNA can be found in circulating leukocytes and may stimulate CD4 cells. Further, one study revealed that infection with HCV genotype 1 was associated with a quicker progression to AIDS and death; but two cross-sectional studies and a large longitudinal study failed to show a relationship between infection, progression to AIDS, speed of CD4 cell decline, or death. HIV infection does appear to impair antibody response to HCV in coinfected patients, making diagnostic testing inaccurate.

Hepatitis E, an enterally transmitted virus that causes acute hepatitis, has an increased incidence among the HIV population, but it does not appear to be clinically significant. Another putative hepatotropic virus, hepatitis G virus, is transmitted parenterally and is likely quite common among HIV-positive patients. No studies have yet defined the impact of hepatitis G virus infection on HIV disease and vice versa, but it appears to be of little clinical importance.

Another viral organism responsible for hepatocellular necrosis in patients with AIDS is cytomegalovirus (CMV), a ubiquitous herpesvirus which commonly involves the liver. Autopsy studies suggest it is actually among the most common pathogens found in the liver of these patients. It is seen in 33–44% of them, almost uniformly in the setting of multiorgan involvement. It is less commonly discovered on antemortem liver biopsy, perhaps due to sampling error. Though the presentation is usually subclinical, patients may present with fever, malaise, weight loss, hepatomegaly, a mild elevation of transaminases, and mild cholestasis. Histologically, CMV is associated with sparse hepatocellular necrosis, typically with a portal and periportal mononuclear cell infiltrate, but more significant inflammation is not atypical (Fig. 2). CMV infects hepatocytes, Kupffer cells, and bile duct epithelial and endothelial cells. Infected cells contain characteristic large intranuclear and small cytoplasmic inclusions. The nuclear inclusions may be surrounded by a halo, forming the characteristic "owl's eye" appearance. Reminiscent of HBV, the immune dysfunction

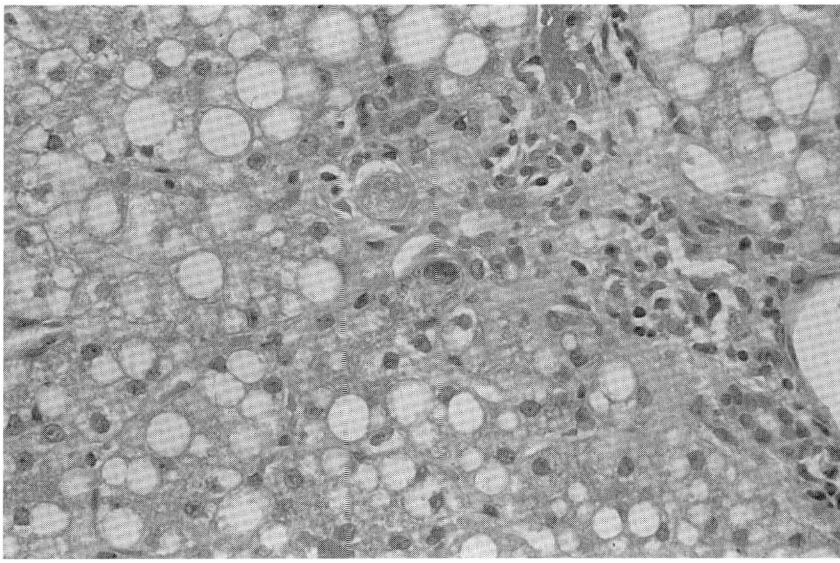

Figure 2 High-power photomicrograph of a needle core biopsy of the liver showing a single periportal markedly enlarged cell with a single eosinophilic nuclear inclusion and granular cytoplasmic inclusions characteristic of CMV. Note the minimal inflammatory infiltrate. Most of the other hepatocytes show macro- and microvesicular steatosis, frequently found in liver biopsies from HIV-positive patients (H&E stain; original magnification ×400.)

induced by HIV may diminish the immune-mediated damage against CMV-infected hepatocytes and result in augmented CMV replication.

Herpes simplex virus (HSV) dissemination to the liver is occasionally reported in patients with AIDS, usually patients with extensive herpetic ulceration elsewhere. AIDS patients with HSV hepatitis usually present with severe aminotransferase elevations. On histology, hepatocytes contain Cowdry type A intranuclear inclusion bodies, but immunopathological staining may be needed to distinguish this entity from CMV. HSV infection may result in submassive hepatic necrosis with coagulopathy, encephalopathy, and shock. Other viral agents implicated in HIV-related hepatic disease include human herpesvirus 6, varicella zoster virus, Epstein-Barr virus, and adenovirus.

Little is known about the direct relationship between HIV and the liver. The liver contains the largest population of tissue macrophages, the Kupffer cells, whose position within the sinusoids allows for contact with infected T cells flowing through the sinusoid and free viral particles in the blood. Immunoreactivity for HIV-1 antigens, predominantly in Kupffer cells, sinusoidal mononuclear cells, and endothelial cells can be shown in 80% of liver biopsies of AIDS patients. Kupffer cells and endothelial cells represent a physical barrier to HIV, preventing infection of the underlying hepatocytes. If this barrier were to be disrupted, could hepatocytes then be infected? Despite a lack of CD4 receptors on these cells, hepatoma cells lines can be productively infected by HIV-1 in vitro. It is not clear what effect these changes have on liver function, morbidity, or mortality, but infection does appear to be associated with Kupffer cell hypertrophy.

Granulomatous Inflammation

Granulomatous inflammation is a common endpoint to a spectrum of hepatic insults including infection, drug reaction, and idiopathic causes. It is the most common histological finding in many studies, most often representing a nonspecific finding without obvious clinical import. Regardless of cause, granulomatous disease is characteristically accompanied by elevated alkaline phosphatase levels, presumably due to infiltration of the hepatic parenchyma and obstruction of the terminal branches of the biliary tree.

The most commonly reported hepatic opportunistic infection is *Mycobacterium avium* complex (MAC). It is found in 20–55% of autopsies and in 10–30% of liver biopsies in patients with AIDS. MAC affects patients with advanced immunosuppression, often with a history of multiple other opportunistic infections. Patients characteristically present with nausea, diarrhea, abdominal pain, and, on exam, may have hepatomegaly or biliary obstruction due to enlarged nodes at the porta hepatis. MAC infection is associated with elevated alkaline phosphatase levels, but abnormal transaminases may be the sole liver-associated enzyme abnormality in this disease. Liver biopsy is required for definitive diagnosis of Hepatic MAC and reveals diffuse, poorly formed granulomas composed primarily of foamy histiocytes, with a paucity of other cells and lack of caseation necrosis. Acid-fast bacilli are found within and surrounding the granulomas. Acid-fast staining must be performed to identify the causative organism, but culture may allow diagnosis of mycobacteria in the absence of acid-fast organisms on biopsy.

Depressed cell-mediated immunity increases the risk of developing hepatic tuberculosis; extrapulmonary *Mycobacterium tuberculosis* (MTB) is seen in greater than half of AIDS patients with lung disease. In one study, 85% of patients with extrapulmonary disease had hepatic infection. Patients typically present with fever, night sweats, weight loss, cough with sputum production, anorexia, lymphadenopathy, and hepatomegaly. Laboratory analysis reveals an elevated alkaline phosphatase, with mildly elevated bilirubin and aminotransferase levels. Hepatic abscesses due to MTB have also been described. Infection often occurs with less immunosuppression than with MAC, so granulomas tend to be well formed, with less tissue load of acid-fast bacilli. Other mycobacteria implicated in hepatic disease include *Mycobacterium xenopi*, *M. genavense*, and *M. kansasii*.

Fungal infections of the liver commonly cause a granulomatous response. These granulomas are poorly formed, with minimal inflammatory response. Fungal infection is often asymptomatic except for fever and right-upper-quadrant pain. Laboratory analysis usually reveals a cholestatic picture and variably elevated bilirubin. Ultrasound and CT scan may reveal focal or diffuse irregularities in the liver parenchyma, but as often it demonstrates a nonspecific, heterogeneous liver texture. Common fungal pathogens include *Cryptococcus neoformans* (Fig. 3), *Histoplasma capsulatum*, *Candida albicans*, and *Coccidiodes immitis*. *Histoplasma* disseminates to the liver in 16% of infected patients. Silver stain of biopsy material will reveal rounded yeast with budding forms. Demonstration of characteristic yeast forms or pseudohyphae on Gomori–methenamine silver stain of biopsy samples is diagnostic for candidal infection. Hepatic infections by *Aspergillus* sp. and *Sporothrix schenckii* have also been described in the literature.

The most common response to protozoal liver infection is granuloma formation. In patients receiving aerosolized pentamidine (Nebupent) for prophylaxis of *Pneumocystic carinii* pneumonia (PCP), extrapulmonary spread of *P. carinii* was not uncommon. One autopsy study reported finding hepatic *Pneumocystis* in 39% of such patients. They may present with mild abdominal pain, associated with variable elevations of transaminases and

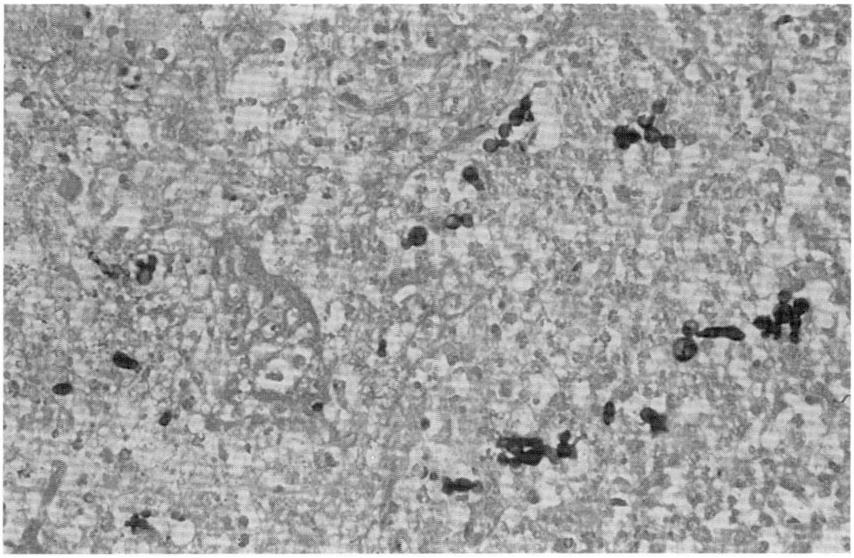

Figure 3 High-power photomicrograph of a needle core biopsy of the liver showing a hepatic abscess with multiple budding yeasts consistent with *Cryptococcus*. The identity of the yeast was further clarified by a positive mucicarmine stain of the thick capsules. (GMS stain; original magnification, ×400.)

alkaline phosphatase. Abdominal computed tomography (CT), and, rarely, plain radiographs may demonstrate diffuse punctate calcifications of the liver. Liver biopsy shows foamy nodules that are periportal or diffuse, containing numerous *Pneumocystis* cysts that stain with methenamine silver. *Toxoplasma gondii* may also disseminate hematogeneously to the liver and may present with granulomatous disease or as a hepatitis. Microsporidial infection of the liver is a rarity but has been associated with elevated bilirubin, transaminase, and especially alkaline phosphatase. Light microscopy reveals focal granulomatous and suppurative necrosis, mainly in the portal area, accompanied by characteristic spores, sporoblasts, and sporonts. *Entamoeba histolytica* may invade the bowel wall and spread to the liver, forming an abscess. Other rare hepatic infections include *Schistosoma* spp. and reactivated *Leishmania donovani*.

Mass Lesions

Neoplasia represents the most common cause of hepatic mass lesions in patients with AIDS. Still, many infectious entities such as CMV, fungi, bacteria, or mycobacteria may present as mass lesions.

Kaposi's sarcoma (KS), the most common hepatic neoplasm seen in AIDS, is found predominantly in homosexual males, but all risk groups may be affected. Despite the presence of hepatic KS in approximately one-third of all patients with cutaneous involvement, it is seldom found on antemortem biopsy. Patients may present with abdominal pain and hepatosplenomegaly with an elevated alkaline phosphatase, but most commonly it is asymptomatic. Diagnosis can be made by directed biopsy of mass lesions, but in the majority of cases, radiographic studies cannot delineate the small lesions. On computed tomography, KS lesions are hypoattenuated, but they enhance after a bolus of contrast. Lesions tend to originate in the capsular, hilar, and portal areas, invading the parenchyma from these sites. Given the vascular nature or KS, the safety of liver biopsy has been questioned. This worry is largely unfounded. Microscopically, KS appears as areas of vascular endothelial cell proliferation with associated spindle-shaped cells, extravasated erythrocytes, and vascular lakes. Hemorrhage and central necrosis within tumorous masses is common. Lesions involving the biliary tree may result in obstructive jaundice and cholangitis. Hepatic KS does not appear to shorten life expectancy.

Non-Hodgkin's lymphoma (NHL) commonly involves the liver. In patients with AIDS, NHL is associated with a high incidence of extranodal disease, the liver representing the most commonly affected abdominal organ. Liver involvement has been reported in 14% of patients with lymphoma elsewhere and in 29% of all patients with intraabdominal involvement. There have been 15 reports of primary hepatic lymphoma occurring in patients with AIDS. Hepatic NHL may remain asymptomatic but commonly presents with weight loss, fever, and night sweats, symptoms similar to those of opportunistic infections. When bulky, hepatic lymphoma may cause dull right-upper-quadrant pain or hepatomegaly with jaundice. Ultrasound examination may show various-sized solitary or multiple mass lesions larger than those due to opportunistic infection of KS. In over 90% of patients with hepatic lesions, abdominal CT shows evidence of lymphomatous involvement of other viscera or lymph nodes. Diagnosis is occasionally made by random liver biopsy (Fig. 4) or at autopsy. Compression of the extrahepatic bile duct by portal or peripancreatic lymphadenopathy may cause intrahepatic biliary dilatation, and patients may present with painless jaundice. Lymphomatous involvement of the gallbladder may result in perforation. Hodgkin's lymphoma is less common but may also involve the liver at an advanced stage.

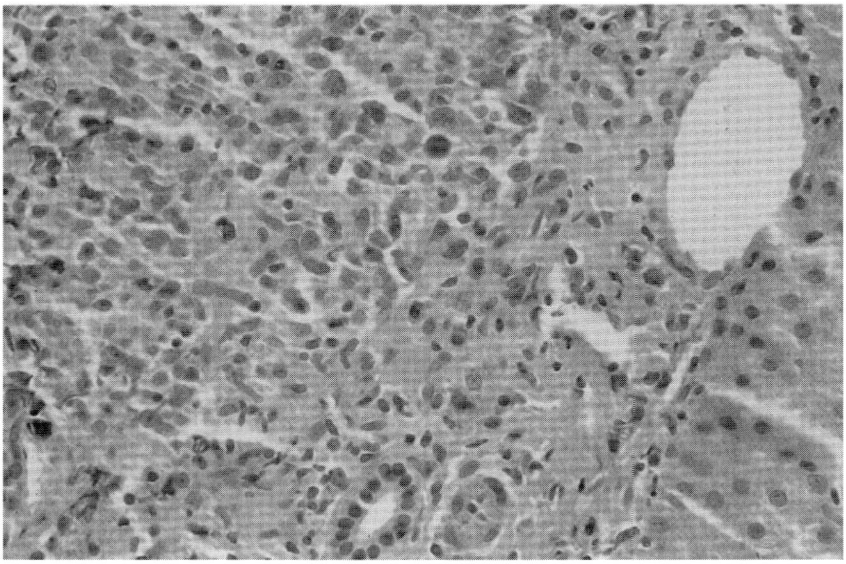

Figure 4 High-power photomicrograph of a portal area showing a lymphoid infiltrate composed predominantly of large atypical lymphocytes, consistent with a high-grade, diffuse, large cell lymphoma. (H&E stain; original magnification, ×400.)

Other neoplastic mass lesions that have been discovered in the livers of AIDS patients include malignant fibrosarcoma, chronic lymphocytic leukemia, leiomyoma, hepatoma, cholangiocarcinoma, and metastatic disease.

Vascular Lesions

The most common vascular lesions seen in patients with AIDS are KS (discussed above), peliosis hepatis and sinusoidal dilation and congestion. Peliosis hepatis may be due to *Bartonella henselae* or *Bartonella quintana*, the organisms previously implicated as causes of bacillary angiomatosis. Sinusoidal dilatation and liver involvement is heralded by fever, weight loss, abdominal pain, and hepatosplenomegaly in patients who are severely immunosuppressed. These patients may or may not have cutaneous lesions of bacillary angiomatosis. Laboratory analysis may reveal mild to moderate elevations of aminotransferase levels and a moderate to severe elevation of alkaline phosphatase. Abdominal CT examination displays multiple, small, low-attenuated lesions throughout the hepatic parenchyma. The liver texture is often heterogeneous and the organ enlarged. Peliosis hepatis is best diagnosed histologically. Biopsy reveals cystic blood-filled spaces a few millimeters in diameter within the liver. These peliotic spaces are often associated with fibromyxoid stroma containing few inflammatory cells, capillaries, and clumps of bacilli. The gram-negative organism can be detected by Warthin-Starry stain or by electron microscopy, both intracellularly in sinusoidal endothelial cells and extracellularly. Cultures are usually negative.

Hepatotoxic Drugs

The use of hepatotoxic medications represents one of the most common causes of enzyme elevations in general (see Chap. 1) and in particular in patients with AIDS. Up to 90% of AIDS patients are treated with at least one drug associated with hepatotoxicity (see Table 2), often necessitating dose reduction or discontinuation. A hepatocellular pattern of liver-associated enzyme abnormalities is related to the use of amphotericin B (Fungizone), isoniazid (Nydrazid), rifampin (Rifadin, Rimactane), ethionamide (Trecator), pyrazinamide, metronidazole (Flagyl), tetracycline (Achromycin V), penicillins, ganciclovir (Cytovene), azole antifungals, pentamidine (Pentam 300), phenytoin (Dilantin), sulfa-containing drugs including trimethoprim/sulfamethoxazole (TMP/SMX) (Bactrim; Septra), and nucleoside analogues. Hepatotoxic drugs associated with a cholestatic pattern include albendazole, azithromycin (Zithromax), erythromycin (E-mycin, Ery-Tab, Ilosone), TMP-SMX, and

Table 2 Potentially Hepatotoxic Drugs Used in Patients with AIDS

Hepatocellular		Cholestatic	Mixed
Zidovudine (AZT)	Penicillins	Albendazole	TMP/SMX
Deoxyinosine (ddI)	Amphotericin B	Azithromycin	Tegretol
Ketoconazole	Ethionamide	Erythromycin	
Isoniazid	Pyrazinamide	Prochlorperazine	
Rifampin	Metronidazole		
Phenytoin	Tetracycline		
Valproic acid	Ganciclovir		
Pentamidine			

prochlorperazine (Compazine). Mixed hepatocellular and cholestatic patterns are often seen, especially with TMP-SMX and carbamazepine (Tegretol). Nucleoside analogues may be toxic to mitochondria, resulting in disturbed oxidative phosphorylation and a fatal syndrome of lactic acidosis and fulminant or subfulminant liver failure. While this is rare, physicians are advised to carefully monitor patients receiving nucleoside analogue therapy who have elevated liver-associated enzymes or hepatomegaly. Most drug-related toxicities can be reversed when the drug is discontinued or the dose lowered. The presence of eosinophils on liver biopsy and the absence of organisms on special stain suggests drug-induced liver disease in patients with a compatible history.

Nonspecific Findings

Hepatic biopsies from AIDS patients are seldom normal; nearly one-third of biopsies yield nonspecific findings. Possible causes of nonspecific liver pathology include malnutrition, use of total parenteral nutrition, exposure to hepatotoxic drugs, increased levels of cytokines, weight loss, disseminated infection, or alcohol abuse. Many may be due to yet unidentified organisms or to HIV itself. Mild to moderate diffuse macrovesicular steatosis is the most common nonspecific finding on liver biopsy. It is commonly associated with hepatomegaly and elevated levels of alkaline phosphatase and has been implicated in liver failure leading to death. Patients with HIV who have high red blood cell transfusion requirements are subject to hepatic iron overload. While the duration of iron overload is likely to be too short to result in secondary hemochromatosis, elevated hepatic iron may exacerbate viral hepatitis. Other nonspecific findings include focal hepatocyte necrosis, granulomas, sinusoidal abnormalities, Kupffer cell hyperplasia, portal inflammation, fibrosis, congestion, bile stasis, piecemeal necrosis, and bile duct proliferation.

BILIARY TRACT DISEASE

The biliary tree, including the gallbladder, is a common site of pathology in HIV-infected patients. The most commonly encountered diseases are acalculous cholecystitis and AIDS cholangiopathy. The major pathogens include cryptosporidia, microsporidia, MAC, and CMV, although in half the patients no organism is found. Acalculous cholecystitis most commonly presents with right-upper-quadrant or epigastric pain, fever, nausea, vomiting, and, commonly, diarrhea and weight loss. Jaundice is a rare symptom, but alkaline phosphatase is markedly elevated most of the time. Ultrasound may show a thickened, dilated gallbladder or may be normal. Gallbladder sludge is often seen. Hepatobiliary scintiscans may be useful for establishing the diagnosis of HIV-associated acalculous cholecystitis (see Chap. 2). These scans will reveal delayed visualization or nonvisualization of the gallbladder. Histology often reveals an edematous, inflamed, and ulcerated gallbladder mucosa but no gangrene or necrosis. Cholangitis is a common accompaniment, occurring in greater than 50% of AIDS patients with acalculous cholecystitis.

AIDS cholangiopathy was first described in three patients complaining of right-upper-quadrant pain and fever. Periductal inflammation affecting the extrahepatic and often the intrahepatic bile ducts, with mural thickening, beading, and nodularity, results in irregular narrowing along the involved bile duct segment. When the papilla of Vater is involved, dilatation of the common bile duct and occasionally the pancreatic duct may result. The presentation of cholangiopathy is the same as that of acalculous cholecystitis:

pain and fever, nausea, vomiting with an elevated alkaline phosphatase, and usually normal bilirubin. The most commonly used classification of the endoscopic retrograde cholangio-pancreatography (ERCP) changes of AIDS cholangiopathy was proposed by Cello. He described four different patterns of disease; type I combined sclerosing cholangitis and papillary stenosis, type II papillary stenosis alone, type III sclerosing cholangitis alone, and type IV long extrahepatic bile duct strictures. If ERCP is performed, abnormalities will be found in 77%. Ultrasonography and CT are not as sensitive but are commonly employed before ERCP. One study found that ultrasound had a sensitivity of 97% and a specificity of 100% in the prediction of an abnormal ERCP exam, suggesting that ERCP should be reserved for patients with ERCP abnormalities. ERCP may also be used for therapeutic interventions such as sphincterotomy or stent placement as well as for obtaining biopsy of the ampulla and distal common bile duct. Ampullary biopsy specimens should be obtained to examine for parasites, protozoa, fungi, and CMV. Immunosuppression predisposes to bacterial cholangitis superimposed on cholangiopathy. AIDS cholangiopathy does not appear to affect survival.

DIAGNOSTIC APPROACH

When an HIV-positive patient presents with abnormalities suggesting liver disease, a rational diagnostic approach can narrow the broad differential diagnosis, permitting a directed evaluation (Fig. 5). Since opportunistic diseases cause liver disease through blood-borne or lymphatic dissemination, a thorough history and physical examination as the starting point may reveal extrahepatic clues to the diagnosis. The clinician should pay particular attention to prior opportunistic infections that may have disseminated to the liver, use of potentially hepatotoxic medications or alcohol, and recent travel. The absolute CD4 cell count is equally important in the determination of a differential diagnosis. An HIV-infected patient with a normal CD4 cell count is unlikely to have an opportunistic infection of the liver but may have MTB or KS, while patients with CD4 cell counts below 100 become susceptible to MAC or CMV infection. The combination of abnormal liver enzyme tests and fever is quite common. Hepatomegaly, right-upper-quadrant pain, and jaundice are less common. The clinician must bear in mind that when CD4 counts are < 50, almost all HIV-infected patients will have some abnormality of liver enzymes. Many will have nonspecific abnormalities on liver biopsy. To biopsy every patient with abnormal liver enzymes is not practical or rewarding and may even be dangerous. Clinicians must always remember that in their zeal to find an opportunistic disease, they should not overlook the fact that HIV-infected persons will also be subjected to nonopportunistic, non-HIV-related processes typical for their age and sex.

Mere biochemical abnormality should not immediately trigger a major clinical investigation unless it is accompanied by symptoms of pain, fever, jaundice, or hepatic decompensation. When these do occur, aggressive diagnostic testing should probably be carried out, because a significant percentage of hepatobiliary disease is potentially treatable and treatment may prolong life and/or improve its quality. Elevated transaminases (more than three to four times normal) usually result from typical and HIV-related viral hepatitides, drug- or toxin-induced liver disease, or ischemic injury. These patients should be screened for viral, immunological, and metabolic diseases. If these tests are negative and the patient is stable, they should be followed for another 6 months, with repeat evaluation of liver chemistries. If abnormalities have not moralized, liver biopsy should be considered.

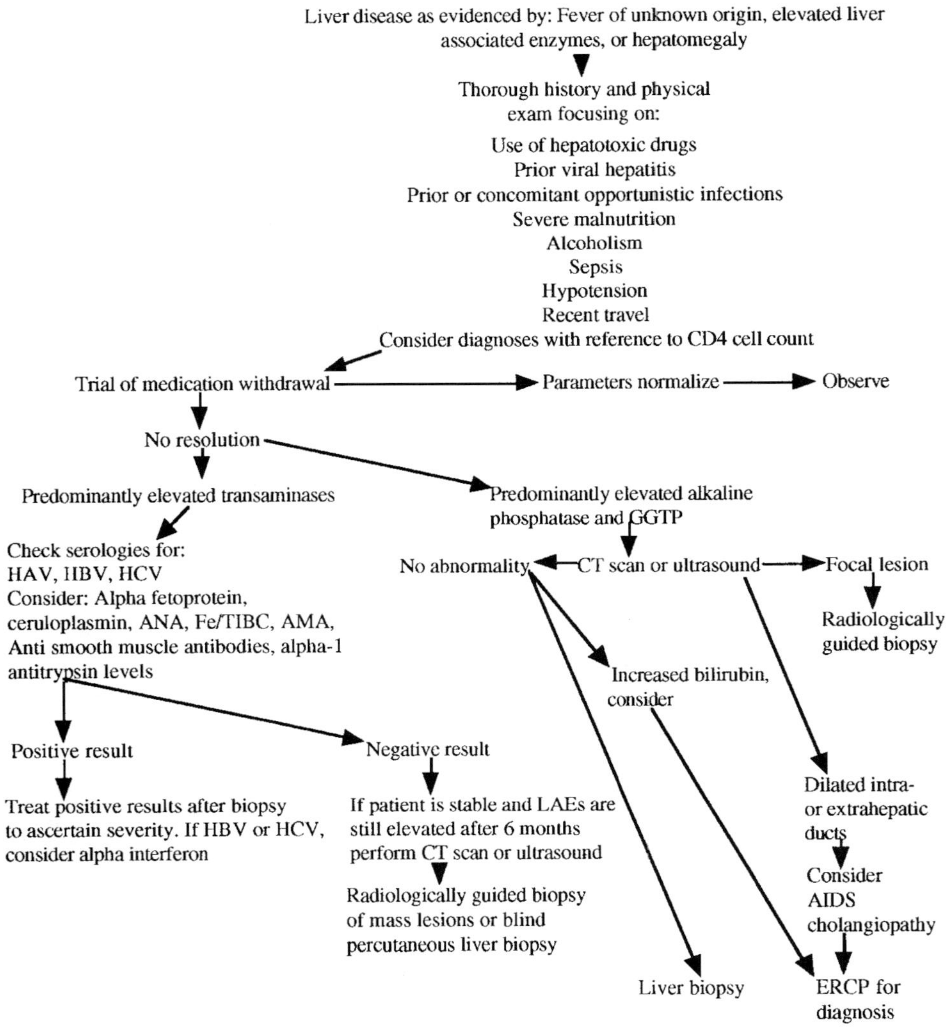

Figure 5 Approach to the patient with HIV-related hepatic disease.

Patients with a predominantly cholestatic pattern (elevated alkaline phosphatase and gamma glutamyl transpeptidase, GTTP) commonly have MAC, MTB, fungal infections, protozoal infections, as well as drug hepatotoxicity, neoplasia, peliosis hepatis, and biliary tract disorders. Jaundice, though rare in HIV, may be caused by an intrahepatic process, such as drug effects or viral hepatitis, or due to extrahepatic biliary obstruction.

The use of liver biopsy is controversial in the evaluation of liver disease in patients with AIDS. Since the liver is commonly involved in systemic disease that has disseminated lymphohematogenously, a diagnosis may often be established through less invasive means. These include biopsy and culture of peripheral sites such as the blood, skin, gastrointestinal mucosa, lymph nodes, and bone marrow. Liver biopsy may be reserved for workup when less invasive procedures and a trial of medication withdrawal have failed to yield a diagnosis. Liver biopsy is safe in immunocompetent patients but may be associated with a slightly higher risk of bleeding in patients with AIDS. We avoid biopsy in patients with a prothrombin time greater than 3 s over control or a platelet count less than 50,000.

Despite an increased risk, liver biopsy is the most specific diagnostic technique for parenchymal liver disease in these patients. Opponents of liver biopsy cite a number of important points. They focus on studies that failed to find a correlation between indications for liver biopsy and histopathological findings and those that concluded that liver biopsy rarely results in new AIDS-specific diagnoses or improved survival. Proponents quote studies that revealed a specific diagnosis in 30–80% of biopsies and that the finding of opportunistic infections or neoplasms on liver biopsy may yield important prognostic information. A recent review compiled autopsy and liver biopsy data from 22 previous studies encompassing 635 HIV patients. It concluded that 34% of liver biopsies and 38% of autopsies yielded important diagnostic information. In a recent retrospective analysis of 501 liver biopsies performed on AIDS patients with abnormalities of liver chemistries, fever, hepatomegaly, or right-upper-quadrant pain, we found that 64% of liver biopsies yielded a histopathological diagnosis, 46% of which were potentially treatable. Furthermore, 58% of patients with fever who had already undergone nondiagnostic workup, including bone marrow biopsy, were diagnosed by liver biopsy. Stratification of biopsy results according to CD4 cell count failed to reveal a significant difference in the yield, nor was there a difference when the data were analyzed according to indication for biopsy. Liver biopsy may be more fruitful when performed on patients with a longer history of HIV infection and with a history of multiple opportunistic infections. Laparoscopy allows for direct visualization of abnormalities in half the AIDS patients with elevated liver enzymes, hepatomegaly, ascites, fever of unknown origin, or right-upper-quadrant pain. When these are coupled with laparoscopic liver biopsy, a diagnosis is made in 70%. As our ability to treat opportunistic infections of the liver improves, liver biopsy will likely assume greater importance in the diagnosis of liver disease in patients with AIDS.

TREATMENT

Viral Hepatitis

The value of treatment of HBV and HCV with alpha interferon in patients with HIV is debatable (Table 3). Interferon alpha (Intron A, Roferon A at a dose of 5 million units once daily or 10 million units thrice weekly) for chronic HBV infection in immunocompetent patients may have a response rate as high as 40–50% after 3–4 months (see Chap. 7). Since it facilitates HBV clearance by modulating the host immune response as well as by direct antiviral effects, one might expect that the beneficial effect of interferon may be limited in HIV-positive patients with depressed cell-mediated immunity. Patients with AIDS have higher levels of HBV DNA, lower pretreatment transaminase levels, and less hepatic inflammation, all of which have been shown to be predictors of poor response to interferon. This has been verified in a number of trials, which revealed that the response to interferon therapy, as judged by seroconversion from HBe antigen seropositivity to negativity, is not as great in the HIV-positive patients. A recent study of HIV-positive patients revealed that they were one-fifth as likely to respond to a 12-week course of alpha interferon (8% response) as compared with homosexual HIV-negative patients (38% response). Azidothymidine (AZT) has been used in combination with interferon in an attempt to improve the seroconversion rate by improving immune function and by suppressing HBV

Table 3 Therapy for Hepatobiliary Pathogens

Pathogen	Therapy	Adverse reactions
Hepatitis B virus	Interferon alpha 5 million units qd	Early: fever, chills, myalgia, arthralgia, headache
	Interferon alpha 10 million units tiw	Late: leukopenia, granulocytopenia, thrombocytopenia, irritability, fatigue, depression, anorexia, nausea, rashes, and alopecia
	Lamivudine 300 mg PO bid	
Hepatitis C virus	Interferon alpha 3 to 5 million units tiw	Same as above
Cytomegalovirus	Ganciclovir 5 mg/kg IV q 12h	Neutropenia, thrombocytopenia, anemia, rash
	Foscarnet 60 to 120 mg/kg IV q8h	Nephrotoxicity, electrolyte disturbances, headache, fatigue, nausea, penile ulceration, seizures
Herpes simplex virus	Acyclovir 30 mg/kg IV qd	Phlebitis, nephrotoxicity, nausea, vomiting
Mycobacterium avium complex	Clarithromycin 500 mg PO bid	Diarrhea, abdominal pain, nausea, vomiting, headache, hepatotoxicity
	Ethambutol 15 mg/kg PO qd	Optic neuritis, neuropathy, abdominal pain, nausea
	Rifampin 10 mg/kg PO qd	Fever, chills, malaise, leukopenia, thrombocytopenia, hemolytic anemia, drug interactions, hepatotoxicity
	Ciprofloxacin 750 mg PO qd	Nausea, diarrhea, central nervous system disturbance, hepatotoxicity
	Clofazamine 100 mg PO qd	Drowsiness, neuropsychiatric disturbances, nausea, constipation, urinary frequency
	Amikacin 7.5 mg/kg IV qd	Auditory, vestibular, and nephrotoxicity
Mycobacterium tuberculosis	Isoniazid 300 mg PO qd	Peripheral neuropathy, nausea, vomiting, abdominal pain, hepatotoxicity
	Pyrazinamide 20 to 30 mg/kg PO qd	Hepatotoxicity, thrombocytopenia, sideroblastic anemia
	Rifampin 600 mg PO qd	See *Mycobacterium avium* complex
	Ethambutol 15 mg/kg PO qd	See *Mycobacterium avium* complex
Bartonella henselae, *Bartonella quinatana*	Erythromycin 500 mg PO qd	Nausea, vomiting, abdominal pain, hepatotoxicity
Cryptococcus neoformans	Fluconazole 200 mg PO qd	Headache, nausea, abdominal pain, rash, hepatotoxicity
	Amphotericin B 0.6 mg/kg IV qd	Fever, chills, anorexia, phlebitis, hypotension, tachypnea, nausea, vomiting, abdominal pain, diarrhea, anemia, headache, nephrotoxicity, hepatotoxicity
Histoplasma capsulatum	Itraconazole 200 mg PO qd	Hepatotoxicity, nausea, vomiting, abdominal pain, drug interactions

Table 3 Continued

Pathogen	Therapy	Adverse reactions
Candida albicans	Fluconazole 200 mg PO qd	See *Cryptococcus*
	Amphotericin B 0.5 mg/kg IV qd	See *Cryptococcus*
Coccidiodes immitis	Fluconazole 200 mg PO qd	See *Cryptococcus*
	Amphotericin B 0.5 mg/kg IV qd	See *Cryptococcus*
Pneumocystis carinii	TMP-SMX (15 mg TMP and 75 mg/kg SMX in four divided doses)	Rash, fever, leukopenia, nausea, vomiting, hepatotoxicity
Toxoplasma gondii	Pyrimethamine 75 mg PO qd	Hypersensitivity, anorexia, vomiting, pancytopenia, hematuria, cardiac arrhythmias
	Sulfadiazine 1.5 g PO q6h	Rash, fever, leukopenia, nausea, vomiting, hepatotoxicity
Microsporidium sp.	Albendazole 400 mg PO bid	Abdominal pain, rash, hepatotoxicity

polymerase, as shown in vitro. While this regimen is well tolerated and does not accelerate HIV progression, the response rate remains poor. Zidovudine has little effect on HBV DNA levels and HBV DNA polymerase activity. One small study suggested that prednisone before interferon may increase the likelihood of HBV clearance in HIV patients, though a randomized, controlled multicenter trial in immunocompetent patients showed no benefit.

Recently, lamivudine, the (-) enantiomer of 2′-deoxy-3′-thiacytidine, a potent inhibitor of HIV reverse transcriptase, has been found to inhibit the reverse transcription of HBV. It has therefore been used to treat chronic HBV infection in immunocomponent as well as HIV patients. A recent trial involving 40 severely immunodeficient HIV patients with chronic HBV who had failed or were intolerant of interferon, revealed that lamivudine, at a dose of 600 mg/day or 600 mg/day followed by 300 mg/day for 1 year, was active against HBV. The majority of (88%) of patients with high HBV replication at baseline cleared HBV DNA (measured by PCR), and 18% lost HBe antigen seropositively. The patients who began the trial with low HBV replication at baseline fared even better. The medication was well tolerated by the patients in this trial with only a few patients experiencing nausea, vomiting, and abdominal pain. It remains to be seen whether the positive effect seen in this trial will be durable, whether maintenance lamivudine will be required, and whether the findings will equate with improved quality or quantity of life. Both ganciclovir and foscarnet, drugs used in the treatment of CMV disease, have been anecdotally shown to have a slight effect on HBV disease.

The response rate of HIV-seropositive patients to HBV vaccination is also poor, since antibody response to HBsAg is CD4 cell-dependent. While immunocompetent patients have a nonresponse rate of ≤5%, the nonresponse rate in HIV-seropositive patients is more than 40%. Vaccination results in significantly lower antibody levels in HIV-seropositive patients, even after repeated doses. Furthermore, patients with AIDS lose protection more frequently. Titers must be checked after the third dose of the vaccine. It is unclear whether booster doses or the initial use of higher or additional doses will improve the response to vaccination. Risk-factor modification as well as vaccination still seems advisable in HIV positive patients without markers of past HBV infection.

Aggressive therapy to prevent progression to advanced liver disease appears to be the optimum approach to dealing with chronic HCV infection. A number of trials have shown the usefulness of alpha-interferon treatment of HCV in the immunocompetent population (see Chap. 9). There have been a number of small studies, presented as abstracts, and four studies published as full-length articles that have evaluated the use of interferon in the treatment of HCV-infected patients who are also HIV-infected. Most of these studies have concluded that treatment of this population results in an initial efficacy and long-term responses similar to those of the HIV-seronegative population. The first full-length article evaluated interferon in 12 HIV-seropositive patients. One-third normalized their aminotransferases, but only one patient (8%) was a long-term responder after 12 months of follow-up. A second study examining 14 patients with HCV and asymptomatic HIV showed that treatment with 9 million units of interferon daily for 6 months, followed by 6 million units, and then 3 million units thrice weekly for 3-month periods resulted in a 55% end-treatment response with a 44% sustained response 6 months after interferon withdrawal. The third study used 5 million units of interferon for 3 months, then 3 million units thrice weekly for 9 months to treat 57 patients and demonstrated an end-treatment response in 38% of HIV-HCV coinfected patients as compared with 47% of HIV-negative patients. This was not a significant difference. Soriano and colleagues showed that treatment with 12 months of interferon alpha (5 million units thrice weekly for 3 months followed by 3 million units thrice weekly for the next 9 months) in 80 coinfected patients resulted in a 32% end-treatment virological response. The response rate was similar to that of HIV-negative controls (37%); 31% of HIV patients relapsed within 12 months as compared with 12% of non-HIV infected patients. Longer follow-up by this group showed that the expected decline of CD4 cell counts 18 months after discontinuation of interferon did not result in more frequent relapse of HCV in the patients who had responded to therapy. Unfortunately, none of the studies evaluated the effect of interferon treatment of HCV on patient morbidity or survival. Ongoing studies are now looking at the use of ribavirin (Virazole) in combination with interferon to treat HCV in HIV patients.

Multiple variables probably modulate the efficacy of interferon in this population. The absolute CD4 cell count appears to be correlated with the responsiveness of patients to interferon therapy. Multiple logistic regression analysis of Soriano's study showed that female sex and a CD4 cell count of greater than 500 were independently associated with a better response to interferon. Most trials have only enrolled patients whose CD4 cell counts were above 200, so it may be difficult to draw firm conclusions about this relationship. The response to interferon therapy may also depend on the infecting strain of HCV. A full response to interferon is seen in fewer patients who harbor HCV genotype 1b and those infected with multiple strains of HCV. In addition, responsiveness to interferon may be decreased in patients with high viral titers in serum. All of these variables are found more commonly in the HIV-infected intravenous drug user with HCV.

Many interferon-treated patients receive AZT in addition to the interferon. AZT may have an independent role in HCV suppression and may be beneficial for treatment of coinfected patients by preserving immune function. One study that specifically analyzed combination therapy revealed that 2 months of treatment with alpha interferon and zidovudine resulted in normalization of ALT activity in some co-infected patients, but this was not confirmed in larger trials. Interferon may also have activity against HIV; in doses used to treat HCV, it may slow the rate of HIV progression.

The adverse effects of interferon therapy are worthy of note. In a large percentage of patients, therapy is associated with mild to moderate adverse effects. Bacterial infection associated with the immunosuppression induced by interferon therapy is among the most worrisome effects of therapy. Urinary tract infections, sinusitis, and bronchitis are seen with increased frequency in patients receiving this drug. More serious infections have also been noted; thus, any sign of fever should be promptly evaluated. Despite the high incidence of adverse effects associated with the use of this agent, there does not seem to be an increase in the incidence of intolerance among the patients who are HIV-infected. A few studies have noted that use of interferon is associated with the risk of a precipitous fall in the CD4 cell count among HIV patients who are so treated. This drop is believed to be due to induction or exacerbation of autoantibodies against certain HLA class II antigens. Despite this, no study has shown that the incidence of opportunistic infections is increased with interferon. The CD4 cell counts may rebound spontaneously during therapy or after discontinuation of therapy in a subset of patients.

Opportunistic Infections

There is a history of therapeutic nihilism surrounding treatment of MAC infection. Early studies did not show a benefit of treatment on survival, but more recent studies have supported the use of antibiotics. While single-drug therapy with clarithromycin, at a dose of 500–2000 mg/day, has been reported to eradicate MAC from blood cultures in the majority of treated patients, long-term monotherapy results in drug resistance. Significant benefit has been achieved with combinations of three or four antimycobacterial agents used for more than 12 weeks. The most common regimens include a macrolide such as clarithromycin or azithromycin and two or three of the following: rifampin, ethambutol, ciprofloxacin, or clofazamine. Amikacin may be used during the initial 3 weeks of therapy. Treatment results in decreased bacterial load and symptomatic improvement as well as improved survival. Lifelong maintenance therapy will be required to prevent recurrence. Gastrointestinal tuberculosis responds to combination antibiotics for 9–12 months. The agents most commonly used include isoniazid, rifampin, ethambutol, and pyrazinamide. In areas where multidrug-resistance tuberculosis is endemic, treatment must be based on culture-determined sensitivities.

The organisms implicated in peliosis hepatis are sensitive to a variety of agents. The drug of first choice is erythromycin, 500 mg PO four times daily. Other options include tetracycline and doxycycline (Doryx; Vibramycin) and possibly gentamicin (Garamycin) or rifampin. Relapse after treatment may occur, necessitating prolonged courses of at least 3 months. The question of chronic maintenance therapy has not yet been answered. Spontaneous resolution may occur without antibiotics.

No controlled trials have examined the use of ganciclovir or foscarnet in the treatment of CMV hepatitis, but given their efficacy for nonhepatic infection, it seems reasonable to treat infected patients. Patients should be induced with either ganciclovir 5 mg/kg twice daily or foscarnet (Foscavir) 90 mg/kg three times daily for 2 weeks. No recommendations can be made regarding the need for daily maintenance therapy. Patients with CMV cholangitis may benefit from anti-CMV therapy as well. Hepatic HSV infections should be treated with intravenous acyclovir (Zovirax), but prognosis remains poor. At present, there are no chemotherapeutics effective against adenovirus, but serum immune globulin or ribavirin (Virazole) are considerations. HHV-6 may be treated with either ganciclovir or foscarnet.

The treatment of fungal and protozoal hepatic pathogens requires standard therapy. Either amphotericin with or without flucytosine (Ancobon) or fluconazole (Diflucan) may be used for cryptococcal and candidal infections, while itraconazole (Sporanox) or amphotericin may be used for *Aspergillus* or *Histoplasma*. Treatment of microsporidian hepatitis and cholangitis has not been studied in a controlled fashion, but evidence suggests that albendazole treatment of one species, *Intestinalis septata*, may be of benefit.

Visceral involvement with KS, though not a likely cause of death, is a poor prognostic sign. KS requires treatment when symptomatic, and the presence of hepatic KS need not alter the multiagent chemotherapy regimens used for disease elsewhere in the body. These can involve radiation, chemotherapy or immunomodulation with interferon. Although tumor stage appears to predict survival, it does not predict response to interferon therapy. Non-Hodgkin's lymphoma behaves in an aggressive fashion in AIDS, with extralymphatic involvement, more B symptoms, and poor survival. Many aggressive chemotherapy regimens for the treatment of hepatic lymphoma have been tried. Each yields a similar response and none has offered a survival advantage. Therapy is limited by bone marrow suppression, especially neutropenia. Colony-stimulating factors can be helpful. While remission rates as high as 50% have been reported, recurrence is high and disease-free intervals short. Prognosis is poor, with median survival of only 2–7.5 months.

Treatment of HIV-related biliary disease is also similar to that for immunocompetent patients. Patients with cholecystitis should undergo cholecystectomy. This procedure will alleviate symptoms, though it is unlikely to help patients with coexistent cholangitis. In one review, open cholecystectomy in 11 AIDS patients with CMV cholecystitis was associated with 9% morbidity but no mortality. Other series have reported mortality as high as 33%. Laparoscopic cholecystectomy may lead to decreased morbidity and mortality in this population. Patients with AIDS cholangiopathy, especially papillary stenosis, may benefit from endoscopic sphincterotomy or stent insertion for focal biliary duct strictures. Sphincterotomy has been shown to significantly reduce long-term pain scores, but laboratory abnormalities commonly remain, perhaps due to progression of the intrahepatic disease. Secondary bacterial infection of the abnormal biliary tree is a significant factor to be considered and it should always be treated with antibiotics even when other pathogens are present.

CONCLUSION

Hepatobiliary involvement with opportunistic infections and neoplasms is a well-recognized component of AIDS and affects many patients. In this chapter we examined the wide range of hepatobiliary disease due to viral, bacterial, protozoal, fungal, neoplastic, and iatrogenic causes and the management thereof. The diagnostic approach to this problem must be thorough. With a rational approach, most patients with AIDS hepatobiliary disease can be diagnosed and treated in a cost-effective manner with low morbidity. Further studies will be required to determine whether diagnosis and treatment of these entities will equate with improved quality of life and increased survival.

BIBLIOGRAPHY

Bodsworth NJ, Cooper DA, Donovan B. The influence of human immunodeficiency virus type 1 infection on the development of hepatitis B virus carrier state. J Infect Dis 1991; 163:1138–1140.

Bonacini M. Hepatobiliary complications in patients with human immunodeficiency virus infection. Am J Med 1992; 92:404–411.

Cappell MS, Schwartz MS, Biempica L. Clinical utility of liver biopsy in patients with serum antibodies to the human immunodeficiency virus. Am J Med 1990; 88:123–130.

Cello JP. Human immunodeficiency virus-associated biliary tract disease. Semin Liver Dis 1992; 12: 213–218.

Eyster ME, Fried MW, Di Bisceglie AM, Goedert JJ. Increasing hepatitis C virus RNA levels in hemophiliacs: relationship to human immunodeficiency virus infection and liver disease. Multicenter Hemophilia Cohort Study. Blood 1994; 84:1020–1023.

Persidsky Y, Steffan AM, Gendrault JL, Hurtrel B, Berger S, Royer C, Stutte HJ, Muchmore E, Aubertin AM, Kirn A. Permissiveness of Kupffer cells for simian immunodeficiency virus (SIV) and morphological changes in the liver of rhesus monkeys at different periods of SIV infection. Hepatology 1995; 21:1215–1225.

Poles MA, Dieterich DT, Schwarz ED, Weinshel EH, Lew EA, Lew R, Scholes JV. Liver biopsy findings in 501 patients infected with human immunodeficiency virus (HIV). J Acquir Immune Defic Syndr Hum Retrovir 1996; 11:170–177.

Prego V, Glatt AE, Roy V, Thelmo W, Dincsoy H, Raufman JP. Comparative yield of blood culture for fungi and mycobacteria, liver biopsy and bone marrow biopsy in the diagnosis of fever of undetermined origin in human immunodeficiency virus-infected patients. Arch Intern Med 1990; 150:333–336.

Soriano V, Garcia-Samaniego J, Bravo R, Gonzalez J, Castro A, Castilla J, Martinez-Odriozola P, Colmenero E, Suarez D, Rodriguez-Pinero FJ, Moreno A, del Romero J, Pedreira J, Gonzalez-Lahoz J. Interferon alpha for the treatment of chronic hepatitis C in patients infected with human immunodeficiency virus: Hepatitis-HIV Spanish Study Group. Clin Infect Dis 1996; 23: 585–591.

Telfer P, Sabin C, Devereux H, Scott F, Dusheiko GM, Lee C. The progression of HCV-associated liver disease in a cohort of haemophiliac patients. Br J Haematol 1994; 87:555–561.

22
Management of Liver Neoplasms

Douglas R. LaBrecque and Azade Çakir-Yedidag
University of Iowa, Iowa City, Iowa

INTRODUCTION

In the fifth century B.C., Hippocrates first distinguished between *scirrhus* and *carcinoma* of the liver. Despite this early recognition of the differences between these two conditions, the terms came to be used interchangeably, creating confusion in the western literature. In the 1700s, Morgagni described hard tumors of the liver as *steatomata*. Bayle, in 1812, published the first description of a solid tumor of the liver, comparing it to solid tumors of the breast. Virchow's dictum that "Organs commonly affected by metastases are rarely the site of primary neoplasia" delayed the recognition of hepatocellular carcinomas (HCC) until 1911, when Goldzieher and von Bokay called carcinomas arising from hepatocytes "*carcinoma hepatocellularie*.

Hepatic tumors are most commonly metastatic and malignant. In the adult population, 80–90% of primary liver neoplasms are HCCs. In this chapter, we first focus on HCC, which is an important public health concern worldwide. Cholangiocarcinomas and cystic/biliary epithelial lesions will be discussed elsewhere. Hepatoblastoma is another epithelium-derived lesion. Rare mesenchymal neoplasms of the liver include malignant hemangioendothelioma (angiosarcoma), epithelioid hemangioendothelioma, and undifferentiated sarcoma. Metastases to the liver are covered in the final part of this chapter, followed by a discussion of the benign liver tumors (Table 1).

HEPATOCELLULAR CARCINOMA

Hepatocellular carcinoma (HCC) constitutes 90% of primary liver tumors and is the leading cause of cancer deaths worldwide. Each year 500,000 to 1 million new cases are diagnosed, mostly in previously cirrhotic livers. The incidence of HCC varies widely according to geography. The highest incidence is seen in the Far East, with 100–150 new cases per 100,000 population per year. The Americas, northern and central Europe, and Australia have comparable rates in the range of 3–7 new patients per 100,000 annually. The rates for Japan and the Mediterranean countries lie between these values. When geographical characteristics are taken into account, several patterns emerge in the areas of high inci-

Table 1 Simplified Classification of Primary Liver Tumors

Malignant	Benign
Epithelial	Epithelial
Hepatocellular carcinoma	Hepatocelluar adenoma
Fibrolamellar carcinoma[a]	Focal nodular hyperplasia
Hepatoblastoma[b]	Nodular regenerative hyperplasia
Cholangiosarcoma	Bile duct adenoma
Biliary cystadenocarcinoma	Biliary cystadenoma
Carinoid tumor	Intrahepatic biliary papillomatosis
Mixed and other carcinomas	
Mesodermal	Mesodermal
Hemangiosarcoma	Hemangioma (cavernous hemangioma)
Epithelial hemangioendothelioma	Infantile hemangioendothelioma[b]
Undifferentiated (embryonal) sarcoma[b]	Lipoma
Embryonal rhabdosarcoma	Other rare tumors and mixed tumors
Leiomyosarcoma	
Lymphoma	
Other sarcomas, rare tumors, and mixed tumors	
Tumor-like	
Peliosis hepatis	
Mesenchymal hamartomas[b]	
Corset liver	
Compensatory lobal hyperplasia	

[a]An important histological variant of hepatocellular carcinoma with a significantly better prognosis.
[b]Occurs in infants and children.
Source: From LaBrecque, 1996, with permission.

dence: namely, lower socioeconomic status, a striking male preponderance, and a more aggressive disease course, with an earlier disease onset (30–50 versus 50–60 years). Cirrhosis is a strong risk factor for HCC; 6–40% of patients with cirrhosis have tumor foci at autopsy. Furthermore, the 3-year cumulative risk of HCC in cirrhotics is reported to be 12.5%.

Etiology and Pathogenesis

A single genetic marker that predisposes a patient to develop HCC has not been found. In most cases, several independent events must occur to produce malignant transformation. The multistep development of carcinogenesis is well described in animal models (Fig. 1). The overwhelming evidence suggests a strong environmental role in the development of the disease (Table 2). This has been emphasized in recent decades by the elucidation of the roles of hepatitis B virus (HBV) and hepatitis C virus (HCV) in hepatic carcinogenesis. Rare genetic abnormalities such as hereditary tyrosinemia predispose to HCC, despite dietary measures. In type I glycogen storage disease, 10 cases of HCC and 50 cases of hepatocellular adenomas (HCA) have been reported, suggesting an initial imbalance in glucose metabolism triggering cellular glycogen overload, which, in turn, leads to proto-oncogene activation. Furthermore, a multistep process linking glycogenosis to steatosis to

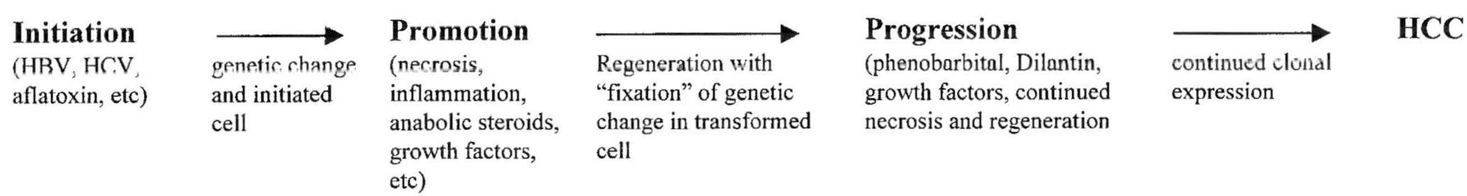

Figure 1 The multistep model of hepatocarcinogenesis.

Table 2 Risk Factors for Development of Hepatocellular Carcinoma

Definite	Possible
Hepatitis B virus (40–50%)[a,b]	Oral contraceptives
Hepatitis C virus (40–50%)[b]	Androgenic/anabolic steroids
Aflatoxin	α_1-antitrypsin deficiency
Macronodular cirrhosis (40–50%)	Ataxia telangiectasia
Micronodular cirrhosis (3–10%)	Alcohol (5–15%)[e]
Hereditary tyrosinemia (40–100%)	Type I glycogen storage disease
Hereditary hemochromatosis (3–27%)[c]	
Vinyl chloride monomer[d]	
Thorotrast[d]	

[a]Percentages in parentheses indicate death rate from HCC in various disease states.
[b]Estimated deaths from HCC, cirrhosis, or both.
[c]Risk if cirrhotic; timely phlebotomy to prevent development of cirrhosis eliminates risk of HCC.
[d]Primarily hemangiosarcomas.
[e]If cirrhotic, due to alcohol.

glycogen-poor HCC is suggested, based on the presence of "preneoplastic" glycogenosis and evidence for a disturbed glucose metabolism in a multitude of explants/biopsies. In idiopathic hemochromatosis, a 20% risk for developing HCC has been noted. These neoplasms developed in a cirrhotic background.

Aflatoxins are a group of ubiquitous mycotoxins found in corn, peanut oil, soy sauce, and fermented soybeans. Aflatoxin B1 (AFB1) has a range of biological activities including mutagenesis, teratogenesis and carcinogenesis. After ingestion, it is converted to its reactive epoxide, AFB1-8,9-oxide, by the cytochrome P-450–dependent mixed oxygenases, chiefly in the liver. This epoxide variant and the concomitantly released reactive oxygen species are highly reactive and can form adducts with DNA, RNA, and proteins, probably explaining its biological effects. Alternative pathways of dealing with AFB1 exist, partially explaining the resistance to AFB1 effects in certain individuals: hydroxylation (to AFQ1 and AFM1) and demethylation (to AFP1). Thus, aflatoxin has been implicated as one of the major environmental factors in the etiology of HCC. Exposure to aflatoxin, bound to peripheral blood albumin, poses a lifetime risk even with intermittent intake. Furthermore, a specific mutation in codon 49 of the tumor suppressor p53 gene has been implicated in 8 of 16 Chinese and 5 of 10 sub-Saharan African HCC patients. These patients were known to be exposed to aflatoxin in their food. Geographic high-aflatoxin exposure translates into an incidence of 25% in the mutant p53 gene. Interestingly, none of 15 HCC patients from Australia had this specific mutation in their p53 genes.

Hepatocellular carcinoma developing in association with HBV infection has been well studied. In Far Eastern countries such as Taiwan, 80–90% of chronic liver disease and HCC are caused by HBV. Several possible oncogenic mechanisms include a role for the hepadnavirus x-gene (HBx), which transactivates regulatory sequences of HBV and heterologous sequences of other viruses as well as a vast array of cellular genes. In addition, HBV sequences are frequently integrated into the cellular DNA. Mice transgenic for HBx develop HCCs. Transfected cells undergo oncogenic transformation in vitro and there is evidence for transactivation of oncogenes c-*myc* and c-*jun* by HBx. Hepatitis B virus transactivating sequences have been amplified from 81% (21/26) of the tissues of HCC obtained from patients with chronic HBV infection.

In the last decade, HCV has emerged as an important factor in the development of HCC. Longitudinal studies following Japanese patients with anti-HCV antibodies (Ab) showed that 16 of 62 patients developed HCC during 5 years of observation. Cirrhosis was found to impose an additional risk for the development of HCC. Some 47–83% of HCC patients in Japan, Italy, and Spain have circulating antibody to HCV. In contrast, areas where HBV is endemic have a low prevalence of HCV Ab. The pathogenesis of HCV-associated HCC is unknown. However, HCV replication intermediates have been documented in HCC explants and a mutation in the p53 gene similar to that seen in HBV has been suggested, with a documented p53 mutation in 30–50% of HCC specimens. In Taiwan, anti-HCV ab and HCV viremia by PCR were present in 70–80% of HCC patients in whom HBsAg was negative. The Far Eastern HCV isolates are dissimilar to the U.S. isolates with only 78% homology. The viral detection rates (serum PCR) were 66–71% in patients with chronic HCV disease and 83% in those with cirrhosis or HCC. The rates of development of HCC in biopsy-proven HBV+, HCV+, HBV+/HCV+, and HBV−/HCV− hepatitis patients were similar in all groups, 3–5%/year. In the United States, the contribution of HCV to the development of HCC is not well established, but there is a strong impression among hepatologists that HCC is becoming increasingly common, especially in association with HCV and HBV. Clinical consequences of the effects of infection with different HCV genotypes are unknown and most of the studies focus on the clinical response—e.g., to interferon—but there is growing evidence of an increased association of HCC with type 1b HCV infection. It is safe to state that most of the "cryptogenic" HCC cases in the United States are probably secondary to HCV infection, with a smaller contribution from HBV.

Another interesting host/agent interface is observed with *Schistosoma japonicum*, a trematode that causes an infestation known to be associated with HCC and colorectal cancer (see Chap. 20). In a mouse model, *S. japonicum* infection reduced the activity of the cytochrome P-450 mixed function oxidase system, theoretically exposing these animals to high levels of nondetoxified substances. The agent most commonly associated with the development of HCC in Western countries is alcohol. Its mechanism of carcinogenesis is unknown. Suggested neoplastic mechanisms include DNA damage from highly reactive adduct formation, alteration of steroid metabolism with resultant developmental abnormalities at the cellular level, and a relative deficiency in retinoid. Experimental studies suggest that the HBV and/or HCV infection–driven regenerative stimulus may predispose the cellular microenvironment to the mutagenic effects of alcohol and its derivatives as well as "fix" and propagate the mutation through the recurrent cycle of damage and repair.

Association between oral contraceptive use and induction of liver tumors was first recognized by Baum et al. in 1973. Despite a slight increase in the incidence of benign liver tumors, a similar trend was not observed for HCC. The most commonly found liver tumors in this group of patients are liver cell adenomas and focal nodular hyperplasia. The impact of pregnancy on HCC is unknown due to the rarity of the disease in pregnant women. Through 1995, 28 cases were recorded, with the common denominators of high parity and long-term use of oral contraceptives. Median patient survival was adversely affected by pregnancy. Furthermore, clinical trials employing sex steroid antagonists such as tamoxifen for HCC were unsuccessful.

Diagnosis and Staging

In its typical Western presentation, HCC is rare (less than 5 per 100,000 per year), associated with alcohol and/or HBV/HCV, insidious in presentation, and more commonly seen in males. Associated cirrhosis is micro- or macronodular and HCC arises late in the course of cirrhosis. One out of three cases is resectable at the time of diagnosis.

Patients usually present with vague complaints of fatigue, weight loss, right-upper-quadrant pain, abdominal mass, or decompensation or cirrhosis. Physical examination may reveal stigmata of chronic liver disease (15–50%), hepatomegaly (62%), ascites (23%) and fever (8%). Infrequently (5%), the patient will present with a constellation of findings such as erythrocytosis, changes in secondary sexual characteristics, hypercalcemia, carcinoid syndrome, hypoglycemia, hypercholesterolemia, cachexia, etc., signifying a paraneoplastic syndrome. Rarely, the patient may present with hepatic rupture, acute abdomen, and hemoperitoneum. Standard laboratory tests offer little help in reaching a diagnosis. An elevation in γ-glutamyl transpeptidase and a prominent rise in alkaline phosphatase with a normal bilirubin and minimally elevated transaminases are suggestive of a focal process. Bilirubin is usually normal in early disease, and jaundice is not a characteristic finding. Presentation may be complicated by direct tumor invasion of vascular structures with the development of hemobilia, Budd-Chiari syndrome, or inferior vena cava syndrome due to involvement of the renal veins.

The serum alpha fetoprotein (α-FP) and abdominal ultrasound (US) are effective screening tools for high-risk patients such as cirrhotics, and HBV and HCV infected patients. Serum α-FP is a useful marker for the diagnosis of HCC despite the fact that moderate increases in the levels of this marker can be observed in association with inflammation and damage due to other liver diseases. With the advent of surveillance by sophisticated liver imaging, the α-FP level at the time of diagnosis is often lower. An α-FP less than 1000 ng/mL is not reliably diagnostic for HCC. Two-thirds of patients with "resectable" small HCCs will have an α-FP below 200 ng/mL. An arbitrary cutoff for high suspicion in the absence of a confirmatory imaging study may be set at 300–500 ng/mL. Lower values must be followed closely, relying heavily on the observation of a rising trend in serial determinations, to push for more aggressive evaluation. A newer approach is the determination of an α-FP fraction that is more HCC-specific and cross-reacts with *Lens culinaris* agglutinin due to the presence of certain carbohydrate epitopes on HCC-elaborated α-FP. Abnormal serum prothrombins such as des-gamma-carboxyprothrombin, when used in combination with α-FP, may increase the diagnostic sensitivity of the combined tests to $> 85\%$ in HCC. Elevated α-FP is also seen in tumors of the embryonic foregut, ataxia telangiectasia, hereditary tyrosinemias, Indian childhood cirrhosis, hepatoblastoma, and pregnancy.

The gamma-glutamyl transpeptidase variant isozyme 2 was present in 87% of cases with HCC in a Chinese study. This isozyme, along with variant 5′-nucleotidase, may be useful in following α-FP–negative patients. Fibrolamellar HCC almost never displays a high α-FP level. However, it is capable of elaborating a series of proteins with high affinity to vitamin B_{12} and neurotensin.

HCC is noted, on rare occasion, as a calcified mass within the liver shadow on plain x-rays of the abdomen. It may appear as an area of low uptake on ^{99m}Tc liver scans, whereas con iminodiacetic acid scans, it shows uptake 50% of the time. A gallium scan is positive 90% of the time. Ultrasound with Doppler flow analysis demonstrates a hypoechoic mass with hypervascularity and shunting. Although used worldwide as a screening tool, ultrasound is less frequently utilized in the United States (see Chap. 2). However, intraoperative ultrasound has the highest sensitivity for detection of liver masses (96% or better). Standard CT demonstrates a hypodense mass. Core and border irregularities are often noted. The tumor mass takes up dense contrast on the contrast CT. Internal areas of low uptake may indicate necrosis. Magnetic resonance imaging reveals hypointense T1 images almost uniformly. A tumor blush is characteristic on celiac angiograms, with prominent arteriovenous shunting apparent.

The conventional CT scan was able to detect HCC in only 68% of patients who were ultimately found to have HCC when transplanted for end-stage liver disease. Furthermore, it identified only 54% of the multifocal nodules that were present in the explants. The advent of faster helical CT and electron-beam CT technologies and the use of dynamic CT scanning allows liver imaging to be completed in less than a minute, with the added advantages of arterial and portal venous phase imaging. Delayed studies can increase the detection rate an additional 40%. Invasive CT (CT portogram) with catheter infusion of celiac, superior mesenteric, and splenic arteries was able to detect 87–96% of the nodules subsequently verified in the explant. The disadvantages of this technique include low specificity, due to a high false-positive rate with benign lesions. Administration of lipiodol through the proper hepatic artery may show a delayed blush of the agent, which has a longer "dwell time" in tumor tissue. Detection rate for this technique is only 50–75%. The recent development of dynamic MRI using an expanding array of liver-specific intravenous contrast agents and rapid sequential scanning techniques, has produced an increasingly valuable role for MRI in the diagnosis of HCC. However, only marginally better results are obtained through MRI, and the much greater expense of this technology makes CT the diagnostic procedure of choice for imaging of liver masses (Table 3).

In a patient with documented HBV/HCV infection, heavy alcohol use, and cirrhosis or cirrhosis due to hemochromatosis, serial α-FP determinations (twice yearly) and US of the liver (at least annually) may be helpful in early diagnosis. If these are abnormal, further attempts at localizing and diagnosing the HCC with dynamic CT, MRI, angiography, and percutaneous biopsy are justified. In interpreting the liver biopsy, malignant lesions that may be diagnosed as benign include well-differentiated HCC, fetal and macrotrabecular hepatoblastoma, well-differentiated cholangiocarcinoma, Kaposi's sarcoma, and epithelioid hemangioendothelioma, making evaluation by a highly experienced hepatopathologist essential. Any combination of the above studies may establish a diagnosis of HCC, and selection must be based on the local expertise available.

Tissue diagnosis and staging are mandatory before a strategy for therapy is planned. An exception to this rule may be made when a typical liver mass is found in a cirrhotic liver and the α-FP is > 1000. This constellation of findings is sufficient to establish a clinical diagnosis of HCC. The AJCC criteria offer a staging system based entirely on pathological findings (Table 4).

Pathology

Hepatocellular carcinoma is multicentric in the majority of cases, especially those with underlying cirrhosis. It is typically located in the right lobe. In "endemic" areas, global hepatomegaly is a common finding. When HCC is observed in a noncirrhotic patient, it is typically a single, large mass with "satellite" nodules. Rarely, a diffuse infiltrative pattern with no distinct capsule is recognized. The typical North American HCC is less well encapsulated than a typical Asian HCC. Gross characteristics do not have an impact on

Table 3 Imaging Techniques and Hepatic Masses

US	Noninvasive, low-cost, readily available; with color Doppler imaging, also provides information on vascular patency, and volume, and direction of flow; demonstrates peritumoral vessels and intratumoral blood flow, indicating hypervascularity, which helps in differential diagnosis; power Doppler is superior in demonstrating tumor vascularity and smaller intrahepatic vessels; sensitivity to 1 cm; ideal screening technique; diagnostic for simple cysts; unable to convincingly determine etiology of solid or mixed masses; excellent technique for guided biopsy; marked obesity or bowel gas interfere with the exam; generally the screening test of first choice but the value of this technique is highly operator-dependent.
CT	Radiation and contrast exposure; readily available and provides "normal anatomy" for nonradiologist; sensitivity to 1 cm; nearly isodense lesions may be missed due to volume averaging or timing of imaging to contrast injection; will screen for extrahepatic lesions simultaneously; thus identifying metastatic disease beyond the liver. Regenerative nodules and uneven distribution of blood flow may produce false positives in cirrhotic liver. Helical (spiral) CT provides arterial and venous (portal) images which maximize the information obtained.
Dynamic bolus CT	Increased radiation exposure (must first localize lesion and then take multiple timed images); correctly identifies two out of three hemangiomas.
CTAP	Invasive, requiring placement of angiography catheter for bolus injection; superior delineation of anatomic location of lesions to help with surgical planning; more sensitive than standard CT and will often save unnecessary surgery by identifying additional tumor nodules not noted on standard CT or US; may produce increase in false-positive findings in presence of severe cirrhosis.
MRI	Totally noninvasive but very expensive; excellent biplanar images with sensitivity to 1.0 cm; accuracy may be a problem in the presence of severe cirrhosis, especially with ascites; problems identifying lesions near the diaphragm due to cardiac motion–induced artifacts; provides additional information on vascular supply and patency; dynamic MR imaging with liver-specific IV contrast materials, and rapid sequential scanning is playing an increasingly valuable role in HCC diagnosis.
Angiography	Most invasive, with high contrast dose and high radiation exposure; most expensive (along with MRI); provides most accurate information on vascular supply, patency, and flow, including pressures if needed.
Nuclear medicine	Minimally invasive, less costly (except for US), and readily available; less sensitive (2-cm minimum); primarily useful to distinguish hepatic adenomas from local nodular hyperplasia (due to the lack of Kupffer cells for colloid uptake in the adenomas) and identifying hemangiomas (with the ^{99m}Tc tagged RBC-SPECT study).
PET scan	Still experimental; limited availability; high cost; accuracy and specificity not yet defined

Key: US, ultrasound; CT, computed tomography; CTAP, computed tomography arterioportogram; MRI, fast spin echo magnetic resonance imaging; RBC-SPECT, technetium 99m–tagged red blood cell study utilizing single-photo emission computed tomography; PET scan, positron-emission tomographic scan.

Table 4 Staging of HCC[a]

Stage		
I	T1	Solitary, <2 cm, no vascular invasion, no nodes or metastases
II	T2	Solitary, <2 cm, with vascular invasion; or multiple tumors <2 cm without vascular invasion, limited to one lobe; or solitary tumor >2 cm without vascular invasion, no nodes or metastases
III	T1 or T2	Plus regional lymph node metastases
	T3	Solitary tumor >2 cm with vascular invasion; or multiple tumors limited to one lobe, none >2 cm, with vascular invasion; or multiple tumors limited to one lobe, with any tumor nodule >2 cm, with or without vascular invasion, with or without nodal metastases
IV A	T4	Multiple tumors in more than one lobe; or tumor(s) involve(s) a major branch of portal or hepatic veins, with or without nodal metastases; no distant metastases
IV B		Tn, with or without nodal metastases, with distant metastases

[a]The Primack modification of staging for African HCC patients introduces serum bilirubin, ascites, weight loss, and portal hypertension into the equation. If all the preceding are normal, the patient is considered stage I. A serum bilirubin above 2.0 mg/dL in a patient with ascites and weight loss of less than 25% of ideal body weight (IBW) in the absence of portal hypertension places the disease in stage II. In a patient with a more than 25% loss of IBW and portal hypertension, stage III is reached. Okuda's modification for eastern HCC characterizes four prognostically important variables: size of the tumor (whether it involves >50% of the liver in two-dimensional imaging), presence or absence of ascites, serum albumin (cutoff, 3.0 g/dL) and bilirubin (cutoff, 3 mg/dL). The presence of one or two of the above indicators places the patient in stage II; when three criteria are abnormal, the patient is in stage III.

prognosis apart from deciding on surgical approach. Vascular or ductular invasion is a common characteristic. On microscopy, a classic trabecular pattern with close resemblance to normal hepatocytes and sinusoidal architecture is observed. Striking characteristics include an absolute lack of Kupffer cells and, if they are present, dilation of bile canaliculi, giving rise to what is termed a pseudotrabecular pattern. Rarely, a strong fibrotic reaction may surround the tissue in the variant called sclerosing hepatic carcinoma.

Pathologic predictors of outcome after hepatic resection for HCC include stage, capsule formation, tumor-free margins of more than 1 cm, associated cirrhosis, vascular invasion, intrahepatic metastases, and DNA ploidy.

The fibrolamellar variant of HCC is an uncommon liver tumor seen in young adults without a previous history of liver disease. In the East, where HCC takes more than 18,000 lives annually, fibrolamellar HCC is very rare. There is no HBV/HCV association. Physical examination and history do not add much to the assessment of α-FP levels are noncontributory. Unlike regular HCC, it is more often seen in the left lobe. Resection is curative more often than with HCC and prognosis is relatively better.

Treatment and Prognosis

"Standard" Therapies

The recent proliferation of therapeutic modalities for HCC enables the clinician to personalize the management of each patient according to each institution's relative strengths (Table 5). However, center-specific expertise in a certain noninvasive or palliative approach

Table 5 Treatment of Hepatocellular Carcinoma—Many Options, None Definitive

Standard therapies—widely available	Experimental therapies
"Curative":	Surgical resection with neoadjuvant (presurgery) and/or adjuvant (post surgery) chemotherapy
1–3 nodules, less than 5 cm in diameter; no metastases	Percutaneous acetic acid or hot saline injection
Surgical resection	Cryosurgery with liquid nitrogen
Percutaneous ethanol injection	Hyperthermia therapies
Chemoembolization ± liver transplantation[a]	Microwave coagulation therapy (MCT)
	Laser therapy
Palliative:	Chemoembolization ± liver transplantation ± adjuvant chemotherapy[a]
More than 3 nodules or 1 nodule greater than 5 cm in diameter; no metastases	Immunotargeting: Mono- or polyclonal antibodies to ferritin, α-fetoprotein, or "tumor-associated antigens"
Percutaneous ethanol injection	Monoclonal antibodies alone
Chemoembolization ± liver transplantation[a]	Antibodies linked to chemotherapeutic agents
Surgical resection in limited cases	Antibodies conjugated with ^{131}I, ^{125}I, ^{90}Y, ^{99m}Tc (radiotherapy and radioimmunodetection)
	Liposome-encased chemotherapeutic agents

[a]Liver transplantation and its various multimodal variations are clearly still experimental and controversial forms of therapy. However, because transplantation is so widely available and is considered by many to be the treatment of choice, it is listed under both standard and experimental therapies.

should not limit a patient's options to palliation, since subtotal hepatectomy offers the best chance for cure of HCC. The resectability rate for western HCC is 20–33%, with an in-hospital mortality rate of 1.5–4%. The mortality rate has significantly diminished over the last decade due to the increased proficiency of liver surgery as well as the development of the techniques of vascular isolation, venovenous bypass, and liver transplantation. Regardless of tumor size, the 5-year survival rate following resection in HCC has improved from 15–24% to 25–49% in American and European centers, approaching the success of Asian groups (24–57%). Perioperative mortality is increased threefold in patients with cirrhosis. Other predictors of failure include hemorrhage and postoperative loss of hepatic function. The most favorable results are obtained after resection of tumors less than 5 cm in diameter, unilocular, and well encapsulated. Three-year survival can approach 50% after liver resection in these patients, even in the presence of cirrhosis. Thus, an ideal candidate for resection should have a noncirrhotic liver, an anatomically accessible lesion less than 5 cm in diameter, and no evidence of vascular invasion or extrahepatic involvement.

Systemic chemotherapy with single-agent or combination regimens is very disappointing in the treatment of HCC. After intraarterial injection met with variable results, chemoembolization was developed as an alternative approach, utilizing various substances that occlude the branches of hepatic arteries. The infused particles produce dearterialization and necrosis of the tumor tissue, at the same time delivering a toxic dose of the drug into the liver. Chemoembolization protocols have several theoretical advantages: tumor-specific toxic drug delivery, ischemia of arterial flow–dependent tumor tissue, prolonged exposure of the tumor to the chemotherapeutic agent, and reduced systemic toxicity. The technical skill of the operator, choice of the embolic agent, and unique patient characteristics should be considered. Numerous reports confirm significant tumor necrosis following any of the published protocols. There appears to be an additional benefit from repeated sessions of embolization. In HCCs less than 4 cm in size, transcatheter arterial (chemo) embolization (TAE) was performed with injection of a mixture of oil and chemotherapeutic agents with Gelfoam particles. Since its introduction in 1983, considerable experience has been gained. In one series of 100 carefully selected patients, the reported local recurrence rates were 18 and 33% at 1 and 4 years, respectively. The survival rate at 4 years was 67%. A surgical approach (liver resection) to tumors of similar size (< 5 cm) yielded a 5-year survival of 44% (n = 362). Despite improvements in survival, TAE has definite risks, including pain and fever, death from liver failure, main hepatic artery thrombosis, terminal hepatic necrosis (delayed anoxic pseudolobular necrosis), superinfection, and bleeding. In multifocal or large HCC in an anatomically disadvantageous location or for treatment of local recurrences, chemoembolization is a viable option, especially in the setting of a patent portal vein.

Percutaneous ethanol injection (PEI) produces necrosis and coagulation of the tumor tissue through ultrasound (US)-guided administration of absolute ethanol (99.8%) into the tumor. Complete necrosis is accomplished in 60% of patients with tumors less than 3 cm in diameter. In a study from Italy, the efficacy of PEI in treating HCC was equal to that of resective surgery, with comparable survival rates of about 65% at 3 years follow-up. Untreated cohorts (treatment refusal or historic controls) had a 10% survival rate. Percutaneous injections of acetic acid (15–50%) and even hot saline have produced similar results to PEI. In a Japanese study, the predictors of failed PEI for HCC were α-FP exceeding 20 ng/mL and the presence of cirrhosis.

Thus, a small HCC (< 3–5 cm) can be treated with the same "published" efficacy by resection, liver transplantation, or, as in Europe and Japan, percutaneous ethanol injection. While the latter offers the safety of a relatively noninvasive procedure and reported 5 year survival rates exceeding 50%, the tendency for multicentricism of HCC dictates the need for a close long-term follow-up, as frequently as every 3 months. The major drawback to any therapy that does not include liver transplantation is that the milieu for the development of HCC (the diseased liver) remains and the likelihood of HCC recurrence or death from progressive liver failure is not alleviated. Unfortunately, the lack of any large prospective trials comparing different treatment modalities and the careful preselection of patients in the published trials of single modalities make it impossible to provide true outcomes-based recommendations. In all cases, the asymptomatic, noncirrhotic or Child's class A cirrhotic patient, with a single lesion < 3.0 cm in diameter, did best, but similar 3–5 year survival rates have even been reported in carefully selected patients who received no treatment. Prospective, randomized, controlled trials are desperately needed.

Experimental Therapies

In advanced disease, combination chemotherapy/surgery/radiation protocols with or without arterial embolization are currently under way in a multitude of centers. Systemic therapy for HCCs not amenable to surgical treatment should take into account prognostic factors influencing survival. These factors are poor performance status, older age, and poor hepatocellular reserve. In cases of large, unresectable, fibrolamellar or nodular HCC, the option of combined chemo/radiotherapy has been suggested. Intrarterial chemotherapy and resection followed by external-beam radiotherapy has been successful in extending the expected survival of 18–24 months to 44 months.

Repeat hepatic resection for recurrent liver tumors should be undertaken when there are limited numbers of metastases, technical ability to resect all the macroscopic disease is present, the patient is physically capable of tolerating the procedure, and an adequate postresection hepatic reserve will remain. Of the approximately 30% primarily resectable cases, 20–50% will have a recurrence within the first 2 years. The majority (80%) of these patients will have liver involvement. HCC behaves very similarly to metachronous colorectal metastases in this context, with a similar 5-year survival rate of 20–40%. However, the median survival rate for secondary liver resection was only 32 months in a European series. For curative intent, liver transplantation is the only alternative to repeat resection.

The ominous scarcity of available donor organs dictates that liver transplantation should be considered only under very limited circumstances for HCC. The best results are obtained in patients with good general functional status, cirrhotic livers, and small, unifocal tumors with no nodal involvement. Patients most likely to benefit from liver transplantation are the young, noncirrhotic patients with large, unresectable fibrolamellar HCCs. Overall, 5-year survival after liver transplantation for HCC, including this type of relatively benign lesion, ranges between 20 and 45%. This is dramatically improved to 75% in patients with stage I and II tumors with cirrhosis. However, in a disease with a very unpredictable natural history such as HCC, these results should be interpreted with caution, since several studies suggest that small HCCs in cirrhotics may have been "dormant" for several years before the diagnosis, and the untreated patients may have a survival rate reaching 50% in the absence of terminal liver disease. The combination of liver transplantation with neoadjuvant chemotherapy (pre-, post- and sometimes intraoperative) is being explored in a few centers, based on the unsatisfactory results obtained with liver transplantation alone. In selected patients with advanced (multifocal disease or stage III or IVA) tumors, the results are encouraging, with 5-year survival rates reaching 50%.

Locoregional immunochemotherapy has been studied by Yamamoto's group in Japan, utilizing intraarterial infusions of interleukin-2 (IL-2) in combination with doxorubicin in 17 Stage IV patients. Clinical efficacy of the IL-2 therapy was monitored by natural killer (NK) and lymphokine-activated killer (LAK) cell activity and tumor response. Complete remission was achieved in four and partial remission in two patients, with 8-month survival of these patients. Direct injection of wild-type p53 DNA into the tumor tissue and transfection work involving sensitization of the tumor by various virally encoded nucleotide kinases appear promising.

In a multivariate analysis, Okuda's grading, serum creatinine, and des-gamma-carboxyprothrombin levels were found to have the most significant effects on prognosis. Pathological indicators of prognosis following resection/transplantation therapy have also been described. Apart from the "R" status or "resection for cure" attempt at the initial operation, the TNM (tumor, node, metastasis) status of the presenting lesion had an impact on survival. Clinically detectable hepatomegaly, age, sex, and the location of the tumor at diagnosis are controversial as prognostic factors. Histological type/degree of differentiation and the presence of cirrhosis were influential on survival only in resected patients. The presence of ascites, hepatorenal syndrome, hyperbilirubinemia, and a low serum albumin were independent predictors of poor survival.

The Complications of Spontaneous Rupture

Spontaneous rupture of an HCC is a rare complication and requires emergency surgery. Typical findings on presentation may range from hypotension and shock to moderate right-upper-quadrant pain and a rapid increase in liver size. The diagnosis can be made by peritoneal lavage, paracentesis, or radiological methods. CT is diagnostic in 100% of cases if the patient is hemodynamically stable enough to undergo the procedure. There is a 10–50% reported mortality even with urgent surgical intervention. The suggested method for hemostasis is transcatheter selective arterial embolization, followed by definitive surgery if indicated. Mean survivals for patients who have undergone angiographic embolization or surgery were 247 and 98 days, respectively.

HEPATOBLASTOMA

Although infrequent in adults, hepatoblastoma is the most common liver tumor in children 0–5 years old, with a peak occurrence before 3 years of age. Sex distribution is not clear, but there is an association with congenital anomalies such as hemihypertrophy, talipes, macroglossia, absence of the right hemidiaphragm, and Meckel's diverticulum, as well as anomalies of the kidneys and the heart. Compared to Wilms' tumor and neuroblastoma, it is rare, with an incidence of 0.2–5.8% in the infant age group. Clinical presentation is characterized by failure to thrive, nonspecific upper GI symptoms, anorexia, and an abdominal mass. Alpha-fetoprotein levels are elevated in up to 90% of the cases and paraneoplastic syndromes such as precocious puberty may be apparent due to elaboration of human chorionic gonadotrophin (hCG) by the tumor tissue. Cystathioninuria, a common finding (50%) in childhood HCC, is less frequent. CT reveals a mass and angiograms show an avascular lesion. Pathology reveals a well-encapsulated solitary mass 10–12 cm in diameter. Under microscopy, mesenchymal connective tissue and embryonic epithelial cells with dedifferentiation characteristics, such as a high nucleocytoplasmic ratio and sprinkle shape, are noted. A better differentiated hepatoblast component with poorly formed hepatic architecture constitutes the "fetal" component. In the connective tissue component, muscle elements are characteristically infrequent. After tissue diagnosis, the prognosis is dismal if surgery is not attempted. A combination of surgery and chemo-radiotherapy has resulted in marginal improvement in the prognosis for these patients in selected centers.

NONPARENCHYMAL TUMORS

Sarcomas

Malignant Hemangioendothelioma (Hepatic Angiosarcoma)

Angiosarcoma of the liver, also known as hemangioendothelial sarcoma or Kupffer cell sarcoma, is rare. Ten to twenty cases are diagnosed each year in the United States. Its pathogenesis has been widely studied and exposure to vinyl chloride, thorium dioxide contrast material (Thorotrast), arsenic and anabolic sex steroids have been established as risk factors, accounting for 25% of these cases. There is a weaker association with oral estrogen and phenelzine intake. The few angiosarcomas observed in children or young adults have been attributed to malignant transformation of benign infantile hemangioendotheliomas.

Angiosarcoma is seen primarily in the elderly, with peak incidence in the sixth and seventh decades. Men are affected three times more often than women. Clinical presentation is insidious, with features similar to those of HCC. The most frequent finding is hepatomegaly (70%). Liver failure and jaundice are less common (25%). Patients with polyvinyl chloride exposure may have associated splenomegaly. Laboratory studies are usually noncontributory, with mild anemia and thrombocytopenia as well as mildly elevated transmianase and bilirubin levels being occasionally seen. Serum α-FP and other markers are usually normal. On radiological examination, plain films may reveal calcific areas or long-standing retention of contrast in Thorotrast-induced cases. Selective angiograms may show characteristic filling defects (70%), caused by displacement of the hepatic arterial tree by tumor mass and "puddling" of the contrast during the midphase of angiography. Liver biopsy is much riskier than in HCC due to the highly vascular nature of the mass.

Angiosarcomas may occur as single masses in either lobe, but the usual presentation is multifocal. The typical appearance is that of multiple nodules with central hemorrhagic necrosis. Multiplying endothelial cells are thought to displace hepatocytes and trigger atrophy, while the cavity is filled with blood. Identification of displaced liver cell plates with reticulin-rich fiber interposition and staining of the malignant cells for factor VIII may aid in the diagnosis. Mean life expectancy in angiosarcoma after the diagnosis is less than a year. Liver failure is the cause of death and most patients have metastases at the time of diagnosis, rendering a surgical approach futile. Intraperitoneal hemorrhage or frank gastrointestinal bleeding may trigger a catastrophic course. Pooling of excessive amounts of blood in the liver and arteriovenous shunting may induce cardiac failure and coagulation disturbances. Attempts at radiotherapy and chemotherapy have been uniformly unsuccessful.

Epithelioid Hemangioendothelioma

Clinically less aggressive than angiosarcoma, epithelioid hemangioendothelioma (EH) has been recognized since the early 1980s. Epithelioid structures within the tumor mass frequently caused diagnostic confusion with metastatic carcinoma. Following electron microscopic and immunohistochemical studies, the endothelial nature of the tumor was recognized. The nomenclature was based on its clinical behavior, which placed it in the spectrum somewhere between angiosarcomas and benign hemangiomas. The pathogenesis is mostly unknown. There have been reported cases related to vinyl chloride exposure and oral contraceptive intake. The tumor is generally multicentric with no clear-cut margins. The central area is solid, similar to cartilage tissue in gross appearance. Histopathology reveals a dense epithelioid stroma with spindle-cell/epithelioid-appearing endothelial tumor cells. Weibel-Palade bodies, an endothelial cell marker recognized on EM, are usually present. These small vesicles contain a glycoprotein core, are physiologically expressed on activated endothelial cells, and are characterized as P-selectin or CD62P. Stains for CD62P or factor VIII confirm the endothelial nature of the tumor. When pseudopapillary growth is pronounced, this lesion may be difficult to distinguish from a carcinoma.

EH appearing in adults differs from infantile HE. The adult form can occur at any age, although the mean age at presentation is late forties to fifties. Approximately 60% of patients are female. The recognition of EH in the last decade led to reviews of records of patients who were previously classified as having metastases and/or angiosarcomas. The incidence of EH was judged to be equal to that of angiosarcoma. Most of the patients are symptomatic, with abdominal pain, nonspecific upper-GI symptoms, and jaundice. Up to 10% of the tumors are diagnosed incidentally during laparotomy performed for other reasons. Laboratory examination is usually not helpful. Calcification may be apparent on x-ray. Ultrasound usually reveals a solid, hyperechoic mass. It may appear hypoechoic when there is central necrosis of a large mass. Multicentricity is so common that radiological examination cannot be relied on to distinguish these lesions from metastases to the liver. Unlike the case in angiosarcoma, bleeding after percutaneous liver biopsy is not a frequent problem. Interpretation of the biopsy is crucial, however, since the recognition of EH as a clinical entity is relatively new.

The clinical course of EH varies, depending on the proximity of the tumor to intrahepatic or extrahepatic structures. Since it is relatively indolent and slow-growing, it may be present for years prior to diagnosis. If it is in a relatively innocuous area of the liver, the patient may have a normal survival. When EH is diagnosed, liver transplantation is the therapeutic modality of choice, due to the tumor's multicentricity and, theoretically, low likelihood of recurrence under immunosuppression based on its well-differentiated nature.

Other Sarcomas

Undifferentiated sarcoma (embryonal sarcoma) affects children and adolescents. There are fewer than 200 cases reported in the literature and synonyms are abundant, including fibrosarcoma, primary sarcoma, mesenchymal sarcoma, and malignant mesenchymoma. The soft, bulky tumors have glycoprotein-rich cores and on microscopy show degenerated, displaced hepatocyte plates in a surrounding connective tissue pattern with multiple mitotic figures and multinucleated cells. This poorly differentiated tumor is thought to be a malignant variant of the "benign mesenchymal hamartomas." The clinical features include equal sex and race distribution, presentation with increased abdominal girth/abdominal mass, and pain. Radiological studies are characteristic for rapid interval growth and septations within the large, solitary mass. At the time of diagnosis, only 25% are resectable, and the common sites for metastases include the bony skeleton and the lungs. Repeated cures were accomplished only by surgical resection. Other sarcomas—such as leiomyosarcoma, rhabdomyosarcoma, and liposarcoma—are exceedingly rare, and the treatment options are limited, with poor survival.

METASTASES TO THE LIVER

Overview

Metastatic tumor masses in the liver are 18–41 times more common than primary liver tumors. While the most common primary malignancies metastasize to the liver more often, anatomic proximity dictates the frequency with which the liver involvement is detected. Thus, gallbladder cancer (78%) leads the list in frequency of histological involvement, followed by pancreatic primaries (70%). Those with portal venous drainage account for almost half of the metastases seen. However, patients with lung cancer (42%), colon cancer (56%), and breast cancer (53%) form the majority of cases encountered in clinical work (Table 6).

Diagnosis

When accompanied by symptoms, most of the tumors are very advanced. Blunt, unrelenting right-upper-quadrant pain with referral to the right subscapular area is present in 30% of patients. Evidence of ascites or liver failure is uncommon. Nonspecific upper-GI symptoms such as nausea and vomiting are present more commonly, with weight loss and anorexia compounding the presentation. Physical findings may include hepatomegaly and, with biliary tract involvement, jaundice. There may be a variety of paraneoplastic syndromes,

Table 6 Frequency of Tumor Metastases to Liver at Time of Autopsy

Tumor	Liver metastases (%)
Gallbladder	77.6
Pancreas	70.4
Unknown primary	57.0
Colon	56.0
Breast	53.2
Melanoma	50.0
Ovary	48.0
Testis	44.4
Stomach	44.0
Bronchogenic	41.8
Urinary bladder and ureter	37.9
Cervix	31.7
Endometrial	31.5
Esophagus	30.3
Kidney	23.9
Thyroid	17.1
Prostate	12.6

Source: Data derived from Craig JR, Peters RL, Edmondson HA. Tumors of the Liver and Intrahepatic Bile Ducts. Washington, DC: Armed Forces Institute of Pathology, 1989:257.

depending on the primary lesion. The most characteristic constellation of findings are seen in patients with neuroendocrine neoplasias. Laboratory studies frequently reveal abnormalities in ALT, serum alkaline phosphatase, gamma-glutamyl transpeptidase, and 5′-nucleotidase. Bilirubin is elevated more often in patients with symptoms. Carcinoembryonic antigen (CEA) levels are frequently elevated with colorectal metastases as well as in certain other conditions. Thus, the sequential determinations of CEA are more reliable in patients with documented colorectal/gastrointestinal malignancies. Depending on the primary, CA19-9, α-FP, CA-125, Du-Pan-2, CA-50, neuron-specific enolase, melanocyte markers, etc., may also be positive.

Imaging modalities are utilized in a similar fashion to HCC, with variable US findings. Nuclear medicine studies using ^{99m}Tc liver scan or iminodiacetic acid derivatives show uptake defects. Plain x-rays and CT on rare occasion demonstrate calcifications. Contrast CT may reveal single or multiple masses with hyperdense peripheral margins surrounding an often necrotic, low-density core. On MRI scan, vascular tumors may "light up" on T2 phase. A tumor blush is characteristic in angiograms. The minimal tumor size detected by each of the techniques depends heavily on the expertise of the examiner, ranging from 0.5 cm for MRI or CT with portal contrast to 1 cm for US and 2 cm for liver scan. The "gold standard" for diagnosis is CT/ultrasound or direct vision-targeted biopsy of the mass. Fine-needle-aspiration biopsies may be interpreted using CytoSpin technology, yielding a diagnosis 90% of the time, but a highly skilled cytologist is required to approach these figures.

Pathology

In many cases the primary source of the cancer can be ascertained, again depending on the expertise of the interpreter. The presence of pseudoglandular structures, mucin, and overall gastrointestinal epithelial appearance with varying degrees of anaplasia suggests a colorectal primary. Poorly differentiated small-cell tumors may originate from lung. Specific markers may be of utility in diagnosing less common tumors. However, it may be impossible to determine the primary when it is an undifferentiated adenocarcinoma.

Management

General Principles

Based on the primary pathology, systemic chemotherapy has variable results. Transcatheter arterial embolization (TAE) methods have been utilized with less encouraging results than those achieved with HCC. The presence of portal vein or hepatic artery thrombosis in a patient with normal arterial anatomy precludes its use. Another difficulty arises from the lower degree of differentiation and lesser dependence on arterial circulation of these tumors. Noncolorectal metastases to the liver are rarely candidates for resection. As a general rule, the less portal system involvement in the drainage of the primary, the less the indication for aggressive surgery. In particular, midgut carcinoid tumors have a very favorable outlook (70% 5-year survival), following multimodality treatment employing aggressive resection of metastases and chemoembolization.

Colorectal Metastases

The role for aggressive therapy in colorectal metastases to the liver has been established over the last few decades. Following resection of colon cancer, 50% of the patients will be lost due to recurrence of the original disease and 25% will have liver involvement. The typical sequence of events for a well-differential colorectal carcinoma involves local, lymphatic, vascular (portal), hepatic, and then systemic metastases. With increased dedifferentiation and/or worsening biological behavior, the individual growth pattern will shift from this scenario, giving rise to synchronous liver metastases and distant metastases at the time of diagnosis of the colorectal primary. In conformity with these concepts, the stage at diagnosis carries prognostic importance when resection for metachronous disease is undertaken: Dukes' B patients have a 35% 5-year survival, as opposed to 28% for those with Dukes' C. Thus, the presence of hilar/extrahepatic lymph nodes, metastatic sites outside the liver, more than four metastases in the liver, surgical margins of less than 1 cm, or involvement of both lobes indicate a poor prognosis for attempted resection. Independent of the size of metastases, the postresection liver volume, required amount of blood transfusions, and residual functional capacity of the liver are important predictors of outcome. Previously performed chemotherapy may adversely affect the regenerative capacity of a noncirrhotic liver. The expertise of the surgical team is also an important variable, since formal anatomic resections are associated with better outcome. Since there have been numerous advances in the surgical armamentarium, it is imperative that local expertise in a certain technique be utilized. Under optimal conditions, with the above criteria met, the expected overall 5-year survival ranges from 30–40%.

Local/regional chemotherapy employing TAE or indwelling arterial pumps is evaluated based on response to therapy, which is defined as a reduction in CEA levels or reduction in the tumor mass on CT scans. The reported median survival in patients who are not candidates for surgical resection ranges from 11–26 months. Newer modalities such as percutaneous US-guided radiofrequency ablation appear promising in selected candidates with tumors not amenable to resection (disease-free survival: 18 months, 8 of 16 patients with multiple metastases).

The limited experience with liver transplantation for metastatic carcinoma comes almost completely from studies at the University of Pittsburgh. Sometimes extending to the level of complete upper abdominal exenteration with liver and pancreatic islet transplantation, the survival rates obtained in patients with neuroendocrine tumors or adenocarcinomas reach 25% at 5 years. However, when adenocarcinomas alone were studied, none of the 12 patients survived beyond 3 years. Thus, the shortage of donor organs and generally poor results should dictate a critical evaluation of the utility of liver transplantation for metastatic liver disease.

BENIGN TUMORS OF THE LIVER

Hepatocellular Adenoma (HCA)

There is a direct relationship between oral estrogen use and the formation of HCA, with an estimated incidence of 3–4 per 100,000 per year. Most patients are females of reproductive age. Anabolic steroids and metabolic diseases such as tyrosinemia and type I glycogen storage disease are less frequent causes. The duration of exposure to oral estrogens and older age (more than 5 years and 30 years, respectively) are associated with increased risk. The role of combination pills in tumorigenesis cannot be ruled out based on the presence of progesterone. Because of their hormonal sensitivity, these tumors may increase dramatically in size during pregnancy (pregnancy is contraindicated in women with untreated HCA). Acute rupture of an HCA may be the only presenting symptom and is seen almost exclusively in women on oral contraceptives. At the other end of the spectrum, HCA may be diagnosed incidentally during liver imaging for other reasons. Laboratory studies are nondiagnostic. On standard abdominal films, no calcification is seen. Nuclear medicine studies show single, large uptake defects, although 20% of the time there may be uptake of the tracer by the lesion. Ultrasound with Doppler flow analysis shows significant enrichment of the flow at the periphery of a large hyperechoic mass. Loss of echogenicity in the center may signify hemorrhage. CT shows a homogenous, hypodense mass. Peripheral "feeder" vessels may be noted after administration of contrast. Due to a high fat/glycogen content, T1 images are usually hyperintense on MRI study. Angiography reveals centrifugal glow and hypervascularity in the periphery.

Grossly, the HCA is a single, often large (10 cm or more) tumor with a tan-gray color. There may be areas of focal hemorrhage and necrosis. The microscopic appearance may be very difficult to distinguish from that of a well-differentiated HCC or normal liver tissue.

Patients present with acute hemoperitoneum, 30% of the time, necessitating urgent resective surgery or hepatic arterial embolization. HCA may undergo malignant transformation. A longitudinal study revealed that 4 patients from a 39-patient group developed HCC over a 30-year period. Patients with multiple growths were at a higher risk. Resection is the recommended therapy in patients who plan to have children or in those with symptoms. Recurrences are common, lending support to transplantation as a therapeutic modality in extreme cases.

Males develop 75% of anabolic steroid-associated HCA. The effects of C-17 alkylated steroids on liver tissue range from the development of cholestasis to HCC and cholangiocarcinoma. The typical patient is an adolescent male who has taken anabolic steroids for more than 4 years. However, it has also been reported in association with C-17 steroid use in Fanconi's anemia, aplastic anemia, impotence, paroxysmal nocturnal hemoglobinuria, renal failure on dialysis, and anemia after renal transplantation. Abdominal pain and mass are common; patients may also present with free abdominal rupture and hemoperitoneom. Presence of high α-FP may indicate an associated HCC or cholangiocarcinoma. On pathological examination, 50% of the patients are found to have multiple tumor foci. Satellite nodules are common in the remaining half, with a primary large mass. Sometimes hemorrhagic, the nodules are usually tan-colored. Peliosis hepatis may be present, as well as bile staining. Microscopy shows tremendous histological variation. Nodules may range from benign-appearing hepatocyte cords to large cells with hyperchromasia. Central cholestasis in acini is a common feature. Differential diagnosis from HCC may be challenging.

After diagnosis, the most important step is discontinuation of the offending agent. Resolution may ensue, although persistence without development of HCC or cholangiocarcinoma for 10–14 years has been observed.

Focal Nodular Hyperplasia

Focal nodular hyperplasia (FNH) is the most common benign hepatic tumor (8% overall of primary hepatic neoplasia) with the exception of vascular tumors. Its pathogenesis is unknown. The equal sex distribution weakens the suggested association with oral estrogens. Some authors suggest a hamartomatous origin rather than a true neoplastic process. Most (75%) of the FNHs are incidental findings during autopsy or laparotomy performed for other reasons. Women on oral contraceptives may have symptoms including abdominal pain, which is a cardinal feature in complications such as free intraperitoneal rupture and/or hemorrhage into the tumor tissue. Laboratory tests are noncontributory. Ultrasound may show a hypoechoic mass and, on CT scan, a characteristic stellate central hyperdense "scar" is often seen. On angiogram, a vessel-rich periphery is seen, with a relatively poorly vascularized core. The central scar will appear as a hyperintense T2 image on MRI scan.

On pathological examination, FNHs are solitary, with a well-demarcated margin but no capsule, and are located in the periphery of the right lobe of the liver. From the central scar tissue, septa radiate peripherally in the mass, giving rise to a microscopic appearance of "focal cirrhosis." They tend to be smaller than hepatic adenomas, with a mean diameter of 5 cm, and show a lesser tendency to bleed. The septa, which are arranged in a spokewheel manner, are invested with thick-walled vascular elements and proliferated bile ducts, without any clear-cut portal units. A premalignant tendency has not been documented. However, individualized treatment plans should address the small likelihood of hemorrhage and a weak potential for growth stimulation by oral contraceptives and pregnancy. In an asymptomatic patient with a confirmed diagnosis of uncomplicated FNH, surgical resection is not recommended. However, if the patient plans to become pregnant, resection may be prudent.

Nodular Regenerative Hyperplasia

Although not a true neoplastic condition, this rare entity is remarkable owing to the fact that it is associated with a variety of diseases, including juvenile rheumatoid arthritis, subacute bacterial endocarditis, the CREST variant of progressive systemic sclerosis, multiple

Table 7 Differential Diagnosis of Hepatic Mass Lesions

	Hepatocellular carcinoma	Metastatic carcinoma	Hepatocellular adenoma	Focal nodular hyperplasia	Cavernous hemangioma	Simple cyst
Incidence/100,000[a]	1–4800[b]	8–20	3–4	3–4	400–7500	170
Solitary	20–40%	5–10%	90%	90%	90%	?
Coexisting liver disease	HBV, HCV, cirrhosis, hemochromatosis	Uncommon in cirrhotic liver	None	None	None	None
Pathogenesis	HBV, HCV, alcohol, aflatoxin, cirrhosis	Hematogenous, lymphatic or direct spread	Estrogens, anabolic steroids	Congenital, estrogens	Congenital, ?estrogens	Congenital
Imaging[c]	US, CT	US, CT, CTAP	US, CT, ^{99m}Tc	US, CT, MRI, ^{99m}Tc	Dynamic bolus CT, ^{99m}Tc-RBC-SPECT scan	US, CT
α-fetoprotein	>300–500 ng/mL	Normal	Normal	Normal	Normal	Normal
Characteristic gross features	Hemorrhage, necrosis, vascular invasion/obstruction	Hemorrhage, necrosis, umbilicated	Hemorrhage, necrosis	Central scar	Blood filled "cyst"	Thin walled cyst with clear fluid
Characteristic microscopic features	"Thick" (>3–4 cells) trabeculae	Replacement of hepatocytes by malignant cells	"Neohepatocytes," normal cord structure, no portal structures	"Focal cirrhosis" with pseudoductules	Blood filled spaces lined by single layer of flat epithelium	Simple cuboidal endothelium
Diagnosis[d]	FNAB or core biopsy	FNAB or core biopsy	Imaging, biopsy	Imaging, biopsy	Imaging	Imaging
Treatment	"Curative resection" or ethanol injection if solitary, <5.0 cm; ?transplantation ± chemoembolization	"Curative resection" if <3.0 cm and 3 or fewer nodules	Discontinue estrogens/androgens; resect if possible, especially if large; otherwise periodic imaging	Discontinue estrogens; periodic imaging	Surgical resection only if symptomatic or >10.0 cm; discontinue estrogens; periodic imaging	Usually no treatment; percutaneous aspiration or surgical enucleation if symptomatic

[a]From autopsy series.
[b]Varies with geographic origin.
[c]Most useful imaging technique with which to obtain a diagnosis.
[d]Definitive test required for confident diagnosis.

Key: US, ultrasound; CT, computed tomography; Dynamic bolus CT: rapid sequential CT images taken at plane of the mass, with delayed images up to 20 min; CTAP, computed tomography arterioportogram; MRI, fast spin-echo magnetic resonance imaging; ^{99m}Tc, technetium 99m–labeled sulfur colloid scan; RBC-SPECT, technetium 99m–tagged red blood cell study utilizing single-photo emission computed tomography; FNAB, fine needle aspiration biopsy for cytology.

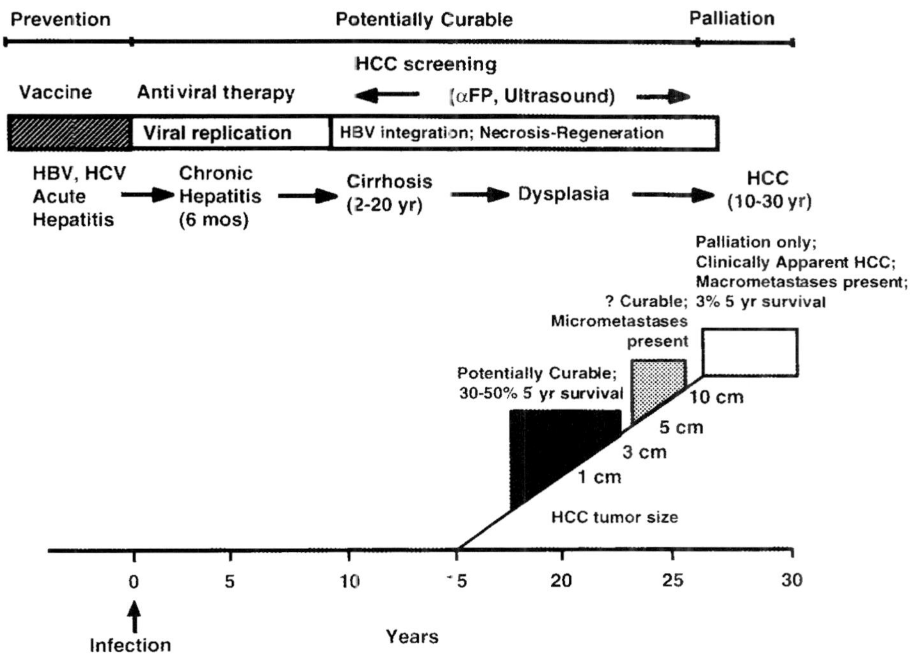

Figure 2 Potential intervention points in the prevention, diagnosis, and treatment of hepatocellular carcinoma associated with viral hepatis. (From LaBrecque, 1996, with permission.)

myeloma, macroglobulinemia, myelofibrosis, polycythemia vera, hereditary hemorrhagic telangiectasia, polyarteritis nodosa, diabetes mellitus, toxic oil syndrome, and certain drugs. Suggested pathogenesis involves occlusion of small intrahepatic portal branches with arterial/portal venous inflammation. Multiple attacks of local ischemia-induced atrophy are followed by regeneration, giving rise to multiple regenerative nodules and compression of the neighboring liver cell plates with minimal surrounding fibrosis. Grossly, the liver is diffusely nodular. The largest nodules may reach 1 cm. The nodules are paler than the surrounding normal liver tissue and on microscopy, consist of hyperplastic hepatocytes. The reticulin stain is diagnostic

Portal hypertension, if it develops, may require specific therapy. However, treatment efforts should be directed at the underlying disease. In some cases, HCC has been shown to develop. Liver failure or rupture are rare. Use of sex steroids is contraindicated.

Cavernous Hemangioma

Patients with these thinly encapsulated, benign, blood-filled tumors are infrequently (15%) symptomatic. Calcification may be apparent 10% of the time. Dynamic CT reveals a hyperechoic, well-defined early defect with late-phase enhancement due to pooling of the blood. Standard CT scans show a hypodense mass with sharp, lobulated borders and contrast enhancement with peripheral filling from large peripheral feeder vessels, which may persist on delayed scans. MRI is sensitive and specific, the latter reaching 100% in some centers. Characteristically, it shows a low signal intensity on T1-weighted images. Single-photon emission computed tomography (SPECT), utilizing red cells tagged with technetium 99-m (^{99m}Tc) can approach MRI's specificity. Since a negative percutaneous needle biopsy does not rule out malignancy, unresected mass lesions should be followed up with an imaging study ever 3–6 months.

The likelihood of pregnancy or oral estrogen intake, tumor size ($>$ 10 cm), and presence or absence of symptoms play a role in the decision regarding resection. If the size and location render the tumor nonresectable, pregnancy should be discouraged.

CONCLUSIONS

Liver masses are a frequently vexing diagnostic problem, producing great anxiety in the patient and physician until the diagnosis is made (see Chap. 2). An understanding of the likely possibilities and the most efficient approach to a diagnosis depends on the initial historical, physical, and risk-factor assessment which will dictate further diagnostic tests (Table 7).

As we learn more about the pathogenesis of HCC, multiple opportunities for intervention in the multistage development of HCC are being identified. This is particularly true of HCC associated with HBV and HCV infections (Fig. 2). Continued basic research into mechanisms of hepatocarcinogenesis and carefully controlled prospective therapeutic trials should lead to better preventive, diagnostic, and therapeutic options.

BIBLIOGRAPHY

Bookstein R, Demers W, Gregory R, Maneval D, Park J, Wills K. P53 gene therapy in vivo of hepatocellular and liver metastatic colorectal cancer. Semin Oncol 1996; 23:66–77.

Farmer DG, Seu P, Swenson K, Economou J, Busuttil RW. Current and future treatment modalities for hepatocellular carcinoma. Clin Liver Dis 1997; 1:361–396.

Ishiguchi T, Shimamoto K, Fukatsu H, Yamakawa K, Ishigaki T. Radiologic diagnosis of hepatocellular carcinoma. Semin Surg Oncol 1996;12:164–169.

Iwatsuki S, Starzl TE, Sheahan DG, Yokoyama I, Demetris AJ, Todo S, Tzakis AG, Van Thiel DH, Carr G, Selby R. Hepatic resection versus transplantation for hepatocellular carcinoma. Ann Surg 1991; 214:221–229.

LaBrecque DR. Neoplasia of the liver. In Kaplowitz N, ed. Liver and Biliary Diseases. Baltimore: Williams & Wilkins, 1996:391–438.

Livraghi T, Bolondi L, Buscarini L, Cottone M, Mazziotti A, Morabito A, Torzilli G. No treatment, resection and ethanol injection in the treatment of hepatocellular carcinoma in cirrhosis. J Hepatol 1995; 22;522–526.

Lygidakis NJ, Stringaris K. Locoregional immuno-chemotherapy transplenic and transtumoral in vivo immunostimulation. Hepatogastroenterology 1996; 43:440–447.

Okuda K, Tabor E. Liver Cancer. New York: Churchill Livingstone, 1997.

Olthoff KM, Rosove MH, Shackleton CR, Imagawa DK, Farmer DG, Northcross P, Pakrasi AL, Martin P, Goldstein LI, Shaked A, Busuttil RW. Adjuvant chemotherapy improves survival after liver transplantation for hepatocellular carcinoma. Ann Surg 1995; 221:734–741.

Pentecost MJ. Transcatheter treatment of hepatic metastases. Am J Roentgenol 1996; 160:1171–1175.

Ros PR, Davis GL. The incidental focal liver lesion: photon, proton, or needle? Hepatology 1998; 27:1183–1190.

23
Management of Cholangiocarcinoma

Frederick C. Johlin, Jr.
University of Iowa, Iowa City, Iowa

Cholangiocarcinoma (CCC) is a rare cancer arising from the extrahepatic bile ducts, which accounts for 15% of the primary neoplasms contained within the liver. The mean survival with aggressive therapy is about 20 months. Therapy designed to improve survival must focus on preventing hepatobiliary infections by maintaining the best possible drainage of the biliary tree. This chapter deals with current understanding of CCC.

BACKGROUND

CCC, a rare tumor, is composed of cells that are similar to bile duct epithelium. This type of cancer is estimated to account for between 7 and 25% of the cancers of the liver in western countries and for about 3% of the cancer deaths. Data from England suggest a crude incidence of 2 patients per 100,000, but autopsy data suggest that this cancer is found in 1 in 10,000 postmortems. Most patients present in the sixth decade of life with the exception of patients who have primary sclerosing cholangitis (PSC) (Fig. 1) or inflammatory bowel disease, who present at a much younger age. A number of risk factors have been suggested. These risk factors include diseases such as sclerosing cholangitis, choledochal cysts, and intrahepatic bile duct stones. In the Far East, the major risk factor for the development of bile duct cancer is infestation with liver flukes. Liver flukes that cause human disease are *Opisthorchis sinensis* (Fig. 2) and *Opisthorchis viverrini*. In countries where hepatocellular carcinoma is prevalent, the relative proportion of liver cancers that are CCC is significantly smaller. This variance in frequency is best typified by the characteristically low frequency of CCC in South Africa; in Hong Kong, the relative frequency of CCC is significantly greater. This endemic prevalence of CCC is also found in all of South China and Thailand. The common variable in most causes of CCC is chronic and recurrent inflammation from stone-related trauma or chronic infections. The role of hepatobiliary cancer and the typhoid carrier state has been well described. This association is best defined for gallbladder cancer. Intrahepatic gallstones have been shown to place patients at risk for CCC. In the vicinity of the intrahepatic gallstones, one can demonstrate atypical bile duct epithelium. Information

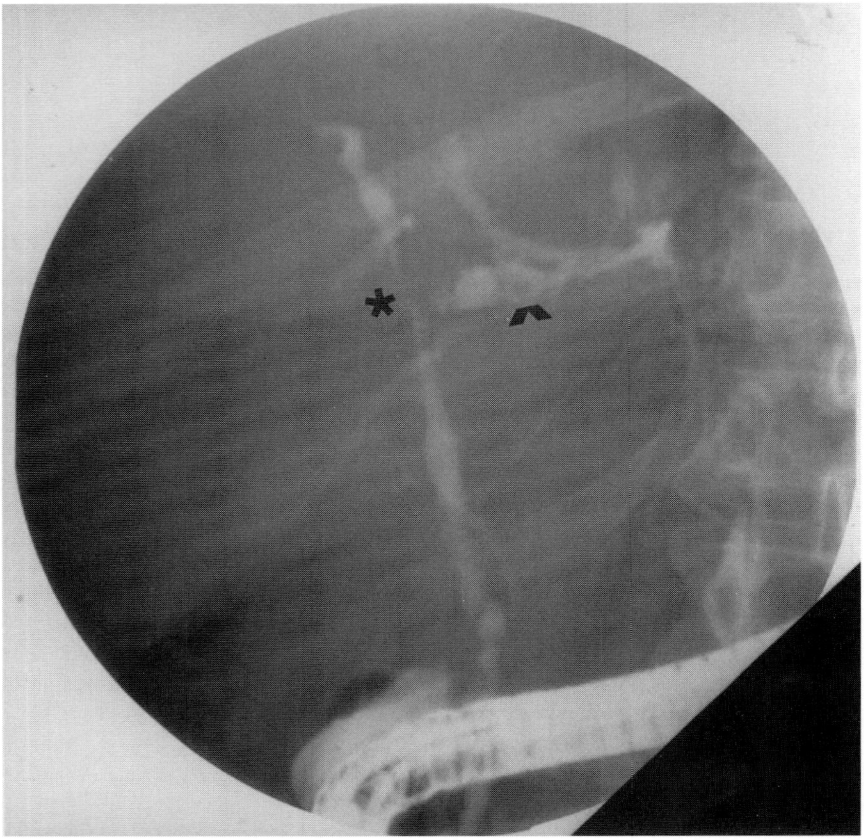

Figure 1 The cholangiogram presented was obtained at the time of endoscopic retrograde cholangiography. The films document not only areas of sacculation and stricture formation but also evidence of a stone in the left hepatic bile duct. The strictures in the common hepatic duct and the right hepatic duct were both malignant, based on brush cytology.

derived from pathological specimens suggests that even the granular tissue contained within the bile duct epithelium can become hyperplastic in the presence of chronic inflammation.

In western countries, the association between CCC and ulcerative colitis or Crohn's disease is now widely accepted. It is estimated that 1 in 256 patients with ulcerative colitis will develop bile duct cancer. Most authorities believe the cause is PSC (see Chap. 13). The availability of serum chemistries has allowed this disease to be detected earlier. When one utilizes screening alkaline phosphatase in patients with ulcerative colitis and Crohn's disease, one can often detect those patients who have either pericholangitis or PSC. The gold standard in detecting this disease remains the cholangiogram. Most major centers perform a retrograde cholangiogram as the test of choice. When patients have inflammatory bowel disease that precedes PSC, the inflammatory bowel disease typically precedes the bile duct cancer by 5 years. The mechanism of carcinogenesis in PSC is most likely chronic injury, yielding inflammation and repeated regeneration of the bile duct and glandular

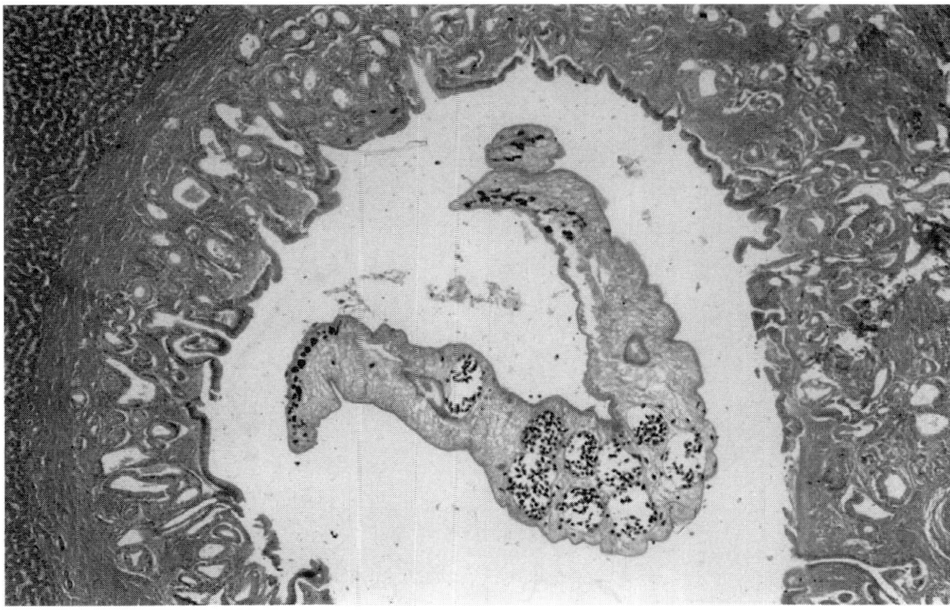

Figure 2 The *Opisthechis sinensis* is contained in a bile duct in this ×10 view of a liver fluke that can cause human disease. (Courtesy of Frank A. Mitros, M.D., University of Iowa.)

tissues. Cystic diseases of the bile duct can also be associated with CCC. These diseases include Caroli's disease, congenital hepatic fibrosis, hepatic cysts, and choledochal cysts.

Thorotrast, a contrast agent used in the earlier part of this century, is the best characterized and most widely documented chemical cause of CCC. The tumors associated with this agent are classically intrahepatic. When one examines these patients with plain radiographs, one is able to demonstrate the dense concentrations of this alpha emitter in reticuloendothelial cell lines (Fig. 3). After decades of exposure to Thorotrast, the bile duct epithelium appears to become dysplastic and can show areas of abnormal papillary growth.

PATHOLOGY

Cholangiocarcinoma can best be classified into categories of nodular, scirrhous, and papillary. These cancers are typically adenocarcinomas, although squamous cell, leiomyosarcoma, carcinoid, and histiocytic lymphomas are also reported. The nodular form of this cancer is characterized by well-demarcated projections from the margins of the bile duct epithelium into the liver parenchyma. Nodular CCC less frequently projects into the lumen of the bile duct than does the papillary form, but both are frequently located in the distal bile duct. The projections of malignant tissue insinuate into the surrounding liver tissue, which can make brush cytology less accurate as a diagnostic tool, as the bulk of the tumor is on the extralumenal side of the bile duct wall. The scirrhous or sclerosing type of CCC is characteristically firm and, on gross histology, is a gray-white tissue (Fig. 4) that can be

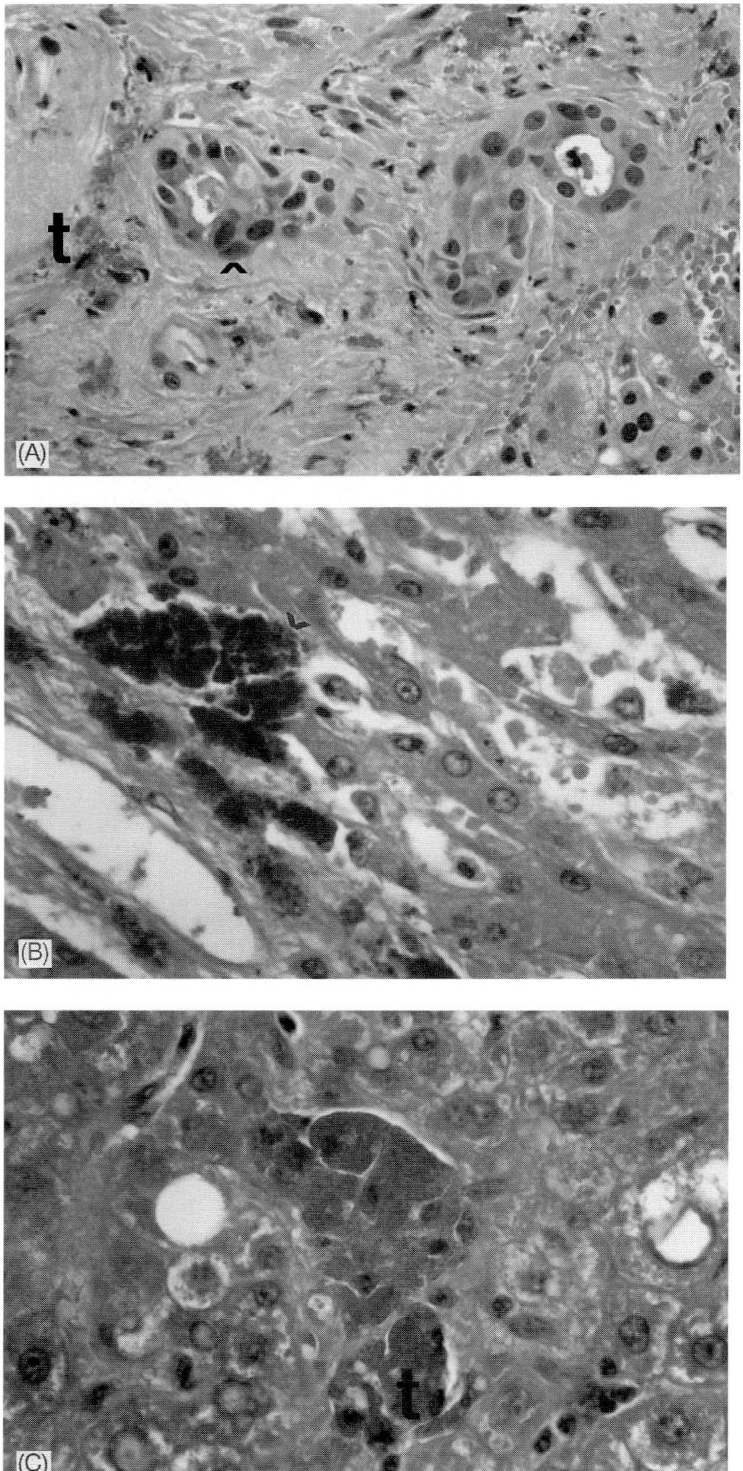
t
(A)
(B)
t
(C)

easily demarcated from the surrounding liver parenchyma. This tumor is classically situated in the hilum of the liver. Papillary CCC can project as an inflammatory mass of friable polypoid tissue directly into the bile duct lumen (Fig. 5). This type of cancer has the best prognosis of CCC. The growth margins of CCC can contain bud-like protrusions into the liver directly surrounding the CCC. Any of these cancers can present as a diffuse or infiltrating type of CCC, but the papillary types are the most likely to be multifocal. These cancers can spread into the liver parenchyma directly or can be located in peripheral segments of the liver with a hematogenous pattern of metastasis, metastasizing along the portal venous structures. The typical mechanism of progression of the cancer is by direct extension or perineural spread in 75% of patients. CCC can also spread by way of lymphatics or by peritoneal seeding. Peritoneal implants frequently yield refractory ascites as a complication. Hematogenous seeding into the systemic circulation is much less common, although bone and lung metastases do occur.

CLINICAL FEATURES

The presenting signs and symptoms of CCC vary greatly, depending on whether the cancer is detected in a symptomatic or an asymptomatic patient. The typical presenting feature in advanced diseases is jaundice with pruritus. Patients can present with concordant fever and chills. The jaundice is typically painless, but pain, cachexia, and weight loss are classically not seen until late in this disease.

A major determinant of the clinical presentation is the location of the CCC. Those tumors that reside in the hilum of the liver can sometimes be difficult to characterize with respect to the extent and location of bile duct involvement, especially in those that occur in the caudate lobe. CCC are best classified by the Bismuth and Corlette classification. Bismuth and Corlette I and II have disease below the confluence of the bile ducts, while Bismuth and Corlette III have involvement of the secondary and tertiary bile ducts. These criteria allow one to suggest and predict the best available therapy and to provide patients with surgical or other drainage options.

Most CCCs that reside in the hilum of the liver will not be visible on computed tomography (CT). CT may provide indirect evidence for the CCC, however, by demonstrating features suggesting (1) asymmetrical atrophy, which signifies loss of portal blood flow to that segment of the liver; (2) dilated bile ducts, which signifies obstruction to biliary flow; (3) collapsed gallbladder, which signifies loss of bile flow into the gallbladder; and (4) low-density lesions, which signify the potential location of the CCC. The isodense characteristics of CCC on plain CT may not be altered even on late-phase enhanced CT. This difficulty is almost never encountered with direct cholangiograms obtained by endoscopic retrograde cholangiography (ERCP) and percutaneous cholangiography (PTC).

Figure 3 (A) The bile ducts in this ×100 photomicrograph demonstrate the dysplastic changes (arrowhead) that underestimate the advanced nature of the cancer damaging this liver after decades of exposure to Thorotrast. The Thorotrast is evident in the cells next to the (**t**). (B) Thorotrast (arrowhead) is evident in this ×160 photomicrograph of damaged bile ducts. (C) Thorotrast is more evident in this ×400 photomicrograph (**t**). (Courtesy of Frank A. Mitros, M.D., University of Iowa.)

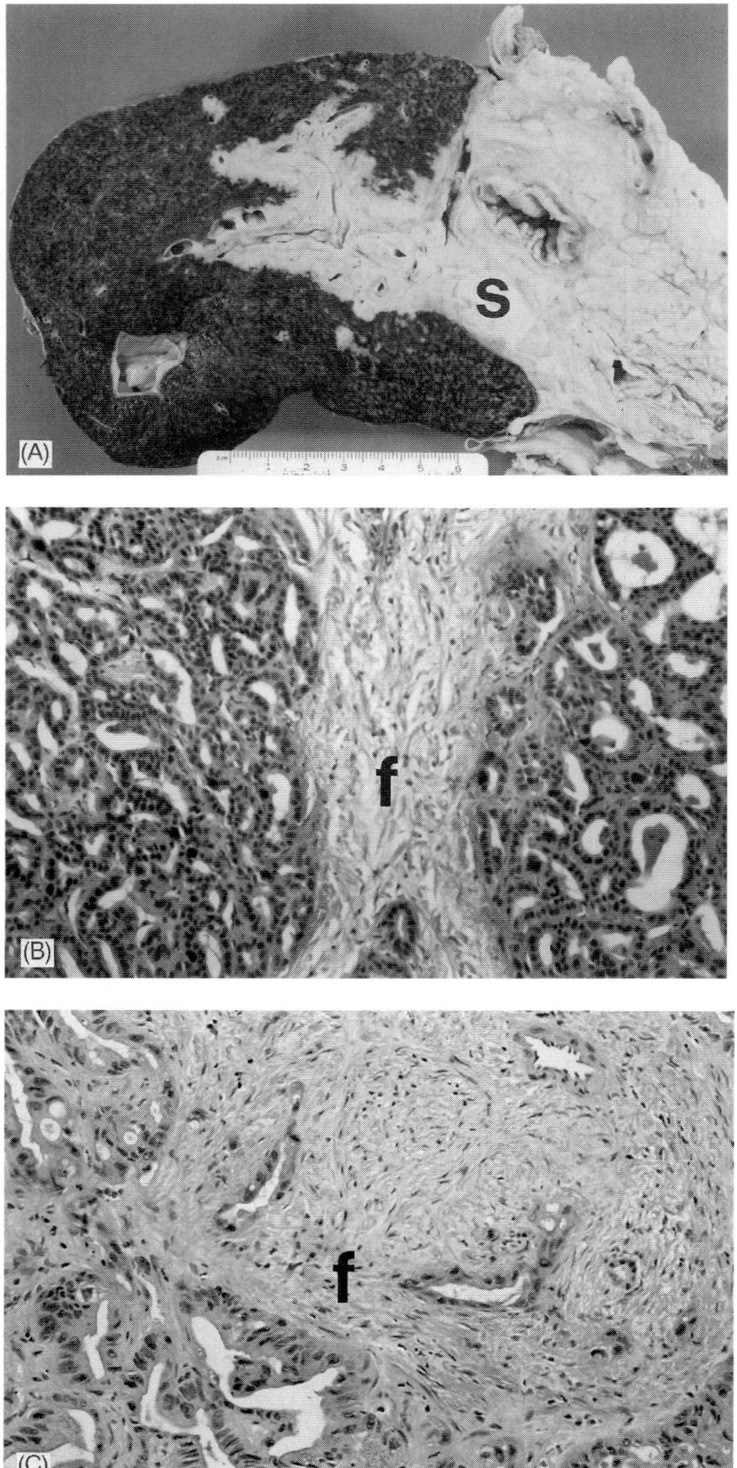
(A)
S
(B)
f
(C)
f

ERCP and PTC allow definition of the anatomic characteristics of the CCC. Cholangiography also frequently provides one with the ability to obtain cytologic and biopsy specimens and to sample bile for certain antigens such as the CEA. ERCP is avoided by some surgeons who care for patients with CCC. They claim that the radiographic definition of the malignant strictures is not adequate with this technique and that better cholangiograms are obtained with percutaneous cholangiography. In addition, data from these centers suggest an increased risk of postoperative bile leaks in those patients in whom preoperative biliary stents have been placed. There are few data suggesting that the patient who is drained preoperatively has an operative advantage; however, some physicians invariably place a stent in any biliary system that they fill with contrast. The ERCP may be difficult to evaluate when the obstructing lesion is composed of a large number of lymph nodes from lymphomas, as demonstrated in Fig. 6, from a young man with Castlemans' syndrome. Cholangiography proves least helpful in peripheral CCC (Fig. 7) but can still allow one to define the anatomy of concern.

Software transformation of MRI data allows one to obtain magnetic resonance cholangiography (MRC)P, a pseudo–three-dimensional reconstruction of the biliary tree. MRC may offer the greatest potential to diagnose CCC without using invasive testing. The scirrhous CCC historically has also posed a problem for MRC diagnosis, as the T 2-weighted spin resonance echoes a signal only slightly more dense than that of normal liver. It has been proposed that this technology might replace diagnostic ERCP in the next decade; however, a false-negative result of over 10% suggests that such a conclusion may be premature.

Angiography has very little role in the diagnosis of CCC. While studies might show a slight increase in vascularity, CCC is more typically a hypovascular lesion. Other features of the CCC seen at angiography may include evidence of encasement, venous or arterial obstruction, and the development of arterial collaterals.

Ultrasonography may provide significant information at essentially no risk to patients and at a reasonable cost. It can define the intrahepatic and the extrahepatic bile duct diameters; provide the definition of the structures in the hilum of the liver; provide information about portal veins, hepatic veins, and hepatic arteries with respect to the flow characteristics within those vessels; and/or identify tumor thrombus or tumor invasion of those vessels. Portal vein involvement is generally considered a contraindication to surgery. The resolution and image management via ultrasonography continue to improve almost at the rate that computer central processing units have improved. The cause of death in most patients is liver failure or secondary sepsis. Sepsis from occluded indwelling stents can be avoided by close attention to the biliary drains. Malignant ascites can create a significant problem with respect to pain and suffering.

Figure 4 (A) A resected liver specimen demonstrates the distinct transition between the malignant scirrhous segments and the more normal liver tissue. (B) The histology of the malignant bile duct tissue has features that are remarkably bland for the aggressive nature of this cancer. The dysplastic and cancerous bile ducts are well differentiated in around the band of fibrosis (**f**). (C) The dense fibrosis (**f**) around the cancerous bile ducts is a very common finding in this type of cancer of the biliary tree. (Courtesy of Frank A. Mitros, M.D., University of Iowa.)

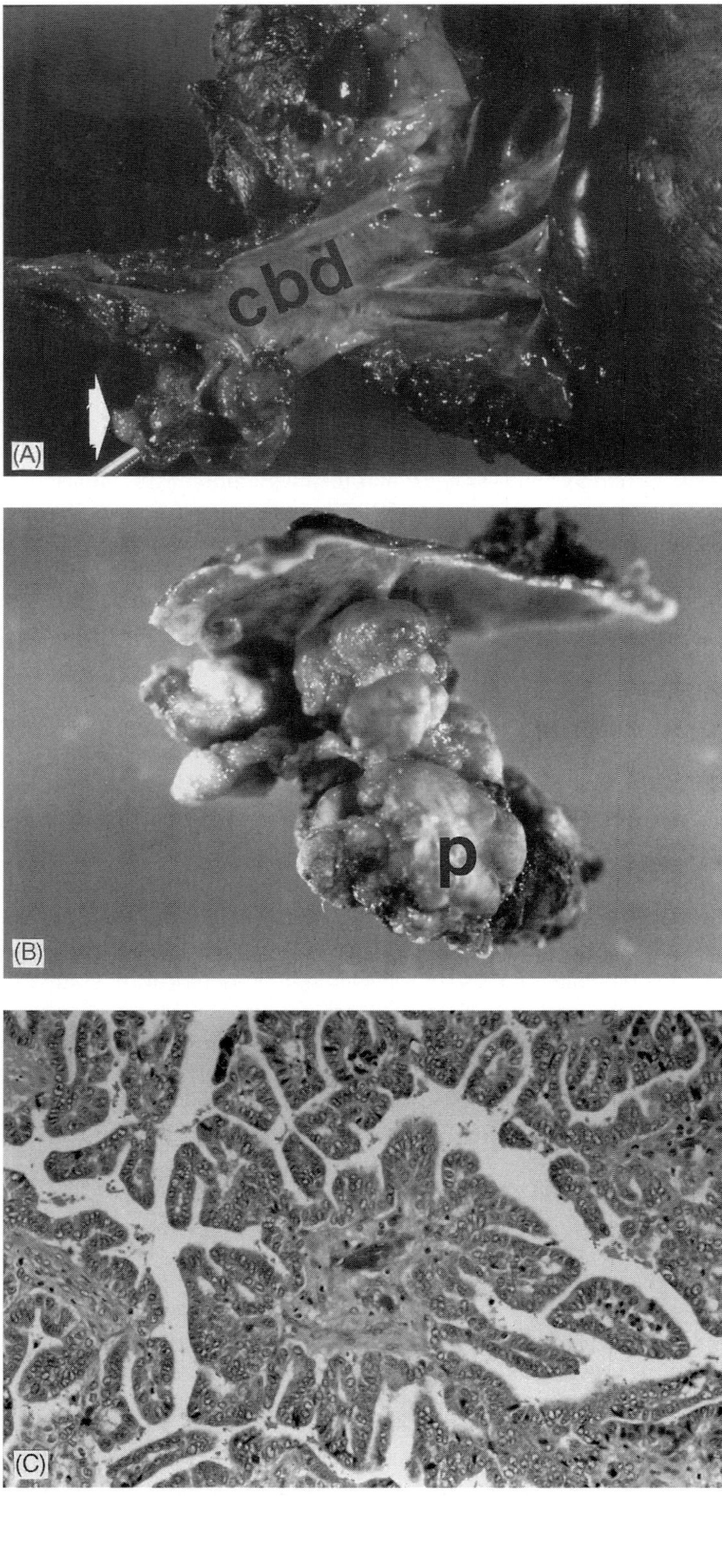
cbd
(A)
p
(B)
(C)

DIAGNOSIS

The diagnosis of CCC invariably requires tissue from the neoplasm or a metastatic lesion. This tissue may at times be difficult to evaluate in cases where the primary neoplasms are well differentiated and the tumor is surrounded by dense fibrous stroma. The clinical scenario can often direct a more aggressive evaluation to provide an accurate diagnosis. The presence of ulcerative colitis or Crohn's disease can encourage the clinician to seek aggressive techniques to obtain tissue by either brush cytology or by fine-needle aspiration, thereby avoiding unnecessary exploratory surgeries. Serum chemistries typically offer little of direct diagnostic value other than encouraging the clinician to increase his or her index of concern. Circulating alkaline phosphatase levels are invariably elevated; however they are also typically elevated in PSC, a disease that is frequently responsible for the development of bile duct cancer. Measurement of the carbohydrate antigen 19-9 (CA-19-9) and alpha fetoprotein (AFP) are often useful in the diagnostic evaluation of patients with hepatobiliary malignancy. CEA levels in bile may also be elevated in this disease but are reported not to be elevated in benign diseases of the biliary tree. Synthetic function is classically preserved in patients with CCC until late in their disease; the exception is the patient with a peripheral bile duct cancer or Thorotrast-induced cancer. The peripheral CCCs are difficult to differentiate from hepatocellular carcinomas without a tissue diagnosis. In the face of hepatocellular carcinoma, AFP is not as frequently positive in those patients that live in the West as it is in those from the Far East or Africa. Therefore, a high AFP is helpful, whereas a normal AFP does not exclude a hepatocellular carcinoma. A very high level of the CA-19-9 suggests that the bile duct cancer will not be resectable, but this has also been noted in benign diseases. The involvement of the dominant bile ducts will invariably cause jaundice in the patient with a central or extrahepatic bile duct cancer.

Cystic neoplasms occur in the biliary tree. These arise from the mucus-secreting glands within the bile duct epithelium. Differentiating benign cystadenomas from cystadenocarcinomas can be very difficult without obtaining the resection specimen. Neither CT scan nor ultrasound is capable of differentiating between the benign and/or the more malignant forms of these neoplasms. These tumors demonstrate papillary invaginations that may contain internal septations. The survival duration typically exceeds that of the scirrhous type of biliary malignancy.

TREATMENT

The goals of treatment are to enhance the quality of life and to provide the greatest chance of a cure. The therapies provided are typically percutaneous drainage, ERCP drainage, or surgical resections with or without adjuvant therapy. Surgery offers the only potential for

---

Figure 5 (A) The resected liver specimen contains a polypoid mass (arrow) that is a papillary cholangiocarcinoma. The metal probe is protruding through the lumen of the common bile duct (**cbd**) where the cancer is evident. (B) The closeup view of this resected bile duct papillary tumor (**p**) demonstrates polyp-like characteristics. (C) The photomicrograph at ×40 demonstrates the well-differentiated nature of this cancer and the frond-like projecting elements. (Courtesy of Frank A. Mitros, M.D., University of Iowa.)

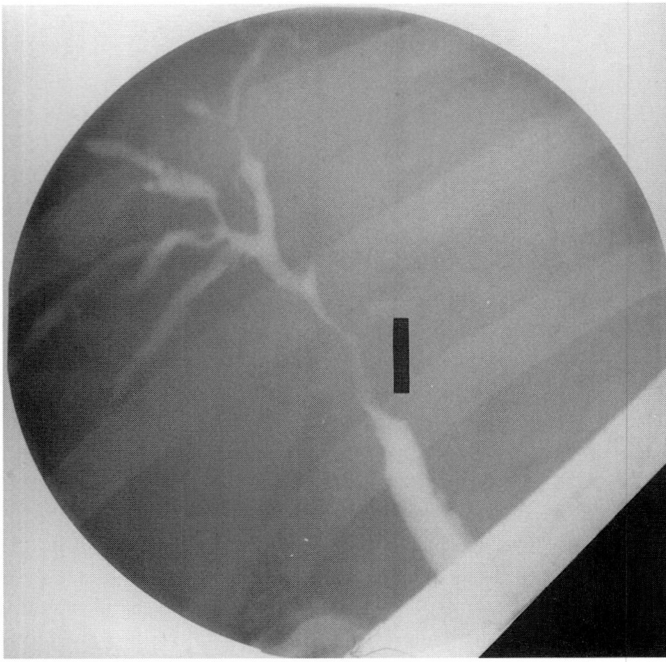

Figure 6 Cholangiogram demonstrating obstruction of a bile duct (1) by a large number of lymph nodes in a young man with Castleman's syndrome.

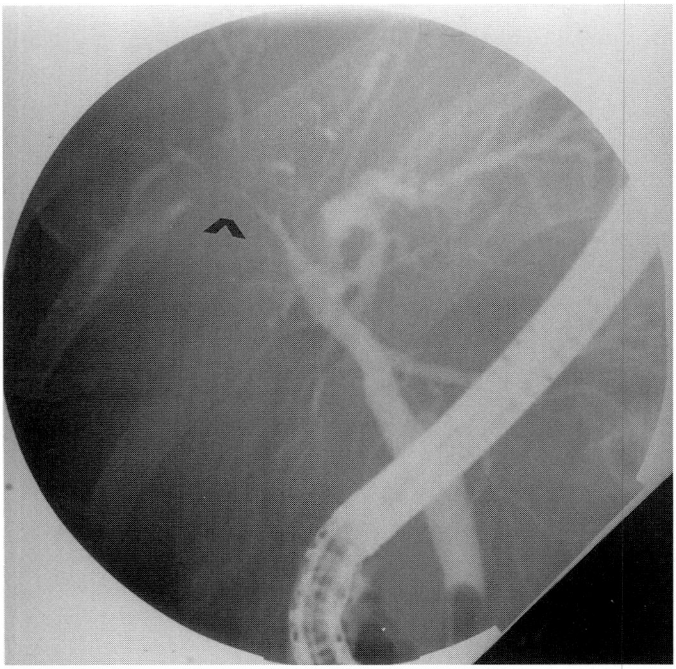

Figure 7 Cholangiogram demonstrating a peripheral cholangiocarcinoma (arrowhead).

cure, but most CCC are not curable at the time of clinical detection. The Bismuth and Corlette classifications can allow one to define who might be a best-suited surgical candidate, but comorbid conditions must also be factored in. Trisegmentectomy, extended lobectomy, lobectomy, and segmental resection are the most common resections recommended in patients with this disease if the cancer is a Klatskin type (hilar) tumor. The main difficulty encountered with surgical resection is being able to detect clean resection margins. The literature suggests that the Japanese have a higher success rate of obtaining clean resection margins as compared with American series. Biliary anastomoses provide the best drainage. There is controversy as to whether U-shaped stenting tubes are useful in patients with biliary anastomoses. When one compares percutaneous drainage with ERCP drainage, the problems of catheter site pain, subcapsular hematoma, and intracavitary bile leaks are essentially nonexistent, although there is a risk of pancreatitis with ERCP drainage. Patients with biliary stents have fewer complications if their drainage includes both right and left hepatic segments. Those patients with unilateral drainage have a poorer survival.

The response to chemotherapy, either by systemic infusion or by direct intraarterial infusion, has demonstrated a disappointing response rate. Thus far, chemotherapy has included 5-fluorouracil (5-FU), mitomycin-C, BCNU, and doxorubicin as agents.

Isolated external-beam radiotherapy provides tumor response, but clear improvement in survival awaits publication of ongoing studies. Survival and quality-of-life measurements when both external beam radiation therapy and brachytherapy are provided appear to be encouraging. The most promising therapy is the use of intracatheter brachyradiotherapy with iridium 192 with supplemental external-beam radiation therapy. Photodynamic therapy is undergoing trials in Bismuth and Corlette type III and IV CCC.

Liver transplantation for patients with symptomatic disease does not promote long-term survival. There may be a role for liver transplantation in the patient in whom a CCC has been detected as part of a surveillance evaluation.

CONCLUSION

CCC is a difficult tumor to diagnose and treat. The main concept involved in treating this disease is to maximize the quality of life and the duration of quality time. In order to accomplish that goal, one must provide each patient with the best possible and most sustainable biliary drainage. This will frequently involve surgical reconstruction of the biliary tree. Liver transplantation offers the potential for prolonged survival in patients in whom a bile duct cancer is found incidentally at the time of transplantation or if discovered via a surveillance protocol.

BIBLIOGRAPHY

Bergquist A, Glaumann H, Persson B, et al. Risk factors and clinical presentation of hepatobiliary carcinoma in patients with primary sclerosing cholangitis: a case-control study. Hepatology 1998; 27:311–316.

Davies W, Matthew C, Nagorney D. Extrahepatic biliary cystadenomas and cystadenocarcinoma. Ann Surg 1995; 222:619–625.

Farmer DG, Shaked A, Colonna JO, et al. Radical resection combined with liver transplantation for foregut tumors. Am Surg 1993; 59:805–812.

Ferrell L. Malignant liver tumors that mimic benign lesions: analysis of five distinct lesions. Semin Diagn Pathol 1995; 12:64–76.

Jay Y-Y, Yeh T-S, Chen M-F. Cholangiocarcinoma presenting as pyogenic liver abscess: is its outcome influenced by concomitant hepatolithiasis? Am J Gastroenterol 1998; 93:253–255.

Klempnauer J, Ridder GJ, Werner M, et al. What constitutes long term survival after surgery for hilar cholangiocarcinoma? Cancer 1997; 79:26–34.

Knechtle SJ, D'Alessandro AM, Harms BA, et al. Relationship between PSC, inflammatory bowel disease and cancer in patients undergoing liver transplantation. Surgery 1995; 118:615–620.

Ortner M-AEJ, Liebetruth J, Schreiber S, et al. Photodynamic therapy of nonresectable cholangiocarcinoma. Gastroenterology 1998; 114:536–542.

Sung JJY, Chung SCS. Endoscopic stenting for palliation of malignant biliary obstruction: a review of progress in the last 15 years. Dig Dis Sci 1995; 40:1167–1173.

Vauthey J-N, Blumgart LH. Recent advances in the management of cholangiocarcinoma. Semin Liver Dis 1994; 14:109–114.

Vijayan B, LaRusso NF. Hepatobiliary disease in inflammatory bowel disease. Gastroenterol Clin North Am 1995; 24:647–669.

24
Management of Acetaminophen Toxicity

Frank V. Schiødt
University of Copenhagen, Copenhagen, Denmark

William M. Lee
University of Texas Southwestern Medical Center, Dallas, Texas

INTRODUCTION

Acetaminophen (paracetamol) is a commonly used over-the-counter drug due to its analgetic and antipyretic characteristics. In contrast to nonsteroidal anti-inflammatory drugs (NSAIDs), it is not prominently associated with gastrointestinal side effects. Acetaminophen was developed more than a hundred years ago and was registered in the United States in 1955. Although it is a safe drug when taken within the recommended dosage (up to 4 g/day) by otherwise healthy individuals, it has a narrow therapeutic window. Acetaminophen is a dose-dependent hepatotoxin and ingestion of as little as 10 g (150 mg/kg body weight) may lead to severe hepatocellular necrosis.

Even when taken within the recommended range, acetaminophen may occasionally be fatal. Alcoholics and fasting or undernourished patients whose glutathione depots are low seem particularly susceptible. Acetaminophen overdose requires adequate therapy initiated shortly after ingestion. Otherwise, the patient may develop fulminant hepatic failure, a condition with a high morbidity and mortality (see Chap. 25).

The incidence of acetaminophen overdose varies between countries, with the highest incidence observed in the United Kingdom. From 1987–1993, the King's College Hospital in London treated 560 patients with severe acetaminophen toxicity, the commonest cause of acute liver failure in that unit. A few other western countries have relatively high incidences. However, in most European countries, the incidence is low, and in other parts of the world, acetaminophen overdose is rarely if ever seen. In the United States, the most recent annual report from U.S. poison control centers, representing 83% of the American population, reported more than 111,000 cases of exposure to acetaminophen (508 cases per million inhabitants per year). Acetaminophen was the only overdose agent in almost 73,000 exposures, 58% in children under 6 years of age; 55 fatal cases were recorded (0.08%). Acetaminophen was taken in combination with other drugs—such as codeine, aspirin, oxycodone, propoxyphene, and so on—in more than 38,000 cases, although only 18% were in children under 6 years of age; 48 fatalities were recorded in this group (0.13%).

Acetaminophen is available in numerous formulations and combinations. Ingestion of two or more different compounds containing acetaminophen may accidentally lead to overdose. Recent British and American studies among adolescents showed limited knowledge of the potential danger of acetaminophen ingestion. Typically, an overestimate of the lethal dose was reported. The warning labels on acetaminophen products remain a problem. With a drug that is perceived to be very safe, the challenge is to alert the public against an overly casual approach without emphasizing its suicide potential.

PHARMACOKINETICS OF ACETAMINOPHEN AND PATHOGENESIS OF HEPATOTOXICITY

The metabolic pathways of acetaminophen have been studied in detail. Following oral administration in the normal individual, acetaminophen is absorbed from the stomach and small intestine within 4 h. Peak plasma acetaminophen levels are observed 30 to 60 min after ingestion of 1 g. Acetaminophen is predominantly metabolized in the liver (96%), and

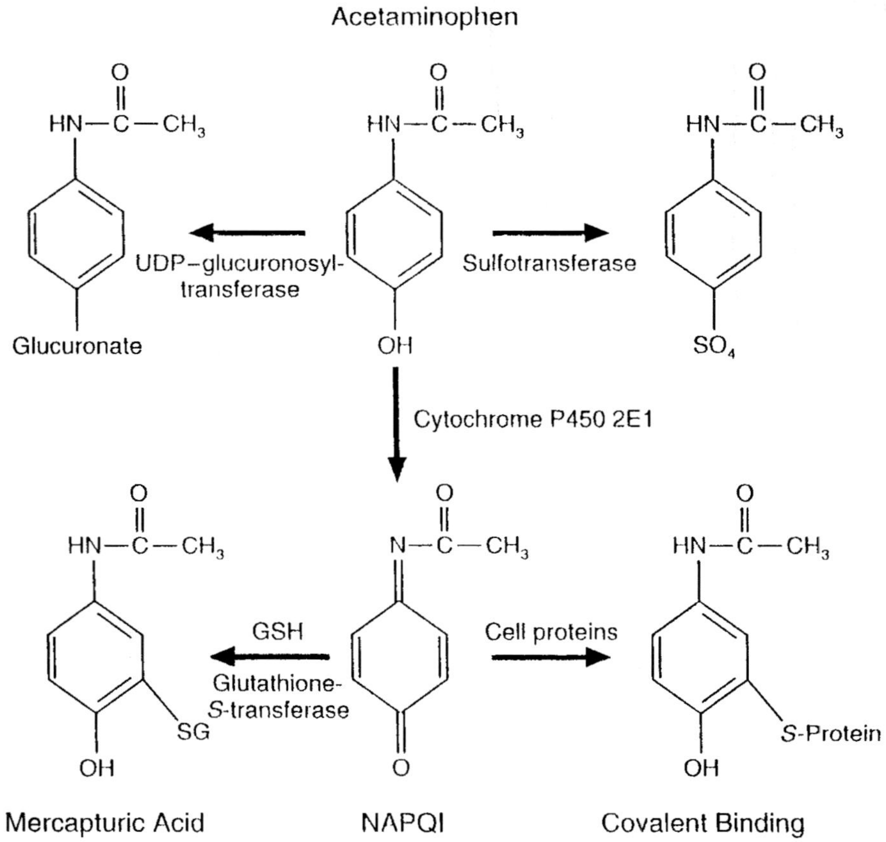

Figure 1 Acetaminophen metabolism.

only a minor portion (2–4%) is excreted in the urine. The major hepatic pathways include glucuronidation or sulfation yielding nontoxic conjugates excreted by the kidney (Fig. 1). Another pathway involves the cytochrome P450 system, especially P450 2E1, by which acetaminophen is metabolized to the highly reactive metabolite *N*-acetyl-*p* benzoquinone-imine (NAPQI). Under normal circumstances, this metabolite is rendered nontoxic by conjugation with reduced glutathione (GSH) from the liver to form mercapturic acid, which is excreted in the urine. NAPQI not conjugated with GSH may bind covalently with proteins and DNA in hepatocytes, causing cell necrosis by mechanisms not yet fully elucidated. Increased cytosolic Ca^{2+} seems to be a terminal phenomenon.

When acetaminophen is taken in therapeutic doses, the major pathways account for 90% of its clearance, whereas the formation of NAPQI accounts for less than 10%. However, with toxic doses, the major pathways become saturated, resulting in increased metabolism via the P450 system, representing up to 50% of the total metabolism.

INCREASED SUSCEPTIBILITY TO ACETAMINOPHEN TOXICITY

Some individuals have an increased risk of developing acetaminophen-induced hepatotoxicity, due either to chronic induction of the P450 system or to low levels of glutathione. This group of high-risk patients includes chronic alcoholics, malnourished or fasting individuals, and patients treated with pharmacological agents that may induce the P450 system.

Chronic Alcohol Use

There is now consistent evidence that chronic use of alcohol may enhance the toxic effects of acetaminophen. Acetaminophen seems to be potentially toxic even in therapeutic doses in some alcoholics. In a recent paper reporting 67 "therapeutic misadventures" in chronic alcoholics, most ingesting > 60 g of alcohol per day, 60% had ingested less than 6 g/day of acetaminophen and 40% had ingested less than 4 g/day. More than 95% of the patients developed transaminase levels > 1000 IU/L. Of the 67 patients, 12 died and 1 underwent liver transplantation. In a volunteer study, acetaminophen disappearance after ingestion of 1 g of the drug was significantly faster in chronic alcoholics than in normal individuals, suggesting enhanced hepatic metabolism in the alcoholics.

The mechanisms behind these observations are not yet fully elucidated. However, some hypotheses exist. Glutathione depletion—due to the often associated alcoholic malnutrition, to fasting, or to inhibited glutathione synthesis—may render the alcoholic individual more susceptible to NAPQI formation. Further, clear evidence of alcohol induction of P450 2E1 seems to be present in animals and in humans.

Acute alcohol intake, on the other hand, seems to have some protective effect with regard to acetaminophen toxicity. This is presumably due to competition of the alcohol and acetaminophen for the P450 system, leading to less formation of NAPQI.

Fasting

Patients who are fasting have an increased susceptibility to acetaminophen toxicity due to depressed levels of glutathione. In one series, the fasting was a result of gastrointestinal disorders of systemic illnesses causing gastrointestinal symptoms (nausea, vomiting). Chronic cardiopulmonary insufficiency has also been reported in one patient to lead to hepatotoxicity after repeated ingestion of small doses (1–3 acetaminophen tablets per day for 3 days). This patient had reduced hepatic and plasma glutathione.

Induction of P450 by Drugs

A number of drugs may induce the P450 system, including phenobarbital and isoniazid. Isoniazid, used in tuberculosis treatment or prophylaxis, often causes hepatic side effects and may significantly increase the toxicity profile of acetaminophen. Ingestion of as little as 3.25 g of acetaminophen has been observed to cause severe toxicity in this setting. Anticonvulsant therapy has also been reported to cause increased acetaminophen toxicity.

OVERDOSE FEATURES

In countries with a high incidence of acetaminophen overdose, the typical adult is intoxicated due to intentional overdose. As in other cases of self-poisoning, the reasons for the acetaminophen overdose are suicidal intent, neurotic disorders, or a "cry for help." Most of these people regret the episode and do not want to die. Accidental overdose in the adult may be due to several factors. People with persistent abdominal pain, toothache pain, back pain, or "flu" symptoms may reduce the interval between each dosage ingested to as little as 1–2 h, adding up to a total of 12–24 g over a 24-h period.

Children

As stated above, acetaminophen overdose in children under 6 years of age is commonly reported to poison control centers. These cases usually involve the accidental ingestion of relatively small amounts of acetaminophen, and fatal cases are rarely reported. Even in children considered to be at risk for toxicity according to the Rumack-Matthew nomogram (see "Treatment" below), severe hepatotoxicity is relatively uncommon. In one series of 417 children under 6 years of age, only 3 of 55 considered at risk (see Fig. 2) developed aminotransferase levels above 1000 IU/L. The mechanism explaining the apparently greater safety margin in children is not known.

Pregnancy

Pregnancy does not seem to affect the outcome or toxicity of acetaminophen overdose for the mother. However, there are reports suggesting that the fetus may be adversely affected. In the largest study to date, 24 pregnant patients with plasma acetaminophen above the treatment line (see Fig. 2) were studied. There was an increased rate of spontaneous abortions/stillbirths in women in whom antidote treatment was begun more than 16 h after overdose. No differences between first-, second-, or third-trimester pregnancies were observed.

CLINICAL FEATURES

The prominent feature of acetaminophen overdose is hepatotoxicity. Other organs may be affected directly by acetaminophen, especially the kidneys, but also the bone marrow and

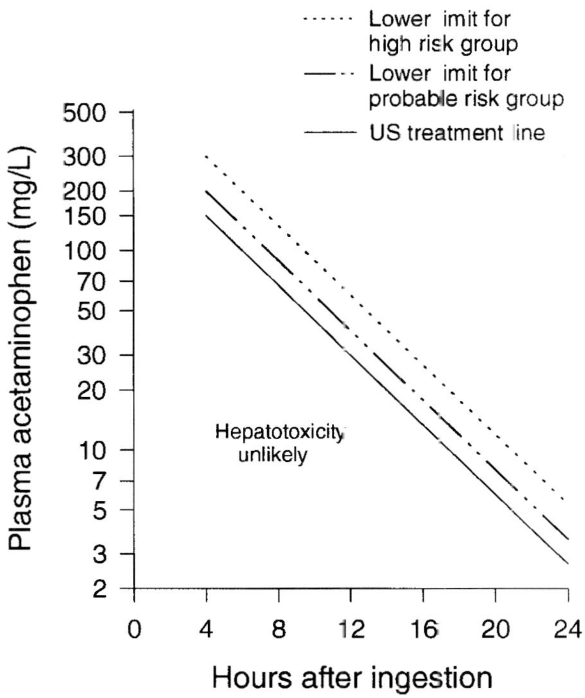

Figure 2 Matthew-Rumack nomogram for plasma acetaminophen and after a single dose acetaminophen. When the result is above the "treatment" line, antidote treatment should be maintained. Plots above the "probable-risk" and "high-risk" lines indicate a 60 and 90 % risk of hepatotoxicity, respectively.

the heart. It is important to note that once hepatic coma has developed (by definition, the onset of fulminant hepatic failure), virtually all organs may be affected. This multiple organ failure is not related to the cause of fulminant hepatic failure but represents a systemic response to the failing liver (see Chap. 25).

Acetaminophen causes a characteristic centrilobular (zone III) hepatocellular necrosis. In the kidney, tubular necrosis is the most prominent finding.

The time sequence in severe acetaminophen toxicity is characteristic (Table 1). During the first 12–24 h after ingestion, the patient may suffer abdominal pain, nausea, and vomiting but does not become drowsy (stage 1). This is followed by a period of relative well-being from 24–48 h after ingestion (stage 2). After 48 h, the symptoms of liver failure become obvious (stage 3). Hepatic coma usually occurs 3–4 days after ingestion but may be delayed up to 6 days. Survivors of stage 3 progress into stage 4, which is the resolution stage. Patients with less toxicity may only experience stage 1 and 2. Once recovery has occurred, full recovery of liver function takes place; no permanent liver damage has been demonstrated after acetaminophen overdose.

Laboratory values in patients with acetaminophen overdose are summarized in Table 2. Patients treated with antidote, usually *N*-acetylcysteine (NAC); within 8–12 h post-ingestion may develop no or only a few biochemical abnormalities. Patients treated later than 12 h will typically have biochemical signs of hepatocellular damage. Levels of

Table 1 Clinical Stages in Acetaminophen Toxicity

Stage 1	0–24 h	Abdominal pain, nausea, vomiting, diaphoresis, general malaise, no drowsiness
Stage 2	24–48 h	Few symptoms, no clinical evidence of liver failure
Stage 3	2–6 days	Evidence of hepatic failure: jaundice, malaise, hepatic encephalopathy, renal failure, multiple organ failure, cerebral edema, sepsis (death)
Stage 4	5–10 days	Symptoms gradually resolve; jaundice and renal failure may be prolonged in severe cases

Table 2 Biochemical Characteristics of Acetaminophen Toxicity

Laboratory values	Minor to moderate toxicity	Severe toxicity
AST/ALT	Normal to mildly elevated (up to 1000 IU/L)	Often very elevated, level > 3000 IU/L may be regarded as almost pathognomonic. Levels typically peak at day 2 to 3 after ingestion.
Bilirubin	Normal to moderately elevated (up to 100 μmol/L = 5.9 mg/dL)	Continue to increase, even after reversal of the condition. Renal failure may add to the hyperbilirubinemia.
Prothrombin time	Normal to moderately prolonged, up to 20 s	Very prolonged, up to >180 s (U.K. standards). Continuous increase at day 4 is a poor prognostic sign.
Plasma coagulation factors (II, V, VII, X)	Decreased moderately (~30–50% of normal)	Markedly reduced, especially factor V.
Creatinine	Usually normal—acute renal failure requiring hemodialysis may occur	Acute renal failure occurs frequently in patients with hepatic encephalopathy. It may be prolonged even after hepatic recovery.
Acid-base disturbances	Respiratory alkalosis, pH normally <7.60	Metabolic acidosis, sometimes uncompensated and severe. Admission arterial pH < 7.30 is a poor prognostic sign.
Platelet counts	Usually normal—occasionally, initial severe thrombocytopenia is observed	Thrombocytopenia ($<100 \times 10^9$ cells per liter) is found in more than 80% of patients with hepatic encephalopathy.
Phosphate	Decreased (<0.8 mM) in two-thirds of patients	Decreased in all patients with fulminant hepatic failure, sometimes to very low levels (<0.4 mM).
Blood glucose	Slightly decreased; 5% dextrose infusion restores normal levels	Severe hypoglycemia may be seen. Continuous 20% dextrose infusion necessary.

aspartate aminotransferase (AST) and alanine aminotransferase (ALT) may become very high up to 50,000 IU/L, peaking at day 2 or 3. In fact, aminotransferase levels can be used for diagnostic confirmation, since levels above 4000 IU/L are rarely seen in conditions other than acetaminophen overdose. The hepatic production of coagulation factors is reduced, resulting in prolongation of prothrombin time, in severe cases more than 180 s (U.K. standards). Plasma levels of coagulation factors II, V, VII, and X are diminished, especially factor V, due to its short half-life. Serum bilirubin is increased and usually peaks late in severe cases, sometimes in stage 4. Hypophosphatemia due to renal loss of phosphate is commonly seen, especially in severe cases. Acid-base disturbances are common. Respiratory alkalosis due to hyperventilation is common in mild cases; metabolic acidosis associated with hyperlactatemia is an ominous sign in patients with hepatic encephalopathy. Alkaline phosphatase, albumin, and total protein levels remain close to normal.

Renal Failure

Acetaminophen may cause acute renal failure, either directly or indirectly. Tubular necrosis, like the hepatic necrosis, is probably due to the effects of NAPQI. Glutathione repletion with NAC prevents tubular necrosis. Renal failure is most commonly seen in patients with progression to hepatic encephalopathy but may be present even in the absence of hepatic coma. Acute renal failure is observed in approximately 50% of fulminant hepatic failure patients with grade III or IV hepatic encephalopathy; it is caused by hepatorenal syndrome, acute tubular necrosis from acetaminophen, prerenal azotemia, or as part of a multiple-system organ failure syndrome.

TREATMENT

As for other cases of intoxication, patients with acetaminophen overdose should be treated according to the following principles: (1) interruption of the absorption of the toxin, (2) use of specific antidote, and (3) supportive care.

Reduction of Acetaminophen Absorption

Within the first 4 h after overdose, acetaminophen may still be present in the stomach. Many patients may have vomited before presentation to hospital, and vomiting or gastric washout within 6 h after overdose has been shown to reduce severe liver disease in untreated patients. Even in the case of vomiting prior to admission, one of the following methods to reduce absorption should be considered.

Gastric Lavage

Lavage produced a substantial reduction in acetaminophen concentration in 14 patients, but less than activated charcoal.

Activated Charcoal

Activated charcoal is thought to bind nonspecifically to substances in the lumen of the stomach and prevent their absorption. After ingestion of 3 g acetaminophen, 50 g of activated charcoal reduced the area under the curve (AUC) for acetaminophen in volunteers. Activated charcoal was superior to gastric lavage and ipecac. Concerns that activated charcoal may interfere with the efficacy of orally administered NAC do not seem justified.

Syrup of Ipecac

Ipecac induces vomiting, usually within 15 min of ingestion. In one study, it reduced AUC when given 5 min after 1 g of acetaminophen but not when given 30 min after. In that study, the effect of ipecac was inferior to that of activated charcoal. However, another study demonstrated similar effects of ipecac and activated charcoal after ingestion of 3 g acetaminophen; in patients, ipecac has reduced acetaminophen concentrations by 41%.

Colyte

Whole gut lavage using Colyte (polyethylene glycol electrolyte solution) has recently been investigated in volunteers after ingestion of 4 g of acetaminophen. Peak plasma acetaminophen was 65% that of controls.

In summary, gastric lavage may be used up to 4 h after an acute ingestion but has no value in chronic ingestion (multiple doses over time). Activated charcoal may be given after gastric lavage. Ipecac and Colyte are not widely used.

Antidotes to Acetaminophen Toxicity

NAC is now established as the main antidote in acetaminophen overdose. It is a safe drug that may be given either orally or intravenously. In the United States, intravenous NAC is not approved by the FDA. Previously, methionine was also used as antidote; however, due to the availability of NAC as Mucomyst, methionine is no longer in use. Three different NAC regimens have been used, one oral and two intravenous, as outlined in Table 3.

None of the studies of NAC were optimal in design, since they were nonrandomized and uncontrolled and the results were compared with historical controls. The inclusion criteria were an acetaminophen level above the treatment line in the Rumack-Matthew nomogram (Fig. 2) and admission to hospital before 24 h after ingestion. Although not directly comparable, the studies did demonstrate a clear protective effect of the regimens when taken within 10 h (Fig. 3, upper panel). Hepatotoxicity, defined as transaminases (ALT or AST) above 1000 IU/L, was seen in less than 10% of the cases with "probable risk," compared with nearly 60% in historical controls. An almost complete protection was seen when NAC was initiated within 8 h. When initiated between 10 and 24 h after ingestion, NAC still offered some protection, although the hepatotoxicity in the 20-h NAC regimen seemed close to that of historical controls (Fig. 3). In the subset of patients at "high

Table 3 N-Acetylcysteine Antidote Regimens

	Oral, 72 h	Intravenous, 20 h	Intravenous, 48 h
Loading dose	140 mg/kg	150 mg/kg in 300 mL 5% dextrose over 15 min	140 mg/kg in 5% dextrose over 1 h
Maintenance dose	70 mg/kg every 4 h for 17 doses, starting 4 h after loading dose; if the patient vomits within 1 h the dose is repeated	50 mg/kg in 500 mL 5% dextrose over 4 h; then 100 mg/kg in 1000 mL 5% dextrose over 16 h	70 mg/kg in 5% dextrose over 1 h, started every 4 h after loading dose started, adding up to a total of 12 doses given 4 h apart
Total dose	1330 mg/kg	300 mg/kg	980 mg/kg

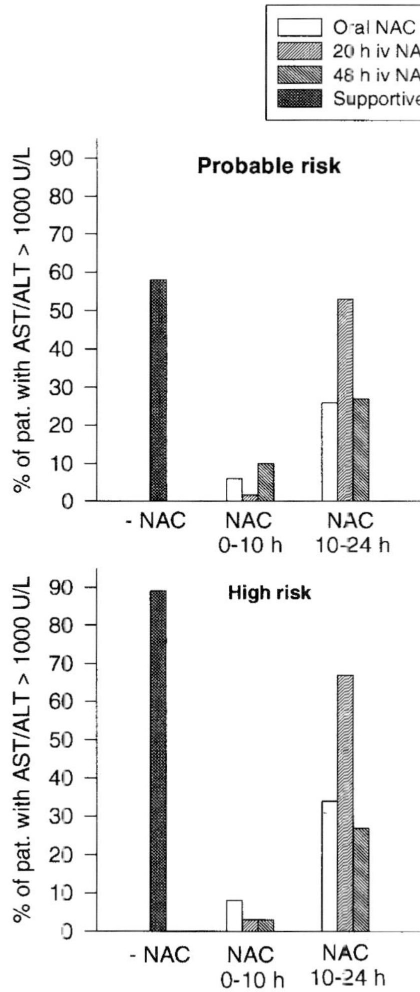

Figure 3 Risk of hepatotoxicity (transaminases > 1000 IU/L) for three different N-acetylcysteine (NAC) treatment regimens and for untreated historic controls ("supportive care"). *Upper panel:* patients with plots above the Matthew-Rumack "probable-risk" line. *Lower panel:* patients with plots above the Matthew-Rumack "high-risk" line.

risk" of hepatotoxicity, defined as acetaminophen levels above the "high-risk" line in the nomogram, NAC was very protective when initiated within 10 h after overdose and still had protective effect when started 10–24 h after overdose (Fig. 3, lower panel). Again, the protective effect seemed less pronounced in the 20-h NAC regimen.

In the two American studies, Smilkstein et al. further divided the 10- to 24-h period in two and found that the probability of hepatotoxicity in patients starting NAC from 16–24 h after overdose was 82% in the 48-h IV regimen and 41% in the oral regimen.

No study to date has compared the efficacy of the different NAC regimens in a controlled fashion.

Nomograms

The Rumack-Matthew nomogram was developed after assessment of a group of untreated patients for hepatotoxicity, defined arbitrarily as an AST or ALT above 1000 IU/L. The nomograms include the plasma acetaminophen concentration on a semilogarithmic Y axis and the time from ingestion of a single dose of acetaminophen on the X axis (Fig. 2). When plotted above the treatment line, NAC treatment should be initiated/continued. Optimally, all patients should promptly receive antidote on admission. When plotted above the line termed "probable-risk" and above "high-risk" denotes a risk of 60 and 90%, respectively, for developing aminotransferases > 1000 IU/L. There are several circumstances under which the nomogran cannot be used to assess the risk for hepatotoxicity sufficiently.

Single Dose Versus Repeated Overdose

Most of the clinical literature so far has concentrated on the effects of a single (over)dose of acetaminophen. However, the potential danger of repeated small doses of acetaminophen is now being recognized, and in these cases the Rumack-Matthew nomogram is of no value.

Extended-Release Acetaminophen

Within recent years, extended-release acetaminophen compounds have become available. No differences in peak plasma-acetaminophen or area-under-curve (AUC) were observed in a recent double-blind crossover study in volunteers given 75 mg/kg body weight of either extended-release or instant-release acetaminophen. However, in patients with acetaminophen overdose, extended-release compounds seem to have a more prolonged absorption period. Thus, the normal assumption that all acetaminophen ingested will be absorbed before 4 h may not be true in the case of ingestion of extended-release products. Misleading "safe" values used in plotting the initial nomogram may lead some physicians to avoid NAC treatment.

High-Risk Patients

As previously stated, chronic alcoholics, fasting individuals, and patients treated with drugs that induce the P450 system may have increased susceptibility to acetaminophen overdose; the nomogram cannot safely be used in these patients.

Therefore, treatment with NAC should be initiated and continued if there is any suspicion of repeated overdose, high-risk circumstances, or ingestion of extended-release acetaminophen regardless of values in the nomogram. We recommend use of biochemical markers, such as aminotransferase or prothrombin time levels, to assess the duration of NAC treatment in these patients. In recent years, the previous belief that NAC may be hepatotoxic and thus contraindicated when given after 24 h after overdose has been discarded. In fact, NAC is now considered safe even in established hepatic disease. Furthermore, both retrospective and prospective studies of late NAC infusion have demonstrated improved hemodynamics and survival in patients with already established hepatic encephalopathy.

N-Acetylcysteine Mechanisms

NAC is the *N*-acetylated derivative of the sulfhydryl amino acid L-cysteine, and its sulfhydryl group is believed to be essential for its early antidote effects. The most important role for NAC is probably in replenishing glutathione stores, which may inhibit the deleterious effects of the toxic acetaminophen breakdown product NAPQI. NAC may restore microcirculatory flow due to its vasodilatatory effects. Furthermore, NAC has a number of other potential beneficial effects. It is a well-known antioxidant, with both extracellular and intracellular actions. Extracellularly, NAC acts directly on oxygen radicals. NAC suppresses the production of TNF-α and influences the pulmonary response to endotoxin. NAC increases soluble guanylate cyclase activity and thereby cGMP, which may account for its vasodilatatory effects.

NAC Side Effects

Given orally, NAC will rarely cause side effects. Intravenous NAC may cause adverse effects in 14% of patients. Usually, the adverse effects are mild, consisting of skin erythemas or mild urticaria, so-called anaphylactoid reactions. These effects can be treated with temporary interruption of the NAC infusion, injection of an antihistamine, and sometimes glucocorticoids. After a few minutes, the NAC infusion can normally be resumed. However, severe adverse reactions have also been observed, including bronchospasm, hypotension, angioedema, tachycardia, respiratory arrest, disseminated intravascular coagulation, and even death. Oral methionine may be considered to replace NAC in case of severe adverse effects.

Other Antidotes

Oral methionine seems to offer protection in the same range as NAC; however, methionine is rarely used now, because no intravenous formulations are available. It may be used in severe cases of NAC adverse effects that do not respond to the treatment mentioned above. Cysteamine had no clinical effect on hepatotoxicity, caused severe side effects, and is no longer used. In animals, a number of antidotes have been studied, many with good protective effects. However, most of these drugs—for instance, iloprost and lobenzarit—protect animals from acetaminophen hepatotoxicity only when given before or shortly after ingestion of the drug.

In summary, *N*-acetylcysteine is the antidote of choice in acetaminophen overdose. Treatment should be initiated promptly on arrival to the medical emergency room and should not await plasma acetaminophen levels. Intravenous and oral NAC seem to offer equal protection, and the protection is almost complete if initiated less than 8–10 h after a single dose ingestion. The physician needs to have a high level of suspicion for the diagnosis of acetaminophen overdose, and suspicion alone should lead to antidote treatment. In some patients, the nomogram may be useless (doubt of exact time of ingestion, fasting individuals, chronic alcoholics, ingestion of extended release acetaminophen, etc.); in these cases, NAC should always be initiated. Even patients presenting more than 24 h after ingestion or in hepatic coma should be given NAC. The duration of antidote therapy should depend on the clinical status of the patient and may be extended until recovery.

Supportive Care

In stages 1 and 2, supportive care consists mainly of correction of electrolytes and blood glucose levels. Blood glucose should be closely monitored (four to six times per day), and intravenous access for 5% dextrose infusion (and NAC infusion) is justified in most patients. Analgesics are generally contraindicated.

Patients who have developed hepatic encephalopathy need to be treated in a specially designed intensive care unit, preferably a liver intensive care unit with access to liver transplantation facilities. The experiences at King's College Hospital in London have demonstrated a significant increase in survival rate in recent decades because of the advent of urgent liver transplantation but also due to improved medical therapy.

Transfer to a specialist liver unit should be considered when (1) INR is > 3.0, or > 2.0 at 24 h, > 4.0 at 48 h, or > 6.0 at 72 h; (2) serum creatinine is > 200 μmol/L (= 2.3 mg/dL); or (3) hepatic encephalopathy, hypotension (mean arterial pressure < 60 mmHg or systolic blood pressure < 90 mmHg), or metabolic acidosis (arterial pH < 7.30) is present.

The treatment of fulminant hepatic failure is discussed in Chapter 25. In brief, intensive monitoring with central venous, arterial, and intracranial catheters is crucial; aggressive and early treatment with respiratory support, prophylactic antibiotics, inotropic drugs, H_2 antagonists, mannitol, and continuous hemodialysis for renal failure improves the chances of survival. The timing of liver transplantation is important because irreversible cerebral complications may develop rapidly.

DIAGNOSIS

Often, the diagnosis is obvious, especially when the patient presents within a few hours after overdose, gives a good history, and plasma acetaminophen levels are found elevated. However, it is important for the physician to maintain a high level of suspicion in cases that are not so clear-cut. The patient may not report repeated small doses unless the physician specifically asks. Chronically alcoholic and fasting patients are more susceptible to acetaminophen toxicity than otherwise healthy individuals. In these patients, levels of plasma acetaminophen may be close to zero. Aminotransferase levels > 4000 IU/L are highly suggestive of acetaminophen toxicity, but these high levels occur relatively late in the course of the disease. As previously stated, NAC is a safe antidote and treatment may be initiated on suspicion alone.

In children, detection of serum 3-(cystein-S-yl)-acetaminophen-protein (3-Cys-A), an adduct of NAPQI and hepatocellular protein, has recently been reported to be a marker of repeated acetaminophen ingestion. However, this observation needs confirmation in larger series and in adults.

PROGNOSIS

Fatal outcome of acetaminophen overdose is relatively rare. In the 1995 annual report from U.S. Poison Control Centers only 103 deaths were recorded (0.093% of the total recorded exposures). In a series from Sydney, Australia, no deaths were observed in 306 patients. Death without hepatic encephalopathy is rarely, if ever, observed. Factors that may contribute to a fatal outcome include unrecognized hypoglycemia and late institution of NAC treatment (> 12 h). Hepatotoxicity (AST or ALT > 1000 IU/L) can be expected in untreated patients with plasma acetaminophen levels above the risk lines in the Rumack-Matthew nomogram. A plasma acetaminophen half-life > 4 h seems to be a good indicator of hepatotoxicity.

In patients with established fulminant hepatic failure, several prognostic indicators associated with a poor outcome have been assessed, among them arterial acidosis, high creatinine and bilirubin, grade III or IV hepatic encephalopathy (the King's College criteria), low plasma coagulation factors V and VIII, and decreased serum levels of the actin scavenger Gc-globulin.

BIBLIOGRAPHY

Gilberston RJ, Harris E, Pandey SK. Kelly P, Myers W. Paracetamol use, availability, and knowledge of toxicity among British and American adolescents. Arch Dis Child 1996; 75:194–198.

Hawton K, Ware C, Mistry H, Hewitt J, Kingsbury S, Roberts D, Weitzel H. Paracetamol self-poisoning: characteristics, prevention and harm reduction. Br J Psychiatry 1996; 168:43–48.

Lee WM. Drug-induced hepatotoxicity. N Engl J Med 1995; 333:1118–1127.

Lee WM. Medical management of acute liver failure. In: Lee WM, Williams R, eds. Acute Liver Failure. Cambridge, UK: Cambridge University Press, 1997:115–131.

Lee WM, Galbraith RM, Watt GH, Hughes RD, McIntire DD, Hoffman BJ, Williams R. Predicting survival in fulminant hepatic failure using serum Gc protein concentrations. Hepatology 1995; 21:101–105.

Litovitz TL, Felberg L, White S, Klein-Schwartz W. 1995 annual report of the American Association of Poison Control Centers Toxic Exposure Surveillance System. Am J Emerg Med 1996; 14:487–537.

O'Grady JG, Wendon J, Tan KC, Potter D, Cottam S, Cohen AT, Gimson AES, Williams R. Liver transplantation after paracetamol overdose. Br Med J 1991; 303:221–223.

Prescott LF, Illingworth RN, Critchley JAJH, Stewart MJ, Adam RD, Proudfoot AT. Intravenous N-acetylcysteine: the treatment of choice for paracetamol poisoning. Br Med J 1979; 2:1097–1100.

Rumack BH, Matthew H. Acetaminophen poisoning and toxicity. Pediatrics 1975; 55:871–876.

Rumack BH, Peterson RG. Acetaminophen overdose: incidence, diagnosis and management in 416 patients. Pediatrics 1978; 62:898–903

Schiødt FV, Atillasoy E, Shakil O, Lee WM, et al. Etiology and outcome for 295 patients with acute liver failure in the United States. Liver Transplant Surg 1999; 5:29–34.

Schiødt FV, Bondesen S, Petersen I, Dalhoff K, Ott P, Tygstrup N. Admission levels of serum Gc-globulin: predictive value in fulminant hepatic failure. Hepatology 1996; 23:713–718.

Schiødt FV, Rochling FJ, Casey DL, Lee WM. Acetaminophen toxicity in an urban county hospital. N Engl J Med 1997; 337:1112–1117.

Smilkstein MJ, Bronstein AC, Linden C, Augenstein WL, Kulig KW, Rumack BH. Acetaminophen overdose: a 48-hour intravenous N-acetylcysteine treatment protocol. Ann Emerg Med 1991; 20:1058–1063.

Smilkstein MJ, Knapp GL, Kulig KW, Rumack BH. Efficacy of oral N-acetylcysteine in the treatment of acetaminophen overdose. Analysis of the national multicenter study (1976 to 1985). N Engl J Med 1988; 319:1557–1562.

Webster PA, Roberts DW, Benson RW, Kearns GL. Acetaminophen toxicity in children: diagnostic confirmation using a specific antigenic biomarker. J Clin Pharmacol 1996; 36:397–402.

Whitcomb DC, Block GD. Association of acetaminophen hepatotoxicity with fasting and ethanol use. JAMA 1994; 272:1845–1850.

Zimmerman HJ, Maddrey WC. Acetaminophen (paracetamol) hepatotoxicity with regular intake of alcohol: analysis of instances of therapeutic misadventure. Hepatology 1995; 22:767–773.

25
Management of Fulminant Hepatic Failure

Norman L. Sussman
Amphioxus Cell Technologies, Inc., Houston, Texas

John R. Lake
University of Minnesota Medical School, Minneapolis, Minnesota

INTRODUCTION

Fulminant hepatic failure (FHF) is one of the most dramatic emergencies in clinical medicine. Without liver transplantation, FHF carries an overall mortality rate of up to 98%, and the patient faces a series of medical challenges, any of which can be lethal. The physician is also in a minefield; every step may lead to disaster. The physician must anticipate problems and respond quickly and appropriately to changes in the patient's status. Every case of FHF is a battle between destruction and regeneration of the liver. The sad truth is that even meticulous medical management by the most experienced physician will not save many patients with severe FHF; liver transplantation will be required in most cases.

The reader may well ask whether aggressive medical care is a pointless exercise. The answer is no; there are strong arguments in favor of aggressive care. First, improved patient care has reduced the overall mortality of FHF over the past decade to about 50% overall. While much of the improved outcome is the result of orthotopic liver transplantation (OLTx), some is due to improved techniques in critical care. OLTx is certainly lifesaving, but the patient must be maintained in relatively good health until an organ is procured. Great skill is often required to keep the patient from slipping beyond help while awaiting a donor. The second, more dramatic reason for good medical care is related to liver biology; the acutely injured liver is capable of full regeneration. The small minority of patients who experience liver regeneration go on to a completely normal life with no sequelae of their disease. There are few medical conditions in which the stakes are so high.

This chapter is meant as a practical guide to the care of patients with FHF; it is organized as follows:

Diagnosis
Establishing the prognosis and assessing the need for liver transplantation

Temporizing measures (dealing with complications)
Liver transplantation
Experimental therapies
Conclusions

DIAGNOSIS

The diagnosis of FHF is based on the development of hepatic encephalopathy after a relatively short illness. Definitions usually give a time frame of 8 weeks after the onset of the first symptom or 2 weeks after the onset of jaundice. Implicit in these time frames is the absence of preexisting liver disease.

Preexisting liver disease changes the entire face of the illness. It renders the patient more sensitive to certain hepatotoxins and reduces further any hope of liver regeneration. Evidence of chronic liver disease must be sought through history and physical findings.

The Importance of Time

The shorter the duration of an episode of FHF, the better the chance of spontaneous recovery. A recent classification of acute liver failure showed a dramatic difference in survival in patients who had been ill for less than seven days (Table 1). This apparent paradox is related to liver biology; the longer the course of the illness, the more it resembles chronic liver disease. Hence, complications of FHF, such as cerebral edema, develop less commonly, and the likelihood of liver regeneration decreases. If the illness persists beyond a few weeks, features of chronic liver disease such as portal hypertension (e.g., variceal bleeding and splenomegaly) can be seen. These patients virtually never recover without transplantation.

Hepatic Encephalopathy

Hepatic encephalopathy in the context of acute liver failure is quite different from the portal-systemic encephalopathy (PSE) that occurs in the course of chronic liver disease. PSE is generally brought on by infections, gastrointestinal bleeding, or fluid and electrolyte

Table 1 Classification of FHF Based on Duration of Illness

	Duration: jaundice to encephalopathy	Survival rate (%)	Cerebral edema (%)
Hyperacute liver failure	7 days	36	69
Acute liver failure	8–28 days	7	56
Subacute liver failure	29–60 days	14	14

A longer period between the onset of jaundice and the onset of encephalopathy brings FHF into the realm of accelerated chronic liver failure. Consequently, spontaneous recovery is rare and the incidence of cerebral edema declines.

Patients with acetaminophen toxicity are not included in Table 1. Acetaminophen-induced liver failure is always hyperacute, and the survival rate of 34% is similar to that seen in other causes of hyperacute liver failure.

Table 2 Clinical Stages of Hepatic Encephalopathy

Grade	Mental state	Tremor	EEG changes
Grade I, prodrome (often diagnosed in retrospect)	Euphoria, occasional depression, mild confusion, slowness of mentation, untidiness, slurred speech, disordered sleep rhythm	Slight	Usually lacking
Grade II, impending coma	Accentuation of stage I; drowsy, but speaking; inappropriate behavior; incontinence	Present (easily elicited)	Abnormal; generalized slowing
Grade III, stupor	Sleeps most of the time but rousable; incoherent or no speech; marked confusion	Usually present (if cooperative)	Always abnormal
Grade IV, coma	Patient may (stage IV A) or may not (stage IV B) respond to painful stimuli	Usually lacking	Always abnormal

Source: Adapted from Trey and Davidson, 1970.

disturbances in a patient with chronic liver disease. It is usually reversed by correcting the precipitating problem.

The encephalopathy that defines FHF has a much more ominous connotation. Four clinical stages have been defined, ranging from subtle personality changes to deep coma (Table 2).

The earliest manifestations of hepatic encephalopathy (grade I) are minor and include subtle personality changes, lethargy, depression, euphoria, slurred speech, and sleep disturbances. As the disease progresses to grade II, the patient becomes more drowsy and may experience periods of restlessness, disorientation, and inappropriate behavior, although simple questions can still be answered appropriately. Grade III is characterized by somnolence, with the patient still rousable by gentle stimulation. The response to questions is inappropriate, and the patient may perseverate or simply stare blankly at the person asking the question. Grade IV encephalopathy is coma with the patient, at best, able to respond to pain.

Progression of encephalopathy from one stage to the next reflects progressive liver dysfunction and can be correlated directly with increasing mortality. This is a multifactorial relationship involving the extent of liver injury, failure of regeneration, and the increasing risk of cerebral edema in grade III and IV encephalopathy.

Other Clinical Findings

The mental changes described in Table 2 are usually accompanied by changes in muscle tone. Hence, additional information can be gained by tracking tendon reflexes, response to stimuli, and pupillary activity. These overlapping clinical signs, as described by Hawker, are shown in Figure 1.

Increasing muscle tone is a typical feature of advancing encephalopathy. Brisk tendon reflexes are usually present by the onset of grade II encephalopathy; with more advanced encephalopathy, the muscle tone may progress to clonus, decerebrate or decorticate posturing, opisthotonus, and, finally, flaccidity, often associated with brain death. Focal neurological findings are exceedingly rare and should suggest an alternative or

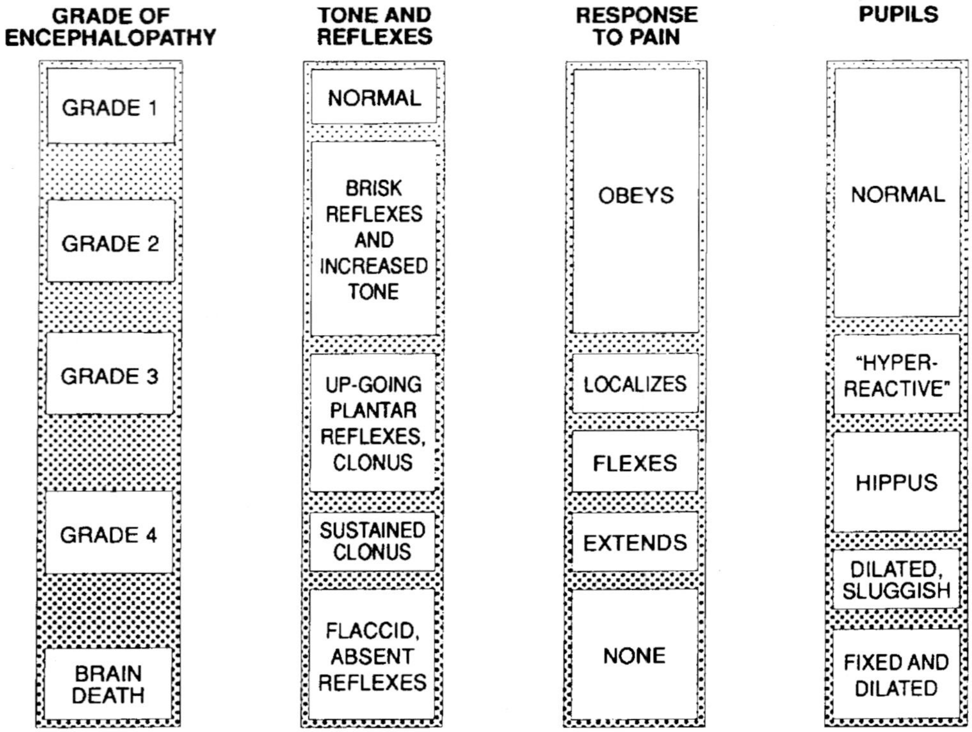

Figure 1 Progression of clinical signs in association with grade of encephalopathy. (From Hawker, 1993.)

complicating problem such as an intracranial bleed or a stroke. Hyperventilation, accompanied by respiratory alkalosis, is almost universal.

Patients with advanced (grade III or IV) encephalopathy require sedation and mechanical ventilation (see "Management," below). Once these are accomplished, brainstem functions become the only clinical parameters left to follow. Absence of pupillary light or corneal reflexes and an elevated blood pressure (Cushing's reflex) are the most useful in this situation. Any of these signs suggests an elevated intracranial pressure and requires an immediate medical response. The signs usually respond to measures that lower the intracranial pressure, but they tend to recur and become refractory to medical measures unless definitive treatment (usually OLTx) or liver regeneration occurs. It is important to recognize that the combination of metabolic brain disease and sedatives preclude the use of an electroencephalogram (EEG) to confirm brain death. A brain blood-flow study such as a technetium scan (see Fig. 2) can diagnose brain death and can be performed without moving the patient.

Cerebral Edema

Cerebral edema leading to intracranial hypertension and ultimately brainstem herniation is one of the leading causes of death in FHF. Some workers have reported that the use of *N*-acetylcysteine (NAC) has drastically reduced the incidence of lethal cerebral edema,

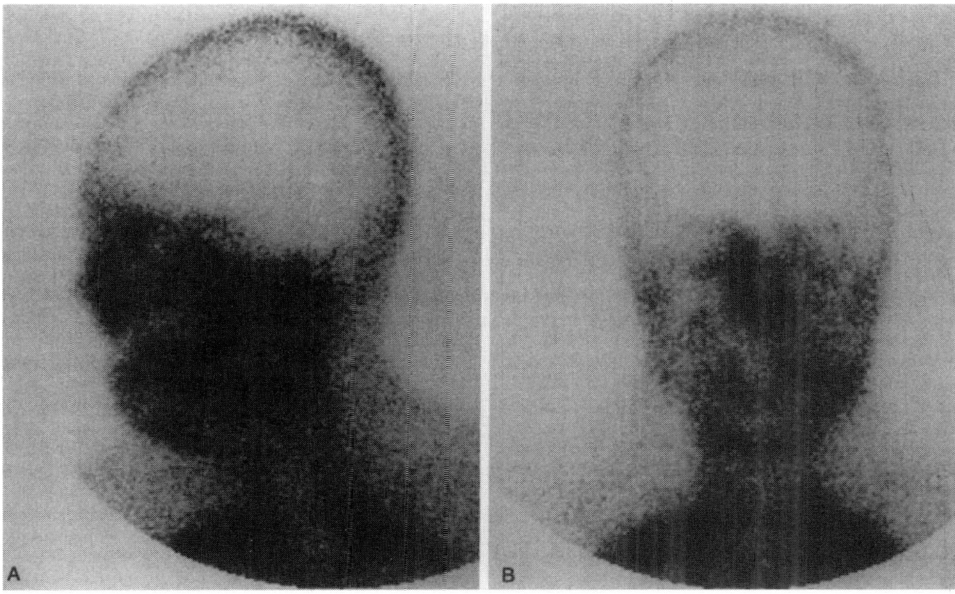

Figure 2 Brain blood-flow study showing absence of brain perfusion, consistent with ischemic brain death. (From Hawker, 1993.)

although this has not been studied prospectively. Historically, cerebral edema has been reported in 75–80% of cases that progress to grade IV encephalopathy.

Brain water starts to increase early in the course of FHF, but it does not become a problem until the volume of the swollen brain begins to exceed the capacity of the cranial vault. Further swelling then leads to one of two complications, brainstem herniation and/or cerebral ischemia. Both conditions are lethal.

The critical measurement in assessing patient status is the cerebral perfusion pressure (CPP), the difference between mean arterial pressure (MAP) and intracranial pressure (ICP). Details of measuring the ICP and managing intracranial hypertension are presented below.

ESTABLISHING THE PROGNOSIS AND ASSESSING THE NEED FOR LIVER TRANSPLANTATION

Once the diagnosis of FHF has been made, the patient's prognosis must be determined. Since most patients will require OLTx in order to survive, the process must be started immediately. The patient must be transferred to a transplant center while able to travel, and the procurement process must be started as early as possible to maximize the chance of locating a suitable donor. This is a relatively small window of opportunity, and many patients rapidly deteriorate beyond salvage. This race against the clock has created the need for early predictors of irreversible FHF.

Advanced encephalopathy (grade III or IV) accurately predicts a poor outcome from FHF but is not helpful in its management. Patients who reach advanced stages of FHF are too unstable to transport, and they rarely survive long enough to undergo OLTx; the period between the onset of grade III encephalopathy and brain death is frequently only a matter of hours. In addition, patients with advanced encephalopathy are at risk for irreversible brain damage during transplant surgery. Thus, huge costs and a valuable organ can be wasted on a patient who ultimately dies or faces long-term institutionalization for organic brain disease.

Predicting outcome early in the course of FHF is difficult because we would like to know, with absolute certainty, who is going to require transplantation and who is going to recover spontaneously. Although this is impossible, we are able to associate certain findings with at least a 90% certainty that the patient will die without a transplant. The tacit understanding is that a small minority of these patients will recover spontaneously, and, by the same token, some of the patients without these predictors will deteriorate and die. In the end this becomes a risk analysis like any other in clinical medicine. We make our initial assessment and continue to reassess the patient until the disease process declares itself unequivocally in one direction or the other. The important thing is to respond as soon as we see objective signs that the patient will require OLTx.

Of the various early predictors that have been proposed, we favor the criteria suggested by the group at King's College Hospital in London. This scheme, commonly known as the King's College criteria, is shown in Table 3.

Our choice of the King's College criteria is based on two factors. First, the scheme

Table 3 King's College Criteria: Predictors of Need for Liver Transplantation in Fulminant Hepatic Failure

Acetaminophen
- pH < 7.3 (irrespective of grade of encephalopathy)
- or *all three* of the following:
  - Grade III–IV encephalopathy
  - PT > 100 s, British reagents (INR > 7.7)[a,b]
  - Serum creatinine > 300 μmol/L (3.4 mg/dL)

Nonacetaminophen
- PT > 100 s, British reagents (INR > 7.7) (irrespective of grade of encephalopathy)
- or *any three* of the following:
  - Age < 10 or > 40 years
  - Any etiology other than hepatitis A or B (i.e., non-A, non-B hepatitis, halothane, idiosyncratic drug reaction, Wilson's disease)
  - Period of jaundice to encephalopathy > 7 days
  - PT > 50 s, British reagents (INR > 3.85)
  - Serum bilirubin > 300 μmol/L (17 mg/dL)

[a]Prothrombin time (PT) is expressed in British units. An additional indicator in patients with acetaminophen overdose is a PT that continues to rise 3 days after the overdose. Patients with this finding have a mortality in excess of 90%.

[b]Prothrombin times reported from Great Britain are longer than those reported from the United States because of a difference in the brain-derived thromboplastin, which is used to initiate the reaction. The International Normalized Ratio (INR) attempts to resolve this discrepancy. Approximate comparisons are shown in the table below.

PT (USA) Rabbit brain-derived thromboplastin	PT (Great Britain) Human brain-derived thromboplastin	INR
25 s	50 s	3.85
35 s	100 s	7.7

Source: From Lee et al., 1995.

measures up exceedingly well against other predictors of prognosis, including serum factor V activity, liver biopsy, measurements of liver volume, and various other specialized tests and schemes. Second and more importantly, the assessment can be performed in most cases within 30 min of the patient's arrival in the emergency room or office. *In fact, the decision to transfer a patient to a transplant center can usually be made in the emergency room before the patient is even admitted to a regional hospital.*

TEMPORIZING MEASURES (DEALING WITH COMPLICATIONS)

Any patient meeting the King's College criteria should be transferred to a transplant center as soon as possible. If encephalopathy is advanced, the benefit of a transfer should be balanced against the danger of precipitating a crisis during transport and the likelihood that the center will locate a donor in time. If the safety of the patient is in doubt, the physician should consult with a transplant center and err on the side of early transfer. If transfer is undertaken, qualified medical personnel should accompany the patient in order to respond to complications *en route*. In this section, we examine general principles, therapeutic measures specific for certain etiologies of FHF, and therapeutic measures that deal with dysfunction of specific organ systems.

General Principles

Upon arrival at the transplant center, the patient should be evaluated by a hepatologist, transplant surgeon, anesthesiologist/intensivist, and transplant coordinator in order to assess suitability for transplantation. This process must be set in motion immediately, while the illness and prognosis are confirmed.

General screening for metabolic disturbances and potential etiologic agents must be done immediately. Our suggested panel of tests is listed in Table 4. From a therapeutic standpoint, several factors deserve special mention. The remainder are either explained in Table 4 or are discussed in the organ-specific section below.

Intubation

Patients who progress beyond stage III encephalopathy must be intubated in order to protect the airway. There has been some opposition to this view, since it precludes the assessment of mental status. On the other hand, the patient is susceptible to two life-threatening problems: aspiration and acute intracerebral hypertension. Intubation prevents the former and helps to control the latter because the patient can be sedated and thus avoid stimuli that may precipitate spikes in the intracerebral pressure.

Electrolyte Abnormalities

FHF is associated with a reduction in free water clearance, so hyponatremia may occur in spite of increased total body sodium. Hypernatremia may also occur, usually as the result of dehydration following mannitol infusion or as a consequence of fresh frozen plasma administration. It is generally wise to avoid saline infusions, since they provide only the most temporary relief of hypotension and may later cause problems in controlling intracerebral pressure.

Hypokalemia is a serious threat in FHF; serum levels and total body potassium are

Table 4 Initial Assessment of Patients with FHF

Parameter	Rationale
Blood glucose	Hypoglycemia is common, continuous glucose infusion is required
Serum electrolytes	Electrolyte imbalance is common—may cause arrhythmia
Serum creatinine	Renal failure is typical
Serum phosphorus	Hypophosphatemia is common in acetaminophen overdose
Leukocyte count	Leukocytosis suggests sepsis—must be treated aggressively
Prothrombin time	Important prognostic factor
Platelet count	Thrombocytopenia is common—predisposes to bleeding
Arterial blood gases	Acidosis is an important prognostic indicator
Blood and urine cultures	Surveillance for sepsis
Chest radiograph	Surveillance for sepsis/adult respiratory distress syndrome
Blood group	Preparation for transplantation
Abdominal ultrasound	Preparation for transplantation
Pulmonary wedge pressure	Filling pressures must be optimized in the event of hypotension, important in cases where cardiopulmonary status is compromised
Intracranial pressure	Intracranial hypertension is a potentially lethal complication, important in cases of advanced (stage III or IV) encephalopathy
Viral hepatitis panel	Diagnosis has prognostic significance
Acetaminophen level	Specific therapy available and prognostic significance
Drug screen	Diagnosis has prognostic significance
Ceruloplasmic and slit-lamp exam	Diagnosis of Wilson disease indicates need for urgent OLTx

Source: From Sussman and Lake, 1996.

usually low. Potassium excretion occurs as a result of renal sodium reabsorption, and it may cause or exacerbate metabolic alkalosis. In addition, the use of mannitol or other diuretics may cause further potassium losses. We measure serum potassium at least twice daily and give potassium intravenously at the first hint that levels are falling. One note of caution: serum potassium may rise abruptly with the onset of renal failure.

Hypoglycemia

Patients with acute liver failure have both an impaired ability to supply glucose (depleted glycogen and limited gluconeogenesis) and impaired clearance of insulin. These two factors make patients susceptible to hypoglycemia. Glucose levels must be monitored closely, and a 5 or 10% glucose drip is essential. We do not administer bolus injections with 50% glucose because the burst of hyperglycemia stimulates further insulin secretion. It is best to avoid this see-saw effect by attending to blood glucose levels early with a continuous infusion of glucose.

Hypophosphatemia

Hypophosphatemia is a recognized complication of acetaminophen poisoning, even in the absence of liver failure. It may also complicate FHF of other causes, e.g., *Amanita phalloides* poisoning, and appears to result from increased renal phosphate losses. Low levels ($<$ 0.3 mmol/L) may, among other things, reduce tissue oxygenation and worsen encephalopathy. Musculoskeletal abnormalities, a hallmark of hypophosphatemia, are masked in comatose patients. Serum levels must therefore be measured at least daily. The recommended dose for phosphorus replacement ranges from 0.0125 mmol/kg/h × 6 h in mild cases to 0.125 mmol/kg/h × 4 h for severe cases (serum phosphorus < 0.5 mg/dL or 0.16 mmol/L). Solutions of sodium and potassium phosphate contain 3 mmol/mL.

The Need for an Intensive Care Unit

Patients with FHF should be admitted to an intensive care unit (ICU), preferably one that is experienced in the management of liver disease. A strong case for specialized care is made by the Liver Failure Unit at King's College Hospital which as reported steadily improving survival rates since its inception in 1973. As shown in Fig. 3, survival for hepatitis A and acetaminophen now exceeds 60%. Transplantation, which is performed on a minority of the patients, appears to have had a minor effect on overall outcome.

Infection Control

General management must include infection control. Reverse isolation has been suggested, although careful attention to hand-washing, line changes, venipuncture sites, and wounds should suffice. Septic complications are usually the result of endogenous organisms. Health care professionals should handle body fluids with appropriate care. Clusters of viral hepatitis have been reported and suggest the need for caution. Vaccination of all personnel against hepatitis A and B is recommended.

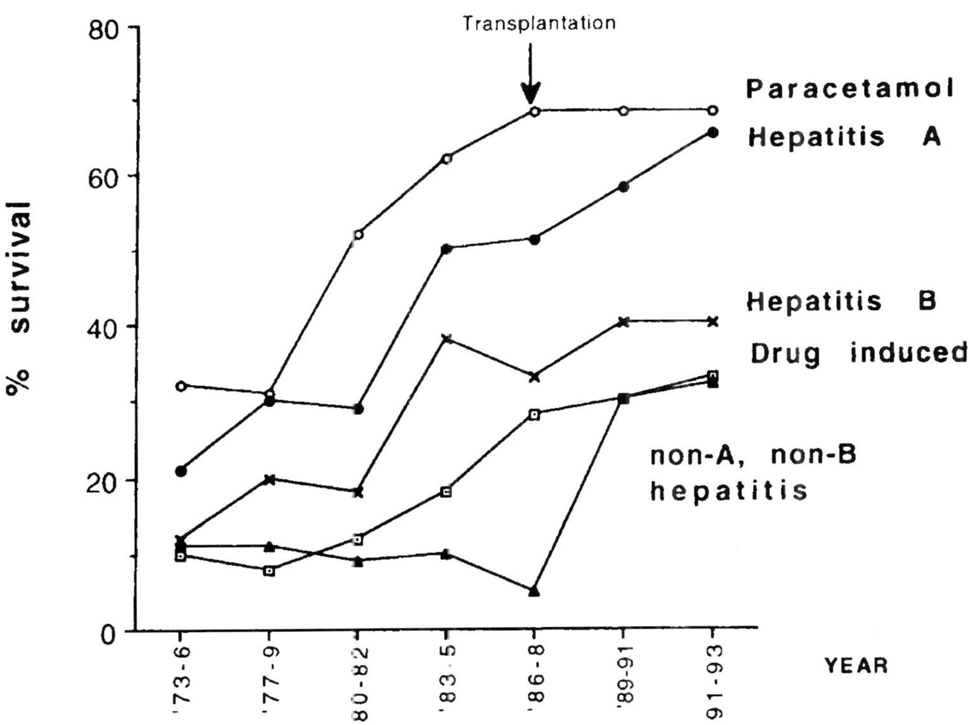

Figure 3 Patient survival (grade III and IV encephalopathy) at King's College Hospital. (From Williams and Wendon, 1994.)

Table 5 Etiology of Fulminant Hepatic Failure

Infections	Drugs/toxins/chemicals	Cardiovascular	Other
Viral hepatitis	Acetaminophen	Portal vein thrombosis	Autoimmune liver disease
Type A	Halothane	Budd-Chiari syndrome	Acute fatty liver of pregnancy
Type B	Isoniazid	Right ventricular failure	Preeclampsia-associated
Type D	Sodium valproate	Cardiac tamponade	Wilson's disease
Type E	Tetracycline	Circulatory shock	Reye's syndrome
Other viruses	NSAIDs	Metastatic tumor	Galactosemia
Yellow fever	Pirprofen	Heat stroke	Hereditary fructose intolerance
Q fever	Ketoconazole		Hereditary tyrosinemia
	Amanita phalloides		
	Yellow phosphorus		

Specific Causes of FHF

There are many courses of FHF (Table 5). Some cases of FHF call for specific measures. Among such cases are acetaminophen overdose, pregnancy-associated liver failure, *Amanita* poisoning, shock liver, and Wilson's disease.

Acetaminophen Overdose

Acetaminophen, normally a very safe drug, has severe consequences if taken in overdose (see Chap. 24). While most of the drug is rendered harmless by conjugation, 5% is converted to *N*-acetyl-*p*-benzoquinonimine (NAPQI) by mixed-function oxidase enzymes, primarily P-450 2E1. NAPQI is a highly reactive molecule whose toxicity is kept in check by liver stores of glutathione. If glutathione stores are depleted by an overdose of acetaminophen or if they are diminished by other factors such as starvation or fasting, NAPQI begins to bind irreversibly to intracellular proteins. This irreversible binding produces cell damage and necrosis (see Fig. 4).

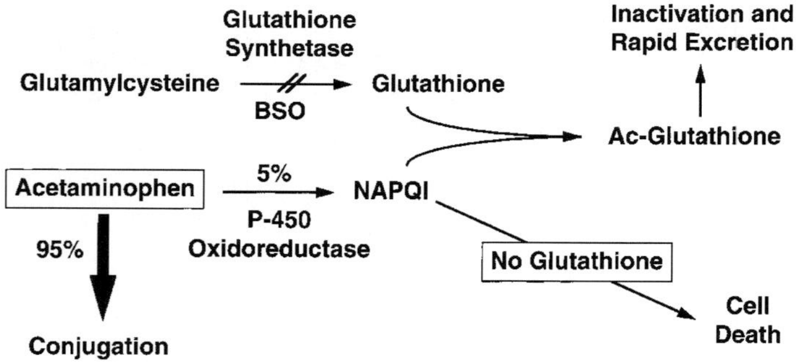

Figure 4 Mechanism of acetaminophen toxicity in the liver. Under normal circumstances, only 5% of acetaminophen is converted into NAPQI, and this is rapidly inactivated by glutathione. Factors that increase P-450 activity may increase toxicity, and factors that inhibit P-450 are known to decrease toxicity. Glutathione stores can be diminished by starvation for as little as 12 h, and by buthionine sulfoximine (BSO), an inhibitor of glutathione synthetase. Low glutathione stores increase the toxicity of acetaminophen.

Acetaminophen ingestion may lead to FHF in the three circumstances of (1) overdose (usually > 15 g for an adult), (2) excessive P450 activity, and (3) glutathione depletion. These three factors are not always easy to distinguish from one another. It may be difficult to establish the amount of acetaminophen actually ingested, and alcohol (acute or chronic consumption), barbiturates, and fasting all increase the toxicity of acetaminophen. At particular risk are alcoholics and babies who have been vomiting in association with a febrile illness.

Many patients have no symptoms or signs immediately following acetaminophen overdose, although a significant number experience nausea and vomiting, followed by abdominal pain and hepatic tenderness. There is usually a symptom-free window that may lull the patient and the physician into a false sense of security. Transaminases begin to increase within 12–24 h and peak at levels of about 10,000 IU/L on about day 3. Jaundice usually becomes clinically apparent after 24 h and progresses in concert with the liver disease. The PT is disproportionately high in cases of acetaminophen toxicity as compared with other causes of FHF. This explains why the PT is not, in itself, an important prognostic indicator in acetaminophen poisoning. The PT is always high in severe cases and usually peaks on day 3; a PT that continues to increase after day 3 is an ominous sign, associated with a 93% mortality.

Oliguric renal failure (urine output < 300 mL/24 h; serum creatinine > 300 μmol/L) occurs in 1–2% of all cases of acetaminophen overdose and in 11% of severe cases, usually within 24–72 h. Acetaminophen is, in fact, a direct nephrotoxin, and renal failure has been reported in the absence of significant liver necrosis. Alcohol may enhance nephrotoxicity.

Several metabolic complications may accompany acetaminophen overdose. Hypophosphatemia as a result of renal phosphate loss is common, and it may occur in the absence of liver damage. Hypoglycemia, a threat in all cases of severe liver failure, is caused by an inability to mobilize glycogen stores, lack of gluconeogenesis, and inappropriately high insulin levels. Transient acidosis may be an early finding and may dominate the clinical picture. This acidosis usually responds to fluid loading and must be distinguished from the lactic acidosis occurring > 24 h after ingestion, which is the result of tissue hypoxia and poor lactate clearance by the failing liver. Like a late-rising prothrombin time, late acidosis is associated with a poor prognosis (Table 3).

The management of acetaminophen overdose in the first few hours is like most drug overdose situations; gastric lavage should be performed to prevent further drug absorption. Also, the early metabolic complications described above must be corrected. Once a few hours have passed, the likelihood of recovering tablets from the stomach diminishes, and the second phase of management, maintenance of glutathione levels, becomes important.

The likelihood of acetaminophen liver disease, and hence of the need for specific therapy, is a function of serum levels and time after overdose. A nomogram relating these two factors is shown in Fig. 5. The utility of this nomogram is, however, questionable. An error in timing makes a big difference in the meaning of any serum level, and the curve does not compensate for factors like alcohol ingestion and fasting. A practical approach is described below.

Liver damage by acetaminophen can be prevented or minimized by glutathione precursors such as *N*-acetyl-cysteine (NAC) or methionine. NAC has the ability to protect against liver damage for at least 24 h after an overdose, although necrosis can be completely averted in the first 8 h. This being the case, NAC should be administered as soon as the diagnosis of acetaminophen overdose is made. It is better to start treatment that is later discontinued than to miss the therapeutic window.

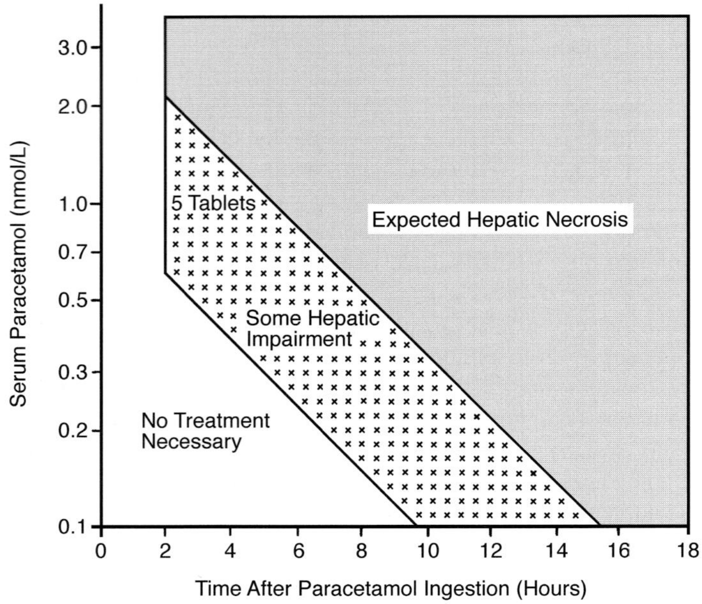

Figure 5 Nomogram for treatment of acetaminophen poisoning with N-acetylcysteine (NAC). (From Hawker, 1993.)

Late administration of NAC (> 24 h after overdose) appears to have some efficacy as well; survival, cerebral edema, and renal failure are all favorably influenced. The reason for the improved outcome does not appear to be related to improved liver function, since no changes in PT or mental status are reported. Rather, tissue oxygen delivery appears to be improved (see "Cardiovascular Disorders," below). In the late studies of NAC, the dose was given intravenously as 150 mg/kg in 200 mL 5% dextrose over 15 min followed by 50 mg/kg in 500 mL 5% dextrose over 4 h followed by 100 mg/kg in 1 L 5% dextrose over 16 h. Side effects such as urticaria, angioneurotic edema, and bronchospasm may occur in response to NAC and should be treated with steroids and antihistamines.

NAC is not available in an intravenous form in the United States and must therefore be given by nasoenteral tube. This route is effective, but the physician must be on the lookout for the nauseated patient who vomits part or all of the medication. Repeat dosing is essential under these circumstances. Placing the tube in the small intestine may lessen the likelihood of this problem with subsequent doses.

NAC is given as a loading dose of 140 mg/kg followed by 17 doses of 70 mg/kd at 4-h intervals. Treatment can be discontinued if serum values are out of the range shown in Fig. 5 (assuming accurate information about time of ingestion) or after 24 h if no abnormalities of clotting or renal function have occurred.

OLTx is indicated in a minority of patients with acetaminophen poisoning. Those who meet transplant criteria (see above) should be transplanted as soon as possible. In a recent study, half of the transplant candidates were referred after developing a medical contraindication to OLTx (refractory hypotension, severe cerebral edema, sepsis) and half of the remainder developed a contraindication before a donor organ was obtained.

Mushroom Poisoning

Mushroom poisoning causes several hundred deaths annually in Europe and the United States. The mushrooms are found in temperate forests in late summer and fall and are usually ingested by overconfident amateur collectors. *Amanita phalloides* accounts for 95% of cases, and one to three mushroom caps are sufficient to cause FHF.

A. phalloides contains two toxins, phalloidin and α-amanitin. Both are hepatotoxic, but phalloidin is not absorbed from the gastrointestinal tract; the entire effect of mushroom poisoning is thus caused by α-amanitin. The mechanism of toxicity is by irreversible inhibition of RNA polymerase II.

Mushroom poisoning is characterized by severe abdominal pain and watery diarrhea, which develops 6–24 h after ingestion and lasts 1–4 days. Aminotransferases usually begin to rise at about the time that the diarrhea subsides, and levels comparable to those arising with acetaminophen are seen. Encephalopathy develops 2–4 days after ingestion, and death occurs 5–7 days after ingestion.

α-Amanitin poisoning can be confirmed by radioimmunoassay of serum and urine samples, although this is usually unnecessary if a clear history of mushroom ingestion is obtained. Early management usually includes fluid and electrolyte replacement to compensate for gastrointestinal losses. Patients usually present too late for primary detoxification by gastric lavage, but extensive enterohepatic recycling suggests that repeated doses of activated charcoal and cathartics may remove some toxin. In addition, forced diuresis may help early in the course. Hemoperfusion and dialysis are not particularly useful.

Specific therapy for *Amanita* poisoning includes silibinin (also known as silymarin, a flavanoid-alcohol from the fruit *Silybum marianum*) and penicillin G. Silibinin has proven efficacy in an animal model of *Amanita* poisoning, although human data are lacking. It is an antioxidant, but its action is probably related to its ability to interfere with α-amanitin uptake by hepatocytes. Silibinin may be useful up to 48 h after ingestion. Thioctic acid and NAC do not appear to influence the course of the illness. Overall mortality is 22%, and OLTx should be considered in cases that meet early transplant criteria (Table 3).

Pregnancy-Related Liver Failure

FHF may occur in association with pregnancy and may require specific treatment in terms of early delivery or cesarean section. (The full spectrum of liver disease in pregnancy is discussed in Chapter 33.) The two conditions that cause FHF are acute fatty liver of pregnancy (AFLP) and liver failure associated with preeclampsia. AFLP is the result of intrahepatic accumulation of fat, which has a histological appearance similar to that of Reye's syndrome, Jamaican vomiting sickness, tetracycline toxicity, valproic acid toxicity, and medium- and long-chain acyl-CoA dehydrogenase deficiency.

AFLP presents late in pregnancy with a mean gestational age of 34 weeks (range 28–39 weeks). The early features are nonspecific: nausea, vomiting, fatigue, malaise, and abdominal distress. Fever, headaches, diarrhea, and back pain may also occur, and progression to typical FHF usually takes 1–2 weeks. Elevated liver enzymes and bilirubin are universal, although transaminases are typically below 300 IU/L and the prothrombin time is usually elevated.

Management of AFLP requires prompt delivery, either induced or by cesarean section. This is not usually a problem; the disease occurs late in pregnancy and prompt delivery is associated with improved maternal and fetal survival. The condition typically begins to resolve after delivery, although it may worsen at first. A few cases have been transplanted postpartum, although this is rarely necessary.

The term *preeclampsia* describes a triad of hypertension, proteinuria, and edema which develops to a greater or lesser degree in 5–10% of pregnancies. The onset of seizures signals the transition to eclampsia. The liver can be affected by preeclampsia/eclampsia, and a substantial proportion of affected women manifest some degree of liver damage, ranging from mild hepatocellular necrosis to hepatic rupture, which may be accompanied by hemolytic anemia and thrombocytopenia.

Eclampsia-related liver disease is more common than AFLP and has several distinguishing features. It usually occurs earlier in pregnancy and may cause extensive liver necrosis with commensurately high transaminase activities. HELLP syndrome (hemolysis, elevated liver enzymes, and low platelets) is the typical clinical manifestation, and the presence of clotting abnormalities and disseminated intravascular coagulopathy (DIC) puts the fetus at risk because of subsequent placental damage.

The management of HELLP syndrome includes close monitoring of platelet levels, coagulation function, and DIC. Antihypertensive agents and volume expansion may be necessary, and fetal monitoring for distress and lung maturity is essential. Delivery, usually by cesarean section, must be undertaken if the fetal lungs are mature, fetal distress is apparent, or the maternal biochemical parameters deteriorate. If the mother is stable and the fetal lungs are immature, corticosteroids may be given in an attempt to hasten lung maturation.

An extension of the HELLP syndrome is hepatic hematoma or rupture. These are probably the result of confluent necrosis and present as acute right-upper-quadrant pain. Hepatic tenderness is common, and shock may ensue within a few hours. Diagnosis is usually made by computed tomography (CT) and must be treated with appropriate fluids and observation. Suspicion of a tear in Glisson's capsule is an indication for emergency laparotomy.

Wilson's Disease

Wilsonian FHF is universally fatal unless treated by OLTx, so an early diagnosis is essential. Wilson's disease should be suspected in all patients under 20 years of age who present with FHF (Table 6). Furthermore, certain clues should alert the clinician to the diagnosis. Among these are low serum ceruloplasmin, low serum alkaline phosphatase activity, low venous uric acid, evidence of hemolysis, and Kayser-Fleischer rings on slit-lamp examination. None of these tests is diagnostic, but the diagnosis is usually made by a preponderance of evidence. If the diagnosis remains questionable, 24-h urinary copper levels are usually diagnostic.

Table 6 Making the Diagnosis of Fulminant Wilson's Disease

Clinical finding	Fulminant Wilson's disease	Other causes of FHF
Hemolysis	Present in 100% of cases	May be present
Low serum ceruloplasmin	Normal serum level in 15% of cases	May be low in non-Wilson's
Low serum alkaline phosphatase activity	Nonspecific, but common	Usually normal or elevated
Kayser-Fleischer rings	May be absent in young patients	May be seen in cholestatic liver disease
Level of 24-h urinary copper	Usually elevated	Usually normal

Effect of Fulminant Hepatic Failure on Specific Organ Systems

Liver failure, especially in its acute form, has far-reaching effects on other organs. With a general failure of acid-base balance, thermoregulation, oxygen delivery, and energy supply, many organs begin to fail. The end result, a combination of cardiovascular collapse, cerebral edema, renal failure, respiratory failure, and pancreatitis, is known as multiorgan failure (MOF). The mechanism of MOF is poorly understood, but it may be related to defective oxygen utilization by the tissues. The role of inadequate oxygen at the tissue level is discussed below.

Cardiovascular Disorders

FHF is accompanied by a severe circulatory disturbance characterized by low systemic and pulmonary vascular resistance and a compensatory increase in cardiac output and metabolic rate. This is a pathological state reminiscent of septic shock and adult respiratory distress syndrome and is associated with abnormal oxygen transport and utilization—i.e., the normal relationship between oxygen delivery (DO_2) and uptake (VO_2) is disrupted. It is quite likely that disordered oxygen uptake is the unifying factor in the development of multiorgan failure; its early recognition and treatment may minimize secondary organ damage and promote liver regeneration. The subject is beyond the scope of this chapter but is discussed in detail in most critical manuals and texts.

As a practical matter, hypotension remains one of the most serious and difficult problems in the management of FHF; its onset is cause for grave concern. Full hemodynamic monitoring is essential in order to maintain an adequate blood pressure and, by extension, normal tissue perfusion. Low blood pressure must be addressed immediately.

The first line in managing hypotension is fluid administration. Colloids are preferred to crystalloids because the latter enter the brain, where their osmotic effect increases brain edema. The blood pressure frequently remains uncontrollably low in spite of an optimized filling pressure. At this point, vasopressors must be used.

Anecdotal evidence suggests that epinephrine and norepinephrine are more effective than dobutamine in the context of FHF; epinephrine and norepinephrine increase both cardiac output and systemic vascular resistance. Unfortunately, they may also worsen tissue hypoxia. Coadministration of prostacyclin or NAC, agents that improve tissue oxygen uptake at the microvascular level, have been suggested as a remedy to this problem. This advice is little help in the United States, where intravenous preparations of prostacyclin and NAC are unavailable for routine use. In any event, restoration of blood pressure must take precedence in the treatment scheme. If microvascular function can be modulated by NAC or other agents, optimized cardiovascular function should include a cardiac index greater than 4.5 $L/min/m^2$, oxygen delivery (DO_2) greater than 800 $mL/min/m^2$, and oxygen consumption greater than 150 $mL/min/m^2$.

Hepatic Encephalopathy and Cerebral Edema

Hepatic encephalopathy is a chemical inhibition of brain function. It is not in itself injurious even though it reflects the extent of liver damage. Cerebral edema, on the other hand, is a physical condition. It results from the accumulation of brain water and becomes a problem when the volume of the swollen brain exceeds the volume of the cranial cavity. Once this limit is reached, small changes in brain volume have profound effects on the intracranial pressure.

FHF is accompanied by a panoply of metabolic problems, any of which could be the cause of hepatic encephalopathy alone or in concert. Theories about a causative agent in hepatic encephalopathy abound. Included in the list are ammonia, glutamine, false neurotransmitters, and benzodiazepine-like compounds (see Chap. 36).

The cause of cerebral edema is also debated. Two general mechanisms have been described: breakdown of the blood-brain barrier (vasogenic edema) and impaired cellular osmoregulation (cellular or cytotoxic edema). It is possible that both mechanisms operate to a greater or lesser degree in any individual case, as discussed briefly below.

Vasogenic edema is typified by head trauma; a favorable response to steroids is thought to result from restoration of the blood-brain barrier. The ineffectiveness of steroids as well as the favorable response to mannitol (an osmotic agent) suggest an intact blood-brain barrier in FHF. On the other hand, the blood-brain barrier becomes more permeable to certain compounds, suggesting at least a partial vasogenic component.

Cytotoxic edema implicates a cellular defect. Several mechanisms have been proposed, including cellular swelling as a primary event, intracellular sodium accumulation as the result of altered membrane Na^+, K^+-ATPase activity, intracellular glutamine accumulation, and the hypoxic consequences of altered cerebral blood flow. The field is rather confusing at present because variables such as body temperature and the choice of experimental model have profound effects on the nature and extent of cerebral edema.

A proposed relationship between hepatic encephalopathy and cerebral edema is shown schematically in Fig. 6.

There is no need to treat hepatic encephalopathy. Recent work on the use of benzodiazepine inhibitors has been more interesting in terms of discovering the basis of encephalopathy than as a therapeutic tool. Lactulose, while useful in the management of chronic hepatic encephalopathy, has no role in the management of acute liver failure. It does not improve brain function, may worsen hypernatremia, and may cause bowel distention, which later interferes with surgery.

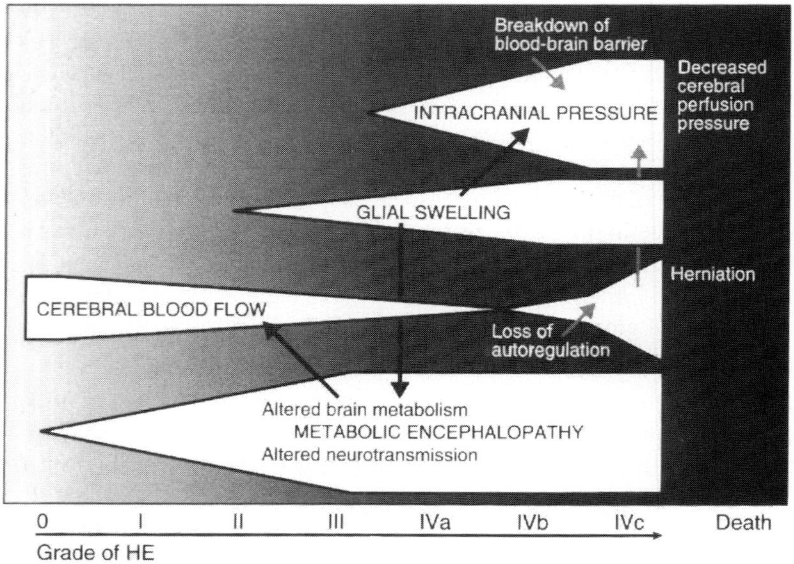

Figure 6 Proposed relationship between encephalopathy, intracranial pressure, and cerebral blood flow in FHF. (From Ferenci, 1994.)

While we do not treat encephalopathy, it is critical as a guide to patient care. The onset of grade III encephalopathy marks a turning point in management; the patient is in danger of both aspirating and developing intracranial hypertension. The first is easily treated by intubation, the second requires skill and experience.

Clinical signs of intracranial hypertension are unreliable. The risk of permanent brain damage increases at about 25 mmHg, and 25% of patients reach this level without displaying typical signs. Systolic hypertension and pupillary abnormalities are not usually seen until the intracranial pressure (ICP) exceeds 30 mmHg. The usual signs, such as headache and vomiting, are completely absent because the patient is comatose.

An abrupt rise in the ICP may be rapidly fatal because of uncal herniation while a slowly increasing ICP may result in cerebral ischemia. Blood flow to the brain is reflected in the cerebral perfusion pressure (CPP), the difference between the mean arterial pressure (MAP) and the ICP:

$$\text{CPP} = \text{MAP} - \text{ICP}$$

The CPP should be kept above 50 mmHg to prevent hypoperfusion.

The importance of a raised ICP and the lack of corroborating clinical findings has led to increasing use of ICP monitoring, usually with an extradural catheter. The danger of precipitating intracerebral bleeding is related to the ICP at the time of catheter insertion. It is thus wise to anticipate the need and place the monitor before the onset of intracranial hypertension. We also correct the prothrombin time to within 5 s of control and ensure that the platelet count is above 75,000/μL.

The role of the ICP monitor is to guide management of intracranial events. The monitor can be used to take specific action in response to a clinically silent elevation of the ICP, to prevent inappropriate liver transplantation, and to guide intraoperative management.

Retrospective analysis of patients with ICP monitors results in more frequent interventions to reduce the ICP, and a prolonged survival time (60 versus 10 h). This difference can be critical in a patient who is waiting for an organ and may even buy the time necessary for liver regeneration to begin. A steady decline in ICP in a patient who is otherwise stable may be an early indication that recovery is taking place.

Postoperative neurological complications, including fatal cerebral edema, have been reported in 10–50% of patients who have reached grade IV encephalopathy prior to OLTx. The ICP monitor can be used to avoid this type of result if patients with refractory intracranial hypertension are denied OLTx. This approach has been criticized because it excludes patients who might benefit from transplantation. The authors have countered that the current shortage of donors necessitates great care in organ allocation and have reported a 93% postoperative survival rate.

Control of ICP is critical during OLTx. The ICP rises during the preclamp and reperfusion phases and rises consistently with isoflurane inhalation. Venovenous bypass may limit the intraoperative rise in ICP, and this, along with alternative anesthetic agents, should be considered in all cases of FHF undergoing OLTx.

While ICP and CPP can be used as guides to management, they should not be used to diagnose brain death. Loss of brainstem function or a cerebral perfusion scan should be used.

Patients with grade III–IV encephalopathy are at risk for a slowly rising ICP as well as sudden bouts of intracranial hypertension. Factors that typically precede an acute increase in ICP include fever, agitation, and arterial hypertension. Any stimulation, especially moving the patient, should be avoided. A major problem is the overzealous use of

CT scans; they rarely provide useful information and should be avoided unless localizing neurological signs are present.

The preferred nursing position is supine, with the head no higher than 20 degrees above the horizontal. Patients with an ICP monitor may have their heads higher if it produces a salutary effect on ICP and CPP. Endotracheal suctioning must be minimized; lidocaine squirted into the endotracheal tube may reduce the cough reflex if pulmonary toilet is needed. Seizures, which are frequently masked by coma or sedation, must be treated aggressively. An electroencephalogram (EEG) may be required to diagnose clinically silent seizures. Hypoxia and hypercapnia must be avoided and blood pressure maintained with pressors if necessary to keep the CPP above 50 mmHg.

The physician has limited options when it comes to lowering an elevated ICP. Head elevation (see above) and hyperventilation are both used early in management.

Moderate hyperventilation (P_{CO_2} of 25–35 mmHg) may cause a transient decrease in the ICP; spontaneous hyperventilation is common in FHF, so forced hyperventilation has a small incremental effect on the P_{CO_2}. This point of view is supported by a controlled trial in which hyperventilation reduced neither the incidence nor the number of episodes of intracranial hypertension. Nevertheless, hyperventilation is used commonly and may be useful as a short-term treatment of acute intracerebral hypertension. If it is used, the P_{CO_2} must not drop below 24 mmHg, because hypocapnia at this level is associated with intense cerebral vasoconstriction and cerebral ischemia. There is another theoretical objection to hyperventilation: it may reduce blood flow and oxygen utilization by the brain.

Osmotic agents (e.g., mannitol) and loop diuretics (e.g., furosemide) may be used to treat intracranial hypertension. Mannitol is the favored agent, usually in a dose of 0.5–1 g/kg over 5 min. It should be given in response to a raised ICP or clinical signs of cerebral edema if an ICP monitor is not available, and the dose may be repeated as necessary until the serum osmolality is about 320 mOsm/L. Mannitol is not as effective if the patient is anuric, and its use should be coupled with renal replacement therapy under these circumstances (see below).

If intracranial hypertension does not respond to the above measures, thiopental or pentobarbital may be useful. These are usually given as a bolus followed by a continuous infusion, and their use is usually limited by systemic hypotension. Great care must be taken to maintain the CPP if these agents are used; pressors may be required. Once barbiturate coma is induced, all brainstem reflexes may be lost, and brain death cannot be diagnosed on clinical or EEG criteria.

There is some thought that barbiturates exert their beneficial effects through their anticonvulsant activity. Seizures increase both the ICP and the brain's consumption of oxygen, and any measure which reduces their incidence or severity is likely to be of benefit.

Kidney Dysfunction

Renal failure complicates FHF in 40–50% of cases and in 70% of cases caused by acetaminophen. Acetaminophen is both hepatotoxic and nephrotoxic; it may cause renal failure with FHF or, occasionally, without severe liver necrosis. Renal failure has even been reported after ingestion of therapeutic doses of acetaminophen and its toxicity is enhanced by alcohol and cardiac failure.

The association between liver failure and renal failure was first described in cirrhotics. It is a functional abnormality in which the kidneys remain structurally normal. The kidneys resume function if the liver recovers, a liver transplant is performed, or even if the kidneys are transplanted into a patient with normal liver function. The condition is known

Table 7 Difference Between Hepatorenal Syndrome and Acute Tubular Necrosis

	Hepatorenal syndrome	Acute tubular necrosis
Pathophysiology	Renal vasoconstriction	Ischemic tubular damage
Urine sodium concentration	<10 mmol/L	50–70 mmol/L
Urine/plasma creatinine	>10	<10
Urine osmolality	>1.010	Approx. 1.010
Urinary casts	Rare	Common

Source: Adapted from Hawker, 1993.

as hepatorenal syndrome (HRS), and it accounts for about 75% of renal failure in FHF. The presence of HRS does not correlate with the severity of the liver disease (see Chap. 39).

HRS may progress to acute tubular necrosis (ATN), a structural injury of the kidney tubules. These two entities are quite different in their pure forms (see Table 7) although they frequently overlap during the transition from HRS to ATN. Urea cannot be used as a marker in the setting of liver dysfunction, as urea synthesis is reduced.

HRS is thought to result from renal vasoconstriction in response to the systemic vasodilatation that accompanies liver failure. The renal blood flow (RBF) is usually about 40% of normal, and patients with clinical renal failure have RBFs and glomerular filtration rates (GFRs) of about one-tenth the values of patients without renal failure. It is important to understand that HRS renders the kidneys exquisitely sensitive to insults, and even trivial sepsis or a short period of hypotension may result in severe renal dysfunction.

Renal failure is best prevented by maintaining the patient's blood pressure and avoiding sepsis. Low-dose dopamine may also help renal perfusion (2–4 μg/kg/h), and nephrotoxic agents such as aminoglycosides should be avoided if possible. These measures will not prevent renal shutdown in advanced FHF, and renal support should be undertaken as soon as volume or electrolyte management becomes a problem, or the patient's urine output drops below 30 mL/h.

If renal support is necessary, it must be continuous. Acute hemodialysis causes an abrupt increase in ICP and reduction in CPP. Continuous arteriovenous (or venovenous) hemoperfusion (CAVH/CVVH) or hemodiafiltration (CAVHD/CVVHD) do not cause these increases and are therefore preferred. It is also important to recognize that most dialysis fluids contain lactate. Some patients may be unable to cope with the lactate load, and a bicarbonate-based dialysis bath will be required.

Several centers anticoagulate patients in the course of CVVH. We endorse this practice because each clotted cartridge consumes platelets and clotting factors, and each cartridge change carries with it the risk of a hypotensive episode. Heparin administration to an activated clotting time of 200–250 as appears to have minimal side effects in our experience. A surprising level of heparin resistance may be encountered as a result of a deficiency of antithrombin III (now known as antithrombin).

Pulmonary Dysfunction

In addition to damage caused by aspiration or mechanical ventilation, patients with FHF are susceptible to specific lung problems. Dilatation of the pulmonary vasculature results in tissue hypoxia and edema, with consequent hypoxemia. Dilated blood vessels and pleural angiomata are seen commonly, and pulmonary edema in the absence of left ventricular failure occurs in almost 40% of patients. Noncardiac pulmonary edema is part of MOF and a frequent cause of death in FHF. Once it develops, patients cannot be rescued with liver transplantation.

Management of lung disease in FHF is nonspecific; once the patient progresses to grade III encephalopathy, intubation is necessary in order to protect the airway. In patients with evidence of lung injury, mechanical ventilation with positive end-expiratory pressure is used to assure adequate tissue oxygenation.

Infections

Infections are common in the setting of FHF. Failure of the immune system occurs because several cell types—including Kupffer cells, neutrophils, and lymphocytes—function poorly, and serum opsonins such as fibronectin are decreased. The significance of infectious complications has grown as ICU care has improved; the longer the patient survives in the ICU, the greater the risk of a life-threatening infection. Sepsis is the most frequent cause of late death from FHF.

The problem is compounded by the absence of typical features of infection. Fever and leukocytosis are frequently absent, and sepsis may present with the onset of renal failure or worsening MOF. Infection should be suspected in any patient whose condition deteriorates after a period of improvement.

Studies have demonstrated that bacterial infections occurs in 80–90% of patients and fungal infections occur in almost one-third in the absence of prophylactic antibiotics. Common fluids that yield positive cultures are sputum, blood, and urine. Pneumonia is always detectable by chest x-ray. Bacterial peritonitis is exceedingly rare and suggests chronic liver disease.

Bacterial infections may be present at the time of admission to the ICU, but fungal infections generally occur later. Fungal infections almost always accompany bacterial infection, with *Candida* spp. being the most frequent organisms. Fungal infection frequently causes late deterioration in a patient who was previously stable or improving and is lethal if not recognized and treated. An empirical, broad-spectrum regimen should be replaced when specific agents and sensitivities are available.

The prevention of sepsis in FHF is not as clearly defined as treatment. Commonsense practices such as careful hand-washing are very important. Prophylactic antibiotics and/or selective bowel decontamination have been shown to decrease the incidence of infection but have not been proven to improve patient survival. In practical terms, most patients receive prophylactic antimicrobials. Amphotericin B by inhalation, though not proven effective, may decrease the risk of fungal superinfection.

Gastrointestinal Bleeding

Gastrointestinal bleeding has become less of a problem with the routine use of intravenous H_2 blockers. The most common cause and site of bleeding is stress ulceration of the stomach. Clotting defects should be corrected as needed, and endoscopic therapy may be required if the bleeding is persistent. While portal hypertension may be present, it rarely causes gastrointestinal bleeding.

Coagulopathy

FHF causes profound abnormalities in clotting. The defects are not uniform and include a mixture of reduced synthesis, increased consumption, variable fibrinolysis, and platelet abnormalities. This mixture makes it rather surprising that the prothrombin time reflects residual liver function so accurately.

The liver synthesizes most of the clotting factors. The damaged liver has a reduced capacity to manufacture these factors, so patients with FHF have defective clotting, which can be monitored by a variety of functional assays. Factors with a short half-life are the first to decline, the reason why factor V is the favored assay of some investigators. The PT, which measures factors I, II, V, VI, and X, is used routinely in most cases. Two important considerations in the use of clotting as a measure of liver injury are the recognition that vitamin K deficiency must be excluded and, as mentioned previously, that acetaminophen toxicity causes a coagulopathy that is disproportionately greater than the extent of liver necrosis.

DIC or localized intravascular coagulopathy, as measured by elevated levels of thrombin-antithrombin (TAT) complex is common in FHF. The condition is usually mild and not a major contributor to the coagulopathy. It is usually seen in association with septicemia.

Fibrinolysis, as measured by the presence of fibrin degradation products, is usually present in FHF. It is not usually severe, although it may cause a problem if the patient has a bleeding site and a concomitant problem with clot stabilization.

Platelet count, morphology, and function can all be abnormal in FHF, but spontaneous bleeding remains rare. Bleeding from incisions and other skin puncture sites may be a nuisance, but the risk of intracranial bleeding does not correlate with platelet count or function.

The coagulopathy of FHF does not require treatment unless clinically significant bleeding has occurred or an invasive procedure is planned. Although the risk of bleeding following placement of an intracranial pressure monitor does not appear to correlate with the platelet count, we infuse platelets to bring the count to 75×10^9/L and give FFP prior to monitor placement.

Nutritional Considerations

FHF is a hypermetabolic state; catabolism increases by up to a factor of four. Yet, despite this obvious imbalance, parenteral nutrition has no proven impact on survival. This may be related to the acute nature of the disease or the fact that the liver has a limited capacity to handle the load. Nevertheless, patients with a prolonged illness or a long convalescent period are likely to benefit from good nutrition. Branched-chain amino acids, despite their theoretical advantages, do not appear to be superior to other forms of parenteral nutrition in the setting of acute liver failure. The added expense is not justifiable.

LIVER TRANSPLANTATION

FHF is occasionally caused by an agent such as a herpesvirus which can be treated specifically with acyclovir. Aside from these rare cases, and for the specific role of NAC in acetaminophen poisoning, no drugs significantly improve the outcome of FHF. Steroids may make matters worse in the case of fulminant hepatitis and must be used with caution. Thus, the only curative therapy for FHF is transplantation.

Orthotopic Liver Transplantation—Partial Orthotopic and Heterotopic Liver Transplantation

Although OLTx has never been subjected to prospective evaluation, it has become the standard of care in most centers. The issue will never be resolved for purists, but it represents a reasonable position given the accuracy of prognostic indicators and the high mortality among patients who are listed for OLTx but do not receive an organ in time.

Postoperative survival in 14 trials published between 1987 and 1993 was 65%, although stringent selection criteria may improve this figure to over 90%. Most of the deaths following OLTx for FHF occur within the first few months; beyond this point, survival is comparable to that of other transplant patients.

One of the most important factors contributing to the success of OLTx for FHF is the rapid assessment of prognosis. If the patient has a poor prognosis with medical therapy alone, immediate transfer to a regional transplant center is mandatory. Most centers can determine within 24 h whether someone is an appropriate candidate for OLTx. This maximizes the time the center has to look for an appropriate donor organ. Recently, the United Network for Organ Sharing (UNOS) changed the definition of status I (the highest priority) patients to be those with FHF, primary nonfunction, and hepatic artery thrombosis occurring in the first 7 days post-OLTx. This should increase the likelihood of patients with FHF receiving OLTx if they are judged to be transplant candidates. However, this will depend in part on whether or not the unit of distribution of donated livers remains the local Organ Procurement Organization (OPO) (see Chap. 43).

It is also important to recognize that not all patients with FHF are candidates for OLTx. Sometimes this is obvious on presentation—e.g., serious comorbid disease or psychosocial contraindications. It is equally important to ask on a daily basis whether the patient is still a candidate for liver transplantation. Contraindications to OLTx that can develop during the course of the disease include uncontrolled intracranial hypertension, uncontrolled systemic hypotension, sepsis, and acute respiratory distress syndrome ($P_{O_2} \cdot 70$ mmHg on $Fi_{O_2} \cdot 0.6$).

The most important posttransplant complications that occur following OLTx are prolonged ICU stay secondary to the need for extended mechanical ventilation, renal insufficiency, and fungal infections. Contrary to what one might believe, immediate graft function does not translate into an immediate improvement in the level of consciousness. These patients commonly take 2–4 days to improve neurologically and may take up to 2 weeks to attain a relatively normal mental status. In addition, patients may sustain lung injury because of the liver failure and/or sepsis. For these reasons, patients with FHF require prolonged airway intubation with or without mechanical ventilation.

Renal insufficiency is common in the setting of FHF. Patients with renal insufficiency should be on CVVH prior to OLTx, and this should be continued during surgery. In general, these patients continue to require CVVH posttransplant for some period, usually < 2 weeks. If renal failure persists postoperatively, CVVH can usually be converted to intermittent hemodialysis after a few days.

Auxiliary Liver Transplantation

An area of interest in OLTx, especially in relationship to FHF, is auxiliary liver transplantation. In this procedure, a partial liver graft is either placed in a heterotopic position or, more commonly, orthotopically in a space provided by a partial hepatectomy of the native liver. The technique offers the advantage of patients potentially recovering native liver function postoperatively. In addition, since only a part of the donated liver is transplanted, one can transplant the rest of the allograft into a second recipient. Live donors, particularly in the case of pediatric recipients, have also been used for procuring a segment of liver.

Approximately 60% of patients recover native liver function when this technique is used. Once the native liver has recovered, one can withdraw immunosuppression and allow rejection of the auxiliary graft, or one can surgically remove the allograft. Recovery of native liver function is generally assessed by HIDA scanning. While this procedure sounds ideal, it is technically demanding, and one must be certain that the auxiliary graft is of adequate size to sustain the patient.

EXPERIMENTAL THERAPIES

Hepatocyte Transplantation

There has been renewed enthusiasm regarding the use of hepatocyte transplantation in the management of FHF. Acute liver failure is lethal in the presence of $\geqslant$ 30% necrosis. If an adult liver weighs about 1500 g, we can assume that roughly 450 g of liver (or 360 g of hepatocytes) are necessary for survival. Cell therapy involves injecting several grams of hepatocytes into the portal circulation. The mass of cells that can be injected is limited by the extent to which the cells obstruct hepatic blood flow as they are trapped in the sinusoids; overaggressive treatment causes death from acute portal hypertension. This therapy is still highly experimental.

Artificial Liver

Liver support modeled after kidney dialysis has been an elusive dream for several decades. A variety of stop-gap measures—including hemodialysis, charcoal hemoperfusion, exchange transfusion, and plasma exchange—have all proven to be ineffective in the treatment of acute liver failure. In the 1960s, it became apparent that a nonfunctioning liver could be replaced only by another liver, and studies with animal cross-perfusion and ex vivo liver perfusion were undertaken. These intrepid workers soon realized that their studies were dangerous and that they afforded the patient a short-lived therapeutic benefit; the animal organ was rapidly destroyed by the patient's immune system. However, it was clear that animal organs provided good albeit short-lived support. More recently, human livers have been shown to work in an ex vivo format. The problem is that the current shortage of human livers is unlikely to improve in the near future, so organs will not be available for extracorporeal use as long as they are needed for transplantation.

Models for Liver Assist

An artificial liver is the optimum therapeutic option for FHF. It can provide the window necessary for the liver to recover and has the potential to keep patients stable in anticipation of liver transplantation if recovery is deemed impossible. The requirements for a liver assist device are similar to those for any artificial organ; it must mimic the function of the native organ with acceptable risk to the patient. Since no liver assist device has yet been proven effective in clinical trials, any discussion of liver support must involve some conjecture. The following are suggested as a hypothetical basis for the successful development of an artificial liver.

Noninvasiveness. Since the goal is temporary support, the device should produce as little trauma as possible. The terms *extracorporeal liver assist device* (ELAD) and *bioartifical liver* (BAL) refer to devices that are perfused outside the body. They are the hepatic equivalent of kidney dialysis and represent the least invasive method of providing liver support (Fig. 7).

Metabolic Capacity. Liver failure is universally fatal if less than 30% of the hepatocytes remain viable on biopsy. The only way to ensure this threshold value is to make a device that provides at least 30% of native function.

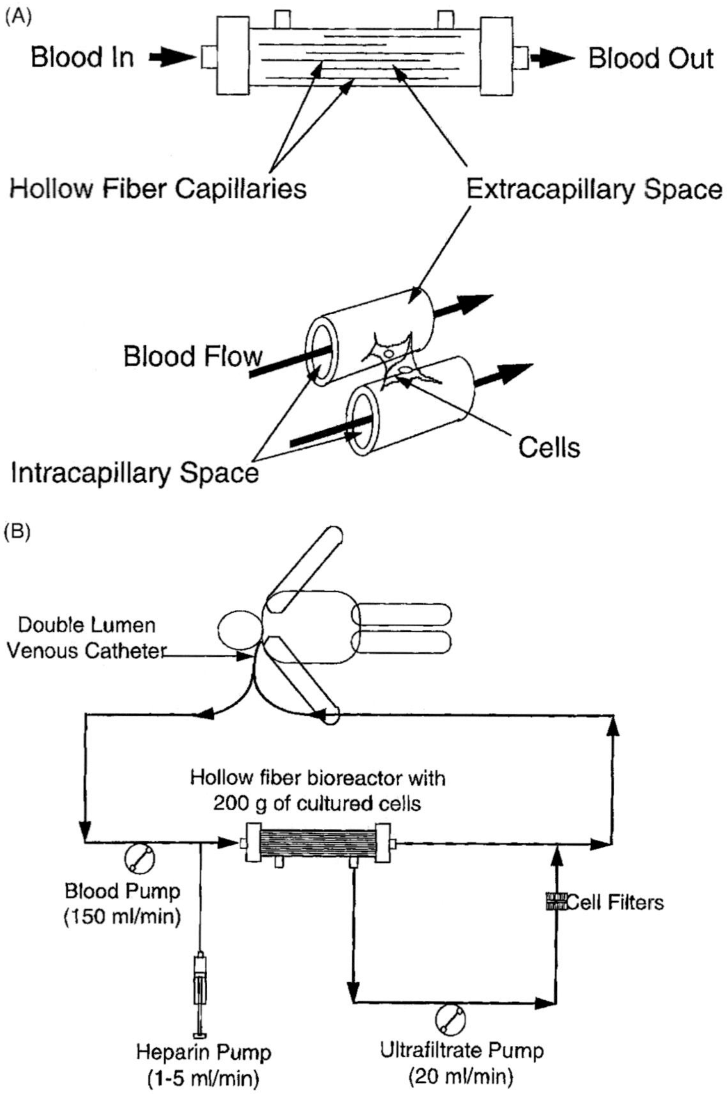

Figure 7 (A) Schematic diagram of an extracorporeal liver assist device. Cultured human liver cells are injected into the extracapillary space of a dialysis cartridge and grown in culture. The cells grow to confluence over 2–3 weeks and reach about 200 g of functional mass. Two cartridges in series supply 30–40% of normal liver function. (From Sussman et al., 1992.) (B) Circuit diagram for using an artificial liver. The cartridge is perfused with blood from a jugular vein catheter. (From Kelly and Sussman, 1994.)

Continuous Treatment. Continuous liver function should be the goal of liver support. Intermittent treatment is not physiological and may leave the patient vulnerable to metabolic complications while they are disconnected from their support device.

Availability. Liver assist is frequently required on an urgent basis; it must be available on short notice.

Ease of Operation. The procedure should be no more complex than hemodialysis. Systems that require concurrent procedures or the manipulation of whole organs are not acceptable.

Safety. This is a relative term, especially in the context of a disease that has an overall mortality rate of 85% and for which standard therapy includes liver transplantation. Nevertheless, liver assist should not expose the patient to unnecessary risk and should not have long-term sequelae in those patients who survive the acute episode.

Cost-Effectiveness. While saving lives should be the primary goal of liver assist, the realities of current medical economics cannot be ignored. Interventions that have the potential to reduce medical costs will be more palatable to both the medical community and third-party payers.

Several groups are currently developing liver assist devices. The extent to which each of them meets the ideals described above is a reasonable basis for studying their strengths and weaknesses. All the devices discussed in this section are extracorporeal. They thus meet the requirement for noninvasiveness.

Metabolic Capacity. How much of a liver mass is required for support is unknown. In addition, whether one can achieve extraordinary support from a relatively small hepatocyte mass by better engineering of the device is uncertain. The current literature contains reports of several liver assist devices that contain less than 10 g of hepatocytes. The reason is related to the technology. Most devices utilize primary hepatocytes, cells isolated from fresh animal livers. Several problems hamper this approach. First, the technique is expensive and time-consuming, and it yields relatively small numbers of cells. Second, the cells do not divide after they have been harvested, so device manufacture relies on repeated cell isolations. Third, the cells have a limited life span once treatment starts. This drives the cost up further by requiring the use of a new device after 6 h of treatment. Finally, the danger of infectious agents is becoming more of a reality. The recent outbreak of bovine spongiform encephalitis in Great Britain has mandated a switch to serum-free production. Careful maintenance of germ-free donor herds will be necessary in the future.

Cell lines, especially those of human origin, circumvent many of the problems of animal primaries. The major problem is that cultured cells generally lack the broad-based metabolic repertoire of normal hepatocytes. Human liver cell lines that retain many of the important properties of a normal hepatocyte exist; however, whether they contain the key function that will prevent the brain from swelling remains uncertain. Cell lines have been used for liver support in animal and human studies. A liver assist device is made by injecting 1–2 g of cells into a hollow fiber dialyzer and feeding it with culture medium. The cells grow to confluence over 2–3 weeks.

Availability. Since the primary cells do not keep well in culture, they must either be frozen or harvested from whole liver when needed. Cryopreservation is clearly the better alternative in this instance. Working with immortalized cells also allows the maintenance of an inventory of devices which are ready for use.

Ease of Operation. Some liver assist devices are perfused with plasma, a process that requires on-line plasma separation. Others use whole blood, but this requires heparin as an anticoagulant.

Safety. Aside from the dangers inherent in any extracorporeal treatment, liver assist adds unknown dangers associated with the brand-new field of cell therapy. In the case of primary hepatocytes, infectious agents remain a concern. A great deal of uncertainty remains in this area, as indicated by a recent report of the potential for infection of human cells by endogenous porcine retroviruses.

The use of immortalized cells gets around several of these issues. First, a master cell bank can be laid down and extensively tested and characterized. Second, strict adherence to standard tissue culture procedures should eliminate detectable contamination. Finally, the growth period (typically 3 weeks) provides sufficient time to track the performance of each device and to exclude common pathogens, endotoxin, and mycoplasma.

One safety issue associated with the use of cultured cells is the theoretical risk of tumor transmission. The actual risk is probably low. First, the patient's blood does not normally come into contact with the cells in the device; blood flows through the interior of the fibers while the cells are located on the outside (the extracapillary space). Second, an inoculum of cultured cells is very unlikely to survive the body's rejection efforts. Third, the treatment system ensures that pressure in the blood space is always positive relative to the extracapillary space. Thus, even in the rare event of a fiber rupture, blood flow into the extracapillary space prevents cells from gaining access to the bloodstream. Finally, the risk-to-benefit ratio is very favorable; the initial target population has a mortality rate of about 90%. In the final analysis, long-term follow-up of surviving patients will be required before this question can be answered definitively.

Cost-Effective. If liver support functions only as a bridge to OLTx, it will add to the overall cost of patient care. On the other hand, if liver assist therapy replaces liver transplantation, the cost savings will be substantial. A patient who avoids OLTx is spared the initial cost of about $250,000 as well as the long-term maintenance costs of immunosuppression. In addition, the current shortage of donor organs must be considered; over 12,000 patients are currently listed for OLTx in the United States. Nonsurgical treatment of FHF could free up several hundred livers, which can be used more appropriately in patients with irreversible liver diseases.

Current State of Liver Assist

Two types of ELAD are likely to see clinical testing in the near future. One is the primary liver cell–based device developed by Demetriou and colleagues; the other is a culture-based device developed by Kelly and Sussman. Both groups have treated over 20 patients with good anecdotal results. However, the caution of previous liver assist devices looms large; many therapies that were touted as great advances in the treatment of FHF failed when they were tested in a rigorous clinical trial. The community of liver physicians is determined not to make the same mistake again.

CONCLUSIONS

FHF is a lethal disease with a very high overall mortality. Careful attention to patient management has resulted in longer survival times for patients after hospitalization. The additional time is often very important; it may spell the difference between death and a successful liver transplant. It may also allow some patients to recover native liver function, although this remains an outside chance.

Liver transplantation is the only lifesaving modality we can currently offer. It is less than ideal because it results in a permanent change of lifestyle and life expectancy. It is also likely to remain donor-limited for the foreseeable future.

Experimental procedures such as partial orthotopic and heterotopic liver transplantation offer the benefits of OLTx along with the possibility of later recovery of native liver function. These procedures are more difficult to perform than standard OLTx, and most patients will not be candidates.

Extracorporeal liver assist devices will be subjected to widespread clinical testing in the near future. Some of these devices are seen only as a bridge to OLTx, but we insist that recovery of native liver function is possible and should be the goal of liver assist programs.

BIBLIOGRAPHY

Ferenci P. Brain dysfunction in fulminant hepatic failure. Hepatol 1994; 21:487–490.

Hawker F. The Liver. In Park GR, ed. Critical Care Management. London: Saunders, 1993:410.

Kelly JH, Sussman NL. The hepatic extracorporeal liver assist device in the treatment of fulminant hepatic failure. ASAIO J 1994; 40:83–85.

Lee WM, Galbraith RM, Watt GH, Hughes RD, McIntire DD, Hoffman BJ, Williams R. Predicting survival in fulminant hepatic failure using serum Gc protein concentrations. Hepatology 1995; 21:101–105.

Marino PL. The ICU Book. Philadelphia: Lea & Febiger, 1991:713.

Munoz SJ. Prothrombin time in fulminant hepatic failure [letter; comment]. Gastroenterology 1991; 100:1480–1481.

O'Grady JG, Schalm SW, Williams R. Acute liver failure: redefining the syndromes [published erratum appears in Lancet 1993; 342:1000, see comments]. Lancet 1993; 342:273–275.

Sussman NL, Chong MG, Koussayer T, et al. Reversal of fulminant hepatic failure using an extracorporeal liver assist device. Hepatology 1992; 16:60–65.

Sussman NL, Lake JR. Treatment of hepatic failure—1996: Current concepts and progress toward liver dialysis. Am J Kidney Dis 1996; 27:605–621.

Trey C, Davidson CS. The management of fulminant hepatic disease. In: Popper H, Schaffner F, eds. Progress in Liver Disease. New York: Grune & Stratton, 1970:282–298.

Williams R, Wendon J. Indications for orthotopic liver transplantation in fulminant liver failure Hepatology 1994; 20:5S–10S.

26

Management of Nonalcoholic Steatohepatitis

Paul Angulo and Keith D. Lindor
Mayo Clinic and Mayo Foundation, Rochester, Minnesota

DEFINITION

Nonalcoholic steatohepatitis (NASH) is a clinicopathological entity characterized by the development of histological changes in the liver that are nearly identical to those induced by excessive alcohol intake, but in the absence of alcohol abuse. NASH is commonly associated with obesity, type II diabetes mellitus, and hyperlipidemia and must be distinguished from other clinical conditions characterized by hepatic steatosis and inflammation, including excessive fasting, jejunoileal bypass, total parenteral nutrition, chronic hepatitis C, Wilson's disease, and liver damage induced by drugs like corticosteroids, calcium channel blockers, high-dose estrogens, chloroquine, and amiodarone among others. A variety of terms have been used to describe this entity, including *fatty liver hepatitis*, *nonalcoholic Laennec's disease*, *diabetes hepatitis*, and *alcoholic-like liver disease*. Even though an alcoholic hepatitis–like histological picture of liver injury in the absence of alcohol intake was described more than three decades ago, the term *nonalcoholic steatohepatitis* was first introduced by Ludwig and colleagues in 1980. Although it is uncertain whether the accumulation of fat in the liver is the cause of inflammation or whether there is another reason for the hepatitis, NASH should be differentiated from the simple accumulation of fat in the liver called *fatty liver* or *hepatic steatosis*, which is frequently found in liver biopsy from patients with and without primary liver disease.

The amount of alcohol intake required for the development of chronic liver disease has not been clearly established. A threshold dose of 80 g/day of ethanol was found in all patients who developed cirrhosis. Alcohol abuse has been defined by some authors as > 20 g/day of ethanol ingested. Diagnosis of NASH is considered by us when ethanol intake has been < 40 g/week in the context of a compatible histological picture. The term *nonalcoholic steatohepatitis* is widely used now to describe those patients with compatible biopsy findings and lack of significant alcohol consumption, previous surgery for weight loss, history of drugs associated with steatohepatitis, evidence of genetic liver disease, or chronic hepatitis C infection.

Table 1 Prevalence of Nonalcoholic Steatohepatitis

Author	Year	Number of liver biopsies[a]	Well-defined NASH, n (%)
Ludwig et al.	1980	535	20 (3.7)
Diehl et al.	1988	298	39 (13)
Lee et al.	1989	515	49 (9.5)
Teli et al.	1995	156	4 (2.5)
Propst et al.	1995	95	30 (31.5)
Pinto et al.	1996	160	32 (20)
Total		1759	174 (9.8)

[a]Histological injury compatible with alcoholic liver disease.

The prevalence of NASH is unknown. Some retrospective studies (Table 1) have reported a prevalence of NASH varying from 2.5%–31.5% (mean 9.8%) in all liver biopsies that showed changes interpreted as diagnostic of or compatible with alcoholic liver disease independent of body weight and diabetic status. However, owing to the high prevalence of obesity, diabetes mellitus, and hyperlipidemia in the general population together with the frequent absence of symptoms of liver disease and liver biochemical abnormalities, the prevalence of this entity may be higher than suspected and actually underestimated. A decrease in the threshold for performing a liver biopsy, influenced by the eventual availability of effective treatment for patients with NASH, will probably lead us to diagnose more patients with this entity.

PATHOGENESIS AND CLUES TO FUTURE TREATMENT STRATEGIES

Fatty acids from diet or adipose tissue are transported to the liver and taken up by hepatocytes, where they are oxidized and used for triglyceride synthesis. Triglycerides are combined with specific proteins (apoproteins), and are secreted into the circulation in the form of very low density lipoproteins (VLDL).

There is a continuous circulation of fatty acids between liver and adipose tissue; the direction of this flow is from adipose tissue to the liver in the fasting state, and it is reversed in the fed state. Since fatty acids may also be synthesized directly from glucose using acetyl coenzyme A as an intermediate, insulin is crucial in the regulation of adipose tissue triglyceride synthesis by promoting glucose entry into adipocytes and by inhibiting cyclic adenosine monophosphate (cAMP) formation. Insulin response to alteration in blood glucose concentration determines whether fat synthesis and storage occur or whether triglyceride lipolysis is dominant in adipose tissue. Glucose calories exceeding those needed to saturate hepatic glycogen stores are converted to fatty acids in the liver as well. Insulin deficiency, by promoting lipolysis, is an important cause of fatty liver and steatohepatitis in patients with poorly controlled diabetes mellitus. In that situation, massive lipolysis results in an enormous mobilization of free fatty acids, which are taken up by the liver and used for triglyceride synthesis. Low glucose availability, as occurs in fasting hypoglycemia, is accompanied by low insulin levels and the inhibition of adipose tissue lipolysis by insulin is removed and an increase in free fatty acid mobilization occurs. Conversely, in states of high glucose availability and increased insulin levels, inhibition of

Table 2 Causes of Nonalcoholic Steatohepatitis

Nutritional	Drugs	Metabolic/genetic	Other
Obesity	Corticosteroids	Wilson's disease	Environmental hepatotoxins
Adult-onset diabetes mellitus	Estrogens	Lipodystrophy	Inflammatory bowel disease
Protein-calorie malnutrition	Salicylates	Dysbetalipoproteinemia	HIV infection
Starvation	Calcium channel blockers	Weber-Christian disease	Small bowel diverticulosis
Total parenteral nutrition	Amiodarone	Wolman's disease	
Rapid weight loss	Tamoxifen	Cholesterol ester storage	
	Tetracycline		
	Chloroquine		
	Perhexiline maleate		

adipose tissue lipolysis occurs and free fatty acid mobilization is decreased. There is a regulation of the rate of synthesis of fatty acids in the fed and fasting states that includes multiple mechanisms, such as the activity of fatty acid–synthesizing enzymes, availability of substrate and pyruvate for acetyl CoA production, effects of different hormones such as glucagon, pituitary trophic hormones, epinephrine, and norepinephrine that activate lipolysis by increasing cAMP concentration in adipose tissue, and insulin, which inhibits lipolysis by reducing cAMP concentration.

An increase in exogenous triglyceride intake increases the quantity of fatty acids available for uptake by the liver. About one-third of the circulating fatty acids is removed by the liver, and this amount of proportional to the free fatty acid concentration in portal venous blood.

There is no known specific cause of NASH. Several conditions are known to be associated with this entity (Table 2). Numerous theories for the development of fatty liver have been proposed; they are based on derangements of the normal physiology of hepatic triglyceride synthesis and secretion. These theories include abnormalities of physiological and biochemical regulation in the series of steps by which the VLDL and apoproteins are synthesized, assembled into nascent particles, transported sequentially through subcellular compartments, and finally secreted. Defects in one or more of these events can be involved in the pathogenesis of fatty liver. Although there are no definitive data concerning the relative importance of these mechanisms, some may be more important than others depending on the agent directly responsible for the production of hepatic steatosis. Fatty liver is a frequent finding in liver biopsy specimens from patients with and without primary disease of the liver characterized by the accumulation of triglyceride-filled vacuoles in the hepatocyte cytoplasm. Pure hepatic steatosis seems to be a largely benign condition, with a favorable outcome in most patients; however, in a subset of these patients, the steatosis alone or in combination with other factors seems to provide the necessary substrates to initiate the inflammatory response, which will end in the development of NASH. The degree of steatosis has been correlated with the degree of inflammation in some clinical and experimental studies.

The pathogenesis of NASH is multifactorial and not completely understood. Free fatty acids are potentially cytotoxic. In vitro studies have shown that free fatty acids cause mitochondrial swelling, increase lysosomal fragility, depress enzyme activity, and impair membrane integrity. This cellular damage with subsequent inflammation may result in cellular death and fibrosis. Levels of circulating free fatty acids and rate of presentation to the liver may contribute to the morphological and functional liver damage in patients with NASH. However, most of our patients with NASH had serum free fatty acid levels within the normal range and, in a preliminary analysis, we did not find any obvious correlation between serum free fatty acid levels and liver damage determined by liver biochemistries and liver biopsy. Other factors associated with increased levels of serum free fatty acids and/or with the rate of presentation to the liver may be necessary for development of NASH. Increased circulating levels of endotoxin, which is a known potent agonist for production of proinflammatory cytokines such as tumor necrosis factor alpha (TNF-α) can play a role in the development of steatohepatitis, as happens in patients with alcoholic liver disease. This hypothesis is supported by experimental studies demonstrating that Kupffer cells function abnormally in obese, diabetic, hyperlipidemic rats with steatosis and this abnormal phagocytic activity can play a permissive role for prolonged exposure to these cytokines, with the consequent development of hepatic inflammation, especially in females. This is also supported by some studies showing that some antibiotics prevent the development of liver damage in animals and humans after jejunoileal bypass performed for the control of morbid obesity and during total parenteral nutrition, suggesting that absorption of bacterial products may be responsible for development of liver damage in these patients. Likewise, intestinal bacteria are involved in a variety of potential hepatotoxic events, including deconjugation of bile salts, endogenous alcohol production, inactivation of hepatic lipotropes such as choline, release of endotoxin and peptidoglycan-polysaccharide polymers. Based on these data, it is tempting to speculate that proinflammatory and acute-phase cytokines serve as a permissive factor for the histological expression of alcohol-like injury in a fatty infiltrated liver. Further studies evaluating the role of endotoxin, cytokines, and, importantly, the immune response in the development of NASH in humans and in those nonobese, nondiabetic females and males are needed.

Cytochrome P450IIE1 (CYP2E1) and P-450 reductase (CYP reductase), which seem to have an important role in the development of clinical and experimental alcoholic liver disease, might also be involved in the development of NASH. CYP2E1 and CYP reductase produce hydroxyl radical, the most potent oxygen-centered radical responsible for initiation of lipid peroxidation, resulting in perpetuation of oxidative stress. Oxidative stress is considered to be a pivotal signal for expression of TNF-α and interleukins-1 (IL-1), 6 (IL-6), and 8 (IL-8). Increased levels of CYP2E1 have been demonstrated in the methionine- and choline-deficient diet model of steatohepatitis and in liver biopsies of patients with NASH. Oxidative stress produced by CYP2E1, as measured by depletion of glutathione and increased thiobarbituric acid reacting substances in the liver, has been demonstrated in this nutritional model of NASH.

Oxidative stress ensues whenever there is an imbalance between the generation of free radicals and the capacity of antioxidant defense. Vitamin E (alpha tocopherol) is a potent antioxidant, particularly against membrane lipid peroxidation and, along with others, is shown to suppress TNF-α, IL-6, and IL-8 expression by monocytes and/or Kupffer cells. The role of vitamin E and other antioxidants such as ascorbate and methionine in the development of NASH demand further evaluation. If any pathogenic role of alpha-tocopherol deficiency in the development of NASH is demonstrated, its adequate supplementation may be important for the prevention of hepatic steatosis and the increased vulnerability of the fatty liver to other factors such as endotoxemia in its progression to NASH (inflammation) and NASH to fibrosis and/or cirrhosis.

The role of nutrition in the development of NASH is suggested by several mechanisms: its apparent higher prevalence in obese patients, the apparent necessity of liver fatty infiltration as a condition for the subsequent development of inflammation, the development of nutritional deficiency during the phase of rapid weight loss and fat mobilization associated with liver damage after intestinal bypass, and the development of liver fatty infiltration during starvation and protein-calorie malnutrition. The critical role that nutrition can play in the pathogenesis of NASH, at least as a cofactor, can be deducted from the effects of specific deficiencies such as proteins, vitamin E, B_6, B_{12}, thiamine, folate, ascorbate, zinc, and selenium in normal hepatic physiology and antioxidant defenses. The actual role of these substances in the development of NASH needs to be further investigated.

Since NASH is seen in a subpopulation of patients with fatty liver and progression of NASH to increased fibrosis or cirrhosis has occurred in around 40% of those patients who had repeated liver biopsy during the follow-up, genetic predisposition for the development of this entity and its progression to a more severe disease cannot be excluded. Presence of autoantibodies and elevated hepatic iron concentration with improvement in aminotransferase level after phlebotomy, reported in a few patients with NASH, suggests a role of autoimmunity and iron in the development of this entity. However, a clear cause-and-effect has not been recognized and increased levels of serum and hepatic iron most likely result from underlying hepatic necroinflammatory activity. Toxic biles acids like lithocholic acid, might play a role in the production of liver damage in patients with NASH. Derived from its normal precursor by bacterial action, this secondary bile acid may well be absorbed in toxic amounts from the colon. Because the small bowel, which normally reabsorbs the primary bile acids, is bypassed, absorption of toxic biles acids has been implicated in the pathogenesis of liver damage after jejunoileal bypass and other conditions characterized by bacterial overgrowth. A potential role for toxic bile acids can be supported by the improvement in liver biochemistries and degree of steatosis after 12 months of treatment with ursodeoxycholic acid (UDCA), which seems to replace hepatotoxic bile acids.

ASSOCIATED CONDITIONS AND RISK FACTORS

It has been recognized for a number of decades that patients with obesity and/or diabetes can sometimes develop hepatic fatty infiltration and inflammation even without alcohol intake. Obesity with or without other factors such as diabetes, malnutrition, drug intake, hyperlipidemia, and female gender has been considered as a major risk factor for the development of NASH. A high prevalence of obesity in patients with NASH has been reported, varying from 60–100% in most series. A lower prevalence of 39% was reported by Bacon and colleagues. NASH has been found in 9–36% of morbidly obese patients. A relationship between the development of NASH and the degree of obesity, the presence of diabetes, and age has been reported in some series.

Prevalence of diabetes in patients with NASH has varied from 0% in children to 21–74% in adults and appears to be higher in NASH than in alcoholic steatohepatitis. About half of adult-onset diabetic patients have hepatic steatosis and most of them are obese women. Fatty liver is less common in insulin-dependent diabetic patients, with a reported incidence of 4.5–17%. Hepatomegaly in these cases is usually due to cytoplasmic glycogen deposition. It appears, therefore, that obesity or any obesity-associated condition is the major factor in the fatty infiltration seen in adult-onset diabetes and not the diabetes mellitus itself.

The reported incidence of hyperlipidemia in patients with NASH has varied from 21–81%, but its role in the development of NASH and the progression to fibrosis and/or cirrhosis has not been clearly evaluated. The increased prevalence of coexistent cardiovascular disease reported in patients with NASH in some series may be due to abnormalities in lipid metabolism in these patients.

The role of gender in the development of NASH is even less clear. Early studies reported a higher prevalence in women varying from 65–83% and leading to speculating that female gender was a permissive factor for the development of NASH. Recent series have reported a higher prevalence in men, 72% in children, and 58% in adults. One of these series found a higher prevalence in nonobese, nondiabetic men, emphasizing that NASH is not confined to obese diabetic women.

PATHOLOGY

The normal liver contains approximately 5 g of lipid per 100 g of wet weight, with phospholipid being the most abundant form. Although fatty acids are incorporated into phospholipids and cholesterol esters, the predominant lipid that accumulates in the liver in patients with NASH is triglyceride. Macroscopically and in the absence of cirrhosis, the liver has a pale yellow, greasy appearance and usually shows a substantial increase in size and weight, up to 6 kg. Lipids account for a greater proportion of the wet weight than in normal liver, up to as much as 50%. NASH reveals the same histological spectrum found in alcoholic hepatitis: hepatocellular steatosis, lobular inflammatory cell infiltrate, and sometimes Mallory bodies, fibrosis, and cirrhosis. Hepatic steatosis in patients with NASH is present primarily as large droplets or macrovesicular fat and is seen at low magnification as cytoplasmic vacuoles or clear holes within hepatocytes that represent the space occupied by the fat dissolved during routine tissue processing. The affected cells appear ballooned, like adipocytes with flattened peripheral nuclei. Appropriate stains, such as oil red O or Sudan black, on frozen sections is essential to visualize the fat, particularly to diagnose lesser degrees or steatosis. Fatty infiltration may be localized focally to the centrilobular region zone 3 of Rapaport's acinus, or it may be diffuse. A periportal distribution (zone 1) is found in some pathological states such as total parenteral nutrition, methotrexate injury, protein-calorie malnutrition, and some toxic states. Not only fatty infiltration but also cellular inflammatory infiltrates accompanying steatosis are required for the diagnosis of NASH. The inflammatory infiltrate may be mixed neutrophils and lymphocytes and seen predominantly in zone 3. Portal tracts are relatively spared from inflammation, and its presence should suggest other causes. Mallory's hyaline has been found in more than 50% of patients with NASH; even though it is most commonly seen in alcoholic liver disease, it is not specific for that condition. Fibrosis, when present, is a concerning histological finding in patients with NASH because it suggests an advanced and irreversible injury. It is first laid down in the pericellular space around the central vein and in the perisinusoidal region. With disease progression, fibrosis increases and the central-to-portal bridging that results leads to cirrhosis, with its consequent complications of portal hypertension and hepatic failure. NASH was previously not believed to progress to cirrhosis, but several studies clearly showed the presence of severe fibrosis or cirrhosis in approximately one-third of patients with NASH at the time of initial evaluation. Likewise, progression to cirrhosis has been documented in patients followed up for several years. Although the degree of inflammation, fatty infiltration, and Mallory bodies in the liver biopsy can suggest one or another diagnosis, no histological features clearly distinguish patients with alcoholic or non-alcoholic steatohepatitis. Bile duct injury is not seen in NASH.

CLINICAL PRESENTATION

Tables 3 and 4 show the clinical, laboratory, and histological data in 70 prospectively evaluated patients with nonalcoholic steatohepatitis seen at Mayo Clinic.

Symptoms and Signs

Most patients with NASH have no symptoms, and this entity is usually suspected in patients with abnormal laboratory tests, radiological findings, or unexplained persistent hepatomegaly. Some patients complain of a sensation of fullness or discomfort in the right upper abdomen that can be continuous or may occur after a large meal or when bending forward. Frequent complaints that are attributed to the liver disease include the nonspecific constitutional symptoms of tiredness, fatigue, diminished physical activity, loss of appetite, and malaise. Palpable hepatomegaly is the only physical finding in most patients with NASH, but it cannot be felt in some patients because of adipose tissue in the abdominal wall. The development of portal fibrosis or cirrhosis in a patient with NASH does not necessarily produce any striking change in the clinical picture. However, jaundice, palmar erythema, spider angiomata, splenomegaly, and ascites highly suggest advanced disease with progression to cirrhosis.

Laboratory

Mild-to-moderate elevation of serum aminotransferases (ALT, AST) is the most common and often the only laboratory abnormality found in patients with NASH. Serum levels are usually less than 300 IU/L or less than three times the upper limit of normal. Isolated elevation of serum aminotransferase in asymptomatic patients suggests NASH, particularly when the ALT level is greater than the AST level in contrast to alcoholic hepatitis. However, serum aminotransferase levels can be in the normal range in patients with morbid obesity and NASH. As in alcoholic steatohepatitis and chronic hepatitis C infection, there is no direct correlation between aminotransferase levels and degree of liver damage in

Table 3 Clinical and Histological Data in 70 Patients with Nonalcoholic Steatohepatitis Seen at the Mayo Clinic[a]

Mean age (years)	45
Gender F/M	47/23
	n (%)
Symptoms attributed to liver disease	35 (50)
Obesity	50 (71)
Adult-onset diabetes mellitus	17 (24)
Hyperlipidemia	28 (40)
Severe fibrosis/cirrhosis	12 (17)

[a]Diagnosis of NASH was based on liver biopsy showing steatosis and inflammation and other causes of liver disease such as alcohol abuse, viral infection (hepatitis virus B and C), and drugs; autoimmune and genetic/metabolic causes were appropriately excluded.

Table 4 Laboratory Data in 70 Patients with Nonalcoholic Steatohepatitis Seen at the Mayo Clinic[a]

Test (normal)	Mean ± SD	Range	% of patients with abnormal values
ALT (9–45 U/L)	97 ± 51	13–237	90
AST (12–31 U/L)	72 ± 47	21–334	86
Alkaline phosphatase (114–309 U/L)	240 ± 138	70–1171	11
GGT (9–48 U/L)	119 ± 139	24–765	72
Total bilirubin (0.1–1.1 mg/dL)	0.7 ± 0.3	0.2–1.5	13
Total protein (6.3–7.9 g/dL)	7.4 ± 0.4	6.1–8.9	15
Albumin (3.5–5 g/dL)	4.4 ± 0.5	2.1–5.4	3
Prothrombin time (8.4–12 s)	11.3 ± 0.9	8.4–13.3	24
Free fatty acids (239–843 μEq/L)[b]	792 ± 254	438–1515	30
Ceruloplasmin (23–43 mg/dL)	41 ± 13	20.7–94.5	2
Serum iron (35–150 μg/dL)	100 ± 46	42–253	12
Ferritin (20–300 μg/L)	294 ± 247	6–1196	38
Transferrin saturation (14–50%)	30 ± 12	10–60	6
TIBC (250–400 μg/dL)	336 ± 78	36–448	12
Autoantibodies > 1:80	6/50		9
Antinuclear	6/50		9
Antismooth muscle	0/50		0

[a]Diagnosis of NASH was based on liver biopsy showing steatosis and inflammation and other causes of liver disease such as alcohol abuse, viral infection (hepatitis virus B and C), and drugs; autoimmune and genetic/metabolic causes were appropriately excluded.
[b]Quantification in 30 patients.

patients with NASH. Although serum aminotransferase level is not an ideal test for identifying patients with NASH or to detect progression of fatty liver to NASH or NASH to cirrhosis, no other blood test has proven better and no test accurately estimates the extent of fatty infiltration, inflammation, or fibrosis. Gamma glutamyltransferase (GGT), alkaline phosphatase, and bilirubin are within the normal range or mildly elevated in the absence of substantial fibrosis or cirrhosis. High level of these enzymes should lead to a suspicion of biliary tract disease. When NASH has progressed to cirrhosis, other abnormalities such as hypoalbuminemia, elevation of the prothrombin time, and hyperbilirubinemia are frequently found. Elevation of fasting blood glucose and serum cholesterol or triglycerides can be seen in patients with poorly controlled diabetes and hyperlipidemia. In general, the severity of abnormalities in liver function tests in patients with NASH is less than that in patients with alcoholic steatohepatitis.

Variable titers of autoantibodies, such as antinuclear antibody and antismooth muscle antibody, can be found in some patients with NASH who do not have conclusive criteria for diagnosis of autoimmune hepatitis or a positive response to corticosteroids. Elevated serum iron, ferritin, and transferrin saturation can also be found. Furthermore, a hepatic iron concentration of more than 1500 μg/g dry weight has been reported in some patients, but with a calculated hepatic iron index that excludes homozygous hemochromatosis.

Imaging

Fatty infiltration of the liver produces a diffusely increased echogenicity that can be detected by ultrasound (US). This can be ascertained when the liver texture is compared with that of the kidney. The normal liver is only slightly more echogenic than the renal parenchyma; however, in patients with NASH, liver texture becomes markedly more echogenic than kidney texture. Cirrhosis is associated with a similar appearance, and in that case clear identification of the intrahepatic vessels—such as the left, middle, and right hepatic veins—concurrently with a regular hepatic surface is highly suggestive of NASH. Fatty infiltration of the liver produces a low-density hepatic parenchyma when it is analyzed by computed tomography (CT). In most patients with NASH, fatty infiltration is diffuse, and it is detected when fatty changes affect more than 50% of the hepatocytes within the imaged region. However, in some cases fatty infiltration may be focal and can be detected by CT as islands of low-density parenchyma or by US as an hyperechoic area relative to the surrounding unaffected liver. Focal fatty infiltration may sometimes be due to regional differences in perfusion with areas of decreased portal flow tending to accumulate less fat than do better perfused areas. Focal fatty infiltration detected by US and/or CT can be misinterpreted as metastases. In these cases, demonstration of a nonspherical mass with indistinct margins that does not produce a mass effect suggests the correct diagnosis of focal fatty infiltration. When one is confronted with the question of whether the focal lesions represent tumors or other masses or are merely regions of normal liver parenchyma embedded within the fatty infiltration, magnetic resonance imaging (MRI) can be an invaluable noninvasive imaging technique that is useful in distinguishing space-occupying lesions from focal fatty infiltration. The most effective technique for detecting regions of fatty liver is opposed-phase (outphase) imaging. A zone of decreased attenuation seen on a CT scan is likely to represent focal fatty infiltration if it appears normal on T2-weighted spin-echo MRI. The level of confidence for diagnosing focal fat is increased greatly by the use of a chemical-shift MRI technique. Although there is no universal agreement as to whether MRI is superior to CT in the evaluation of the liver, a number of reports have found MRI superior to CT. In addition, greater incremental improvement in MRI compared with CT is expected. Radionuclide imaging is no longer a primary method for detecting the presence of focal liver defects. Uptake of colloid sulfur in technetium-99m (^{99m}Tc) sulfur colloid study reflects the number of Kupffer cells within the liver parenchyma. In patients with focal fatty infiltration, the sulfur colloid study will demonstrate that the lesions seen on CT have normal uptake of colloid; but when single-photon-emission tomography (SPECT) is performed, these lesions can produce defects on the sulfur colloid study with normal uptake by the normal parenchyma. In these cases, sulfur colloid studies do not separate benign from malignant lesions. Studies with xenon^{133} have been recommended to confirm the presence of fatty infiltration, since its high partition coefficient causes xenon to be taken up by fat; however, xenon uptake occurs much less consistently than sulfur colloid defects

Natural History

The natural history of NASH has not been well defined. It is clear that NASH is not a benign disorder but one that can progress to irreversible liver disease. Some patients present with advanced fibrosis or cirrhosis at the time of diagnosis. In other instances the disease remains stable or progresses over many years. The actual progression of NASH to severe fibrosis and/or cirrhosis has not been completely evaluated, since only a few patients have been followed with liver biopsy performed over time. Taking these results together, it seems that progression to fibrosis or cirrhosis occurs in around 40% of patients during the first 10 years of follow-up, with steatohepatitis unchanged in most of the remainder and even improvement or resolution in a few of them. Even though obesity is clearly a risk factor for the development of NASH, specific risk factors for the progression of NASH to fibrosis and/or cirrhosis have not been clearly identified. Presence of pericentral and perisinusoidal fibrosis have been recognized as precursor lesions for progression to severe fibrosis and cirrhosis. Female gender and obesity did appear to be linked to the more severe form of the disease in a recent report. Survival probability in 30 patients with NASH has been reported to be 67% and 59% by 5 and 10 years, respectively. This survival is significantly higher when compared with the survival of patients with alcoholic steatohepatitis but not significantly lower than that of an age- and sex-matched normal population. Pure nonalcoholic fatty liver has a more benign course when inflammation and fibrosis are absent, as has been shown in a long-term follow-up study.

DIAGNOSIS

The typical patient with NASH is a middle-age woman with adult-onset diabetes and obesity, defined as a body weight more than 10% above expected (ideal) weight. However, because NASH affects not only obese women with diabetes, it should be suspected in any individual with otherwise unexplained elevation of serum aminotransferase levels, no matter the gender, diabetic status, or body habitus. Evaluation of patients with liver biochemical abnormalities should begin with blood tests to exclude infectious, autoimmune and metabolic causes. US and/or CT are the noninvasive imaging techniques most used in the evaluation of patients with unexplained elevation of aminotransferase and/or hepatomegaly, and one or the other should be performed when NASH is a diagnostic consideration. When other causes of liver disease have been excluded and fatty infiltration is revealed by US or CT in a patient with an elevation of serum aminotransferase, a liver biopsy can be considered unless a drug or environmental factor is considered to be responsible, in which case a diagnostic trial of avoidance is warranted. The diagnosis of NASH should be made based on the correct histopathological appearance previously described. Because fatty infiltration frequently exists in the presence of concurrent hepatic pathology in the setting of abnormalities in serum biochemistries, a biopsy may be warranted to determine the presence or absence of inflammation, fibrosis, and cirrhosis, particularly when medical management will be affected.

Incidental imaging detection of fatty infiltration with normal liver enzymes probably does not warrant percutaneous biopsy, although normal liver enzymes in obese patients do not exclude the presence of steatohepatitis or fibrosis progressing to a more severe disease. Liver biopsy is not needed in patients with fatty infiltration during total parenteral nutrition or with hepatomegaly in poorly controlled diabetic patients unless warranted by lack of resolution of the hepatic abnormality.

Differential Diagnosis

Some disease states are associated with hepatic fatty infiltration and inflammation. Among them, alcoholic steatohepatitis should always be considered as a diagnostic possibility when the histological picture previously described is found in the liver biopsy. Lack of antecedent alcohol history or alcohol abuse confirmed by the patient and sometimes through interviews with family members who are in close contact with the patient will be helpful in excluding alcoholic liver disease. Symptoms such as fever, anorexia, nausea and vomiting, and signs of portal hypertension and liver failure such as spider angiomata, jaundice, splenomegaly, and ascites are more often found in patients with alcoholic steatohepatitis than NASH. A cholestatic picture in the liver function tests with elevation of alkaline phosphatase, GGT, and serum bilirubin in conjunction with a AST/ALT ratio higher than two highly suggest alcoholic liver disease. In particularly difficult cases, blood alcohol levels can be helpful. Ingestion of any drug associated with steatohepatitis—such as corticosteroids, high-dose estrogens, amiodarone, calcium channel blockers, tamoxifen, salicylates, or tetracycline in the previous months—should be excluded. Because fatty infiltration, inflammation, and Mallory-like cytoplasmic inclusions resembling NASH can be found in patients with chronic hepatitis C, this hepatic infection should always be excluded and not considered a form of NASH. Autoimmune hepatitis should be excluded in patients with autoantibodies, particularly with titers to nuclei or smooth muscle > 1:80 for adults or > 1:20 for children. In these cases, other laboratory and histological criteria for the diagnosis of autoimmune hepatitis should be sought. In some patients, however, a therapeutic trial with corticosteroids may be necessary. Wilson's disease and sometimes alpha-1 antitrypsin deficiency and hemochromatosis should be considered in the differential diagnosis of NASH. These genetic diseases must be confidently excluded because of different effective therapies and important familial implications. A careful clinical history, disease-specific laboratory tests, and expert histological examination of the liver biopsy exclude alternative diagnoses in most instances.

TREATMENT

No medical treatment has proven to be totally effective for all patients with NASH. Obese patients with NASH should be enrolled in a weight-reduction program. Several studies demonstrating normalization of liver biochemistries resulting from weight reduction have been reported. Weight reduction is accompanied by improvement in fatty infiltration in obese patients taking a low-calorie diet. However, in patients with a high degree of fatty infiltration, pronounced reduction of fatty change and faster weight loss seem to promote portal inflammation or fibrosis as a complication of weight loss. Rate and exact quantification of degree of weight loss required for normalization of liver histology have not been established. Weight reduction ($\geqslant$ 10%) corrected abnormal liver biochemistries in adults and children; however, no histological data were available. Aminotransferase levels are insensitive markers of liver damage and of progression to a more severe disease. The resolution of fatty infiltration cannot be detected by using only conventional liver biochemistries. Weight loss < 1.6 kg/week has been recommended, since none of the patients losing less than 230 g/day developed fibrosis. Weight loss of about 500 g/week has been used in children to normalize persistent elevation of aminotransferase. The means by which weight loss is achieved is important and can play a critical role in developing more severe liver damage. Starvation or total fasting seems not to be effective. In contrast, it has been associated with development of pericellular and portal fibrosis, bile stasis, and focal necrosis. This paradoxical effect can be due to a high amount of fat mobilization with an important increase in the level of circulating free fatty acids from adipose tissue. Thus, maintenance of weight loss may lead to marked improvement in liver histology in some patients but may also have adverse effects on liver histology in others. In addition, achieving an ideal weight is virtually impossible for many patients.

Because low-calorie diets are not without risk, patients should be carefully evaluated prior to treatment. Different caloric restrictions have been used. A formula providing 600–800 calories per day with 45–100 g of high-quality animal protein, less than 100 g carbohydrate, and less than 10 g fat in adults seems to be reasonable, particularly for patients who are $\geqslant$ 30% overweight. Prescription of this low-calorie diet has been recommended by some authors only after more conventional 1200 calorie per day diets have been tried and proven unsuccessful. Diet to produce weight loss should always be prescribed on an individual basis, with some modifications according to overall patient health. Individuals who have obesity-related disease such as diabetes mellitus, hyperlipidemia, or cardiovascular disease will require close medical supervision during weight loss to adjust the medication dosage as needed.

Gradual and sustained weight loss but not total starvation seems to be necessary to reduce the amount of fat in the liver; if fatty infiltration per se is the sine qua non for NASH development and progression to cirrhosis, maintenance of an ideal body weight should be the main therapeutic goal. However, further investigation is needed to determine the adequate quantity and rate of weight loss as well as the content of the formula to be recommended for obese patients with NASH.

Although no correlation exists between the degree of control of the diabetes and fatty infiltration, all obese patients with adult-onset diabetes and NASH should be enrolled in a weight-reduction program with a low-carbohydrate, high-protein diet and considered for therapy with an oral hypoglycemic agent. Patients with insulin-dependent diabetes and hepatomegaly will show improvement in symptoms due to hepatomegaly when appropriate control of hyperglycemia is achieved.

Metronidazole and polymyxin B have been shown to prevent and sometimes reverse the development of fatty infiltration after intestinal bypass in obese patients and during total parenteral nutrition, respectively. Beneficial effects of intestinal decontamination in order to reduce proinflammatory cytokine production in NASH has not been evaluated. Specific nutritional deficiencies such as plasma-free choline deficiency during total parenteral nutrition has been implicated as a cause of fatty infiltration, and its supplementation was associated with resolution of hepatic steatosis. Several drugs (see Table 2) and environmental exposure to hepatotoxins—such as petrochemical substances and, rarely, carbon tetrachloride and phosphorus compounds, which have long been known to cause NASH or hepatic steatosis—should be sought in these patients, since their withdrawal may be accompanied by resolution of the liver disease.

The decision to intervene with pharmacological therapy aimed at the underlying steatohepatitis is based on the anticipated risks of progression to severe liver disease. The usefulness of different drugs in the treatment of NASH needs to be evaluated in controlled trials. This is particularly true for those patients who do not achieve ideal body weight and for nonobese patients with NASH. However, pilot studies evaluating new treatments and drugs may be necessary as a first step before organizing larger studies.

Clofibrate is a lipid-lowering drug that decrease the content of hepatic triglyceride in rats with ethanol-induced hepatic steatosis. Based on this, a pilot study was performed to evaluate the usefulness of clofibrate 2 g/day in the treatment of NASH, but after 12 months of therapy there was no significant change from baseline in liver biochemistries, or degree of fatty infiltration, inflammation, or fibrosis.

Ursodeoxycholic acid (UDCA) is the epimer of chenodeoxycholic acid and appears to replace endogenous bile acids, of which some may be hepatotoxic, with the non-hepatotoxic UDCA. UDCA has membrane-stabilizing or cytoprotective and immunological effects, with symptomatic and biochemical improvement in patients with primary biliary cirrhosis and autoimmune hepatitis. In a pilot study performed in 24 patients with well-defined NASH, UDCA 13–15 mg/kg/day for 12 months was associated with significant improvement in ALT, alkaline phosphatase, GGT, and hepatic steatosis compared to baseline. The possible benefit of UDCA is now being investigated in the context of a randomized controlled trial.

A better understanding of pathogenic mechanisms will certainly lead us to evaluate different drugs blocking essential steps in the development and progression of NASH, such as agents that decrease cytokine release or block cytokine actions, agents that reduce oxidative stress, and those that can supplement endogenous antioxidant stores.

If NASH progresses to cirrhosis, with its consequent complications of portal hypertension and liver failure, orthotopic liver transplantation remains a potential lifesaving therapeutic alternative.

BIBLIOGRAPHY

Anderson T, Gluud C, Franzmann MB, Christoffersen P. Hepatic effects of dietary weight loss in morbidly obese subjects. J Hepatol 1991; 12:224–229.

Bacon BR, Farahvash MJ, Janney CG, Neuschwander-Tetri BA. Nonalcoholic steatohepatitis: an expanded clinical entity. Gastroenterology 1994; 107:1103–1109.

Buchman AL, Dubin MD, Moukarzel A, Jenden JD, Roch M, Rice KM, Gornbein J, Ament ME. Choline deficiency: a cause of hepatic steatosis during parenteral nutrition that can be reversed by intravenous choline supplementation. Hepatology 1995; 22:1399–1043.

Drenick EJ, Fisler J, Johnson D. Hepatic steatosis after intestinal bypass: prevention and reversal by metronidazole, irrespective of protein-calorie malnutrition. Gastroenterology 1982; 82:532–548.

Kanders BS, Blackburn GL. Very-low-calorie diets for the treatment of obesity. In: Blackburn GL, Kanders BS, eds. Obesity: Pathophysiology, Psychology and Treatment. New York: Chapman and Hall 1994:197–215.

Laurin J, Lindor KD, Crippin JS, Gossard A, Gores GJ, Ludwig J, Rakela J, McGill D. Ursodeoxycholic acid or clofibrate in the treatment of non-alcohol-induced steatohepatitis: a pilot study. Hepatology 1996; 23:1464–1467.

Ludwig J, Viggiano TR, McGill DB, Ott BJ. Nonalcoholic steatohepatitis: Mayo Clinic experience with a hitherto unnamed disease. Mayo Clin Proc 1980; 55:434–438.

Pappo I, Becovier H, Berry EM, Freund HR. Polymyxin B reduces cecal flora, TNF production and hepatic steatosis during total parenteral nutrition in the rat. J Surg Res 1991; 51:106–112.

Vajro P, Fontanella A, Perna C, Orso G, Tadesco M, De Vincenso A. Persistent hyperaminotransferasemia resolving after weight reduction in obese children. J Pediatr 1994; 125:239–241.

27

Management of Hemochromatosis

Bruce Y. Tung and Kris V. Kowdley
University of Washington, Seattle, Washington

INTRODUCTION AND CLASSIFICATION

Hemochromatosis is defined as the abnormal accumulation of iron in parenchymal tissues, especially the liver, heart, pancreas, and other organs. The term *hemochromatosis* is used most commonly to denote *hereditary hemochromatosis* (HHC, primary hemochromatosis, genetic hemochromatosis), the HLA-linked disorder caused by abnormally increased intestinal iron absorption. HHC should be distinguished from other forms of iron overload, specifically *secondary iron overload* and *parenteral iron overload* (Table 1). Secondary iron overload may occur in disorders of ineffective erythropoiesis, including thalassemia major and sideroblastic anemia, and in chronic liver diseases, particularly alcoholic liver disease and chronic viral hepatitis. Parenteral iron overload is caused by multiple red blood cell transfusions or other forms of parenteral iron.

There is increased intestinal iron absorption in secondary iron overload, which is stimulated by the underlying disorder. In addition, these patients may receive multiple transfusions that contribute to excess total body iron. Parenteral iron overload is distinguished by initial accumulation of iron in cells of the reticuloendothelial system; in contrast, iron loading occurs primarily in hepatocytes in HHC. Over time, many of the end-organ effects of secondary iron overload may be similar to those in HHC. Parenchymal iron accumulation may also occur in parenteral iron overload once the reticuloendothelial system becomes saturated with iron, leading to clinical manifestations of iron overload. This chapter focuses on the pathogenesis, clinical presentation, diagnosis, and management of HHC and its complications, with a brief discussion of iron chelation therapy for secondary and parenteral iron overload.

EPIDEMIOLOGY AND GENETICS

Hereditary hemochromatosis (HHC) is the most common genetic disorder in persons of Northern European descent, with a gene frequency of approximately 5–7% and an esti-

Table 1 Classification of Iron Overload

Hereditary hemochromatosis (genetic, primary)
Secondary iron overload
Ineffective erythropoiesis
Thalassemia major
Sideroblastic anemia
Chronic liver disease
Alcoholic cirrhosis
Chronic viral hepatitis
Postportacaval shunt
Porphyria cutanea tarda
Parenteral iron overload
Transfusional iron overload
Excess parenteral iron
Neonatal hemochromatosis
African iron overload

Source: Adapted from Bacon and Tavill, 1996.

mated disease prevalence of 1 in 300. It is inherited as an autosomal recessive trait; penetrance is age-related and may be incomplete.

The putative gene for HHC is known to exist on the short arm of chromosome 6, in linkage with the locus for HLA-A of the major histocompatibility complex. Furthermore, HHC is associated with specific HLA-A and B phenotypes; HLA-A3 occurs in 73% of HHC patients, HLA-B7 in 47%, and HLA-B14 in 29%. A putative gene for HHC, termed *HFE* (formerly known as HLA-H), has recently been identified. A specific G-to-A missense mutation at nucleotide 845 of *HFE*, which leads to a cysteine to tyrosine substitution at amino acid 282 (C282Y), has been found to be homozygous in 82–100% of HHC patients. A second missense mutation, with substitution of histidine to aspartate at amino acid 63 (H63D), has also been described, but is of unclear clinical significance. Only C282Y homozygotes and some C282Y/H63D compound heterozygotes appear to be at risk of significant iron overload. Genetic testing for the C282Y mutation is very useful in the diagnosis and screening of HHC, although further study in this area is needed to more precisely define its role.

PATHOPHYSIOLOGY

The underlying metabolic defect in HHC appears to be abnormally regulated iron absorption in the proximal small intestine. In normal persons, iron deficiency leads to enhanced intestinal absorption of iron, and iron repletion is followed by a resultant decline in iron absorption. In HHC patients, absorption of iron is inappropriately elevated despite high body iron stores and high circulating iron levels. The potential role of the *HFE* gene product in the regulation of iron absorption has not yet been discovered.

The liver serves as a major site of iron storage, in the normal state as well as in cases of iron overload. In HHC, hepatic iron deposition occurs primarily in hepatocytes (Fig. 1). The characteristic pattern of iron staining in HHC reveals prominent iron deposition in

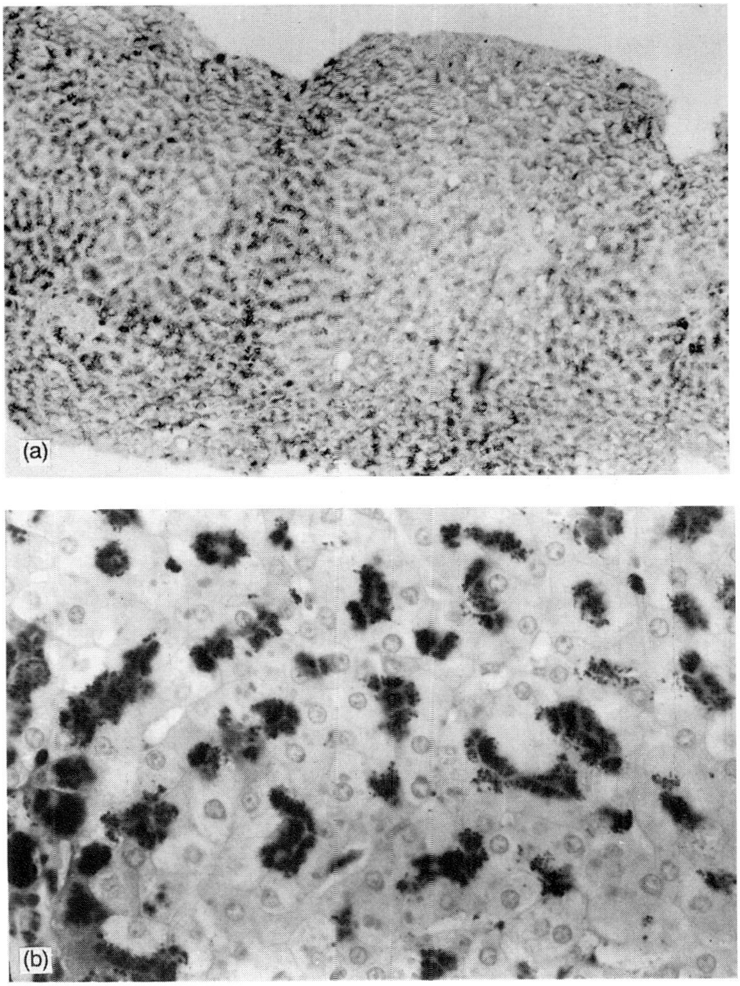

Figure 1 (a) Liver biopsy in hereditary hemochromatosis. Iron staining is predominantly confined to periportal hepatocytes, with a decreasing intensity of staining in pericentral hepatocytes. (Perls' Prussian blue stain.) (b) Liver biopsy in transfusional iron overload. Iron staining is panlobular and confined to Kupffer cells, with sparing of hepatocytes. (Perls' Prussian blue stain.)

periportal hepatocytes (zone 1 of Rappaport), with decreasing intensity of iron staining in pericentral hepatocytes (zone 3). Fibrosis begins in the portal triads and may lead to micronodular cirrhosis. This progression of hepatic involvement is often seen without significant infiltration of inflammatory cells or active hepatitis.

The exact mechanism by which iron accumulation leads to liver damage is unknown. Most experimental evidence points to an important role for iron-induced generation of free radical species. These free radical species may have wide-ranging deleterious effects on hepatocytes, especially the initiation of lipid peroxidation of membrane phospholipids, with subsequent mitochondrial and lysosomal dysfunction. It has also been postulated that iron-induced oxidative damage to hepatic DNA may play an important role in hepatocarcinogenesis. These potentially cytotoxic effects of iron-induced free radical species most likely overwhelm cytoprotective mechanisms—such as antioxidants, scavenging enzymes, and repair processes—in order for cellular damage to occur. Hepatic fibrogenesis is thought to be triggered by activation of hepatic stellate cells, which may, in turn, be stimulated directly or indirectly by iron-induced lipid peroxidation.

CLINICAL FEATURES

The classic clinical features of HHC may not present until the fourth or fifth decades of life. Phenotypic expression of the disease is influenced by dietary intake of iron, alcohol intake, and pathological or physiological blood loss. Accordingly, men present earlier than women, as menstruation delays iron loading in women. Dietary heme iron is usually well absorbed, although absorption of nonheme iron can be increased (vitamin C, meat-containing diets) or decreased (dietary fiber, tannins) by other dietary components. In areas where consumption of meat and alcohol is high, phenotypic expression of HHC is probably very common and may be complete.

With earlier diagnosis through population and family screening, the clinical presentation of HHC is changing. Identification of patients with HHC from abnormal serum iron studies or liver function tests before the development of symptoms is increasingly common. The classical description of "bronze diabetes" is now uncommonly seen. The most common presenting symptoms of HHC are shown in Table 2. Impotence, weakness, and arthralgias are frequent in men, and weakness, arthralgias, and symptoms related to liver disease are frequent in women. The most common clinical findings of HHC at diagnosis are shown in Table 3. Hepatomegaly is present in > 50% of newly diagnosed HHC patients; skin pigmentation and arthritis are also frequently observed. Cirrhosis and/or overt diabetes mellitus are seen more commonly than congestive heart failure or cardiac arrhythmias.

DIAGNOSIS

Serum iron studies—including the serum iron concentration, total iron binding capacity (TIBC), and serum ferritin—are usually the first tests ordered when the diagnosis of HHC is considered. Several large studies have confirmed that a threshold transferrin saturation

Table 2 Frequency of Symptoms in Patients Diagnosed with Hereditary Hemochromatosis

Symptom (%)	Edwards et al. $n = 35$	Adams et al. $n = 120$	Niederau et al. $n = 251$
Weakness/lethargy	20	62	82
Impotence/amenorrhea	29	46	34
Abdominal pain	23	22	56
Arthralgia	57	54	44
Shortness of breath	—	19	12
Asymptomatic	37	12	—

Table 3 Frequency of Clinical Findings in Patients Diagnosed with Hereditary Hemochromatosis

Clinical finding (%)	Edwards et al. $n = 35$	Adams et al. $n = 120$	Niederau et al. $n = 251$
Hepatomegaly	54	61	81
Skin pigmentation	43	46	72
Splenomegaly	40	—	10
Arthropathy	31	45	—
Testicular atrophy	24	24	—
Loss of body hair	6	—	16
Cardiac failure	0	19	—
Diabetes mellitus	6	33	48
Cirrhosis (biopsy)	40	42	57
None	29	13	—

(serum iron/TIBC) $\geqslant$ 60% in males and $\geqslant$ 50% in females is sensitive and specific in identifying asymptomatic individuals with HHC. Serum ferritin is usually > 400 ng/mL but is nonspecific for the diagnosis of HHC.

Patients with abnormal serum iron studies should undergo liver biopsy for histological evaluation with iron staining, as well as quantitative measurement of hepatic iron concentration (HIC) (Fig. 2). A pattern of excess iron deposition in periportal hepatocytes with a decreasing concentration of iron deposition in pericentral hepatocytes is consistent with a diagnosis of HHC. Liver biopsy is essential not only in establishing a diagnosis of HHC but also in determining prognosis. Evidence of established cirrhosis has important implications for prognosis as well as the need to screen patients for the development of hepatocellular carcinoma.

Determination of the HIC remains the gold standard in the diagnosis of HHC. Hepatic iron is best measured from fresh tissue that is sent dry, in an iron-free container. Immersion of the biopsy specimen in saline has been shown to artifactually lower the measured iron concentration and should be avoided. When necessary, HIC can also be determined from formalin-fixed, paraffin-embedded specimens. In homozygotes for HHC, HIC is almost always greater than 4000 μg/g dry weight. In addition to HIC, the hepatic iron index (HII) is also helpful in distinguishing patients with homozygous HHC from those with lesser degrees of iron loading, such as heterozygotes for HHC or patients with alcoholic or chronic viral liver disease. The HII is calculated by dividing HIC (in micromoles per gram of dry weight) by patient age (in years) and is based on the concept that HHC homozygotes continue to accumulate iron over time, whereas heterozygotes and those with other causes of mild iron overload do not. Therefore, HII is usually $\geqslant$ 1.9 in HHC homozygotes and < 1.9 in iron loading from these other causes (Fig. 3). However, an HII $\geqslant$ 1.9 is not reliable in distinguishing HHC from parental iron overload; the pattern of iron staining on histological specimens is the most useful in making this distinction (Fig. 1).

The diagnosis of HHC may be equivocal when the HII is between 1.5 and 1.9. In this situation, quantitative phlebotomy can help confirm the diagnosis of HHC. Homozygotes for HHC almost always have more than 4 g of excess body iron; as each unit of blood contains approximately 250 mg of elemental iron, a minimum of 16–20 phlebotomies may

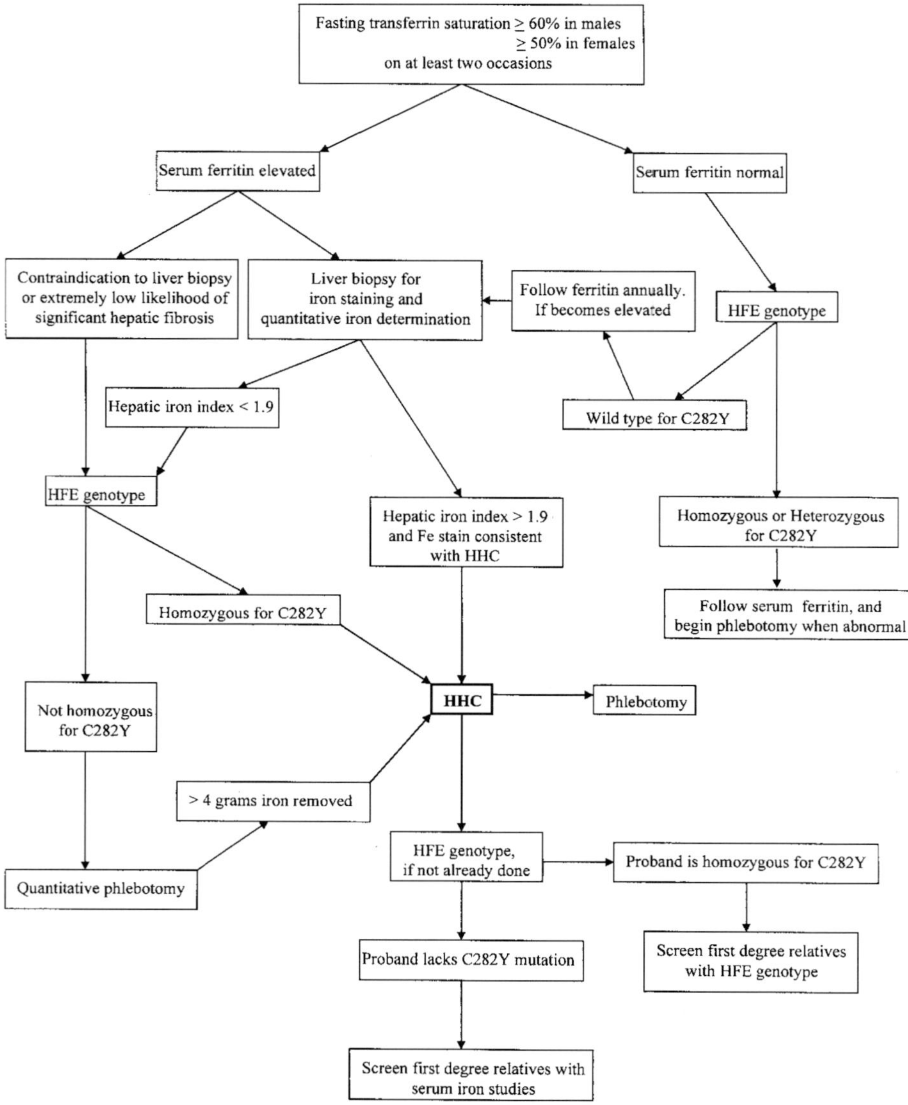

Figure 2 Suggested algorithm for the diagnosis and family screening of patients with hereditary hemochromatosis. (Reprinted from Tung and Kowdley, 1998.)

be needed to achieve iron depletion. Those patients who become iron-depleted after only a few phlebotomies are unlikely to be homozygotes for HHC.

Genetic testing for the C282Y mutation of *HFE* is available as a diagnostic test for HHC. This mutation is present in 82–100% of patients clinically diagnosed with HHC and is likely to be the causative mutation in most HHC patients. Genetic testing for a second mutation in *HFE*, H63D, is also available, although it is unclear if this mutation alone is a cause of HHC. The precise role of genetic testing in HHC is not yet defined, although it is likely to become an extremely important tool in the diagnosis and screening of patients and

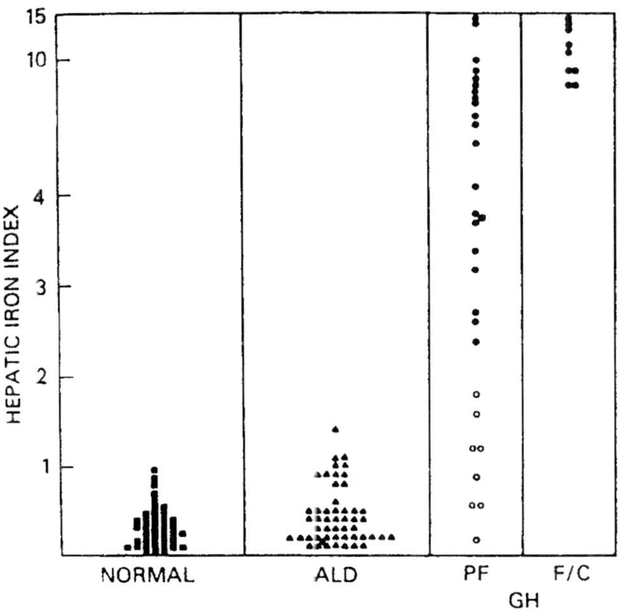

Figure 3 Hepatic iron index in normal subjects, alcoholic liver disease subjects (ALD), and hereditary hemochromatosis subjects (GH). PF = prefibrotic, F/C = fibrotic or cirrhotic. GH heterozygotes are shown by open circles and GH homozygotes are shown by closed circles. (From Bassett et al., 1986.)

their families. Further clinical studies and the potential identification of other significant mutations will help to further define the role of genetic testing in HHC. A suggested algorithm for the diagnosis and family screening of HHC utilizing genetic testing is shown in Figure 2.

In patients with advanced liver disease and cirrhosis, establishing a diagnosis of HHC is extremely difficult. Patients with cirrhosis from any cause often have reduced hepatic synthesis of serum proteins such as transferrin. Decreased serum transferrin levels may therefore elevate transferrin saturation into the range usually seen in HHC. Liver biopsy is often difficult to perform in this setting because of coagulopathy, ascites, and thrombocytopenia. Furthermore, liver biopsy may not be diagnostic, because the specificity of HIC and HII for the diagnosis of HHC is reduced in the setting of cirrhosis. Genetic testing may prove to be useful for the diagnosis of HHC in the setting of end-stage liver disease.

Because of the small but finite risks associated with percutaneous liver biopsy, much interest has been focused on the development of noninvasive measures of hepatic iron. Computed tomography (CT) scanning is neither sensitive nor specific for the detection of hepatic iron overload, especially when hepatic iron is only mildly to moderately elevated. Magnetic resonance imaging (MRI) has shown some promise, as iron overload leads to enhancement of the transverse relaxation (T2) rate. Several studies have demonstrated that the T2 relaxation rate correlates well with measured hepatic iron concentration. If MRI can be proved to correlate with HIC through a broad range of iron concentrations in clinical studies and can be inexpensively performed, it may provide an important noninvasive means of confirming the diagnosis of HHC.

SCREENING

Family screening is an important part of the care of patients with HHC, as discovery of the disease in the presymptomatic period is associated with a normal life expectancy if patients are compliant with phlebotomy. Because the disorder is inherited as an autosomal recessive trait, all first-degree relatives (especially siblings) should be screened. Serum iron studies should be obtained on all first-degree relatives and liver biopsy performed if these studies are abnormal. For siblings of HHC probands, HLA-typing at the A and B loci may be useful. Siblings who share no HLA-A or B hepatocytes with the proband have negligible risk for the development of significant iron accumulation. Siblings who share both HLA-A and B haplotypes with the proband are presumed HHC homozygotes and are at risk of developing clinical iron overload. In rare cases where these putative homozygotes do not show evidence of iron loading, genetic crossover events that disrupt the linkage between the HHC gene and HLA loci are possible causes. Siblings who share one HLA-A or B haplotype with HHC probands are putative heterozygotes for HHC. These putative heterozygotes may have mildly abnormal serum iron studies or mildly elevated hepatic iron but do not accumulate iron over time and do not develop clinically significant iron overload. It may be prudent to check serum iron studies every 2–3 years in these putative heterozygotes to exclude progressive iron accumulation suggestive of such a genetic crossover event. Detection of the C282Y mutation of the putative HHC gene *HFE* is more precise than HLA typing in identifying HHC patients and their asymptomatic family members. Testing of probands and all first-degree relatives for C282Y has supplanted HLA testing for screening family members of HHC patients (Fig. 2), and is not susceptible to errors due to genetic crossover.

HHC is an ideal disease for population-based screening because it is a common disorder, has a long asymptomatic period, is treatable if detected early, leads to significant morbidity and mortality if untreated, and has a readily available screening test. Despite the demonstration in several studies that population screening with transferrin saturation is both feasible and cost-effective, it has yet to be accepted into widespread use. The measurement of the unsaturated iron-binding capacity (UIBC) has also been proposed as an accurate and less expensive test for population screening.

THERAPY OF IRON OVERLOAD

The goal of therapy in HHC is to prevent or reverse the organ damage associated with excess iron accumulation. Part of this goal must be achieved through making a timely diagnosis, as cirrhosis of the liver and diabetes mellitus are irreversible complications of HHC and do not improve with iron-reduction therapy. In contrast, some degree of hepatic fibrosis may improve with iron reduction, and patients who begin phlebotomy therapy prior to the development of cirrhosis have a normal life expectancy (Fig. 4). Once cirrhosis is present, life expectancy is reduced, and the risk of developing hepatocellular carcinoma is increased roughly 200-fold.

Phlebotomy is the mainstay of iron reduction therapy. Most patients tolerate phlebotomy of 500 mL of blood once or twice per week, removing 250 mg of iron per phlebotomy. Weekly phlebotomy is continued until iron depletion is attained, confirmed by the presence of mild anemia, decreased transferrin saturation ($< 45\%$), and decreased serum ferritin (< 50 ng/mL). Some physicians will continue phlebotomy until iron defi-

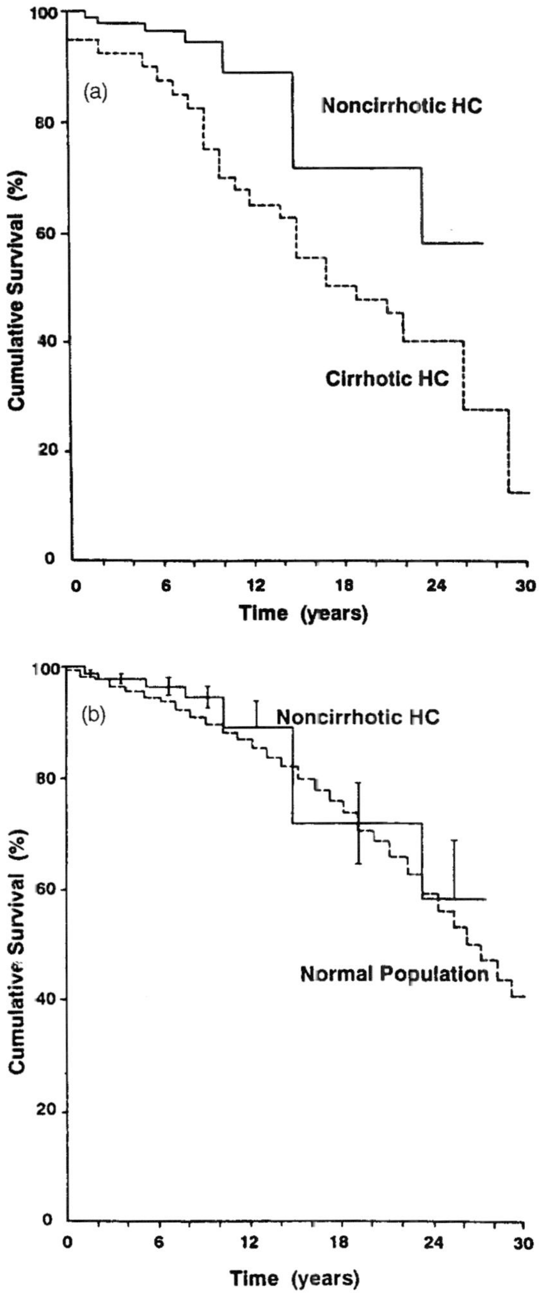

Figure 4 (a) Cumulative survival in patients with hereditary hemochromatosis (HHC). Survival is significantly reduced in the cirrhotic patients as compared with the noncirrhotic patients. (b) Cumulative survival in noncirrhotic patients with HHC. Survival in noncirrhotic patients with HHC matches the rate expected for an age- and sex-matched normal population. (From Niederau et al., 1996.)

ciency is reached, i.e., ferritin < 10 ng/mL, or transferrin saturation is < 10%. Depending on the initial body iron load, iron depletion may take 1–2 years to achieve in some HHC patients. After a state of iron depletion is reached, lifelong maintenance phlebotomy is necessary but may require only 0–4 phlebotomies per year, with a goal of keeping serum ferritin < 50 ng/mL.

Iron chelation therapy with deferoxamine mesylate (desferrioxamine) has a limited role in the treatment of patients with HHC. Chelation therapy removes substantially less iron than phlebotomy, with a maximum of approximately 100 mg of iron per week. In HHC patients, chelation therapy with deferoxamine is reserved for those with severe cardiomyopathy or cardiac arrhythmias. In these selected patients, combination therapy of chelation and phlebotomy promotes accelerated iron reduction.

Chelation therapy is used most commonly in patients with iron overload in the setting of anemia, since these patients cannot tolerate phlebotomy. Thalassemia major is the most frequent indication, but iron chelation may be beneficial in many other hematological disorders that lead to secondary or parenteral iron overload. The main drawback of chelation with deferoxamine is that it must be given either subcutaenously or intravenously as a daily infusion in order to maximize its efficacy. Deferoxamine is a complex hydroxylamine that binds ferris ions, forming ferrioxamine, which is mostly excreted in the urine. However, up to 30–40% of deferoxamine-bound iron is excreted in bile and ultimately in feces; thus 24-h urine collections alone are not accurate in calculating daily iron balance.

Deferoxamine is typically given as a continuous subcutaneous infusion, usually 20–50 mg/kg/day over 10–12 h. This can be accomplished on an outpatient basis with a battery-powered portable infusion pump. In patients with more extensive end-organ damage or those who are noncompliant with subcutaneous infusion, continuous intravenous infusion allows higher doses of deferoxamine and more aggressive iron reduction. Up to 16 g deferoxamine can be given over 24 h in a continuous intravenous infusion.

Deferoxamine is generally well tolerated, although some patients may develop local inflammation at the site of subcutaneous infusion; this is dependent on the deferoxamine concentration in the infusate. In addition, cataracts, retinal toxicity, and ototoxicity have been described and tend to occur when body iron stores are low. This ocular and ototoxicity usually improves when chelation therapy is stopped or when the dose is reduced. Anaphylactic reactions to deferoxamine are rare but have been reported with intravenous and intramuscular administration.

Although vitamin C administration augments the iron chelation response to deferoxamine, it must be used cautiously to prevent enhancement of cardiac toxicity and intestinal iron absorption. Current recommendations are to withhold vitamin C supplementation until cardiac abnormalities have been corrected with chelation and then to limit vitamin C dose to no more than 200 mg daily in patients who are receiving ongoing chelation therapy. In addition, vitamin C should be taken on an empty stomach in order to minimize its enhancement of dietary nonheme iron absorption.

Because chelation therapy with deferoxamine is time-consuming, invasive, and costly, much interest has been focused the development of oral iron chelators. The most widely studied of these is 1,2,dimethyl-3-hydroxypyrid-4-one (L, deferiprone). Although this agent has been shown to be an effective and relatively selective iron chelator, there has been a high incidence of significant adverse effects (agranulocytosis, arthropathy, development of autoantibodies, and death) in preliminary studies. Ongoing clinical studies will hopefully clarify the safety of this agent. Other oral iron chelators are currently being developed, although none has yet shown an acceptable combination of efficacy, selectivity, and safety.

MANAGEMENT OF THE COMPLICATIONS OF HHC

Liver Disease

Excess iron deposition in hepatocytes may continue for years without development of symptoms. Hepatomegaly is a common finding and may be accompanied by splenomegaly if cirrhosis has developed. The presence or absence of cirrhosis is the most important prognostic indicator in HHC. As discussed above, institution of phlebotomy therapy prior to the development of cirrhosis can provide normal life expectancy. In contrast, life expectancy is reduced in patients with cirrhosis, even if iron reduction therapy is begun (Fig. 4).

If cirrhosis is already present at the time of HHC diagnosis, phlebotomy is still indicated provided that patients can tolerate it. Portal hypertension and its complications may improve with iron depletion. In addition, there is a theoretical advantage to iron reduction if liver transplantation becomes necessary. Pretransplant iron depletion could potentially decrease the risk of perioperative cardiac and infectious complications. In HHC patients with cirrhosis, close monitoring for the development of hepatocellular carcinoma is also important. Serial measurements of alpha fetoprotein coupled with abdominal ultrasonography and possibly high-resolution CT scanning are indicated.

HHC patients with cirrhosis are at high risk for the development of hepatocellular carcinoma, which may account for up to 30–45% of deaths in these patients. The presence of cirrhosis, increasing age, alcoholism, smoking, and presence of hepatitis B surface antigen are all independent risk factors for the development of hepatocellular carcinoma in HHC patients. Hepatocellular carcinoma has also been reported to develop in cirrhotic livers after iron-reduction therapy and in a few patients with precirrhotic liver disease. Early diagnosis of hepatocellular carcinoma remains a challenge; unsuspected hepatocellular carcinoma has been found in almost 20% of patients undergoing liver transplantation for HHC.

For end-stage liver disease associated with HHC, orthotopic liver transplantation (OLT) is the only effective therapy. Results of OLT for HHC have so far been disappointing. The survival rates 1 and 5 years after OLT for HHC are 54 and 43%, respectively, which is significantly lower than for other indicators. Although the prevalence of unsuspected primary liver cancer in patients receiving OLT for HHC is high, the short-term survival after liver transplantation is equal to that in patients with and without primary liver cancer. The poor survival after OLT appears to be due more to infectious and cardiac complications. Inadequate diagnosis of HHC prior to liver transplantation plays an important role, as close to 35% of these patients are not appropriately diagnosed pretransplant. Failure to make this diagnosis leads to failure to institute iron-reduction therapy; untreated parenchymal iron overload likely contributes to post-OLT infectious and cardiac complications.

Arthropathy

Articular complications are very common in HHC and may be the major symptom affecting quality of life. Typically, an osteoarthritis-like degeneration of the metacarpophalangeal joints is seen, although symmetrical polyarthropathy involving the proximal and distal interphalangeals, wrists, knees, and hips may also occur. The most common radiological findings are joint space narrowing, with osteophyte and subchondral cyst formation. Chondrocalcinosis is seen in some patients, most commonly involving the wrists, knees, and symphysis pubis.

Although the precise mechanism by which iron accumulation leads to arthropathy is not well understood, hemosiderin deposits are seen in synovial lining cells, with resultant chondrocyte proliferation and fibrosis. Iron deposition appears to stimulate accumulation of calcium pyrophosphate crystals, which coat the surface of the eroded cartilage. Clinical and radiological distinction between the arthropathy of HHC and calcium pyrophosphate dehydrate (CPPD) deposition disease is therefore quite difficult.

Management of arthropathy associated with HHC does not differ significantly from the therapy of degenerative osteoarthritis. Nonsteroidal anti-inflammatory drugs (NSAIDs) provide some degree of relief to most patients. In those in whom joint destruction progresses despite medical therapy, surgical arthroplasty may be necessary.

Cardiac Disease

Cardiac failure is an important cause of death, especially in young patients with HHC or secondary iron overload. Histopathological studies have shown that the majority of myocardial iron accumulates in the sarcoplasm and not in the interstitium, reflecting a storage abnormality rather than an infiltrative disorder. These iron deposits are more marked in the ventricles, lower in atrial muscle, and lowest in cells of the conduction system. There is also significant variability of stainable cardiac iron from endomyocardial biopsies taken from different locations of the same heart. Therefore, when endomyocardial biopsies are to be taken for confirmation of iron overload, multiple areas should be sampled.

Initially, iron accumulation results in clinically silent increases in the thickness of the left ventricular wall. This may progress over time to dilated cardiomyopathy, diagnosed echocardiographically by left ventricular enlargement and reduced ejection fraction. Less commonly, a pattern of predominantly restrictive cardiomyopathy may be seen, characterized echocardiographically by normal left ventricular size but impaired ventricular filling. Despite little histological involvement of the conduction system, electrocardiographic abnormalities have been described in up to 30% of patients with HHC; typically these include low voltage or nonspecific ST- and T-wave changes. The most common arrhythmias associated with cardiac iron overload are atrial tachyarrhythmias, followed by ventricular premature beats and, rarely, ventricular tachycardia.

Phlebotomy therapy has been shown to improve structural and functional cardiac abnormalities, although improvements in cardiac disease are more pronounced if iron reduction is undertaken prior to the development of dilated cardiomyopathy. In patients with dilated cardiomyopathy, phlebotomy therapy has been shown to decrease left ventricular dimensions, decrease the thickness of the left ventricular wall, and improve ejection fraction. The effects of phlebotomy therapy on the incidence of cardiac arrhythmias has not been well studied, although many electrocardiographic abnormalities improve with iron reduction. The effects of deferoxamine on the cardiac complications of secondary iron overload, primarily thalassemia major, have been extensively evaluated. In thalassemia patients, deferoxamine therapy clearly leads to improvements in left ventricular function and reduces the risk of symptomatic congestive heart failure or cardiac arrhythmias.

Frequent postoperative cardiac complications explain in part the relatively poor survival of HHC patients undergoing liver transplantation. In addition, cardiac complications may occur in these patients despite unremarkable preoperative testing such as echocardiography and coronary angiography. More accurate pretransplant diagnosis of HHC may lead to timely institution of iron-reduction therapy, which could reduce post-transplant cardiac complications.

Diabetes Mellitus

Diabetes is typically a late manifestation of HHC, being present in 70% of cirrhotic patients but in only 10% of noncirrhotics. With earier diagnosis and treatment of HHC through family and population screening, the prevalence of overt diabetes in newly diagnosed HHC patients is declining. Although islet cell damage from iron deposition is an important factor in the development of diabetes in HHC, these patients also have a high prevalence of glucose intolerance. As with other causes of cirrhosis, impaired hepatic clearance of insulin coupled with peripheral insulin resistance also play a role in the development of diabetes in HHC patients. The precise mechanism behind this insulin resistance is incompletely understood.

Medical therapy of the diabetes associated with HHC does not differ significantly from the therapy of adult-onset diabetes mellitus. Although more than 50% of diabetics with HHC will require insulin therapy. the usual stepwise approach—using diet and exercise, oral hypoglycemic agents, and insulin—should be undertaken. Phlebotomy therapy does not reverse insulin dependence, but approximately one-third of patients are able to reduce their insulin dose. Noninsulin-dependent diabetes is usually stabilized or improved with phlebotomy, but some patients may progress to insulin dependence if the process of islet cell destruction starts prior to attainment of iron depletion.

All of the complications of diabetes mellitus—including vascular disease, retinopathy, nephropathy, and neuropathy—have been reported in HHC patients with diabetes. All appear to occur with equal frequency in non-HHC diabetics matched for age and duration of disease, although diabetic retinopathy in HHC patients may be less severe.

Other Endocrine Abnormalities

Impotence and amenorrhea are common symptoms of HHC and are usually caused by secondary hypogonadism. In men, serum testosterone levels are low and testicular atrophy is common. Serum luteinizing hormone (LH) and follicle-stimulating hormone (FSH) levels are inappropriately low in both men and women. Histopathological studies have revealed significant iron deposition in the anterior pituitary, with a predilection for gonadotropic cells and relative sparing of thyrotropic, corticotropic, and somatotropic cells. Examination of testicular tissue reveals varying degrees of atrophy, typically with absent spermatozoa and reduced numbers of Leydig cells. Significant iron deposition in testicular tissue is rarely seen. Unfortunately, phlebotomy therapy does not lead to improvements in serum LH, FSH, testosterone, pituitary responsiveness to luteinizing hormone releasing hormone (LHRH), or impotence. Therapy with intramuscular testosterone injections may be beneficial. Clinical hypothyroidism or adrenal failure are uncommon and due to involvement of the pituitary, although cases of iron accumulation in the thyroid or adrenal glands have been reported.

Skin Pigmentation

Bronze pigmentation of the skin is present to some degree in most patients; it is caused by melanin deposition in the basal layers of the epidermis. The mechanism for this process is incompletely understood, but it is felt to be due directly or indirectly to iron-induced activation of melanocytes. Pigmentation is most prominent in sun-exposed areas, but it may also occur in mucous membranes and sun-protected regions. Direct accumulation of iron in macrophages may also occur around sweat glands, imparting a grayish hue to the skin. Skin pigmentation typically improves with phlebotomy therapy.

Infectious Complications

Patients with iron overload have an increased susceptibility to certain bacterial infections. This susceptibility is due in part to the availability of excess free iron, which promotes bacterial proliferation. Defects in the phagocytic activity of mononuclear cells have also been demonstrated in HHC patients; they are potentially reversible with phlebotomy therapy. Although *Yersinia enterocolitica* is a frequent cause of self-limited enterocolitis in normal hosts, it may, in patients with iron overload, cause septicemia and multiple hepatic abscesses. Septicemia with unusual organisms such as *Yersinia pseudotuberculosis*, *Vibrio vulnificus*, and *Listeria monocytogenes* has also been reported in HHC and in patients with secondary overload. Documented infections with these unusual pathogens should prompt a search for the diagnosis of HHC in these patients. Infectious complications also appear to play an important role in the poor survival of HHC patients after liver transplantation. The incidence of markers of chronic viral hepatitis, specifically HBsAg and anti-HCV, has been reported to be increased in patients with HHC. Screening all HHC patients for chronic viral hepatitis may be indicated, since the coexistence of these conditions may act synergistically to accelerate liver damage and increase the risk of hepatocellular carcinoma.

ALCOHOL AND IRON OVERLOAD

The role of alcohol intake in the natural history of iron overload in HHC has been controversial. Even in the absence of HHC, histological evidence of hepatic iron overload is relatively common in patients with alcoholic liver disease (ALD). Although serum iron studies and hepatic iron concentration are elevated in ALD, hepatic iron levels do not usually reach a level suggestive of HHC. Intestinal iron absorption may be increased in ALD, but progressive hepatic iron accumulation over time is not usually seen.

A significant proportion of HHC patients, perhaps as high as 20–30%, have a significant history of alcohol intake. Alcohol is no longer thought to be necessary for the development of the clinical manifestations of HHC, but significant alcohol intake does accelerate the clinical expression of HHC, presumably through synergistic hepatocellular damage and/or cumulative intestinal iron absorption. All HHC patients should be strongly encouraged to avoid or at least severely limit alcohol intake.

DIETARY FACTORS

It is difficult to assess how large a role dietary iron plays in the iron accumulation of HHC. Once patients have been started on phlebotomy therapy, the effect of changes in dietary iron are likely to be negligible. Patients who have been diagnosed with HHC and started on phlebotomy therapy, therefore, should be counseled to avoid supplemental iron, but significant changes in diet to reduce iron intake are unnecessary. Caffeinated beverages may act as iron chelators and reduce iron absorption, but vitamin C supplements increase iron absorption and should be avoided in HHC.

HHC HETEROZYGOTES

Heterozygotes for HHC account for approximately 10–12% of the Caucasian population. Most heterozygotes have normal serum iron studies, although on average the serum iron, transferrin saturation, and serum ferritin are higher in heterozygotes than in matched controls. Elevations of transferrin saturation and serum ferritin occur in approximately 10–20% of heterozygotes. Although the hepatic iron concentration is also higher in heterozygotes than in controls, progressive iron accumulation in the liver does not occur overtime. Clinical evidence if iron overload is unusual in heterozygotes and usually signifies the presence of another disorder, such as sideroblastic anemia or hereditary spherocytosis.

Heterozygotes who are identified through genetic testing for mutations in *HFE* can be reassured that they have a low risk of developing clinical iron overload. Heterozygotes identified through HLA-typing may require serum iron studies every 2–3 years to exclude progressive iron loading; such iron accumulation would indicate that they have been falsely classified as heterozygotes, probably due to a rare genetic crossover event. Alternatively, the heterozygote state can easily be confirmed in these patients with genotype analysis.

BIBLIOGRAPHY

Adams PC, Valberg LS. Evolving expression of hereditary hemochromatosis. Semin Liver Dis 1996; 16:47–54.

Bacon BR, Tavill AS. Hemochromatosis and the iron overload syndromes. In: Zakim D and Boyer TD, eds. Hepatology: a Textbook of Liver Disease, 3d ed. Philadelphia: Saunders, 1996:1439–1472.

Bassett ML, Halliday JW, Powell LW. Value of hepatic iron measurements in early hemochromatosis and determination of the critical iron level associated with fibrosis. Hepatology 1986; 6:24–29.

Edwards CQ, Cartwright GE, Skolnick MH, Amos DB. Homozygosity for hemochromatosis: clinical manifestations. Ann Intern Med 1980; 93:519–525.

Edwards CQ, Kushner JP. Screening for hemochromatosis. N Engl J Med 1993; 328:1616–1620.

Feder JN, Gnirke A, Thomas W, Tsuchihashi Z, Ruddy DA, Basava A, Dormishian F, Domingo Jr., R, Ellis MC, Fullan A, Hinton LM, Jones NL, Kimmel BE, Kronmal GS, Lauer P, Lee VK, Loeb DB, Mapa FA, McClelland E, Meyer NC, Mintier GA, Moeller N, Moore T, Morikang E, Prass CE, Quintana L, Starnes SM, Schatzman RC, Brunke KJ, Drayna DT, Risch NJ, Bacon BR, Wolff RK. A novel MHC class I-like gene is mutated in patients with hereditary haemochromatosis. Nature Genet 1996; 13:399–408.

Hershko C, Pinson A, Link G. Iron chelation. Blood Rev 1990; 4:1–8.

Kowdley KV, Trainer T, Krawitt EL, Knox TA, Susskind K, Pratt D, Kaplan MM, Rubin R, Saltzman JR, Bonkovsky HL, Grace ND. Utility of hepatic iron index in American patients with hereditary hemochromatosis: A multicenter study. Gastroenterology 1997; 113:1270–1277.

Kowdley KV, Hassanein T, Kaur S, Farrell FJ, Van Thiel DH, Keeffe E, Sorrell MF, Bacon BR, Weber Jr. FL, Tavill AS. Primary liver cancer and survival in patients undergoing liver transplantation for hemochromatosis. Liver Transplant Surg 1995; 1:237–241.

Niederau C, Fischer R, Purschel A, Stremmel W, Haussinger D, Strohmeyer G. Long-term survival in patients with hereditary hemochromatosis. Gastroenterology 1996; 110:1107–1119.

Tung BY, Kowdley KV. Clinical management of iron overload. Gastroenterology Clin North Am 1998; 27:637–654.

28
Management of Wilson's Disease

Michael L. Schilsky
Albert Einstein College of Medicine, Bronx, New York

Irmin Sternlieb
St. Luke's/Roosevelt Hospital Center, New York, New York

INTRODUCTION

Wilson's disease is a genetic disorder of copper metabolism in which copper accumulates primarily in the liver due to its reduced biliary excretion and secondarily in the central nervous system and other tissues. Unless specific treatment is initiated, progressive copper accumulation and its toxicity are ultimately fatal. The timely and appropriate treatment of these patients results in prevention of disease progression and often reversal of symptoms and excellent long-term survival.

Wilson's disease affects ≈ 1:30,000 individuals in almost all populations. The Wilson's disease gene, designated ATP7B, resides on chromosome 13. The gene product appears to be an ATPase that transports copper into bile and is involved in the delivery of this metal to the protein biosynthetic pathway for incorporation into ceruloplasmin. Wilson's disease is inherited in an autosomal recessive fashion, and only those individuals with mutations of both alleles encoding the ATP7B gene express the disease.

The three key concepts governing the management of Wilson's disease are (1) establishing the correct diagnosis, (2) initiating appropriate therapy and monitoring for effect and compliance, and (3) screening of first-degree relatives for this disorder.

DIAGNOSIS

The clinical presentation of Wilson's disease ranges widely. However, this disorder should be considered in patients with unexplained liver disease or neurological or psychiatric symptoms. Most patients present manifestations of the disease within the first three decades of life. Very rarely, patients may present in their fifties and sixties.

The diagnosis of Wilson's disease is established by a combination of physical and biochemical findings (see Table 1). The three main tests utilized include determination of

Table 1 Diagnostic Tests for Wilson's Disease

Serum ceruloplasmin
Slit-lamp exam for Kayser-Fleischer rings
Clinical examination for signs of liver disease or neurological impairment
Biochemical screening for evidenec of liver disease
Liver biopsy for quantitative copper determination, histology, histochemistry, ultrastructure
24-h urinary copper excretion
Radiocopper loading test
MRI of brain
Molecular genetic testing

serum ceruloplasmin, measured by ceruloplasmin oxidase activity, a slit-lamp examination for the presence of corneal copper deposits known as Kayser-Fleischer rings, determination of hepatic copper content, and appropriate histology of liver biopsy specimens. Other adjunctive testing includes urinary copper excretion and radiocopper loading tests. In patients with neurological or psychiatric manifestations, abnormalities on MRI of the brain may suggest this diagnosis.

The serum ceruloplasmin concentration is decreased below 20 mg/dL in 90–95% of patients with Wilson's disease. Unfortunately, however, such a result alone does not establish the diagnosis, because 20% of heterozygotes who do not develop the disease, rare individuals with congenital hypoceruloplasminemia, individuals with severe protein-losing enteropathy or nephropathy, and subjects suffering from severe hepatic insufficiency, when the biosynthetic capacity of the liver is markedly impaired, may also exhibit ceruloplasmin deficiency. Levels of ceruloplasmin are also reduced physiologically in newborns and during the first 6 months of life. Moreover, in patients with Wilson's disease, ceruloplasmin levels may be elevated from low to normal ranges because of the presence of an inflammatory process (ceruloplasmin being an acute-phase reactant) or because of hormonal modulation following the ingestion of estrogen-containing birth control pills or by pregnancy.

A slit-lamp examination should be performed on every patient in whom the diagnosis is considered. The presence of Kayser-Fleischer rings is diagnostic of Wilson's disease with only extremely rare exceptions of their presence in individuals with chronic cholestatic disorders such as primary biliary cirrhosis. Kayser-Fleischer rings may not be evident in younger patients but are almost invariably present in patients with central nervous system involvement. Infrequently, sunflower cataracts may be seen.

The combination of reduced ceruloplasmin concentration in the serum and the presence of Kayser-Fleischer rings establishes the diagnosis of Wilson's disease with certainty, and often no further testing is required for these individuals. In the absence of Kayser-Fleischer rings, a liver biopsy should be performed in order to evaluate for histological and histochemical changes compatible with Wilson's disease and, importantly, for determination of hepatic copper content. A concentration of > 250 μg/g copper is diagnostic for Wilson's disease. However, the same levels are present in disorders with long-standing cholestasis, as in primary biliary cirrhosis and sclerosing cholangitis as well as in Indian childhood cirrhosis and in the rare individuals with idiopathic inherited copper toxicosis. Infrequently, sampling error may yield low values of copper if the biopsy consists mainly of connective tissue in the presence of cirrhosis. In young patients, light microscopic findings may be limited, mostly of micro- and macrovesicular steatosis. In others, severe parenchymal cell damage with hepatocellular dropout or inflammatory changes with piecemeal necrosis ranging to cirrhosis can be present. Histochemical staining for copper-binding protein with rhodamine is helpful only if the pattern typical for Wilson's disease—namely, staining throughout individual nodules and absence of staining in adjacent parenchymal nodules—is found. Because of this irregular staining pattern, absence of rhodanine staining on a needle biopsy specimen does not exclude a diagnosis of Wilson's disease. When there is difficulty distinguishing a heterozygote (who may have elevated hepatic copper above the normal range but < 250 μg/g dry weight) from a patient, ultrastructural analysis may be useful. The presence of characteristic abnormal mitochondria with dilated cristae and various inclusions suggests the diagnosis of Wilson's disease. These changes are stage-dependent and are found earlier in the disease at a time when steatosis is prominent. Later in the progression of the disease, dense lysosomes may be visible while mitochondria may appear normal.

When liver biopsy is contraindicated, measurement of 24-h urinary copper excretion may be helpful. Values greater than 100 μg/24 h are present in many symptomatic patients. Normal or intermediate values do not exclude the diagnosis, especially in asymptomatic patients. In individuals with Wilsonian fulminant hepatic failure, urinary copper excretion is markedly elevated. Urinary copper excretion can also be elevated in patients with protein-losing nephropathy if ceruloplasmin is present in the urine. In untreated patients with Wilson's disease, urinary copper excretion dramatically increases following the administration of chelating agents like penicillamine, trientine, British anti-Lewisite (BAL), or tetrathiomolybdate. Administration of penicillamine, 500 mg orally before and 12 h later during a 24-h urine collection for copper is helpful in diagnosing Wilson's disease in children who lack Kayser-Fleischer rings.

Radiocopper loading tests are useful for helping to distinguish patients with Wilson's disease from individuals with other neurological or chronic liver disease when a normal level of serum ceruloplasmin is present. The lack of a secondary rise of radiocopper in the circulation at 24–48 h after its oral administration, representing the incorporation of copper into newly synthesized ceruloplasmin, occurs uniquely in patients with Wilson's disease.

The identification of the gene for Wilson's disease has enabled molecular genetic testing of family members of affected individuals. Since numerous disease specific-mutations have been identified, and no single mutation occurs with a high enough frequency except in rare isolated populations, de novo identification of affected individuals is difficult. Genetic analysis of haplotypes surrounding the Wilson's disease gene may be utilized to identify other affected family members once a proband is identified. Currently molecular genetic testing is experimental and is being performed in only a few centers worldwide. Therefore, clinical and reliable biochemical analysis should be utilized in all suspected cases until appropriately validated testing becomes available.

The diagnosis of Wilson's disease in the setting of acute fulminant hepatitis deserves special mention because of several unique features. In this setting, fulminant hepatitis is associated with a nonimmune hemolytic anemia and markedly elevated serum and urinary copper levels. Most of these patients are in their second decade of life and Kayser-Fleischer rings may not yet be apparent. Paradoxically, levels of serum alkaline phosphatase are frequently depressed in these youngsters, which led to the observation that a ratio of alkaline phosphatase to bilirubin less than 2 may be diagnostic of Wilsonian fulminant hepatitis. We and others have observed patients with Wilsonian fulminant hepatitis in whom this ratio was greater than 2.

Table 2 Therapy for Wilson's Disease

Chelating agents	Penicillamine (Cuprimine)
	Trientine (Syprine)
	British anti-Lewisite (BAL)
	Tetrathiomolybdate
Other	Zinc salts (zinc sulfate, gluconate, acetate)
	Orthotopic liver transplantation

TREATMENT AND MONITORING OF PATIENTS

Treatment goals are to prevent disease progression and to reverse or stabilize symptoms if they are present. Only two modes of therapy are effective, pharmacological treatment and orthotopic liver transplantation (see Table 2). Restrictions on the intake of copper-containing food is adjunctive and not sufficient therapy by itself.

Treatment may be divided into two categories: (1) treatment of symptomatic patients and (2) treatment of asymptomatic patients and maintenance therapy. Most experts on the care of Wilson's disease believe that symptomatic patients should be treated initially with chelating agents, the exception being patients with Wilsonian fulminant hepatitis, who should immediately be considered as candidates for orthotopic liver transplantation. Once symptomatic patients show stabilization of their disease clinically and biochemically, they should receive maintenance therapy with either a chelating agent or zinc salts. The time course for this stabilization is variable, with patients taking months to years to achieve complete stabilization of their disease. Asymptomatic patients should receive maintenance therapy from the outset. Treatment is lifelong, and it is important to be vigilant in monitoring for side effects and compliance. For patients on chelation therapy undergoing surgery or during pregnancy, dose reductions are necessary so as to avoid interference with wound healing.

D-Penicillamine (Cuprimine, Depen, Trolovol)

Penicillamine is a metal chelating agent forming soluble metal complexes that are readily excreted by the kidneys. This drug acts by promoting cupriuresis, reducing tissue copper stores, and possibly promoting the induction of cellular metallothionein. Penicillamine may interfere with fibrogenesis and modulate the immune system.

The initial adult dose is 1 g daily administered in four divided doses about ½ h before meals or 2 h after eating. Once the dosage of 1 g is well tolerated, the dosage of penicillamine should be adjusted in accord with the patient's clinical and biochemical responses. A useful laboratory index for adequacy of the dose and for compliance is the concentration of non-ceruloplasmin-bound serum copper (see "Monitoring of Pharmacotherapy" below). The dose should also be reduced temporarily prior to elective surgery or delivery (see below). For children weighing less than 40 kg, 0.02 g/kg body weight (rounded to the nearest 125 mg) should be administered orally in divided doses about ½ h before meals or 2 h after eating. Pyridoxine, 25 mg daily administered orally, should be given to all patients taking penicillamine due to the drug's weak antipyridoxine action.

Early Side Effects

Sensitivity reactions, almost always reversible, may occur in up to 20% of patients within the first few weeks of penicillamine therapy. Signs and symptoms include fever; diffuse, erythematous, macular, slightly papular, pruritic rash; lymphadenopathy, most commonly localized to the nodes of the neck, and leukopenia or thrombocytopenia. The medication should be discontinued immediately if any of these occurs. Desensitization starting with low doses, with or without the addition of prednisone, usually succeeds in overcoming the sensitivity reaction (see below).

In about 10% of patients with neurological manifestations prior to treatment, symptoms may worsen temporarily during the first weeks or months following the initiation of therapy. Penicillamine can be continued, barring occurrence of other adverse reactions, since the neurological condition will often remit with time. In some patients the deterioration is progressive and alternative treatments, including possible adjunctive therapy with BAL, should be considered (see below). Unfortunately, there are no prognostic criteria that permit the early identification of such individuals.

Late Effects

Renal toxicity typically follows the onset of proteinuria, occurring in fewer than 5% of penicillamine-treated patients with Wilson's disease. When proteinuria exceeds 1.0 g in a 24-h period, an alternative medication should be used.

A lupus-like syndrome may develop in rare patients with Wilson's disease. This syndrome is usually preceded by hematuria and proteinuria and often accompanied by arthralgias. Serum titers of antinuclear antibodies are frequently elevated. Though corticosteroids and reduction of the penicillamine dose may control this reaction, the use of alternate medication should be considered. Goodpasture's syndrome, marked by pulmonary and renal hemorrhages, has been reported to occur in patients with Wilson's disease who had received in excess of 1 g per day penicillamine, but it has not been reported in recent years.

Skin lesions may occur after years of continued penicillamine therapy. The most common is the increased wrinkling of the skin, particularly on the neck, giving a progeric appearance. Less frequent and unrelated to this are the raised, arcuate lesions of elastosis perforans serpingosa, which appear singly or in groups, most commonly on the axillae, neck and buttocks but rarely at other sites. No specific treatment exists for these; however, the lesions may disappear spontaneously irrespective of whether or not penicillamine therapy is discontinued. Penicillamine dermatopathy manifesting as friability with milia-like lesions and weakening of subcutaneous tissue due to interference of cross-linking of elastin and collagen, were seen when daily doses of 3–4 g of penicillamine were used for prolonged periods. Pemphigus or pemphigoid lesions, lichen planus, and aphthous stomatitis have also been reported in several patients receiving penicillamine.

Very rare late and typically reversible side effects occurring in patients with Wilson's disease include anaphylaxis, myasthenia gravis, polymyositis, loss of taste, depression of IgA, and serous retinitis.

Desensitization

Desensitization to penicillamine is infrequently utilized owing to the availability of alternative agents. When necessary, early reactions to penicillamine (except for severe leukopenia) are managed by stopping the medication, waiting for a few days for the reaction to disappear, and then starting prednisone, 30 mg, daily for 3 days prior to readministration of the penicillamine. Penicillamine should be restarted at a dosage of 125 mg, to be increased slowly over weeks to 1 g daily. Prednisone is reduced to 20 mg daily and ultimately tapered and discontinued if no recurrence of the adverse reaction develops.

Pregnancy and Elective Surgery

The regular dose of penicillamine should be continued during the first two trimesters and can be reduced to 500 mg/day during the last trimester. In over 150 pregnancies carried by women with Wilson's disease, no toxicity of the drug to either mother or fetus was seen. For elective surgery or if a cesarean section is contemplated, the dose should be reduced to 250 mg daily for 6 weeks before and until normal wound healing has occurred.

Trientine (Syprine, Trientine Hydrochloride)

Trientine is a metal chelating agent that removes copper from tissue stores and promotes cupriuresis. Trientine seems to be clinically as effective as penicillamine for maintenance therapy and appears to be as effective when utilized as primary treatment for patients presenting with severe liver disease or marked neurological or psychiatric manifestations.

Dosage

The adult dosage is 1–1.5 g orally administered daily in divided doses ½ h before meals or 2 h after eating. In children, 0.5–0.75 g is administered daily in two divided doses.

Side Effects

No hypersensitivity reactions to trientine have been reported; however, in patients with penicillamine-induced lupus, a recurrence with trientine was rarely seen. Few patients have developed a sideroblastic anemia, thought to be the result of drug-induced copper deficiency, which inhibits the effective utilization of iron in the erythropoietic stem cells.

Pregnancy and Elective Surgery

A daily dosage of 1 g of Trientine maintained during pregnancy has not resulted in any known complications to date. For elective surgery and if cesarean section is contemplated, dosage should be reduced to 250–500 mg daily 6 weeks before and until wound healing.

Zinc (Zinc Sulfate, Zinc Gluconate, Zinc Acetate)

Orally ingested zinc reduces the intestinal absorption of copper by stimulating the synthesis of metallothionein in enterocytes, which binds the copper and prevents it from entering the circulation. Zinc may also be hepatoprotective by stimulating metallothionein synthesis in hepatocytes.

Zinc was shown to be effective maintenance therapy for asymptomatic Wilson's disease and for patients who have previously been treated with chelating agents. The role of this agent in the primary treatment of patients with severe liver disease or with neurological or psychiatric manifestations is not clear. Zinc may be utilized concurrently with chelating agents; however, it must be temporally spaced from these drugs in order to be absorbed.

Dosage

The daily adult dosage is 150–200 mg of metallic zinc as zinc sulfate, zinc acetate, or gluconate, given in divided doses, at least 1 h before meals. The dosage is not as well established in pediatric patients; however, 25 mg may be utilized three times daily.

Side Effects

Gastric irritation is the only common side effect that may be in part dependent upon the chemical form of the zinc compound (more likely to occur with sulfate). Biochemical pancreatitis may result following overdosage with zinc salts.

Pregnancy and Elective Surgery

Zinc therapy during pregnancy has not resulted in known complications to date. No dose reduction is necessary for pregnancy or for elective surgery.

British Anti-Lewisite (BAL, Dimercaprol, Dimercaptopropanol)

BAL was the first chelating agent successfully utilized for the treatment of Wilson's disease. This drug removes tissue copper and increases urinary copper excretion. Its present role is restricted to that of an adjunct to oral chelation therapy for patients with Wilson's disease with severe neurological involvement. Since BAL is an uncharged, hydrophobic molecule, it is thought to be able to cross the blood-brain barrier as well as cellular plasma membranes.

Dosage

Following successful use of a 1-mL test dosage, 3 mL of 10% BAL in peanut oil is injected intramuscularly daily in repeated 5-day courses up to 40–60 doses. Because of local pain caused by the injections, not all patients tolerate this treatment. BAL should not be administered in conjunction with medicinal iron due to possible formation of complexes with BAL, which are highly nephrotoxic.

Side Effects

Intravenous injection should be strictly avoided by aspirating before injection of BAL. The incidence of sterile abscesses (which may develop at injection sites) can be reduced by carefully alternating injection sites. Other side effects include tachycardia and anaphylaxis, probably related to an allergic reaction to the vehicle for BAL, and hemolysis in patients with glucose-6-phosphate dehydrogenase deficiency. Administration should be discontinued in the presence of adverse effects.

Tetrathiomolybdate

Tetrathiomolybdate, utilized for decades by farmers and veterinarians for treatment of copper toxicosis in sheep, is being evaluated as an investigational drug for its role as initial treatment for Wilson's disease in the hope of avoiding the initial clinical deterioration that occurs in some penicillamine-treated patients. It is a more effective chelator of copper than penicillamine or trientine. Tetrathiomolybdate reduces intestinal copper absorption and, administered parenterally, enhances cupriuresis.

Dosage

Initial studies utilized a dose of 20 mg six times daily with three daily doses administered between meals and three with meals. The between-meal dosages were increased up to 30 mg until the non-ceruloplasmin-bound copper and plasma molybdenum levels were equal.

Side Effects

A reversible anemia may develop as a consequence of depletion of erythropoietic stem cell copper, which interferes with iron utilization. Initial increases in serum transaminases occurred in some patients, but there was a return to normal with continued therapy.

Pregnancy and Elective Surgery

There are no reports on the use of this agent in pregnancy. Given the effectiveness of thiomolybdate as a copper chelator, dose reduction is likely necessary if elective surgery is contemplated.

Transplantation

Hepatic transplantation plays an important role in the treatment of patients with Wilsonian fulminant hepatitis and those with severe hepatic failure refractory to pharmacological treatment or due to noncompliance with their pharmacologic regimen. In two recent surveys of the outcome of hepatic transplantation for Wilson's disease, survival was 80–82%, comparable to that of other patients with liver disease. The role of liver transplantation for neurological Wilson's disease without hepatic insufficiency is uncertain.

Hemofiltration and Plasmapheresis

Hemofiltration and plasmapheresis have been utilized in few patients with Wilsonian fulminant hepatitis awaiting suitable donor livers. These treatments may delay but do not stay the need for transplantation.

MONITORING OF PHARMACOTHERAPY

There are three major goals: (1) determination of the adequacy of therapy, (2) recognition and screening for side effects or intolerance, and (3) determination of therapeutic compliance.

Adequacy of therapy is determined foremost by the patient's clinical response; the normalization of abnormal laboratory tests; the reduction of the concentration of non-ceruloplasmin-bound copper in the serum to less than 10 μg/dL; and, for patients on chelation therapy, by maintaining the 24-h urinary copper excretion above or close to 500 μg/day. For patients on zinc therapy, urinary copper excretion may remain near or just above 100 μg/day, and sudden rises in urinary copper excretion above this level should suggest the possibility of noncompliance. For patients with neurological or psychiatric symptoms, response is judged by stabilization or reversal of symptoms. Most clinical abnormalities, as well as the biochemical parameters of liver dysfunction improve within 6 months to a year after initiation of therapy. However, normalization of the prothrombin time may take longer or may be delayed indefinitely.

Patients should be alerted to look out for side effects specific to the agent utilized (see above). Following initiation of chelation therapy for symptomatic patients, complete blood counts should be obtained at weekly intervals, then biweekly, and periodically thereafter, and urine should be routinely tested for protein and cellular sediment.

Monitoring of patient compliance is critical to successful management. A patient's refusal to take the prescribed doses of medication may result in lack of improvement, and discontinuation of therapy after intervals of apparent well-being may result in the sudden appearance of severe hepatic insufficiency requiring liver transplantation. Compliance is best achieved if the importance of taking medication regularly is reinforced repeatedly, by counting pills, periodic slit-lamp examinations for documentation of the disappearance of Kayser Fleischer rings, serum testing for biochemical evidence of liver disease, determinations of the fraction of non-ceruloplasmin-bound serum copper, and measurements of urinary copper excretion or zinc content for patients on this therapy. Imaging studies (including magnetic resonance imaging), neurophysiological investigations (visual and auditory evoked potentials), and serial hepatic copper determinations may be of interest but contribute little to a thorough clinical and biochemical examination.

FAMILY SCREENING

Once patients are diagnosed, first-degree relatives should undergo screening. This should include clinical examination for signs of liver or neurological disease, determination of serum ceruloplasmin oxidase activity, slit-lamp examination to exclude the presence of Kayser-Fleischer rings, and biochemical screening for liver disease, which should include assays of serum albumin, aminotransferases, bilirubin, alkaline phosphatase and prothrombin time. If the serum ceruloplasmin concentration is > 20 mg/dL and these individuals are either heterozygotes or homozygously normal, they do not require treatment or monitoring. Children should be screened beginning at age 3. If the serum ceruloplasmin is < 20 mg/dL, further studies are indicated. Urinary copper determinations are not reliable for early detection of Wilson's disease. When reliable molecular genetic studies become available, screening by this method should eliminate the necessity for serial examinations.

With improved technology, it may someday be possible to utilize molecular testing to diagnose Wilson's disease without having first to identify an affected family member. When this is possible, screening of family members for the same disease-specific mutations will make the process cost-effective. With the advent of molecular testing, physicians who recommend this mode must be capable of performing genetic counseling or must refer patients to assure that test results are correctly interpreted and understood.

BIBLIOGRAPHY

Alt E, Sternlieb I, Goldfischer S. The cytopathology of metal overload (review). Int Rev Exp Pathol 1990; 31:165–188.

Cox DW. Molecular advances in Wilson disease. In: Boyer JL, Ockner RK, eds. Progress in Liver Disease. Philadelphia: Saunders, 1996:245–264.

Hoogenraad T. Wilson's disease. In Warlow CP, Van Gijn J, eds. Major Problems in Neurology 30. Philadelphia: Saunders, 1996.

Petrukhin K, Lutsenko S, Chernov I, Ross BM, Kaplan JH, Gilliam TC. Characterization of the Wilson's disease gene encoding a P-type copper transporting ATPase: genomic organization, alternative splicing, and structure/function predictions. Hum Mol Genet 1994; 3:1647–1656.

Scheinberg IH, Sternlieb I. Wilson's Disease. Philadelphia: Saunders, 1984.

Schilsky ML. Wilson's disease: Genetic basis of copper toxicity and natural history. Semin Liver Dis 1996; 16:83–95.

Schilsky ML, Scheinberg IH, Sternlieb I. Prognosis of Wilsonian chronic active hepatitis. Gastroenterology 1991; 100:762–767.

Schilsky ML, Scheinberg IH, Sternlieb I. Liver transplantation for Wilson's disease: indications and outcome. Hepatology 1994; 19:583–587.

Sternlieb I. Copper and zinc. In: Arias IM, Boyer JL, Fausto N, Jakoby WB, Schachter D, Shafritz DA, eds. The Liver: Biology and Pathobiology. New York: Raven Press, 1994:585–596.

29
Management of Porphyrias

Herbert L. Bonkovsky
University of Massachusetts Medical Center, Worcester, Massachusetts

OVERVIEW OF THE PORPHYRIAS

The porphyrias have been termed the "royal malady" because it has been proposed that several members of the royal houses of Stuart and Windsor of the United Kingdom suffered from a form of acute porphyria (variegate porphyria). The term *porphyria* is derived from the Greek word *porphyra*, which means purple, a color often associated with royalty. The derivation is fitting because aqueous solutions of porphyrins are a dark red to purple color.

It is now clear that this group of diseases is due to defects in normal heme synthesis. Accordingly, in order to have an understanding of the basic pathogenesis of these diseases and their treatment, it is necessary to review the pathway of porphyrin and heme biosynthesis and the regulation of the pathway, particularly in the liver.

The Heme Biosynthetic Pathway

As summarized in Fig. 1, the pathway of heme biosynthesis involves eight enzymes. The building blocks are glycine and succinyl-CoA. In the liver, the first step of the pathway, namely, the condensation of glycine and succinyl-CoA in the presence of pyridoxal phosphate (vitamin B_6) is the rate-controlling step of the overall pathway. It is catalyzed by the enzyme 5-aminolevulinate (ALA) synthase, an intramitochondrial enzyme.

After formation of ALA within mitochondria, this intermediate is transported out of mitochondria into the soluble cytoplasmic fraction of the cell. Here the second enzyme, ALA dehydratase (sometimes called porphobilinogen synthase), carries out the condensation of two molecules of ALA to form the monopyrrole porphobilinogen (PBG). The next enzyme of the pathway, PBG deaminase (sometimes called hydroxymethylbilane synthase), carries out the polymerization of four molecules of PBG to form the linear tetrapyrrole hydroxymethylbilane. This intermediate is very unstable in physiologic aqueous solutions. It rapidly undergoes nonenzymatic cyclization with ring closure to form uroporphyrinogen I. Under normal conditions, however, the next enzyme of the pathway, namely, uroporphyrinogen III cosynthase, is present in large excess, such that virtually all of the hydroxymethylbilane that is formed by PBG deaminase undergoes an isomerization

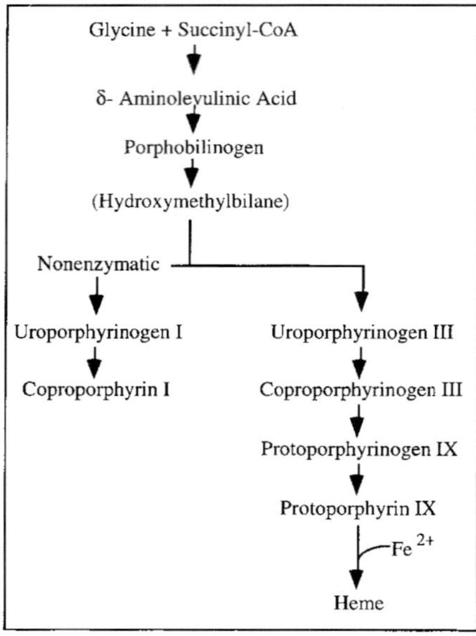

ENZYME	DISEASE
ALA Synthase	
ALA Dehydratase	ALA Dehydratase Deficiency
Porphobilinogen Deaminase	Acute Intermittent Porphyria
Uroporphyrinogen III Synthase (Cosynthase)	Congenital Erythropoietic Porphyria
Uroporphyrinogen Decarboxylase	Porphyria Cutanea Tarda; Hepatoerythropoietic Porphyria
Coproporphyrinogen Oxidase	Hereditary Coproporphyria
Protoporphyrinogen Oxidase	Variegate Porphyria
Ferrochelatase	Protoporphyria

Figure 1 The pathway of heme biosynthesis and the enzymatic defects in the porphyrias.

reaction with ring closure to form the intermediate uroporphyrinogen III. Only uroporphyrinogen or uroporphyrinogen isomers I and III are found in nature.

The enzyme uroporphyrinogen decarboxylase (uro-D), also found in the soluble cytoplasmic fraction of the cell, is capable of carrying out the stepwise decarboxylation of the acetate side chains of either uroporphyrinogen I or uroporphyrinogen III, with the eventual formation of coproporphyrinogen I or III. The enzyme has higher activity with the III as compared with the I isomer as substrate. Measurable amounts of intermediates with 7, 6, and 5 carboxyl groups (hepta, hexa, and pentacarboxy porphyrinogens and porphyrins) accumulate, but, under normal conditions, their amounts are much less than those of uro (octacarboxy) and copro (tetracarboxy) porphyrins.

For further metabolism, coproporphyrinogen III must again be transported into mitochondria, where the next enzyme, coproporphyrinogen oxidase, carries out the oxidative decarboxylation of two of the four remaining propionate side chains. These side chains are converted to vinyl groups, leading to the formation of protoporphyrinogen IX. In the penultimate step of heme synthesis, protoporphyrinogen IX is oxidized to its corresponding porphyrin by the enzyme protoporphyrinogen oxidase. This reaction involves the removal of six hydrogen atoms and leads to the formation of a much more stable, resonating, planar structure typical of all of the porphyrins. It is important to recall that the intermediates in heme biosynthesis are, for the most part, porphyrinogens and not porphyrins. In fact, it is not until this second last step of heme synthesis that a porphyrin intermediate (protoporphyrin IX) is actually synthesized.

The final enzyme of the pathway, ferrochelatase, inserts ferrous iron into protoporphyrin IX to form heme. This enzyme is also located only in mitochondria.

The heme that is formed as a result of the above pathway is utilized in a variety of hemoproteins. In quantitative terms, in hepatocytes, most of the heme is utilized for the formation of cytochromes P450 the superfamily of related hemoproteins that are collectively responsible for the phase I metabolism of an astonishing array of endogenous and exogenous chemicals. Lesser amounts of heme are utilized for the formation of mitochondrial cytochromes; catalase; peroxidase; cytochrome b5, another hemoprotein found primarily in smooth endoplasmic reticulum that plays an ancillary role in drug metabolism; and tryptophan pyrrolase, the rate-controlling enzyme for tryptophan breakdown.

As shown in Fig. 1, defects in one of the enzymes of the heme synthetic pathway are the basic underlying biochemical causes of the porphyrias. However, for most of these diseases, the presence of such a defect in and of itself is not sufficient to produce clinical disease. Rather, other factors are also important.

Regulation of Hepatic Heme Metabolism

The major site of regulation of the pathway resides at the level of activity of the first enzyme, ALA synthase. This enzyme is normally present in low amounts, but its activity can rapidly be increased manyfold, particularly by certain drugs and chemicals that have the potential for producing porphyria. Much experimental and clinical evidence now supports the concept that the major factor controlling the level of activity of hepatic ALA synthase is a small but critical pool of "regulatory" heme within hepatocytes. This pool is envisioned to be depleted by conditions that cause the induction of increased amounts of cytochromes P450 or, even more strongly, by conditions that lead to a rapid breakdown of the heme of cytochrome P450. For example, a variety of potent porphyrogenic chemicals cause such breakdown and often also induce levels of the apoproteins of the cytochromes P450. Thus they can lead to profound depletion of the regulatory heme pool. In contrast, parenteral administration of heme to animals or patients can lead to a repletion or restoration of the regulatory heme pool of hepatocytes and thus to a downregulation of ALA synthase.

The mechanisms whereby the regulatory heme pool decreases activity of ALA synthase include enhancement of the rate of degradation of the mRNA of ALA synthase and blockage of the uptake of enzyme molecules themselves into mitochondria. In some experimental systems, it has also been proposed that heme is capable of decreasing levels of mRNA of ALA synthase by downregulating the rate of transcription of the ALA synthase gene.

The size of the regulatory heme pool may also be affected by the level of activity of heme oxygenase, the enzyme responsible for the breakdown of heme within hepatocytes and other cells. Heme oxygenase can be rapidly and markedly induced by increased amounts of heme in hepatocytes. These increased amounts can be due to the administration of heme to host animals or to a marked induction of ALA synthase, leading to an increased formation of all of the intermediates of the pathway and finally leading to increased levels of heme itself. The central role of the regulatory heme pool in controlling hepatic heme metabolism is summarized in Fig. 2.

Classification of the Porphyrias

Porphyrias are usually classified as being acute or chronic and as being hepatic or erythropoietic. The acute or "inducible" porphyrias are those in which marked induction of hepatic ALA synthase may occur, leading to marked overproduction and overexcretion of ALA and PBG. The major clinical feature of such diseases is the acute porphyric attack, a

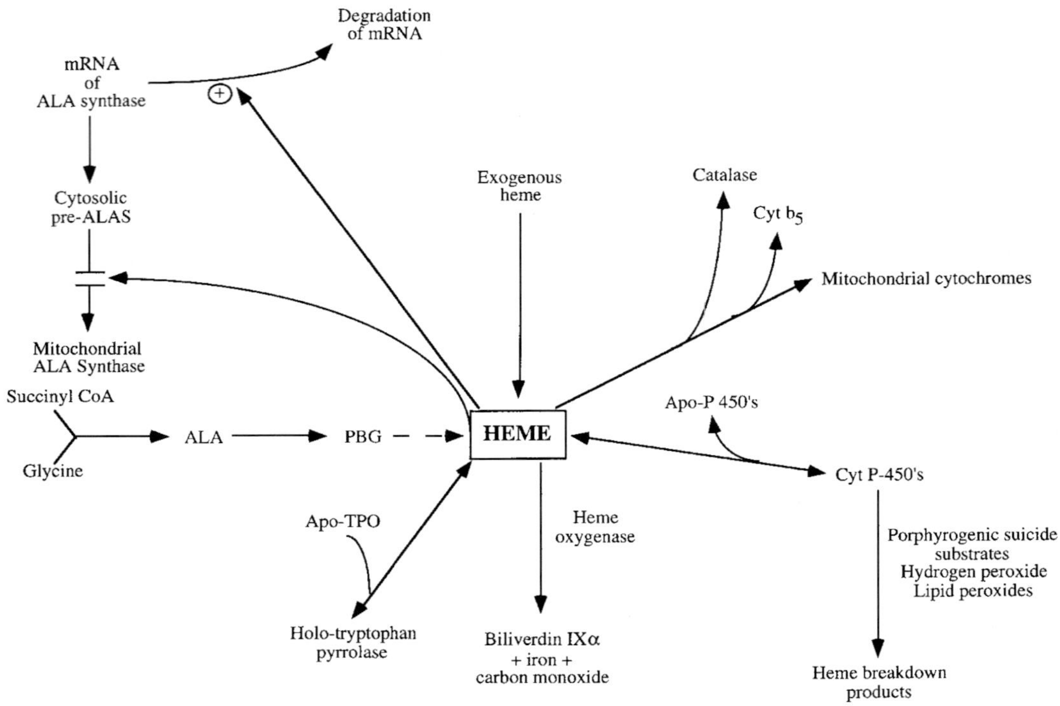

Figure 2 The regulation of hepatic heme metabolism. The key feature is the regulatory heme pool, which provides heme to cellular hemoproteins, particularly the cytochromes P450, and downregulates levels of intramitochondrial ALA synthase. This downregulation is accomplished by increasing the rate of degradation of the mRNA of ALA synthase and by blocking the mitochondrial uptake of the enzyme.

condition characterized biochemically by uncontrolled induction of ALA synthase and clinically by dysfunction of neurons of the autonomic, peripheral, and central nervous systems. As shown in Table 1, the acute porphyrias include acute intermittent porphyria (AIP), porphyria due to severe deficiency of ALA dehydratase, hereditary coproporphyria (HCP), and variegate porphyria (VP). In addition, similar porphyric syndromes may occur in hereditary tyrosinemia type 1 or in lead poisoning. In the latter two diseases, the underlying metabolic disorders may lead to a secondary, profound inhibition of ALA dehydratase, with subsequent marked overproduction and overexcretion of ALA.

The chronic hepatic porphyrias are porphyria cutanea tarda (PCT) and hepatoerythropoietic porphyria. At times, protoporphyria may also be complicated by serious hepatic dysfunction and cirrhosis, even though the actual site of overproduction of protoporphyrin is chiefly the bone marrow. Because such serious or even fatal liver disease may complicate protoporphyria, a case can be made for including protoporphyria as one of the so-called chronic hepatic porphyrias.

The other major classification of the porphyrias is according to the major site of overproduction of porphyrins and porphyrin precursors. According to our current understanding, this overproduction occurs chiefly in the liver or in the bone marrow, the two

Table 1 Classification and Genetics of the Porphyrias

Type of porphyria	Abbreviation	Inheritance	Comments
Acute porphyrias			
Porphyria due to severe deficiency of ALA dehydratase	ADP	Recessive	Rare acquired cases described. Similar syndrome in hereditary tyrosinemia, type I, and lead poisoning
Acute intermittent porphyria	AIP	Dominant	
Hereditary coproporphyria	HCP	Dominant	Rare compound heterozygotes described
Variegate porphyria	VP	Dominant	Rare compound heterozygotes described
Chronic hepatic porphyrias			
Porphyria cutanea tarda	PCT	Dominant or none (acquired)	Associated with liver disease (alcohol, chronic hepatitis C) and iron overload
Hepatoerythropoietic porphyria	HEP	Dominant or intermediate	Homozygous or compound heterozygous form of PCT
Erythropoietic porphyrias			
Congenital erythropoietic porphyria	CEP	Recessive	Severe form; usually manifest in infancy
Protoporphyria	PP	Dominant or recessive	Multigenic inheritance proposed

organs where heme synthesis is most active. According to this classification scheme, the erythropoietic porphyrias are made up of congenital erythropoietic porphyria (CEP), sometimes called hereditary erythropoietic uroporphyria, and protoporphyria. In all of the other forms of porphyria already mentioned, the liver is believed to be the major site of overproduction of porphyrins and/or the porphyrin precursors ALA and PBG.

Pathogenesis of Major Manifestations of the Porphyrias

Porphyrias present clinically either as acute attacks with evidence of neurovisceral and neuronal dysfunction or with cutaneous manifestations. In some of the diseases, notably HCP and VP, there may be features of both acute attacks and the cutaneous features. Although the pathogenesis of the neurovisceral dysfunction in the acute porphyrias has not been established with certainty, it likely involves the factors summarized in Fig. 3. The critical factors are believed to be a marked increase in ALA production, an increase in tryptophan supply from the liver, and a block in heme synthesis, perhaps leading to depletion of neuronal ATP and/or the inability of neurons and their supporting elements to maintain adequate levels of ATP. These factors, perhaps acting in concert, may cause dysfunction of neurons and lead to the clinical manifestations recognized as the acute porphyric attack.

Pathogenesis of Cutaneous Manifestations

Photocutaneous lesions, caused by excess porphyrin deposition in the skin with subsequent secondary reactions may occur in all of the porphyrias, with the exception of AIP and porphyria due to severe deficiency of ALA dehydratase. In these two diseases (and in

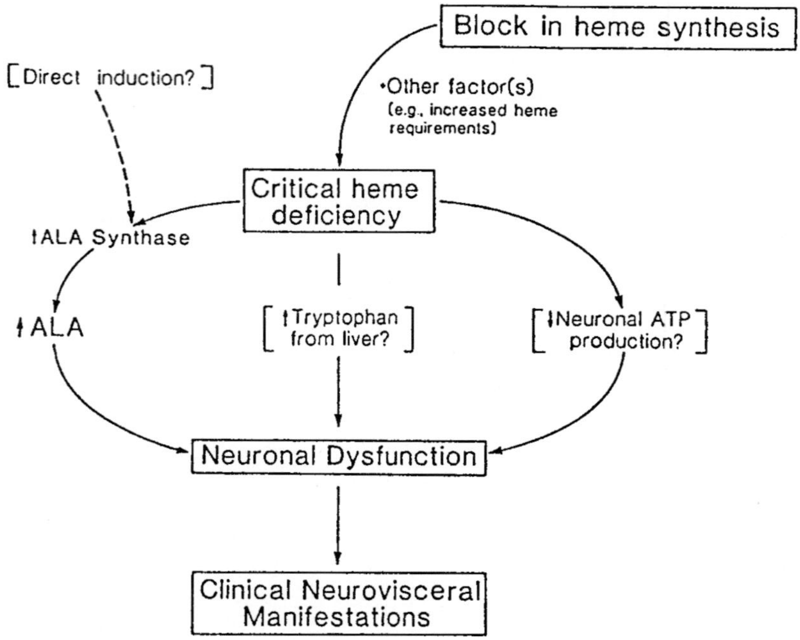

Figure 3 Pathogenesis of neurovisceral features of acute porphyric attacks. (From Bloomer and Bonkovsky, 1989.)

hereditary tyrosinemia type 1 and lead poisoning), marked increases in porphyrins do not occur because the enzymatic defects precede the steps in which porphyrinogens or porphyrins are formed (see Fig. 1).

Photosensitivity caused by porphyrins manifests itself in one of two quite different ways: (1) increased fragility of light-exposed skin, particularly the skin covering the dorsal aspects of the hands and forearms. This type of injury occurs in porphyria cutanea tarda HCP, VP, HEP, and CEP. (2) Acute erythema, burning, and itching of light-exposed skin, particularly the face, the back of the neck, and the dorsal aspects of hands and forearms. This type of reaction is observed in protoporphyria. The difference is probably ascribable chiefly to the fact that protoporphyrin is extremely hydrophobic compared with the more hydrophilic uroporphyrin or coproporphyrin. Protoporphyrin accumulation occurs first and foremost in mitochondria, the subcellular organelle in which, normally, iron is inserted into protoporphyrin to form heme. Protoporphyrin is also thought to "dissolve" into biological membranes. In contrast, accumulation of uroporphyrin occurs predominantly in lysosomes, and the more hydrophilic uroporphyrin and other porphyrins with higher number of carboxyl groups (4–8) do not dissolve into membranes.

The photosensitizing effects of porphyrins in the skin are due to their ability to absorb light and require the presence of molecular oxygen. The current view of pathogenesis is summarized in Fig. 4. Light energy excites electrons of the porphyrins to elevated energy levels, forming a "triplet state." As these electrons return to their ground state, some of the energy is transferred to molecular oxygen, forming highly reactive "singlet" oxygen. Singlet oxygen is capable of damaging tissue by several mechanisms, including peroxidation of unsaturated membrane lipids, direct oxidation and cross-linking of membrane proteins, and oxidative damage to nucleic acids. Peroxidative damage to membranes of

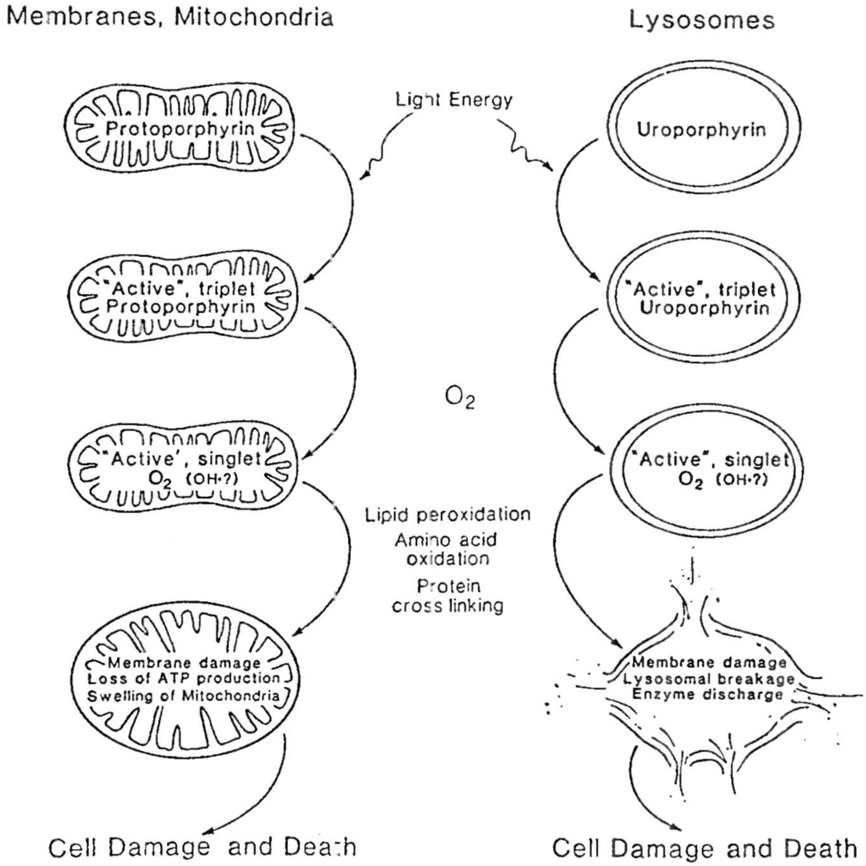

Figure 4 Pathogenesis of cutaneous features of the porphyrias. (From Bloomer and Bonkovsky, 1989.)

lysosomes containing uroporphyrin probably leads to the release of hydrolytic and proteolytic enzymes into the cell, causing cellular autodigestion.

There is probably also a role for activation of the complement cascade in the pathogenesis of porphyric skin lesions, because high levels of several components of the complement pathway and/or products of their cleavage have been detected in blister fluids from patients with cutaneous porphyrias. It has also been found that in the presence of light and oxygen, porphyrins produce a decrease of titers of complement in sera in vitro.

Diagnosis of the Porphyrias

Because of the protean manifestations of the porphyrias, these diseases are frequently misdiagnosed. A full account of the appropriate strategies for making a diagnosis is beyond the scope of this chapter, which is focused principally upon management. For cost-effective diagnostic strategies, the reader is referred to the recent review of Bonkovsky and Barnard (Semin Liver Dis 1998; 18:57–65.). Useful diagnostic algorithms are summarized in Figs. 5 and 6. The following points deserve particular emphasis:

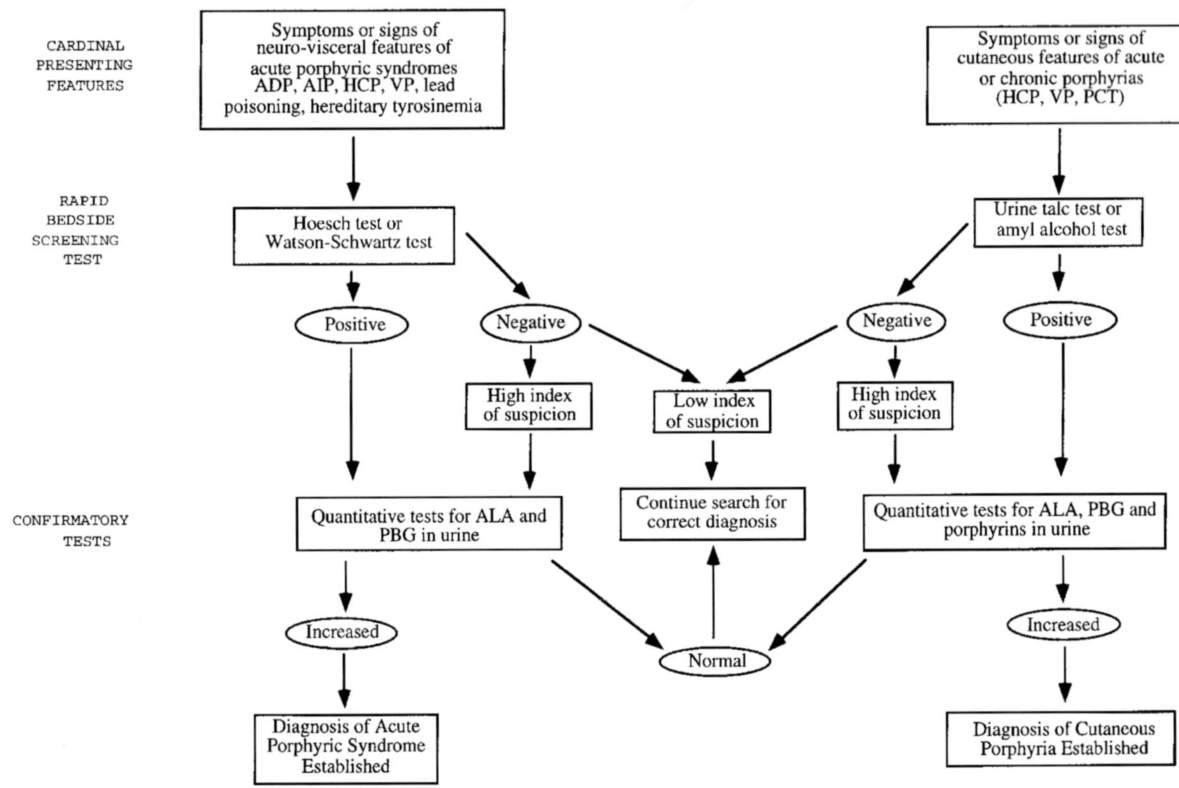

Figure 5 Recommended diagnostic algorithm for patients with features suggesting acute porphyria or porphyria cutanea tarda. (From Bonkovsky and Barnard, 1998.)

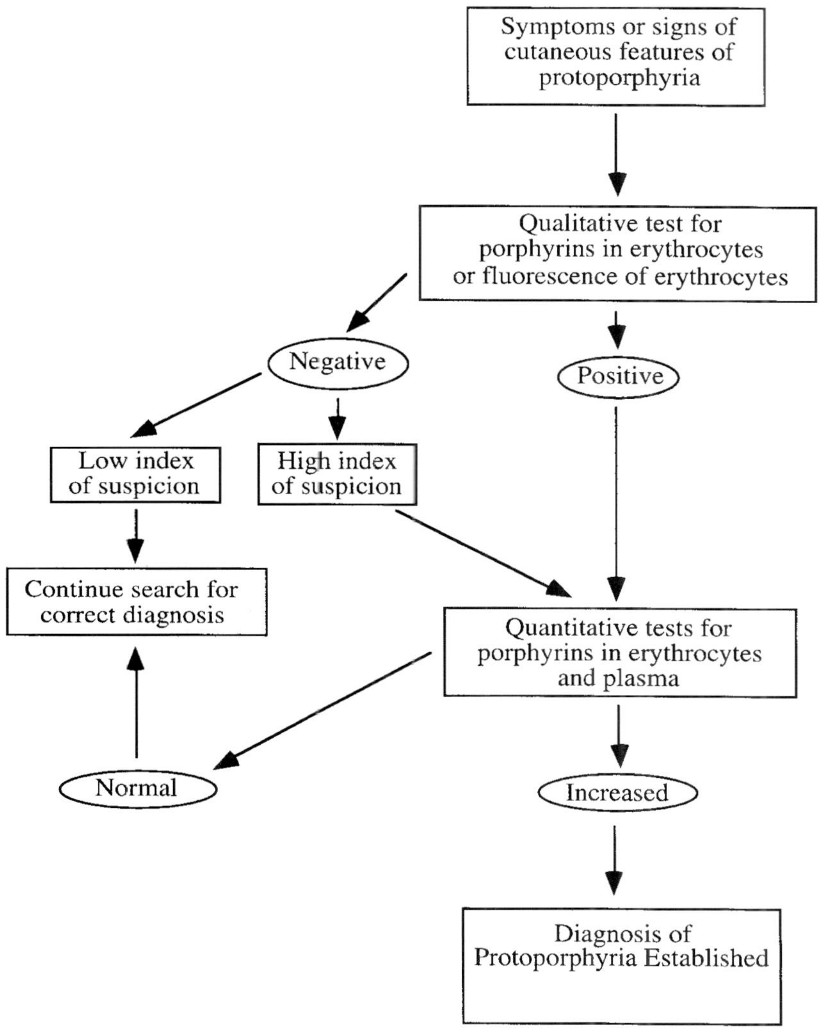

Figure 6 Recommended diagnostic algorithm for patients with features suggesting protoporphyria. (From Bonkovsky and Barnard, 1998.)

1. All patients with acute porphyria in relapse have marked induction of ALA synthase, with subsequent overproduction and overexcretion of ALA (and usually PBG). PBG can be detected rapidly by bedside screening tests, either the Hoesch or the Watson-Schwartz test. If a patient is suspected of having acute porphyria but has a negative screening test, other diagnostic possibilities should be entertained. Nevertheless, if the index of suspicion is very high, quantitative and specific testing for ALA and PBG in the urine should still be carried out, because there may occasionally be false-positive or false-negative screening tests.
2. All patients with cutaneous porphyrias that are clinically manifest will have

definite, measurable increases in plasma porphyrin concentrations. With the exception of those with protoporphyria, such patients will also have increases in porphyrins in the urine. Protoporphyria is the exception, because, due to the marked lipophilicity of protoporphyrin, it cannot be excreted in urine, but only in stool. Accordingly, screening only for urinary porphyrins is not sufficient completely to exclude the possibility of cutaneous porphyria.

3. The excitation and emission fluorescent spectra of plasma porphyrins are useful in the differential diagnosis of cutaneous porphyrias. In particular, the porphyrins that accumulate in clinically manifest variegate porphyria and protoporphyria have characteristic excitation and emission maxima that are useful in differential diagnosis (Table 2).
4. Because of the relative rarity of the porphyrias and the complexities involved in differential diagnosis and in making a firm diagnosis, it is usually a good idea to refer patients suspected of having porphyria to a center where there is special expertise in diagnosing and managing these diseases and/or to discuss patients with physicians associated with one of these centers.

MANAGEMENT OF THE ACUTE PORPHYRIAS

Management of the Acute Attack

General and Nutritional and Analgesic Measures

Attention to the general care of the patient with an acute attack of porphyria is of the utmost importance. This includes maintenance of adequate nutrition, so that negative nitrogen and energy balance is avoided. A generous daily intake of carbohydrate, for adults (at least 300 g of glucose per day) is essential, not only to have a protein-sparing effect and to provide calories and energy but also to repress the overactivity of hepatic ALA synthase. ALA

Table 2 Fluorescent Spectra of Plasma Porphyrins in the Porphyrias[a]

Maximal excitation wavelength (nm)	Maximal emission wavelength (nm)	Type of porphyria
398	619	Hereditary erythropoietic uroporphyria Hepatoerythropoietic porphyria Hereditary coproporphyria Porphyria cutanea tarda (Acute intermittent porphyria[b])
409	634	Protoporphyria
405	626	Variegate porphyria

[a]Measurement of plasma total porphyrin and assessment of the fluorescent spectra are most useful in establishing a diagnosis of porphyria with cutaneous features. In the cases of protoporphyria and variegate porphyria, the characteristic wavelengths for peak emission and excitation are also valuable for making a specific diagnosis.

[b]Plasma porphyrins in biochemically active AIP may be normal or only minimally increased. In AIP, urine testing is essential. Similarly, in the other types of porphyria that produce elevations in plasma porphyrins that fluoresce maximally at 619 nm, testing of urine and stool are important for establishing a specific diagnosis.

Source: From Bonkovsky and Barnard, Semin Liver Dis, 1998.

synthase is one of several hepatic enzymes that is subject to a "glucose effect." This means that the administration of large amounts of glucose or other readily metabolizable carbohydrate is capable of downregulating activity of ALA synthase. The exact molecular mechanism by which this action of glucose is mediated remains unclear. It may have to do with an alteration in the stability of the mRNA for ALA synthase, with the blocking of uptake of the enzyme into mitochondria (these actions are similar to those of heme), or to an indirect effect whereby a generous supply of glucose leads to a repletion of the regulatory heme pool. For example, starvation has been reported to produce an increase in the activity of hepatic heme oxygenase. Perhaps this increase is blunted or prevented by the administration of large doses of glucose and thus the regulatory heme pool is stabilized.

It is also important that patients have frequent checks of their neurological status, because occasionally they may develop rapidly progressive or even fatal weakness. Weakness of the muscles of respiration may lead to development of atelectasis, pneumonia, and respiratory failure. Patients who become paralyzed may require mechanical ventilation and intensive nursing care to prevent complications of the paralyzed state.

The pain associated with acute porphyric attacks can safely be treated with opiate analgesics. Those that have been used most often are meperidine and morphine. Their actions can be enhanced with the addition of a phenothiazine. The phenothiazine that has been used most often is chlorpromazine, which may be given as a long-acting preparation if desired. The usual dose of chlorpromazine has been in the range of 50–400 mg/day. Doses of meperidine may need to be as high as 1000 mg/day. Propranolol is the drug of choice for therapy of systemic arterial hypertension or other manifestations of increased sympathetic tone. It is usually well tolerated, although rare exceptions of severe hypotension and bradycardia have been reported. Cimetidine has been reported to blunt experimental porphyria in rodents and has been used without apparent harm in humans, although whether it is of particular benefit is not established.

Avoidance of Porphyrogenic Drugs

A large number of drugs are known to be porphyrogenic and have been reported to precipitate or exacerbate acute attacks of porphyria. The major ones are listed in Table 3, which also lists a number of drugs that have been found to be porphyrogenic in experimental models of the acute porphyrias (and thus are at least theoretically risky) and drugs that are safe for use, based upon their lack of porphyrogenicity in experimental models and previous experience with their safe use in porphyric patients. Of course, the list of drugs in Table 3 is far from complete, because most drugs have not been tested, nor have they been reported to worsen acute porphyria. If at all possible, drugs that are known to induce one or more forms of cytochromes P450 should be avoided because of the likelihood that they will produce depletion of the regulatory heme pool in hepatocytes and therefore may worsen acute porphyria. In general, it is best to give patients few drugs except for those known to be safe for use.

Monitoring for Hyponatremia and Hypomagnesemia

Patients with acute porphyric attacks are particularly prone to develop hyponatremia and/or hypomagnesemia, which may cause symptoms or signs on their own. The hyponatremia has often been ascribed to high levels of antidiuretic hormone (ADH), which certainly occur in patients with symptomatic acute porphyria. Although it is often said that this is due to a syndrome of inappropriate ADH release, measurements of blood volumes of patients with biochemically active acute porphyria have shown decreases, which are often substan-

Table 3 Drugs and Chemical in Acute Hepatic Porphyrias

Reported to exacerbate disease[a]	Theoretically risky	Believed to be safe
Aminoglutethimide	Alcuronium	Acetaminophen
Antipyrine	Alfadolone acetate[b]	Amitryptyline
Aminopyrine	Alfaxalone[b]	Aspirin
Barbiturates	Allyl-containing compounds	Atropine
Bemegride	Amphetamines	Bromides
N-Butylscopolammonium bromide	Bupivacaine	Calcium salts
Barbamazepine	Bupropion	Captopril
Carbamazepine	Camphor	Chloral hydrate
Carbromal	Chloroform	Chlorpromazine
Chloramphenicol	Clonazepam (large doses)	Colchicine
Chlordiazepoxide	Clonidine	Corticosteroids
Chloroquine	Colistin	Cyclopropane
Chlorpropamide	Diazepam (large doses)	Dicumarol
Danazol	Dramamine	Digoxin
Dapsone	Enalapril	Diphenhydramine
Diclofenac	Etidocaine	Droperidol
Enflurane	Etomidate	EDTA
Ergot preparations	Erythromycin	Epinephrine
Estrogens	Felbamate	Ether
Ethanol excess	Fluroxene[b]	Fentanyl
Ethchlorvynol	Food additives (selected)	Fluoxetine
Ethinamate	Furosemide	Gabapentin
Eucalyptol (in mouthwash)	Heavy metals	Gallamine
Glutethimide	Hydralazine	Guanethidine
Griseofulvin	Lamotrigine	Heparin
Halothane	Lidocaine	Hyoscine
Hydantoins	Mepivacaine	Ibuprofen
Imipramine	Methychlothiazide	Indomethacin
Isopropylmeprobamate	Metoclopramide	Insulin
Mephenytoin	Metyrapone	Labetalol
Meprobamate	Mitotane (o,p′-DDD)	Lisinopril
Methyldopa	Nalidixic acid	Lithium
Methylprylon	Nitrazepam	Losartan
Methsuximide	Nortriptyline	Mandelamine
Nikethamide	o,p′-DDD	Mefenamic acid
Novobiocin	Pargyline	Meperidine
Oral contraceptives	Pentylenetetrazole	Methadone
Pentazocine	Phenoxybenzamine	Methylphenidate
Phensuximide	Prilocaine	Morphine
Phenylbutazone	Pyrocaine	Naproxen
Phenytoin	Rifampicin	Narcotic analgesics
Primidone	Sulfonylureas	Neostigmine
Progestogens	Spironolactone	Nitrofurantoin
Pyrazinamide	Terpenes	Nitrous oxide
Pyrazolone derivatives	Tiagabine	Oxazepam
Succinimides	Tramadol	Oxylate/sodium
Sulfonamides	Tranylcypromine	Pancuronium
Sulfonethylmethane[b]		Paraldehyde
Theophylline and its derivatives		Paroxetine
Tolazamide		Penicillamine

Table 3 Continued

Reported to exacerbate disease[a]	Theoretically risky	Believed to be safe
Tolbutamide	All agents known to induce cytochromes P450 or to increase hepatic heme turnover	Penicillin
Trimethadione		Pentamethonium[b]
Troxidone		Phenothiazines
Valproate		Procaine
		Promazine
		Promethazine
		Propanidid[b]
		Propoxyphene
		Propranolol
		Prostigmine
		Rauwolfia alkaloids
		Reserpine
		Streptomycin
		Succinylcholine
		Tetracycline
		Thiouracil
		Thyroxine
		Vigabatrin
		Vitamins A, B, C, D, and E

[a]Among agents reported to exacerbate disease, those in *italics* have been incriminated most often. Those listed as theoretically risky have not been reported to exacerbate human porphyria, but they are porphyrogenic in experimental systems and probably in humans also. Those believed to be safe have been used in human acute porphyria without apparent ill effects and are not theoretically risky.
[b]Not available in the United States.
Source: Adapted from Bonkovsky, 1990.

tial. In such patients, an increase in ADH production is, in fact, appropriate, as the effort is made to maintain and protect an adequate effective circulating volume. Thus, the increase in ADH in acute porphyria may be "appropriate" rather than "inappropriate."

Specific Therapy with Intravenous Heme (Hematin)

The specific therapy for the acute porphyric attack is intravenous heme. As shown in Fig. 2, heme administered exogenously by the parenteral route is capable of gaining access to and repleting the size of the regulatory heme pool of hepatocytes. It will produce a rapid and profound downregulation of hepatic ALA synthase, and elevated levels of ALA and PBG in plasma and urine typically return to normal within 2–4 days of the initiation of intravenous heme therapy. In the United States, the only currently approved preparation of intravenous heme is hydroxyheme or hematin (Panhematin, Abbott Laboratories, Abbott Park, Illinois; Panhematin hot-line 1-800-622-2688). The usual dose is 3–5 mg/kg per day. There is evidence that lower doses may also be effective. Some authorities prefer to administer hematin every 12 h, but hematin given once daily is equally effective, both clinically and biochemically. A difficulty with hematin is that, once the lyophilized powder has been reconstituted in sterile water (as is recommended in the package insert), the preparation is very unstable. It undergoes a rather ill-defined series of polymerization and oxidation reactions. For this reason, once the powder has been redissolved in water, it needs to be administered as rapidly as possible, preferably within 1 h. In addition, and perhaps in part because of the degradation reactions, solutions of hematin cause a coagulopathy, with decreases in platelet count and prolongation of prothrombin time, partial thromboplastin time, and other measures of the function of soluble clotting factors. Aqueous solutions of hematin are also irritating to veins and may cause thrombophlebitis. If excessive doses of hematin are administered, patients may suffer from hemolysis or transient acute renal failure.

Some of the potential adverse effects of solutions of hematin can be averted or mitigated if the powder is reconstituted in human serum albumin rather than sterile water. A solution with a 1:1 molar ratio of hematin to human serum albumin is stable for an extended period of time and less prone to cause thrombophlebitis. To prepare such a solution, exactly 132 mL of 25% human serum albumin should be added to one 313-mg vial of lyophilized hematin. The resultant solution will contain an equal number of millimoles of albumin and of heme.

Another form of heme for intravenous use (heme arginate), which comes in vials as a rather concentrated solution, is available in many other countries. Its therapeutic effects are similar to those of hematin. It is less irritating to veins than hematin dissolved in sterile water. It is currently undergoing testing in the United States, and the manufacturer (Leiras Oy, Helsinki, Finland) hopes to receive FDA approval for it to be marketed in the United States.

Management of Seizures in Patients with Acute Porphyria

Seizures may complicate acute porphyric attacks, or they may occur in patients with acute porphyria. Therapy of such seizures has been particularly problematic, because most of the drugs used as anticonvulsants are highly porphyrogenic and therefore contraindicated in acute porphyria (Table 3).

Acute seizures can be treated successfully with parenteral magnesium sulfate or benzodiazepines, such as diazepam. However, such treatments are not effective for chronic use. The benzodiazepine clonazepam has been useful, although high doses are somewhat porphyrogenic. Bromides have been used and are not porphyrogenic, but they are quite toxic and have a low ratio of therapeutic to toxic dose levels.

In the past few years, a large number of new anticonvulsants have been developed and tested. Among these newer anticonvulsants, it has recently been shown that gabapentin and vigabatrin are not porphyrogenic and thus appear to be safe for use in patients with acute porphyria. In contrast, felbamate, lamotrigine, and especially tiagabine are highly porphyrogenic and should be avoided if at all possible.

Management of Frequent Recurrent Acute Porphyric Attacks

Some patients, particularly women, suffer monthly attacks of acute porphyria during the luteal phase of their menstrual cycles. These attacks appear to be related to the surge of progesterone that occurs during this phase of the cycle. Such women may be treated by oral contraceptives to suppress their own endogenous cycles. The lowest effective dose estrogen or estrogen-progesterone combination should be used. The reason is that estrogens and progestogens are themselves porphyrogenic and thus represent a potential two-edged sword.

An alternative approach is the use of analogues of luteinizing hormone–releasing hormone (LHRH). Such agents produce a marked downregulation of the production and release of FSH and LH from the pituitary, such that ovarian stimulation ceases and a "medical menopause" ensues, characterized by typical menopausal symptoms such as vasomotor instability and endometrial atrophy. The LHRH analogue that has been used most widely is leuprolide (Lupron, TAP Pharmaceuticals, Chicago). Leuprolide is generally given in a dose of 1 mg (0 2 mL) subcutaneously daily. Occasionally, higher doses may be required. Leuprolide can also be administered as a once-a-month depo preparation. Nearly all women with bona fide cyclical attacks of porphyria will have an excellent response to LHRH analogues. After they have been treated for 6–12 months, efforts should be made to taper and discontinue the LHRH analogue, because there is a great risk that osteoporosis will develop. For this reason, all patients who require LHRH analogues for more than 6 months should have regular measurements of bone mineral density, should take at least 1 g of supplemental calcium per day, should have measurements of serum 25-hydroxy vitamin D levels to ensure that their levels of vitamin D are adequate, and, if osteopenia is present or seen to be developing, should be treated with one of the new bisphosphonate preparations to retard or stop progression of osteoporosis.

Prevention of Acute Attacks of Porphyria

Secondary Prevention

Patients who have had one or more acute attacks of porphyria should be counseled to absolutely avoid drugs or chemicals that are known to be porphyrogenic. This includes alcohol, particularly the forms of alcohol found in dark-colored liquors, such as scotch, bourbon, and red wine. Such forms of alcohol contain appreciable concentrations of 3–5 carbon alcohols, which are even more porphyrogenic than is ethanol itself. They may also contain nonalcohol components that are porphyrogenic. Such patients should also be counseled to avoid starvation or any severe calorie restriction, e.g., diets with extremely low calorie intakes. Negative energy balance in general should be avoided. If such patients need to reduce, they should do so gradually and with close medical supervision. Other factors that may precipitate acute attacks of porphyria are overtiredness, severe physical or emotional stress, and intercurrent illness. If such illness occurs, it is essential that patients seek immediate effective therapy.

Patients should also be counseled to take steps to prevent acute illnesses from occurring. Such steps include vaccination against pneumococcal pneumonia, yearly influenza vaccination, and vaccination against all the usual childhood and adult diseases for which effective vaccines are available. This should include vaccination against hepatitis A and B.

Patients should also be urged to wear Medic Alert bracelets and to carry Medic Alert cards, indicating that they have acute porphyria and are sensitive to barbiturates, hydantoins, and sulfa drugs.

Some patients require regular infusions of hematin to prevent recurrent attacks. The hematin may need to be given one to three times per week or occasionally less often, perhaps every 2–3 weeks.

In those with frequent attacks, for whom heme is often required, the addition of an inhibitor of heme oxygenase, to enhance and/or prolong the effectiveness of heme, is rational. Indeed, it has been shown that although such inhibitors alone have little effect (at least at the doses used), their administration with heme can significantly prolong the biochemical and clinical effects of the latter (Dover et al., *Gastroenterology*, 1994).

Primary Prevention

Whenever a diagnosis of an acute porphyria has been made, the first-degree relatives of the patient should undergo testing to see if they too may harbor the metabolic defect that can lead to the development of symptomatic porphyria. Depending upon the specific type of porphyria, investigation may involve measurements of plasma, stool, urine, or enzymatic activities. The latter are particularly useful in the case of AIP and ADP, in both of which the enzymatic defect is usually expressed in erythrocytes. In the case of AIP, however, there is a form of the disease in which the enzymatic defect is limited to the housekeeping form of the enzyme. Approximately 15% of patients and families have this type of AIP. In them, assay of activity of PBG deaminase in erythrocytes is entirely normal, and the diagnosis cannot be made by such an erythrocytic assay. An additional difficulty is that about 10% of patients and normals will have activities of erythrocytic PBG deaminase that fall into an "indeterminate zone," which is between activities that are clearly normal and activities that are clearly abnormal. In such kindreds, study of the entire kindred may provide clarification of status.

In the case of hereditary coproporphyria and variegate porphyria, assay of erythrocytic enzyme activities is not rational or reliable because the relevant enzymes are intramitochondrial and the adult erythrocytes do not contain mitochondria. Although one large reference laboratory in the United States (The Mayo Medical Laboratory, Rochester, Minnesota) has offered a test for "erythrocytic" coproporphyrinogen oxidase, the assay is fundamentally flawed and unreliable. It should not be used (Hahn and Bonkovsky, *Arch Intern Med*, 1997).

Because all of the genes for the enzymes of heme synthesis have been cloned and sequenced, it is theoretically possible to make the diagnosis of porphyria or of the carrier state for acute porphyria by DNA testing. However, such testing is not generally available. Furthermore, because of marked heterogeneity of specific defects, it may be difficult, time-consuming, and expensive to make a diagnosis by DNA testing unless the defect for at least one member of the family has already been established.

MANAGEMENT OF PORPHYRIA CUTANEA TARDA (PCT)

The pathogenesis of the chronic hepatic porphyrias, particularly PCT, is complex. Patients often have a history of heavy alcohol use, and some degree of iron overload is also common. At times, patients give a history of estrogen ingestion. Management of the disease should always include cessation of the use of alcohol, estrogens, and iron.

Iron Reduction

The cornerstone of therapy continues to be a reduction of iron in the liver. This is generally accomplished by therapeutic phlebotomy, following a schedule as for the treatment of hereditary homozygous hemochromatosis. Indeed, 30–45% of patients with sporadic PCT have been found to be heterozygous for HLA-linked hereditary hemochromatosis.

Antimalarial Medications

Antimalarial medications, such as chloroquine or hydroxychloroquine, are also effective. They act by forming water-soluble complexes with uroporphyrin and heptacarboxy porphyrin, which are then cleared from the liver and excreted in the urine. Initial doses of such medications should be low (125 mg two to three times per week) because high doses may lead to an acute hepatitis with fever and right-upper-quadrant pain. This seems to be due to a rapid and marked clearing of porphyrins from the liver.

Role of Hepatitis C Infection and Its Therapy

In the United States, approximately 50–60% of patients with PCT are infected with the hepatitis C virus. The prevalence of chronic hepatitis C is even higher in countries in southern Europe, where 75–90% of patients with PCT have been found to have evidence of HCV infection. In contrast, the prevalence of HCV infection in patients from northern Europe, Australia, or New Zealand is much lower (0–25%). It is not known how or why HCV infection predisposes to the development of PCT. It is of interest that iron in the liver is also able to exacerbate chronic hepatitis C infection and is associated with a decreased likelihood of response to interferon therapy. Probably, HCV infection and iron both act to increase oxidative stress in hepatocytes, thus favoring the oxidation of uroporphyrinogen to uroporphyrin, which cannot be metabolized further by uroporphyrinogen decarboxylase (Fig. 1) and which, therefore, accumulates in the liver and eventually spills into the plasma. If the PCT is relatively mild (urinary porphyrin excretion less than 2000 μg/24 h), the disease may be treated simply with cessation of alcohol and interferon, targeting the hepatitis C infection. However, because of the evidence that iron reduction improves the response to interferon in chronic hepatitis C, it seems wiser to deplete iron prior to interferon therapy.

Local Skin Protection

All patients with PCT or with any of the other porphyrias in which there are cutaneous manifestations should be advised to avoid strong sunlight or other light sources, to wear opaque protective clothing, and to apply opaque sunscreens, such as zinc oxide or titanium dioxide paste, particularly to areas that are likely to receive sun exposure, such as the nose or the backs of the hands. Sunscreens that protect against sunburn are unfortunately of little or no use because they do not screen out light of 400–410 nm, which is the light that activates porphyrins.

Long-Term Follow-up

It typically takes several (4–9) months for patients with PCT to show a biochemical and clinical response. After they have achieved remission with iron reduction and/or antimalarial therapy, they will often remain in remission for a number of years, particularly if they do not have active hepatitis C and if they avoid alcohol intake. Many such patients will remain in remission for many years after a remission has been achieved. It seems wise to check urinary porphyrin excretion in such patients once a year, in the late winter or early spring. If they demonstrate an increase in urinary porphyrin excretion again, a further course of iron-reduction therapy should be instituted promptly.

MANAGEMENT OF HEPATOERYTHROPOIETIC PORPHYRIA (HEP)

As already described, this disease represents the severe homozygous (or compound heterozygous) form of PCT. Patients typically present in infancy with severe photo-induced skin damage, fragility, and vesiculobullous eruptions. Uroporphyrin overproduction is extremely high, and therapy, which is as for PCT, is not very effective.

Fortunately, the disease is rare. Those who are severely affected should be considered for liver and/or bone marrow transplantation. In future, targeted gene therapy may prove effective.

MANAGEMENT OF PROTOPORPHYRIA

Local Skin Protection and Beta-Carotene

The symptom most often requiring treatment in protoporphyria is the acute photosensitivity with solar urticaria. In mild cases, opaque clothing and avoidance of bright sunlight may suffice. For those who are more severely affected, a variety of topical and systemic agents have been tried, and benefit has been claimed for a number of preparations. The most effective of these appears to be beta-carotene. The usual adult dose is 60–180 mg orally per day. Therapeutic effectiveness is assessed from the patient's symptoms and signs and by measurements of levels of carotene in the plasma. Optimal levels are considered to be 600–800 μg/dL. Such treatment is generally well tolerated, although the skin becomes distinctly yellow, which for some is cosmetically unacceptable.

Reducing Protoporphyrin Production

Efforts should also be directed towards identifying and ameliorating factors that may increase protoporphyrin production or accumulation. In particular, treatment of iron deficiency may have gratifying results. Some patients suffer from increased hemolysis, and in such rare patients splenectomy can alleviate both the hemolysis and a large measure of protoporphyrin overproduction. Hypertransfusion therapy with normal erythrocytes has been beneficial in a few patients in whom it has been used. In theory, it should be effective in virtually all patients with protoporphyria, because developing erythroid cells are the major sources of protoporphyrin and their production can be downregulated by regular transfusions. However, such frequent transfusions are expensive and inconvenient, and they carry with them low but unavoidable risk of transmission of infection. They also will tend, with time, to produce iron overload.

As for the acute porphyrias, high carbohydrate intakes have been reported to decrease fecal and plasma levels of protoporphyrin in protoporphyria. Therefore, starvation or crash dieting should be avoided, and severely affected patients should maintain a daily carbohydrate intake of at least 300 g. Intravenous infusions of hematin have also been described to be of benefit in patients with protoporphyria, particularly those with very high levels of circulating porphyrins and liver injury.

Increasing Protoporphyrin Excretion

Another therapeutic approach is to increase fecal excretion of protoporphyrin by interruption of the enterohepatic circulation. Cholestyramine (12–16 g per day), which binds porphyrins, has often been used, although clinical benefit has been equivocal, at best. Activated charcoal (30 g orally every 3–6 h) has also been reported to be of benefit, but it is really not feasible for patients to take such doses on a chronic basis. Bile salts that form micelles may play a role in secretion of protoporphyrin from the liver and solubilization of the porphyrin in the bile. There have been anecdotal reports of apparent benefit of administration of chenodeoxycholic acid for therapy of severe protoporphyria. In contrast, ursodeoxycholic acid is not of benefit and may actually do harm.

Pigment Gallstones and Their Management

Patients with protoporphyria also are at increased risk to develop pigment gallstones. If such stones become symptomatic, patients should undergo laparoscopic cholecystectomy unless there are strong contraindications to the surgery.

Cirrhosis: The Major Complication of Protoporphyria

The major potential complication of protoporphyria is the development of hepatic fibrosis, cirrhosis, and liver failure. The pathogenesis involves progressive accumulation of protoporphyrin in the liver. Such accumulation can be precipitated or exacerbated by any condition that causes cholestasis. Examples include alcoholic liver disease or acute or chronic viral hepatitis. The development of jaundice without biliary obstruction portends a grave prognosis, often imminent death, although there are exceptions. Nevertheless, any patient with protoporphyria and cirrhosis, especially with hyperbilirubinemia, should be considered for liver transplantation. The management of such patients during and after transplantation is complicated because of their severe photosensitivity and high levels of blood and tissue protoporphyrin. Some of these patients have developed neuronopathic syndromes that resemble the acute porphyrias. Thus, it is better to transplant patients with protoporphyria and cirrhosis before they have reached an end stage of very severe disease. Liver transplantation clearly has been lifesaving, although it has not cured the abnormal protoporphyrin overproduction, which arises principally from the bone marrow. Thus, a true cure of the metabolic disorder requires either bone marrow transplantation or, in the future, perhaps some other, lesser form of effective gene therapy.

MANAGEMENT OF CONGENITAL ERYTHROPOIETIC PORPHYRIA (CEP)

Like HEP, CEP is due to a severe, homozygous (or compound heterozygous) enzymatic defect that causes a very severe form of porphyria, usually manifest early in infancy. It is quite rare, with fewer than two hundred cases having been described thus far.

Local therapy to the skin is as for PCT. Patients with evidence of splenomegaly and hemolysis usually benefit somewhat from splenectomy, which decreases the demand for marrow red blood cell production. Intravenous hematin has benefited some, indicating that hematin can get into erythroblasts as well as into hepatocytes and can downregulate overproduction of porphyrins.

Bone marrow transplantation has been curative in a few, and specific gene therapy is appealing but, to date, unrealized.

ACKNOWLEDGMENTS

I thank Rebecca Silver for typing the manuscript and otherwise assisting in its completion. Supported by a grant from NIH (DK 38825). The opinions expressed in this paper are those of the author; they do not necessarily reflect the official views of the U.S. Public Health Service or the National Institutes of Health.

BIBLIOGRAPHY

Bissell DM. Treatment of acute hepatic porphyria with hematin. J Hepatol 1988; 6:1–7.

Bloomer JR, Bonkovsky HL. The porphyrias. Disease-a-Month 1989; 35:5–54.

Bonkovsky HL. Porphyrin and heme metabolism and the porphyrias. In: Zakim D, Boyer TD, eds. Hepatology: A Textbook of Liver Disease, 2d ed. Philadelphia: Saunders, 1990:378–424.

Bonkovsky HL. The porphyrias. In: Conn RB, ed. Current Diagnosis, 8th ed. Philadelphia: Saunders, 1991:799–804.

Bonkovsky HL. The porphyrias. In: Rakel RE, ed. Conn's Current Therapy. Philadelphia: Saunders, 1993:427–433.

Bonkovsky HL. Advances in understanding and treating "the little imitator," acute porphyria. Gastroenterology 1993; 105:590–594.

Bonkovsky HL, Barnard GF. The hepatic porphyrias. In: Brandt L, ed. Practice of Clinical Gastroenterology. Philadelphia: Current Medicine, 1998:947–960.

Bonkovsky HL, Barnard GF. Diagnosis of porphyric syndromes: a practical approach in the era of molecular biology. Semin Liver Dis 1998; 18:57–65.

Hahn M, Bonkovsky HL. Disorders of porphyrin metabolism. In: Wu G, Israel J, eds. Disease of the Liver and Bile Ducts: A Practical Guide to Diagnosis and Treatment. Totowa, NJ: Humana, 1998:249–272.

Hahn M, Gildemeister OS, Krauss GL, Pepe JA, Lambrecht RW, Donohue S, Bonkovsky HL. Effects of new anticonvulsant medications on porphyrin synthesis in cultured liver cells—potential implications for patients with acute porphyria. Neurology, 1997; 49:97–106.

Hahn M, Bonkovsky HL. Multiple chemical sensitivity syndrome and porphyria: a note of caution and concern. Arch Intern Med 1997; 157:281–285.

Kalman DR, Bonkovsky HL. Management of acute attacks in the porphyrias. Clin Dermatol 1998; 16:299–306.

Lamon JM, Frykholm BC, Hess RA, Tschudy DP. Hematin therapy for acute porphyria. Medicine 1979; 58:252–269.

Pierach CA. Hematin therapy for the porphyric attack. Semin Liver Dis 1982; 2:125–131.

Russo S, Pepe JA, Cable EE, Lambrecht RW, Bonkovsky HL. Synergistic repression of ALA synthase by heme and zinc-mesoporphyrin in a chick embryo liver cell culture model of acute porphyria. Eur J Clin Invest 1994; 24:406–415.

Windebank AJ, Bonkovsky HL. Porphyric neuropathy. In: Dyck PJ, Thomas PK, Griffin JW, Low PA, Poduslo JF, eds. Peripheral Neuropathy, 3d ed. Philadelphia: Saunders, 1992:1161–1168.

30
Management of Alpha$_1$-Antitrypsin Deficiency

David H. Perlmutter
Washington University School of Medicine and St. Louis Children's Hospital, St. Louis, Missouri

INTRODUCTION

Alpha$_1$-antitrypsin (α_1-AT) deficiency is a relatively common genetic disorder, affecting 1 in 1600 to 1800 live births, but prospective natural history studies indicate that only 10–15% of the affected population develop clinically significant liver disease. In most cases this liver disease is first detected by cholestasis in the neonatal period. In some cases it presents later in childhood or early adolescence with complications of portal hypertension. It has also been associated with chronic liver injury and hepatocellular carcinoma in adults. Although it is not entirely clear what proportion of the α_1-AT–deficient population is affected, a substantial number of these individuals develop destructive lung disease and emphysema beginning in the third decade of life. Cigarette smoking markedly increases the rate and severity of this destructive lung disease.

Most data in the literature indicate that the pathogenesis of liver and lung disease in this deficiency involves distinct mechanisms. Liver disease is thought to result from hepatotoxic effects of the mutant α_1-AT molecule retained in the endoplasmic reticulum (ER) of liver cells. Recent studies have suggested that the 85% of α_1-AT–deficient individuals who are "protected" from liver injury can degrade the mutant α_1-AT molecule within the ER. In contrast, there is a lag in ER degradation of the mutant α_1-AT protein in "susceptible" hosts, leading to even greater net retention of the presumably hepatotoxic molecule. Lung disease is thought to result from the decrease in α_1-AT in the circulation and body fluids, particularly the lung fluid. Because α_1-AT is the predominant elastase inhibitor in the circulation and the lower airways, this deficiency allows elastases to destroy the connective tissue integrity of the lung, particularly its elastic properties. By generating an increase in the release of active oxygen intermediates by macrophages and neutrophils, cigarette smoking indirectly facilitates oxidative inactivation of the residual α_1-AT molecules in the lung and thereby accelerates the elastolytic damage.

Management of the liver disease associated with α_1-AT deficiency is for the most part supportive. Children and adults with this deficiency have been successfully treated for liver failure by liver replacement therapy. Although conventional protein replacement or gene replacement therapy is unlikely to be successful in preventing or treating α_1-AT deficiency–associated liver disease, several novel types of gene therapy have been discussed in the literature. Recent studies of hepatocyte transplantation in animal models of liver injury provide some hope that this form of therapy may be useful for α_1-AT deficiency–associated liver disease in the future.

CLINICAL ASSOCIATIONS (Table 1)

α_1-AT deficiency is associated with the neonatal hepatitis syndrome. The infant is evaluated in the first 8 weeks of life for jaundice or hepatomegaly and found to have elevated levels of conjugated bilirubin and transaminases. Only 25% of these infants develop clinically significant liver disease. In some cases, this is manifest by poor growth and progressive liver failure. In other cases, there is slow progression of liver disease over several years. The remaining 75% of the infants who are discovered in the neonatal period may have elevated transaminase levels for many years but never develop significant liver disease. In the only prospective study of α_1-AT deficiency, Sveger identified 127 PIZZ (protease inhibitor phenotype Z homozygous) children by screening 200,000 newborns in Sweden. Of these 127 patients, 14 had prolonged obstructive jaundice and 9 of the 14 had severe liver disease by clinical and laboratory criteria. Another 8 of the 127 PIZZ infants had mild abnormalities of serum bilirubin, transaminases, or hepatomegaly. Approximately 50% of the remainder of the 127 had only abnormalities of the transaminase levels. Published follow-up studies at 18 years of age of the original cohort have shown that more than 85% have persistently normal serum transaminase levels with no evidence of liver dysfunction.

α_1-AT deficiency may also present later in childhood or early in adolescence with complications of portal hypertension, such as ascites, edema, esophageal/gastric variceal bleeding, or hypersplenism. In some of these patients there is a history of jaundice during infancy, indicating that there has been a "honeymoon period" and that this can last for years. In others there is no history of jaundice, hepatomegaly, or even incidentally observed elevation in serum transaminases.

In adults, α_1-AT deficiency can cause chronic hepatitis, cirrhosis, and/or hepatocellular carcinoma. On clinical grounds alone, it may be difficult to distinguish between α_1-AT deficiency and other chronic liver diseases in the differential diagnosis, including autoimmune hepatitis, drug-induced hepatitis, chronic viral hepatitis, and Wilson's disease.

It is well established in the literature that homozygous PIZZ α_1-AT deficiency alone can be the only explanation for liver disease in each of the above clinical situations. It is not clear whether the heterozygous PIZ α_1-AT state by itself can account for clinically signifi-

Table 1 Liver Disease in Alpha$_1$-Antitrypsin Deficiency

Newborn infant	Jaundice, elevated transaminases; poor growth, chronic liver dysfunction
Older child, adolescent	Portal hypertension, bleeding from varices
Adult	Chronic hepatitis Cryptogenic cirrhosis Hepatocellular carcinoma

Table 2 Diagnosis of Alpha$_1$-Antitrypsin Deficiency-Associated Liver Disease

α_1-AT level	10–15% of normal levels
Pi type	Abnormally rapid migration of major isoforms of α_1-AT (PIZZ)
Liver biopsy	Periodic-acid Schiff-positive, diastase-resistant globules in ER of liver cells

cant liver disease of any kind. In fact, most of the evidence suggests that other etiologies such as alcohol, autoimmune hepatitis, or viral hepatitis provide an explanation for liver injury in the heterozygote. It is also possible that other etiologies contribute to the development of liver disease in homozygotes who would have otherwise been "protected" from α_1-AT deficiency–associated liver disease (see below).

DIAGNOSIS (Table 2)

The diagnosis of α_1-AT deficiency is based on the phenotype of the α_1-AT protein present in a patient's serum, as determined by isoelectric focusing or by agarose electrophoresis at acidic pH. The determination of the α_1-AT level in a patient's serum should not be the sole basis of the diagnosis, because α_1-AT is an acute-phase reactant and therefore, may be transiently elevated, even in PIZZ patients, during the host response to tissue injury or inflammation. However, the α_1-AT level may sometimes be useful as a supplemental test to help differentiate family members who are compound heterozygotes and to detect carriers of the rare M phenotype allelic variants, such as M_{malton} and M_{duarte}, which can be associated with liver abnormalities. A research tool that will become more widely available in the future is the detection of specific α_1-AT variants by amplification of genomic DNA using the polymerase chain reaction. This rapid and sensitive technique requires only a small amount of cellular material and can be useful in screening, research studies, and prenatal diagnosis.

The diagnosis of the PIZZ α_1-AT deficiency can be substantiated by the characteristic histological appearance of periodic acid-Schiff–positive, diastase-resistant globules in the ER of hepatocytes. However, this finding alone, or its absence, is not regarded as diagnostic, because the globules can be difficult to detect in the first few months of life and also because similar structures can be observed in PIMM individuals with other liver diseases. The inclusions, 1- to 40-μm round-to-oval eosinophilic bodies, are most prominent in the periportal hepatocytes, although they can sometimes be seen in other hepatic cell types. The liver biopsy may also be characterized by a variable degree of cholestasis, hepatocellular necrosis, inflammatory cell infiltrate, bile duct epithelial cell destruction, and periportal fibrosis or cirrhosis. In some cases, there is bile duct proliferation; in a few, there is paucity of intrahepatic bile ducts.

PATHOGENESIS

The α_1-AT molecule is a ~55-kDa plasma glycoprotein. Its major physiological function is inhibition of neutrophil proteases, including elastase, cathepsin G, and proteinase 3. As an acute-phase protein, its plasma concentration increases three- to fourfold during the host response to tissue injury or inflammation. It is predominantly secreted by hepatocytes in the liver but is also secreted by several different extrahepatic cell types in several different tissues.

The mutant α_1-AT Z molecule is characterized by a single nucleotide substitution of lys for glu 342. It is synthesized normally but is retained early in the secretory pathway in endoplasmic reticulum (ER). The defect is not specific for liver cells—it affects other sites of α_1-AT synthesis, such as macrophages, and is observed in several types of transfected cell lines. Site-directed mutagenesis studies have shown that this single amino acid substitution is sufficient to produce the cellular defect. Structural studies have shown that the mutant α_1-AT Z molecule folds very slowly, leading to accumulation of an intermediate that has a tendency to polymerize, presumably within the ER.

In contrast to the pathogenesis of lung injury in α_1-AT deficiency, which involves an uninhibited proteolytic attack on lung elastin, there is no evidence that the pathophysiology of liver injury in this condition is due to a deficiency of elastase inhibitory capacity. Most evidence favors the concept that the accumulation of α_1-AT in the ER is directly related to liver cell injury. Experiments in transgenic mice carrying the mutant Z α_1-AT allele have provided direct experimental support for this "accumulation theory." These mice have intrahepatocytic globules of α_1-AT; they develop liver disease and, ultimately, hepatocellular carcinoma. Because there are normal levels of α_1-AT and presumably other antielastases in these animals, as directed by the endogenous murine genes, liver injury cannot be attributed to diminished serum or tissue levels of α_1-AT.

Several recent studies have indicated that PIZZ individuals who are "protected" from liver disease are able to degrade the mutant α_1-AT Z molecules that are retained in the ER. Presumably, this reduces the burden of mutant molecules in the ER. The mechanism for ER degradation appears to be complex requiring at least three general steps: binding to a transmembrane ER molecule chaperone calnexin; induction of ubiquitin conjugation to the cytoplasmic tail of calnexin; degradation of the α_1-AT Z-polyubiquitinated calnexin complex from the cytoplasmic aspect of the ER by the 26S proteasome. These studies also provide evidence that PIZZ individuals who are "susceptible" to liver disease have a lag in ER degradation and that different steps in the ER degradation pathway can be altered in a single "susceptible" PIZZ individual (Fig. 1). The combined effect of the abnormal folding of α_1-AT Z in the ER and the lag in ER degradation is marked accumulation of mutant protein within the ER.

MANAGEMENT

The most important principle in the treatment of α_1-AT deficiency is the avoidance of cigarette smoking, which markedly accelerates the destructive lung disease associated with α_1-AT deficiency, reduces the quality of life, and significantly shortens the lives of these individuals.

It is also important that families of affected infants and children understand the implications of the Sveger studies. Most infants/children with α_1-AT deficiency will never develop clinically significant liver disease. Even children who had cholestasis in the first 6 months of life had a low likelihood ($< 25\%$) of developing clinical liver disease.

There is no specific therapy for α_1-AT deficiency–associated liver disease; therefore, clinical care largely involves supportive management for liver dysfunction and prevention of complications (Table 3). This will include special attention to poor feeding, growth failure, and fat-soluble vitamin stores. During infancy, formulas may be supplemented with

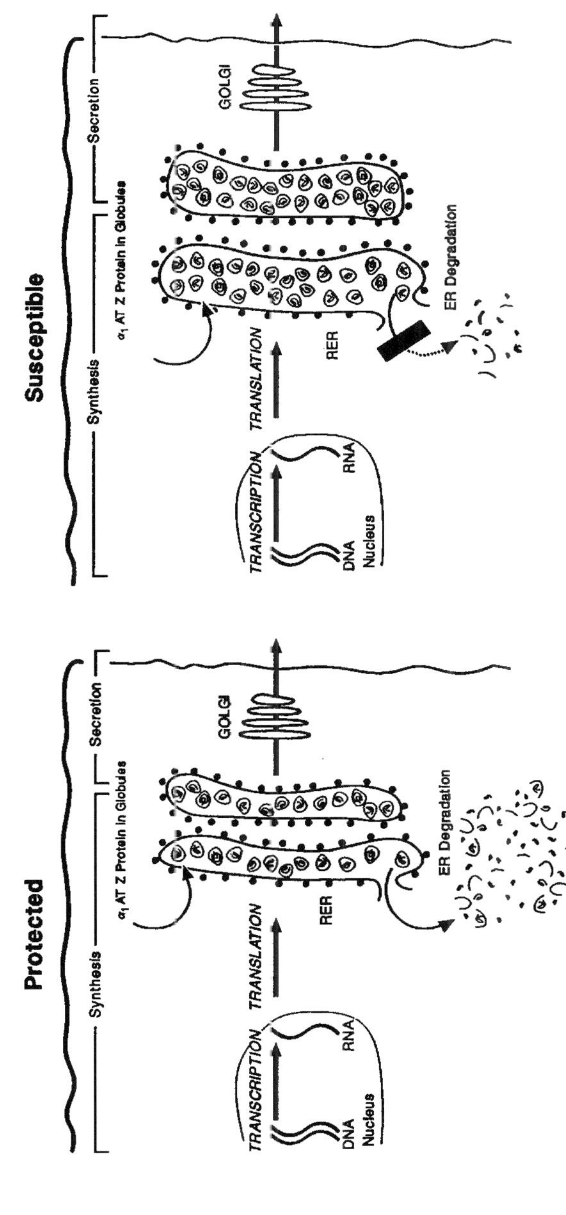

Figure 1 Difference in ER degradation of α_1-AT Z in protected and susceptible hosts. The block in ER degradation in susceptible hosts is represented by a small dark bar. (From Teckman et al., 1996, with permission.)

Table 3 Supportive Management of Alpha$_1$-Antitrypsin Deficiency-Associated Liver Disease

Avoidance of cigarette smoking
Supplementation of feedings with increased calories (MCT oil, polycose, NG tube feedings, TPN)
Vitamin K, sometimes vitamin D, vitamin E
Diuretics: spironolactone ± thiazide
H_2-receptor antagonist during intercurrent illnesses
Ursodeoxycholic acid for cholestatic symptoms
Sclerotherapy/banding for intractable variceal bleeding
Lactulose ± neomycin for encephalopathy

additional calories. Medium-chain triglycerides are recommended because of better absorption in the presence of low intraluminal concentration of bile acids. Glucose polymers may also be added to standard formulas to increase caloric density. Occasionally enteral feedings by nasogastric tube or even home parenteral alimentation therapy may be necessary. Most of the infants with severe liver disease need to be on vitamin K. If the liver disease is associated with cholestasis, vitamin E and vitamin D supplementation may be necessary. A spironolactone diuretic, sometimes together with a thiazide, will be used for children with edema or ascites. Families are given prescriptions for an H_2-receptor blocking agent to start when patients develop a viral respiratory illness, since this is the time when they tend to have bleeding from esophageal and sometimes gastric varices. In contrast to variceal bleeding in adults, variceal bleeding in children often remits spontaneously with expectant therapy. If persistent, however, sclerotherapy and banding therapy may be indicated. Beta blockers have not been effective in most children with liver disease. A small number of children with α_1-AT deficiency develop pruritus, xanthomas, and hypercholesterolemia. We usually put these children on ursodeoxycholic acid. If pruritus becomes severe, it may be necessary to try phenobarbital and/or rifampin. In our experience children are generally unwilling to take cholestyramine or other "relatively unpalatable" bile acid–binding resins. Most of the time this cholestatic picture will "burn out" over time except for relapses during viral infections. Encephalopathy is not common, but when it develops, it is treated with lactulose with or without neomycin. In general, liver dysfunction becomes more pronounced when the child develops an upper respiratory illness or other viral/bacterial infections.

Progressive liver dysfunction and failure in children has been treated by orthotopic liver transplantation, with survival rates approaching 90% at 1 year and 80% at 5 years (Table 4). Nevertheless, a number of PIZZ individuals with severe liver disease, even cirrhosis and/or portal hypertension, may have a relatively low rate of disease progression and lead fairly normal lives for extended periods of time. With the availability of living-

Table 4 Major Treatment Strategies for α_1-AT Deficiency–Associated Liver Disease

Supportive
Shunt surgery (rare)
Orthotopic liver transplantation

related donor transplantation techniques, it may be possible to manage these patients expectantly for some time. Children with α_1-AT deficiency and mild liver dysfunction (elevated transaminases and/or hepatomegaly), without functional impairment do not necessarily have a poor prognosis and may never need liver transplantation. The optimism associated with early transplantation before the onset of complications of chronic liver disease should be accompanied by the recognition that there may be little or no progression of the liver injury in these patients for many years.

Most α_1-AT–deficient individuals with liver disease are not candidates for alternative surgical interventions. However, there are rare, specific clinical situations in which a portacaval or splenorenal shunt might be considered, e.g., in an individual with only mild liver synthetic dysfunction and mild parenchymal liver injury but severe portal hypertension. Several children with severe liver disease and α_1-AT deficiency have survived 10–15 years after shunt surgery before requiring liver transplantation. Moreover, previous hepatobiliary surgery is not a statistically significant risk factor for poor outcome of subsequent liver transplantation.

Patients with α_1-AT deficiency and emphysema have undergone replacement therapy with purified and recombinant plasma α_1-AT either by intravenous or intratracheal aerosol administration. This therapy is associated with improvement in serum concentrations of α_1-AT, in bronchoalveolar lavage fluid concentrations of α_1-AT, and in neutrophil elastase-inhibitory capacity without significant side effects. Although studies have demonstrated only biochemical efficacy, purified plasma α_1-AT has been licensed for clinical use in the α_1-AT–deficient individuals with emphysema because it is thought that data regarding clinical efficacy are virtually impossible to collect. This therapy is designed only for individuals with established and progressive emphysema. Protein replacement therapy is not being used for individuals with liver disease because there is no information to support the notion that deficient serum levels of α_1-AT are mechanistically related to liver injury.

Replacement of α_1-AT by somatic gene therapy has also been discussed in the literature. This strategy is potentially less expensive than replacement therapy with purified proteins and would alleviate the need for intravenous or inhalation therapy. Again, this form of therapy would be useful only in ameliorating emphysema, because liver disease associated with α_1-AT deficiency is not caused by deficient levels of α_1-AT in the serum or tissues. Of course, it would be helpful to know that replacement therapy with purified α_1-AT as it is currently applied is effective in ameliorating emphysema associated with α_1-AT deficiency before embarking on clinical trials involving gene therapy. There are also still major issues that need to be addressed before gene therapy becomes a realistic alternative. In all of the methods that have been described in the literature to date, the levels of the transferred gene product have been low and have been sustained for only short intervals. Enthusiasm for the use of retroviral vectors has been tempered by difficulties in purifying and concentrating the viral particles and also because retroviral infection and therefore transduction of the recombinant gene requires active division of the target cell. The use of adenoviral vectors has been considered more attractive, but recent studies have shown that the host responds with a vigorous, troublesome immune response in the target tissue. A recent study has suggested that lentiviral vectors are an attractive alternative because they can transduce genes into nondividing and terminally differentiated cells.

There is one potential major complication in replacement therapy with either purified α_1-AT or α_1-AT gene. This relates to the fact that α_1-AT is being infused into a host with high levels of free elastase and, if effective, would be expected to generate high levels of elastase-α_1-AT complexes. Such complexes, through the serpin-enzyme complex receptor,

Table 5 Potential Treatment Strategies for α_1-AT Deficiency–Associated Liver Disease

Homologous recombination
Antisense ribozyme
Trans-splicing ribozymes
Chimeric oligonucleotides
Hepatocyte transplantation
Pharmacological treatment to increase ER degradation of α_1-ATZ in selected hosts (e.g., interferon γ)

mediate increases in the synthesis of α_1-AT and in intracellular retention of α_1-AT, thereby predisposing the α_1-AT–deficient host to liver injury.

Several novel types of gene therapy (Table 5), such as homologous recombination for targeted gene disruption and use of ribozymes for targeted RNA destruction, are theoretically attractive strategies for the liver disease in α_1-AT deficiency because they would prevent the synthesis of the mutant α_1-ATZ protein and ER retention. Recent studies have also shown that *trans*-splicing ribozymes can emend a mutant transcript and that chimeric oligonucleotides composed of DNA and modified RNA can correct mutant transcripts. However, there has been very little consideration of the clinical and ethical issues involved in these strategies, which make it unlikely that they will have therapeutic application in the near future.

A very interesting series of studies over the last several years has shown that transplanted adult hepatocytes can replicate and replace a diseased mouse liver. This was originally shown only for an unusual liver abnormality, nodular change induced by targeted transgenic expression of urokinase-type plasminogen activator in the liver. However, it has recently also been shown to occur in an animal model that recapitulates a human liver disease, hereditary tyrosinemia. These data imply that hepatocyte transplantation may permit repair of any metabolic liver disease in which the defect is cell-autonomous, injuring mutant liver cells but not neighboring wild-type cells. Thus, α_1-AT deficiency would be an excellent candidate for such a strategy.

Studies of the mechanism by which α_1-ATZ is retained and degraded in the ER of the subpopulation of α_1-AT–deficient individuals who develop liver injury and use of the transgenic animal model of α_1-AT deficiency type Z should also allow premorbid identification of the target population and suggest several additional strategies for the treatment of this target population.

BIBLIOGRAPHY

Dycaico JM, Grant SGN, Felts K, Nichols WS, Geller SA, Hager JH, Pollard AJ, et al. Neonatal hepatitis induced by α1-antitrypsin: a transgenic mice model. Science 1988; 242:1404–1412.

Eriksson S, Carlson J, Velez R. Risk of cirrhosis and primary liver cancer in α_1-antitrypsin deficiency. N Engl J Med 1989; 314:736–739.

Geller SA, Nichols WS, Kim SS, Tolmachoff T, Lee S, Dycaico MJ, Felts K, Sorge JA. Hepatocarcinogenesis is the sequel to hepatitis in Z #2 α_1-antitrypsin transgenic mice: histopathological and DNA ploidy studies. Hepatology 1994; 19:389–397.

Lomas DA, Evans DL, Finch JJ, Carrell RW. The mechanism of Z α_1-antitrypsin accumulation in the liver. Nature 1992; 357:605–607.

Naldini L, Blomer U, Gallay P, Ory D, Mulligan R, Gage FH, Verma IM, Trono D. In vivo gene delivery and stable transduction of nondividing cells by a lentiviral vector. Science 1996; 272:263–267.

Overturf K, Al-Dhalimy M, Tanguay R, Brantly M, Ou C-N, Finegold M, Grompe M. Hepatocytes corrected by gene therapy are selected in vivo in a murine model of hereditary tyrosinemia type I. Nature Genet 1996; 12:266–273.

Propst T, Propst A, Dietze O, Judmaier G, Braunsteiner H, Vogel W. High prevalence of viral infections in adults with homozygous and heterozygous α_1-antitrypsin deficiency and chronic liver disease. Ann Intern Med 1992; 117:641–645.

Qu D, Teckman TH, Omura S, Perlmutter DH. Degradation of mutant secretory protein, α_1-antitrypsin Z, in the endoplasmic reticulum requires proteasome activity. J Biol Chem 1996; 271:22791–22795.

Rhim JA, Sandgren EP, Degen JL, Palmiter RD, Brinster RL. Replacement of diseased mouse liver by hepatic cell transplantation. Science 1994; 263:1149–1152.

Sidhar SK, Lomas DA, Carrell RW, Foreman RC. Mutations which impede loop-sheet polymerization enhance the secretion of human α_1-antitrypsin deficiency variants. J Biol Chem 1995; 270:8393–8396.

Sveger T, Eriksson S. The liver in adolescents with α_1-antitrypsin deficiency. Hepatology 1995; 22:514–517.

Wu Y, Whitman I, Molmenti E, Moore K, Hippenmeyer P, Perlmutter DH. A lag in intracellular degradation of mutant α_1-antitrypsin correlates with the liver disease phenotype in homozygous PiZZ α_1-antitrypsin deficiency. Proc Natl Acad Sci USA 1994; 91:9014–9018.

Yu M-H, Lee KN, Kim J. The Z type variation of human α_1-antitrypsin causes a protein folding defect. Nature Struct Biol 1995; 2:363–367.

31
Management of Granulomatous Hepatitis

Gerd H. Sauter and Gerd R. Pape
University of Munich, Munich, Germany

Granulomas may appear in the liver in the course of many infectious, toxic, allergic, autoimmune and neoplastic disease processes, but they are also observed in conditions of unknown etiology. The diagnosis of the underlying illness is often obvious. In other instances, hepatic granulomas may be the only clear-cut manifestations of disease activity apart from nonspecific signs and symptoms. In the latter situation, the demonstration of granulomas in the liver should give rise to a diagnostic workup in order to disclose or exclude underlying disease processes that require further treatment.

Hepatic granulomas are manifestations of a circumscribed inflammatory response within the liver. In contrast to most other forms of hepatitis, there is usually no diffuse inflammatory infiltration in the portal tracts or in the liver parenchyma. It has therefore been suggested by some investigators that the occurrence of granulomas in the liver is better designated by the terms *hepatic granulomatosis*, *granulomas of the liver*, or *granulomatous disease of the liver* than *granulomatous hepatitis*. However, the term *granulomatous hepatitis* is widely accepted and broadly used. It was introduced by Eliakim et al. and Simon and Wolff to describe idiopathic forms of granulomatous hepatitis, and it has also been used more loosely to designate the occurrence of hepatic granulomas secondary to other disease processes. In this chapter the term *granulomatous hepatitis* refers to liver diseases characterized by the appearance of granulomas in the liver.

PATHOGENESIS OF GRANULOMATOUS HEPATITIS

Granulomas are small accumulations of modified macrophages or histiocytes surrounded by a rim of mononuclear cells, predominantly lymphocytes of the T-helper type. During granuloma formation, macrophages may take on the appearance of epithelioid cells and multinucleated giant cells.

Macrophages can ingest a broad variety of substances into membrane-bound vacuoles (endocytosis) representing pinocytosis of soluble molecules and phagocytosis of larger particles such as microorganisms. Intracellular degradation or killing of microorganisms is enhanced by the phenomenon of macrophage activation, which is accompanied by morphological changes and by several functional alterations, including production of radicals, secretion of enzymes, enzyme inhibitors, complement inhibitors, cytokines, and enhanced phagocytic activity. Activated macrophages are capable of destroying and processing most of the ingested substances rapidly, and only small portions of proteins (antigenic peptides of varying lengths) are presented in the context of major histocompatibility complex (MHC) molecules to lymphocytes. The sequent immune response is characterized by complex interactions between $CD4^+$ T lymphocytes and antigen-presenting macrophages showing increased expression of MHC class II molecules and increased production of cytokines such as interleukin (IL)-1. Production of interferon (IFN)-γ by T cells further increases expression of MHC class II antigens on activated macrophages. Depending upon the nature of the invading antigen and specific host factors, granulomas may form as a result of the persistence of nondegradable products or hypersensitivity reactions. In a stepwise series of events, an accumulation of activated macrophages, B cells, T cells, and fibroblasts develops. These cells actively produce a vast pattern of enzymes, mediators, and cytokines such as platelet-derived growth factor, transforming growth factor (TGF)-β, insulin-like growth factor, and tumor necrosis factor (TNF)-α.

The $CD4^+$ helper (Th) cells involved in the formation of granulomas may be divided into two functional groups, Thl and Th2. Thl-type cells produce IL-2, IFN-γ, and TNF upon stimulation with antigen and also participate in delayed-type hypersensitivity reactions, while Th2-type cells produce IL-4, IL-5, IL-6, IL-9, IL-10, and IL-13, which are important in the development of B cells and eosinophils. Moreover, the Th2-type response appears to account for certain pathological features of granulomatous reactions such as deposition of connective tissue matrix. Certain granulomas, especially those that develop in response to parasite ova, produce predominantly Th2 cytokines but only small quantities of Thl cytokines. On the other hand, production of large quantities of Thl cytokines and to a lesser degree Th2 cytokines is observed in granulomas of tuberculoid leprosy. At present, the complex interrelationships and regulation of these different T-cell subsets are incompletely understood.

CAUSES OF HEPATIC GRANULOMAS

Infectious diseases are the most common cause of both caseating and noncaseating granulomas in the liver, while noncaseating granulomas are most frequently found in sarcoidosis. Moreover, many other etiologies such as drugs, chemicals, neoplasia, immunological aberrations, and enzyme defects must be taken into account in patients presenting with granulomas in the liver (Tables 1 and 2).

Infections

Extrapulmonary tuberculosis may be associated with both caseating and noncaseating granulomas of the liver. Granulomas are often found within the liver parenchyma in the area of the central vein. The yield of granulomas on liver biopsy in extrapulmonary tuberculosis ranges from 23–80%. Demonstration of tuberculous bacilli by histological staining or by liver tissue cultures is highly specific but insensitive. The sensitivity of detection of *Mycobacterium tuberculosis* in liver tissue by use of the polymerase chain reaction (PCR) is about 60%.

Table 1 Causes of Granulomatous Hepatitis

- Infections
  - Bacterial
    - *M. tuberculosis*
    - Atypical mycobacteria
    - *M. leprae* (lepromatous leprosy)
    - *Brucella* sp. (brucellosis)
    - *Francisella tularensis* (tularemia)
    - *Listeria monocytogenes* (listeriosis)
    - *Tropheryma whippelii* (Whipple's disease)
    - *Bartonella henselae* (cat-scratch fever)
    - *Burkholderia pseudomallei* (melioidosis)
    - *Yersinia enterocolitica* (yersiniosis)
    - Donovan bodies (lymphogranuloma inguinale)
  - Rickettsial
    - *Coxiella burnetii* (Q fever)
    - *Rickettsia coroni* (fièvre boutonneuse)
  - Spirochetal
    - *Treponema pallidum* (syphilis)
- Infections (continued)
  - Fungal
    - *Histoplasma capsulatum* (histoplasmosis)
    - *Coccidioides immitis* (coccidioidomycosis)
    - *Cryptococcus neoformans* (cryptococcosis)
    - *Blastomyces dermatitidis* (North American blastomycosis)
  - Helminthic
    - *Schistosoma* species (schistosomiasis)
    - *Toxocara* (visceral larva migrans)
  - Protozoan
    - *Leishmania* (leishmaniasis)
    - *Toxoplasma gondii* (toxoplasmosis)
  - Viral
    - Epstein-Barr virus (mononucleosis)
    - Cytomegalovirus (cytomegaly)
    - Hepatitis viruses A and C
- Chemical
  - Beryllium
  - Copper
  - Drugs (see Table 3)
- Host defense defects
  - Chronic granulomatous disease of childhood
  - Hypogammaglobulinemia
- Neoplasia
  - Hodgkin's disease, other lymphomas
  - Carcinomas
- Miscellaneous
  - Sarcoidosis
  - Crohn's disease
  - Primary biliary cirrhosis
  - Autoimmune hepatitis
  - Immune complexes
  - BCG vaccine
  - Polymyalgia rheumatica
  - Allergic granulomatosis
  - Fatty liver
  - Chronic viral hepatitis
  - Liver cirrhosis
  - Idiopathic

Source: Modified from Fauci and Wolff, 1976.

Table 2 Frequencies of Underlying Disease Processes in Granulomatous Hepatitis

Unknown	23–50%
Sarcoidosis	11–22%
Tuberculosis	3–50%
Brucellosis	0–26%
Histoplasmosis	0–12%
Drug-related	0–28%
Q fever	0–4%
Primary biliary cirrhosis	5–6%
Hodgkin's disease, lymphomas	3–6%
Cirrhosis of unknown etiology	1–8%
Primary sclerosing cholangitis	0–1%
Hypogammaglobulinemia	0–1%

Granulomatous hepatitis has also been observed following bacille Calmette-Guérin (BCG) vaccination as well as after BCG immunotherapy for neoplastic disease. Hypersensitivity reactions to antigens from the BCG vaccine or persistence of indigestible antigens have been proposed as pathophysiological mechanisms. Disseminated atypical mycobacterial disease as well as leprosy may further be associated with granulomatous hepatitis.

Hepatic granulomas are common in brucellosis. Unpasteurized dairy products and exposure to infected animals continue to be common modes of transmission of *Brucella* sp. Impressive histological alterations may not be reflected by the mild alterations in liver function tests or in liver-specific symptoms. Discrete granulomas indistinguishable from sarcoidosis are seen with *B. abortus*, while areas of necrosis without cellular reaction occur with *B. suis* and *B. melitensis*.

Infections due to *Francisella tularensis* should be considered in persons who have had contact with game or rodents in endemic areas of the northern hemisphere. If microorganisms invade through cutaneous lesions, ulcerative primary complexes of the skin and mucous membranes may precede the development of granulomas in the liver. Granulomas in tularemia typically consist of necrotic nodules, while giant cells are rare. An abundance of polymorphonuclear cells may be seen in the periphery of these nodules.

Infections due to *Coxiella burnetii* (Q fever) may result in divergent pictures of acute and chronic liver disease, including granulomatous hepatitis. In patients presenting with undiagnosed hepatitis or granulomatous hepatitis, especially from rural areas, serological testing for Q fever should therefore be implemented in the diagnostic workup. The hepatic granuloma in Q fever typically contains a fibrin ring surrounding a central area of fat, necrosis, and inflammatory cells.

When hepatic granulomas are associated with joint disease and diarrhea, Whipple's disease should be considered. Examples of other bacterial diseases associated with hepatic granulomas are granuloma inguinale, meliosis, and secondary or tertiary syphilis. Alterations of the liver, however, are rarely predominant features in these disease processes.

Schistosomiasis is an important cause of hepatic granuloma in patients who originate from endemic areas (see Chap. 26). About 200 million people are currently thought to be infected with human-blood flukes of the genus *Schistosoma*: *S. haematobium*, *S. mansoni*, *S. japonicum*, *S. intercalatum*, and *S. mekongi*. Diagnosis can be made by serological testing and examination of feces and urine. However, the identification of ova in granulomata may sometimes be diagnostic. Granuloma formation seems to be the result of a foreign-body reaction to deposited ova and a cell-mediated delayed-type hypersensitivity response to antigenic substances released by larvae of the parasite. The granulomatous response appears to involve both Th1- and Th2-type cytokine reactions, with a preference for the latter. Other parasitic diseases associated with hepatic granulomas are infections due to *Toxocara canis* and *T. cati*. Children are especially at risk of acquiring infections through close contact with dogs and cats or contaminated playgrounds. Liver specimens may reveal part of the larvae with surrounding eosinophilia. Clinically, high counts of eosinophils in the blood, focal posterior uveitis, and endophthalmitis may be found.

Histoplasmosis is an important cause of granulomatous hepatitis in endemic areas, which comprise the Middle West of the United States, Middle and South America, and Africa. In a retrospective study of 50 cases of noncaseating hepatic granulomas from Cleveland, histoplasmosis was found to be the second most common etiology. Histoplasmosis can closely mimic sarcoidosis both clinically and histologically. *Histoplasma gondii* may be cultured from liver specimens. In a prospective study of 26 patients with disseminated histoplasmosis, cultures of liver specimens, along with cultures from blood and bone marrow, produced a definitive diagnosis in almost all cases.

There are several reports of granulomatous hepatitis associated with viral infections due to cytomegalovirus, Epstein-Barr virus, hepatitis A virus, and hepatitis C virus However, in view of the high prevalence of viral diseases in western societies, granulomatous hepatitis is obviously rarely associated with them.

Noninfectious Causes of Hepatic Granulomas

Hepatic granulomas have been reported in 21–79% of patients with established sarcoidosis. Although hepatic involvement usually causes no clinical problems, hepatic decompensation has been described. Granulomas in sarcoidosis often form well-delineated clusters of multinucleated giant cells with inclusion bodies. Older lesions may display an acellular mass of hyaline material and may be surrounded by dense fibrous tissue. Unlike the case in tuberculosis, granulomas in sarcoidosis are preferentially located in the portal tracts. Granulomas in the smaller portal venous radicles may occasionally result in portal hypertension.

Hepatic granulomas may also be seen in primary biliary cirrhosis. They are rare in autoimmune hepatitis.

There is a broad spectrum of drugs and environmental toxins that have been implicated in the production of hepatic granulomas. The mechanisms underlying the pathogenesis of drug-induced formation of granulomas is considered to be a delayed hypersensitivity response that evolves from the stimulation of antigen-reactive T cells by activated macrophages. Presumably, the causative antigen is an unaltered drug or one of its metabolites acting as a hapten. Hepatic granulomas do not usually appear earlier than 2 weeks after the initiation of drug therapy. Granulomatous hepatitis may have an acute onset, particularly when related to therapeutic drugs. On the other hand, granulomas caused by materials retained in reticuloendothelial cells are often asymptomatic. A list of the substances associated with granulomatous hepatitis is given in Table 3.

Hepatic granulomas have also been reported in Crohn's disease, polymyalgia rheumatica, giant cell arteritis, allergic granulomatosis, and various hypogammaglobulinemias. Hepatic granulomas are rare in typical Wegener's granulomatosis. The spectrum of underlying disease processes further includes neoplastic diseases, particularly Hodgkin's disease.

Table 3 Drugs Most Frequently Involved in the Formation of Hepatic Granulomas[a]

Allopurinol	Halothane	Phenylbutazone
Aminosalicylic acid	Hydralazine	Phenytoin
Amoxicillin	Hydrochlorothiazide	Procainamide
Bacille Calmette-Guérin (BCG)	Methyldopa	Quinidine
Carbamazepine	Mineral oil	Quinine
Clavulanic acid	Nitrofurantoin	Salicylazosulfapyridine
Clofibrate	Nomifensine	Sulfonamides
Contraceptive steroids	Papaverine	Tolbutamide
Diazepam	Penicillin	

[a]Some agents that have been reported anecdotally have been omitted.

Chronic granulomatous disease of childhood represents a distinct nosopathological entity that is based on the inability of granulocytes to form the oxygen metabolites needed to degrade ingested microorganisms.

Despite extensive workup, the etiology of granulomatous hepatitis remains unknown in up 50% of patients. These cases probably represent hypersensivity states that manifest themselves primarily or exclusively in the liver while the responsible factors remain obscure. When an acute febrile disease characterized by respiratory symptoms, splenomegaly and a high lymphocyte count occurs, idiopathic granulomatous hepatitis should be considered. Moreover, Simon and Wolff have described 13 patients with high spiking fevers, rigors, severe sweating, and weight loss. This illness lasted months to years and was often disabling. The familial occurrence of this condition has been described.

INVESTIGATIVE ROUTINE

A careful history is essential in patients presenting with granulomatous hepatitis and should include inquiries about proprietary as well as prescription drugs, travel abroad, and contact with animals. Patients should be asked about nonspecific complaints such as weight loss, fever, and malaise. Liver function tests should be performed, although no specific profile of laboratory abnormalities exists. Most frequently, serum alkaline phosphatase is elevated, but gamma-glutamyl-transpeptidase and aminotransferases may also be increased. Physical examination often reveals hepatic tenderness with or without hepatomegaly; splenomegaly may be present. Although tuberculosis seems to occur less frequently nowadays, a tuberculin skin test should be performed. A chest film is helpful to assess hilar adenopathy, nodular lesions within the lung parenchyma, and pulmonary features of tuberculosis. Liver biopsy should be performed to establish the granulomatous nature of the disease and may provide information about its cause. Possibly the diagnostic yield of liver biopsies increases with the size of the liver specimens and may be improved by performing serial sections of the liver biopsy. Part of the specimens should be preserved for culture of bacteria, mycobacteria, and fungi. Moreover, there is an increasing number of microorganisms that can now be identified more sensitively by PCR analysis of tissue specimens.

Serologies for Q fever, histoplasmosis, brucellosis, syphilis, hepatitis A, hepatitis C, and mononucleosis should be obtained routinely. Further laboratory testing should include determination of angiotensin converting enzyme, calcium in serum and urine, and serologies for antinuclear antibodies, antimitochondrial antibodies, and rheumatoid factor.

TREATMENT OF GRANULOMATOUS HEPATITIS

Treatment of granulomatous hepatitis must be directed toward the underlying cause and should not be initiated without a firm diagnosis. The broad variety of different causes of granulomatous hepatitis requires the design of individual treatment regimens, which may be of an antibiotic, immunosuppressive, or cytostatic nature or may just consist in omitting the causative agent.

Selection of treatment may be more difficult in granulomatous hepatitis of unknown etiology. When clinical symptoms like fever, weight loss, or malaise are absent or only mildly expressed, little more than continued observation and treatment of symptoms may be appropriate. The same would apply to acute forms of idiopathic granulomatous hepatitis, which usually resolve spontaneously. Sometimes, the diagnosis of the underlying disease becomes apparent during follow up. Guckian and Perry reported 7 patients with granulomatous hepatitis of unknown etiology who were prospectively followed for at least 2 years. In 4 of these patients, a definitive diagnosis could be established during follow-up (sarcoidosis in 1, tuberculosis in 1, Q fever in 1, syphilis in 1), while 3 patients were assumed to have tuberculosis or sarcoidosis. Withdrawal of drugs should further be considered, especially when granulomatous hepatitis occurs during the first 4–6 months of taking a new drug. In some instances, withdrawal of drugs may lead to a rapid recovery, with subsequent normalization of liver tests and histological changes and thus may uncover drug-induced granulomatous hepatitis.

In the face of continuous deterioration associated with granulomatous hepatitis, several therapeutic approaches have been suggested. Some authors feel that the possibility of tuberculosis must especially be considered in this situation and a "therapeutic trial" with antituberculous drugs should be initiated. For several reasons, this approach has now come into question. The prevalence of tuberculosis has decreased considerably during the last 30 years, some antituberculous drugs are hepatotoxic, and spontaneous remission during antituberculous therapy could incorrectly label a person as having tuberculosis. However, there is a place for such a decision after prolonged and extensive evaluation, but only if the patient is rapidly deteriorating clinically. The effectiveness of glucocorticoids in idiopathic granulomatous hepatitis and allergic conditions as well as in sarcoidosis is well established. Moreover, low-dose oral pulse therapy with methotrexate has recently been reported to be effective in patients with granulomatous hepatitis who did not respond to or did not tolerate glucocorticoid therapy. However, the possibility of an infectious cause must be kept in mind when immunosuppressive drugs are administered to patients with granulomatous hepatitis of unknown etiology, and clinical evaluation should be repeated in the case of deterioration.

BIBLIOGRAPHY

Berk JE, Cohen M. Hepatic granulomas. In: Berk JE, Haubrich WS, Kalser MH, Roth JL, Schaffner F, eds. Bockus Gastroenterology, 4th ed. Philadelphia: Saunders, 1985:3189–3202.

Biest S, Schubert TT. Chronic Epstein-Barr virus infection: a cause of granulomatous hepatitis? J Clin Gastroenterol 1989; 11:343–346.

Diaz ML, Herrera T, Lopez-Vidal Y, Calva JJ, Hernandez R, Palacios GR, Sada E. Polymerase chain reaction for the detection of Mycobacterium tuberculosis DNA in tissue and assessment of its utility in the diagnosis of hepatic granulomas. J Lab Clin Med 1996; 127:359–363.

Eliakim M, Eisenberg S, Levij IS, Sacks G. Granulomatous hepatitis accompanying a self-limited febrile disease. Lancet 1968; I:1348–1352.

Emile JF, Sebagh M, Feray C, David F, Reynes M. The presence of epithelioid granulomas in hepatitis C virus-related cirrhosis. Hum Pathol 1993; 24:1095–1097.

Fauci AS, Wolff SM. Granulomatous hepatitis. Prog Liver Dis 1976; 5:609–621.

Guckian JC, Perry JE. Granulomatous hepatitis. An analysis of 63 cases and review of the literature. Ann Intern Med 1966;65:1081–1100.

Guckian JC, Perry JE. Granulomatous hepatitis of unknown etiology. Am J Med 1968; 44:207–215.

Ishak KG, Zimmerman HJ. Drug-induced and toxic granulomatous hepatitis. Baillières Clin Gastroenterol 1988; 2:463–480.

Klatskin G. Hepatic granulomata: problems in interpretation. Mt Sinai J Med 1977; 44:798–812.

Knox TA, Kaplan MM, Gelfand JA, Wolff SM. Methotrexate treatment of idiopathic granulomatous hepatitis. Ann Intern Med 1995; 122:592–595.

Mahida Y, Palmer KR, Lovell D, Silk DBA. Familial granulomatous hepatitis: a hitherto unrecognized entity. Am J Gastroenterol 1988; 83:42–45.

Marans HY. Granulomatous hepatitis following intravesical bacillus Calmette-Guérin therapy for bladder carcinoma. J Urol 1987; 137:111–112.

Marazuela M, Moreno A, Yebra M, Cerezo E, Gomez Gesto C, Vargas JA. Hepatic fibrin-ring granulomas: a clinicopathologic study of 23 patients. Hum Pathol 1991; 22:607–613.

Mir-Madjlessi SH, Farmer RG, Hawk WA. Granulomatous hepatitis: a review of 50 cases. Am J Gastroenterol 1973; 60:122–133.

Sartin JS, Walker RC. Granulomatous hepatitis: a retrospective review of 88 cases at the Mayo Clinic. Mayo Clin Proc 1991; 66:914–918.

Simon HB, Wolff SM. Granulomatous hepatitis and prolonged fever of unknown origin: a study of 13 patients. Medicine 1973; 52:1–21.

Smith JW, Utz JP. Progressive disseminated histoplasmosis: a prospective study of 26 patients. Ann Intern Med 1972; 76:557–565.

Williams GT, Williams WJ. Granulomatous inflammation—a review. J Clin Pathol 1983; 36: 723–733.

Yamamoto T, Ishii M, Nagura H, Miyazaki Y, Miura M, Igarashi T, Toyata T. Transient hepatic fibrin-ring granulomas in a patient with acute hepatitis A. Liver 1995; 15:276–279.

Zumla A, James DG. Granulomatous infections: etiology and classification. Clin Infect Dis 1996; 23:146–158.

32
Management of Fibrocystic Disease of the Liver

Gregory T. Everson and Roshan Shrestha
University of Colorado School of Medicine, Denver, Colorado

INTRODUCTION

This chapter introduces the reader to the clinical management of the fibrocystic diseases of the liver. The diseases included in this category of hepatic disorders are autosomal dominant polycystic disease, solitary hepatic cysts, congenital hepatic fibrosis, choledochal cysts, and Caroli's disease. Histopathologically, they are characterized by ectasia of intrahepatic bile ducts, cysts of biliary epithelial cell origin, portal fibrosis, and persistence or lack of remodeling of the embryonic ductal plate (ductal plate malformation). The clinical spectrum ranges from an asymptomatic state to cholangitis or manifestations of liver failure. Polycystic liver disease is highlighted, since there have been many recent advances in its natural history, genetics, and treatment.

POLYCYSTIC LIVER DISEASE

Background

Autosomal dominant polycystic kidney disease (ADPKD) is one of the most common inherited disorders (10 times more common than sickle cell disease and 15 times more common than cystic fibrosis) and second only to hemochromatosis among inherited disorders involving the liver. As polycystic patients survive for longer periods of time—owing to improvements in the management of renal cystic disease, dialysis, and transplantation—complications arising in hepatic cysts are recognized with increasing frequency. Many patients may be completely asymptomatic, with normal renal function, and unaware of their underlying disease. Others develop abdominal complaints, infections in cysts, cyst hemorrhage, or, rarely, hepatic decompensation.

Natural History

Hepatic cysts occur uncommonly prior to puberty, but their occurrence increases dramatically from the onset of puberty through the early, childbearing years of adult life (Fig. 1). Most patients are asymptomatic and without clinical consequences; they possess only a few hepatic cysts or have hepatic cysts whose diameters range from a few millimeters to 1 or 2 cm. Some patients develop massive hepatic cystic disease (almost exclusively restricted to women) during early adult life, and many of these patients will become symptomatic, usually with abdominal pain or discomfort, early postprandial fullness, or shortness of breath. Rarely, patients experience complications of advanced liver disease, such as portal hypertension with variceal hemorrhage. As patients live into late adult life, there is risk of renal failure due to renal cystic disease and need for either hemodialysis or renal transplantation. Complications arising in hepatic cysts may occur more frequently in this population. In series of hemodialysis patients, 10–15% experienced complications in hepatic cysts, usually hemorrhage or infection and, rarely, cyst carcinoma.

Risk Factors

Increasing age, female gender, severity of renal cystic disease, and severity of renal dysfunction are the four major risk factors for development of hepatic cysts in ADPKD. Hepatic cysts are rarely detected prior to puberty, but the prevalence increases dramatically during the childbearing years of adult life. By age 60 nearly 80% of patients with ADPKD have hepatic cysts (Fig. 1). Although the age-related prevalence of hepatic cysts is similar in men and women, women experience greater numbers and larger sizes of hepatic cysts. This

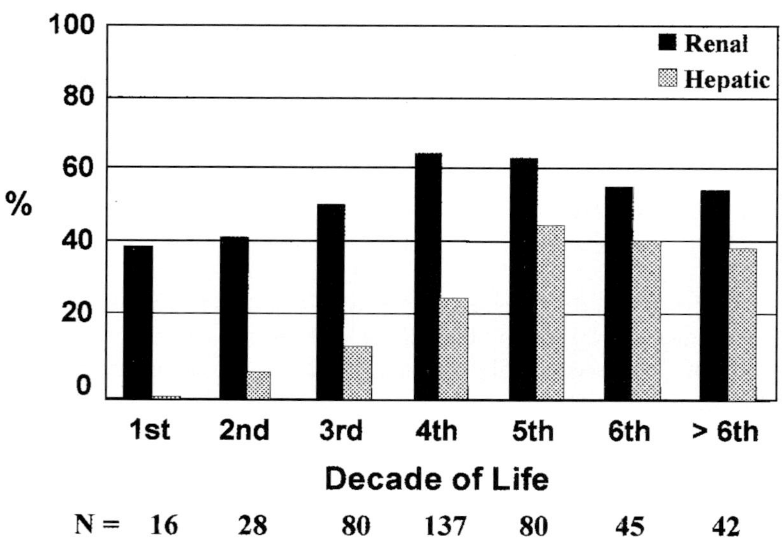

Figure 1 The frequency of renal and hepatic cysts is displayed by age in a population at risk for autosomal dominant polycystic kidney disease (ADPKD). Cysts were detected by real-time ultrasonography. The population at risk included 239 patients with ADPKD and 189 unaffected family members. The number of subjects in each decade is indicated at the bottom. (Adapted from Everson, 1990.)

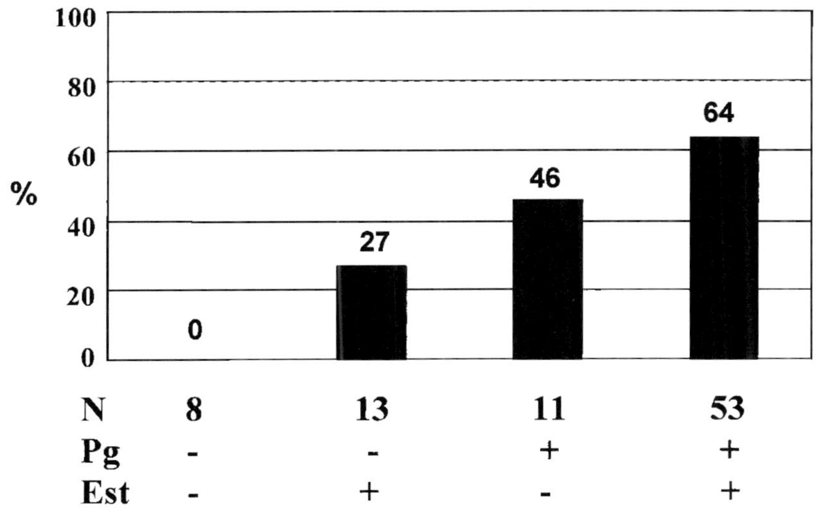

Figure 2 The prevalence of hepatic cystic disease as detected by screening ultrasonography is shown for women stratified by history of prior pregnancy (Pg) or prior use of female steroid hormones (Est). The number above each bar is the percent prevalence and N = number of subjects in each group. (Adapted from Shrestha et al., 1997.)

female tendency to develop extensive hepatic cystic disease correlates with both pregnancy and use of exogenous female steroid hormones (Fig. 2).

The severity of hepatic cystic disease also correlates independently with both the severity of renal cystic disease and the degree of renal dysfunction. The correlation with renal cystic disease likely represents the parallel organ expression of the underlying genetic defect. However, the correlation with renal dysfunction suggests that the progression of hepatic cystic disease may be modified by toxic or metabolic factors that accumulate because of renal failure.

Genetics

ADPKD1

The autosomal dominant inheritance of polycystic disease was established by Dalgaard in 1957 in a study of 284 patients and their family members. Subsequent reports confirmed this pattern of inheritance and indicated that spontaneous mutations accounted for only a minority of cases, < 10%. However, it was not until nearly 30 years later, in 1985, that Reeders and colleagues localized the first gene for ADPKD, ADPKD1, to the short arm of chromosome 16 by linkage techniques. Eight years later, the same group of investigators had identified, cloned, and sequenced the ADPKD1 gene. The protein encoded by this gene is designated as polycystin-1. The amino acid sequence for polycystin-1 has been determined from knowledge of the nucleotide sequence of the ADPKD1 gene, and protein structure has been inferred from the amino acid sequence. This analysis has suggested that polycystin-1 is an ubiquitous protein found in nearly all tissues in the body and that it is likely to be an integral membrane protein involved with calcium flux and cell signaling.

ADPKD2

In 1988, some 3 years after the discovery of the chromosomal localization of ADPKD1, two publications described polycystic families that did not exhibit linkage to markers on the short arm of chromosome 16. Five years later, the location of the ADPKD2 gene was assigned to chromosome 4q[10]; in 1996, the ADPKD2 gene was identified, sequenced, and cloned. The protein encoded by the ADPKD2 gene is called polycystin-2. It shares little sequence homology with polycystin-1 but is ubiquitous and also thought to be a membrane-embedded protein that works in concert with polycystin-1 to regulate calcium flux and cell signaling.

Isolated ADPLD

It was long suspected that some families had a form of polycystic disease uniquely restricted to the liver. Affected family members had extensive hepatic cystic disease with either no or only a few renal cysts. Proof of a liver-restricted form of autosomal dominant polycystic disease was provided in a 1996 study by Pirson and colleagues. They described a Dutch family with isolated polycystic liver disease that was transmitted through three generations. None of the affected family members exhibited linkage to the genetic markers for either ADPKD1 or ADPKD2. As of this writing, the chromosomal location, gene, and encoded protein have not been identified.

Clinical Features

Symptoms

Most patients with polycystic liver are asymptomatic or may note only a protuberant abdomen. In our studies we arbitrarily divided patients with polycystic liver disease into two groups, massive or minimal, based upon a definition for *massive* of a total liver cyst:parenchymal volume ratio greater than 1. Using this definition, we found that most symptomatic cases were restricted to patients with massive hepatic cystic disease. In a recent study, we reported that both abdominal pain and discomfort and shortness of breath correlated with severity of hepatic cystic disease. Pain related to hepatic cystic disease is dull and aching and may be positional. Patients commonly describe abdominal fullness and often resort to ingestion of frequent small meals, since they experience early postprandial fullness when they eat larger meals. Although serum gamma glutamyl transpeptidase (GGT) may be slightly increased in those with massive disease, liver enzymes are typically normal and patients rarely exhibit any features of hepatic decompensation. Likewise, biliary complications are rare.

The major consequence of growth of hepatic cysts is the development of abdominal symptoms without any major clinical manifestations of hepatic failure. Rarely, a patient with polycystic liver disease will experience hepatic decompensation and variceal hemorrhage, ascites, or encephalopathy. Quantitative tests of hepatic function have indicated that nearly all patients with polycystic disease, including those with massive hepatic cystic disease, have preserved hepatic metabolic capacity as judged from the clearance of caffeine and antipyrine. In contrast, there is a slight but significant increase in portal systemic shunting in those with massive hepatic cystic disease (Fig. 3). The increase in portal-systemic shunt is modest and not usually associated with either variceal bleeding or other features of portal hypertension.

The most common clinically relevant complications arising in hepatic cysts are intracystic hemorrhage, infection, and posttraumatic rupture. Rare reports of cyst adenocar-

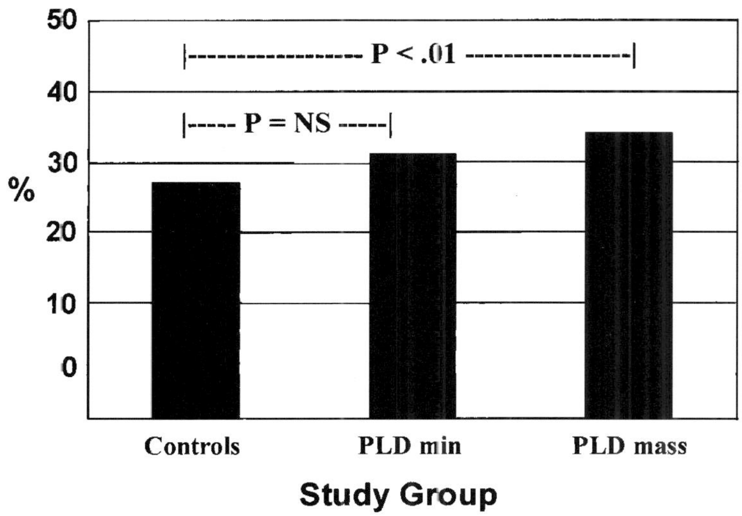

Figure 3 Portal-systemic shunt is slightly increased in patients with the most severe hepatic cystic disease (mean ± SD). (Adapted from Everson, 1993.)

cinoma, biliary obstruction, Budd-Chiari syndrome, and hepatic failure exist. Table 1 lists the complications, the preferred method of diagnosis, and options for medical or surgical management.

In addition to these complications, patients with polycystic disease may have a variety of other associated conditions, including mitral valve prolapse, diverticulosis, inguinal hernias, and berry aneurysms of the cerebral circulation.

Laboratory

Blood counts and standard biochemical tests of liver disease are usually normal. Some patients with hepatic cystic disease exhibit elevations in GGT; there is a weak but signifi-

Table 1 Clinical Complications Arising in Polycystic Liver Disease

Complication	Dx	Rx
Cyst infection	CT, MRI, In-WBC scan	Antibiotics (fluoroquinolones) Drainage if not responding
Cyst hemorrhage	CT, MRI	Medical management, pain control
Cyst adenocarcinoma	CT, MRI, aspiration cytology	Surgical resection
Portal hypertension, hepatic failure	Endoscopy, hepatic angiography	EST/EVL, P-S shunt, OLTx
Budd-Chiari syndrome	Hepatic venography	Cyst decompression; if unsuccessful, resection or OLTx
Rupture of cyst	Clinical suspicion	Medical management, pain control
Biliary obstruction	ERCP	Stent placement, cyst decompression

Key: CT, computed tomography; MRI, magnetic resonance imaging; In-WBC scan, Indium-labeled WBC scan; EST, endoscopic sclerotherapy; EVL, endoscopic variceal ligation; P-S shunt, portosystemic shunt; OLTx, orthotopic liver transplantation; ERCP, endoscopic retrograde cholangiopancreatography.

cant correlation of GGT with severity of hepatic cystic disease. Plain radiographs of the chest and abdomen are usually normal except for elevation of the right hemidiaphragm in those with massive disease. Barium studies are unremarkable except for mass effect of the enlarged liver and kidneys to extrinsically compress the column of barium in the colon. Polycystic patients may have extensive diverticular disease that is expressed at a relatively early age.

Modern imaging methods [ultrasonography, computed tomography (CT), nuclear scans, and magnetic resonance imaging] easily demonstrate hepatic cysts. Ultrasonography is preferred as the initial screening test and other scans are reserved for specific indications or research applications. Hepatic cysts appear as thin-walled cavities without intraluminal echogenicity on ultrasonography. CT scans reveal similar findings, with minor differences in Hounsfield's units between cysts. In contrast, CT scans may exhibit significant heterogeneity between uncomplicated cysts (Fig. 4). Standard liver-spleen scans are of little diagnostic value; scans with dimethyl iminodiacetic acid (HIDA) are normal; and indium-labeled white blood cell scans may be useful in diagnosing hepatic cyst infection.

Cyst Fluid

There have been several analyses of hepatic cyst fluid, and all demonstrate that the composition is consistent with a biliary origin for hepatic cysts. Electrolytes reflect plasma levels, glucose is low to nondetectable, secretary IgA is present, and cyst fluid is relatively enriched in GGT. In vivo, cyst secretion studies suggest that hepatic cysts may secrete fluid

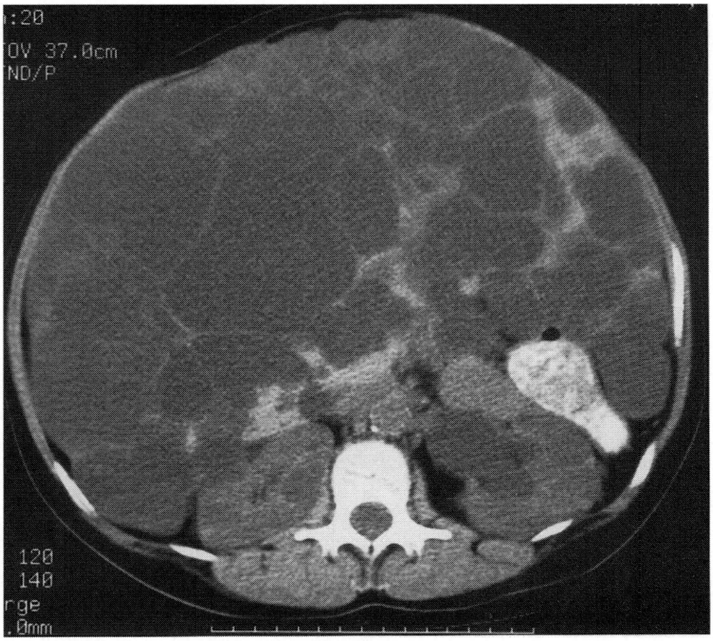

Figure 4 An abdominal CT image from a patient with ADPKD1 and massive hepatic cystic disease is shown. The liver with cysts exhibiting highly variable CT densities extends to the lateral aspect of the left side of the abdomen.

in response to intravenously administered secretin. In vitro studies have further confirmed the biliary origin and nature of hepatic cystic epithelium.

Therapy

Medical Treatments

There are no medical therapies for polycystic liver disease that are effective in causing cyst involution or preventing cyst formation. The finding of secretin-induced secretion by hepatic cysts prompted clinicians to attempt to reduce cyst volume using a long-acting somatostatin analogue. This anecdotal experience failed to demonstrate any significant effect on the growth or size of hepatic cysts.

One of the more intriguing observations is the finding that hepatic cystic disease may be influenced by female gender, pregnancy, or use of exogenous female steroid hormones. A recent prospective study quantitated liver (cyst and parenchymal) and kidney volumes at baseline and after 1 year of follow-up in ADPKD women on and off estrogen replacement therapy. Exogenous estrogen did not influence the growth of renal cysts, but the growth of hepatic cysts was significantly greater on estrogen therapy (Fig. 5).

Should women with polycystic liver disease take estrogen replacement therapy despite the risk of accelerating their hepatic cystic disease? The clinician must individualize treatment by weighing this potentially deleterious effect against the potential for other benefits (bone metabolism, amelioration of estrogen-withdrawal symptoms, lipid metabolism) or other risks (thromboembolism, uterine or breast cancer).

Radiologic Cyst Aspiration and Sclerosis

Symptomatic patients with polycystic disease are often referred to interventional radiologists for cyst aspiration and cyst sclerotherapy (alcohol, doxycycline). This approach should be restricted to patients with one or a few dominant cysts. Most patients with polycystic disease have too many cysts or the cysts that they have are of insufficient size to warrant percutaneous aspiration and sclerotherapy. Cyst sclerotherapy requires ultra-

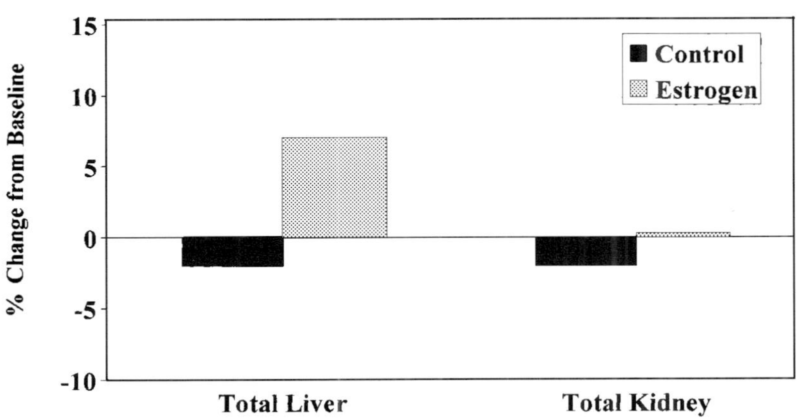

Figure 5 Percentage of volume change in liver and kidney at the end of 1 year of follow-up is shown. Estrogen treated patients are depicted by shaded bar and nontreated controls by solid bar (Adapted from Shrestha, 1997.)

sonographic or CT-guided percutaneous puncture of the targeted cyst and placement of an intracystic drainage catheter (see below, under "Solitary Hepatic Cyst"). Fluid is aspirated from the cyst and then a sclerosant, usually ethanol or a tetracycline derivative (doxycycline), is infused. The patient is moved to ensure contact of the sclerosant with the entire epithelial lining of the cyst cavity. The goal of treatment is destruction of the epithelial surface. The sclerosant is then aspirated and the catheter either removed or placed to gravity drainage or low intermittent suction. For large cysts (> 100 mL or diameter of ⩾ 6 cm), we prefer to leave the catheter to drainage for 24 h and perform a second treatment the next day, prior to removing the catheter. Success in obliterating individual cysts in polycystic patients is approximately 90%.

Cyst Fenestration

Cyst fenestration is the most commonly applied surgical treatment in the management of symptomatic massive hepatic cystic disease. Two approaches have been used: open laparotomy and, more recently, laparoscopy. Several series of open laparotomy, encompassing large numbers of patients, indicate that this approach results in satisfactory resolution of symptoms. However, open laparotomy is associated with prolonged hospitalization and the morbidity of major abdominal surgery. Operative mortality is low (< 1%), and reported rates of postoperative complications (bleeding, infection, bile leak, ascites) range from 0–50%. Because of its less invasive nature, laparoscopic cyst fenestration is gaining increasing acceptance as an alternative surgical technique. Advantages of laparoscopic surgery include less morbidity, reduced hospital stay, and the potential for outpatient surgical management. Individual center experience with laparoscopic cyst decompression is rather limited, but the sum of the results in the reported literature suggests that this approach is effective and associated with low mortality (< 1%) and morbidity (0–25%). At Colorado, we have performed nine laparoscopic cyst fenestrations in five patients (unpublished data). Two patients experienced significant complications during the procedure: gallbladder trauma, resulting in biliary leak and cholecystectomy, and cyst hemorrhage requiring conversion from laparoscopy to open laparotomy with completion of the fenestration. The other three have had successful amelioration of symptoms and reduction in liver volume (Fig. 6).

Liver Resection

One center recently reported its experience with partial liver resection in the management of 31 patients with highly symptomatic, massive hepatic cystic disease. Their ages ranged from 34–69, the gender ratio (M:F) was 3:28, and renal function varied from normal to dialysis-dependent. Nearly all patients experienced significant relief of symptoms, and long-term sustained reduction in symptoms was common (> 95%). However, over 50% experienced significant perioperative morbidity, and there was one perioperative death (due to rupture of an intracranial aneurysm). Although resection is promising for some patients, we would currently reserve hepatic resection for those patients who fail to respond to or are refractory to cyst decompression.

Liver Transplantation

Patients with polycystic disease and hepatic failure may be considered for hepatic transplantation using standard criteria applied to all patients with end-stage liver disease. However, as noted above, the vast majority of patients with polycystic liver disease have preserved hepatic function; hepatic failure sufficient to warrant transplantation is rarely encountered. The patient with massive hepatic cystic disease should be considered for

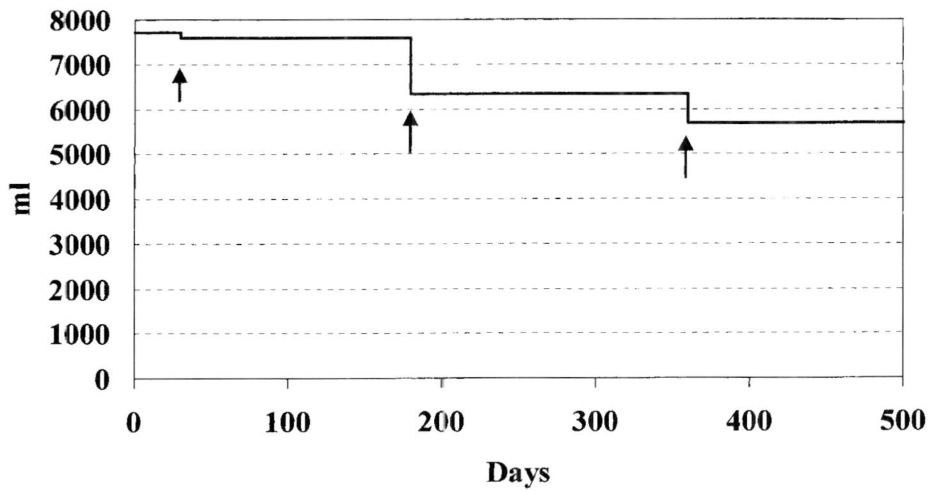

Figure 6 The reduction in liver volume achieved by sequential laparoscopic cyst fenestration in a single patient is shown. Initial liver volume was 7710 mL and final, after three procedures (green ↑ indicates the days of laparoscopic cyst decompression), was 5677 mL.

hepatic transplantation only when other options are unavailable or have failed. Isolated liver transplantation is considered for those patients with preserved renal function but massive hepatic cystic disease with symptoms or complications not amenable to other interventions. Combined liver and kidney transplantation should be considered for those patients with end-stage renal disease (ESRD), on or near dialysis, with symptomatic massive hepatic cystic disease not amenable to radiological, laparoscopic, or alternative surgical interventions. Cyst infection, hemorrhage, and adenocarcinoma are not indications for hepatic transplantation. Cyst reduction procedures (fenestration, resection, sclerosis) are preferred in the initial management of Budd-Chiari syndrome or biliary obstruction due to hepatic cysts.

SOLITARY HEPATIC CYST

Background

Solitary hepatic cysts are relatively common, usually asymptomatic, and most often discovered incidentally during the evaluation of a wide variety of abdominal symptoms or disorders. The exact prevalence of solitary hepatic cysts in the U.S. population is unknown, but the female-to-male ratio is approximately 4:1. A recent Taiwanese study used ultrasonography in a large-scale community-based screening for simple hepatic cysts to explore the age- and sex-specific prevalence and also in a hospital-based study to record the size of simple hepatic cysts. A total of 3600 subjects in eight communities underwent screening ultrasonography and 156 simple hepatic cysts in 132 study subjects were detected. The overall prevalence was, therefore, 3.60%. Prevalence increased with age, ranging from 0.83% below age 40–7.81% in subjects over 60 years of age. The sizes of 219 hepatic cysts in 167 hospitalized patients were measured; 53% had diameters from 1–3 cm and only 7% were larger than 5 cm. Cysts occurred more commonly in the right lobe and were twice as prevalent in women. All of these cysts were asymptomatic and none of the patients suffered clinical consequences.

Clinical Features

Solitary cysts that become symptomatic typically have diameters > 5 cm and present with localized pain in the right upper quadrant of the abdomen. Rarely, solitary hepatic cysts may develop intracystic hemorrhage, infection, or neoplasia. These complications may be diagnosed by radiological imaging studies or cyst aspiration, culture, or cytological and chemical analysis of cyst fluid.

Treatment

Asymptomatic solitary hepatic cysts are best managed conservatively using a "watch and wait" approach. The preferred treatment of symptomatic cysts is ultrasound- or CT-guided percutaneous cyst aspiration followed by alcohol (or doxycycline) sclerotherapy (Fig. 7A and B). This approach is more than 90% effective in controlling symptoms and ablating the cyst cavity. The recurrence rate after successful ablation is only 5–15%. If the radiologically guided percutaneous approach is ineffective or unavailable, treatment may include either laparoscopic or open surgical cyst fenestration. The laparoscopic approach is increasingly utilized for anatomically accessible cysts, and greater than 90% efficacy is reported.

CONGENITAL HEPATIC FIBROSIS

Background

Congenital hepatic fibrosis is a rare inherited autosomal recessive disorder that is most often associated with autosomal recessive polycystic kidney disease. Other clinical associations include adult autosomal dominant polycystic kidney disease, renal dysplasia, nephronophthisis, Meckel-Gruber syndrome, Ivemark syndrome, Jeune syndrome, vaginal atresia, and tuberous sclerosis. Congenital hepatic fibrosis can coexist with other fibrocystic liver diseases such as Caroli's disease and choledochal cyst. The histopathological features may vary, but in nearly all cases there is fibrous enlargement of the portal tracts, which contain abnormally shaped bile ducts. Congenital hepatic fibrosis typically involves all lobes of the liver equally, but on occasion one lobe of the liver may be preferentially affected. Von Meyenburg complexes (VMCs), also referred to as bile duct microhamartomas, are dilated, ectatic, intra- and interlobular bile ducts embedded in a fibrous stroma and occur in nearly all patients with congenital hepatic fibrosis (VMCs are also commonly found in both ADPKD and Caroli's disease).

Clinical Features

Congenital hepatic fibrosis presents in three clinical forms: portal hypertension, recurrent cholangitis, and asymptomatic or latent disease. The first two forms are usually diagnosed in early childhood in patients who present with variceal hemorrhage or unexplained biliary sepsis, respectively. In contrast, some patients will be diagnosed later, during their adult years, when they are evaluated for unexplained hepatomegaly or portal hypertension. Rarely, patients present with evidence of both portal hypertension and cholestasis, the latter

(A)

(B)

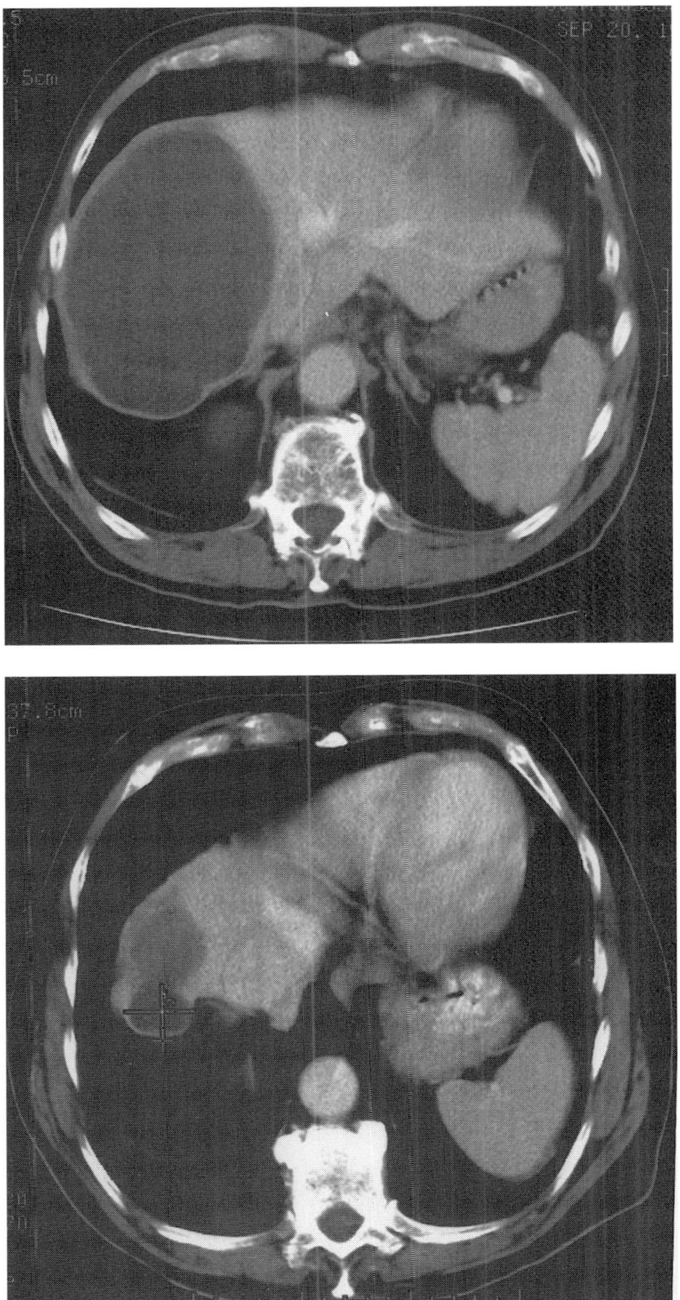

Figure 7 Panel A shows a large solitary hepatic cyst and panel B shows the residual after successful alcohol sclerotherapy.

due either to associated biliary anomalies (Caroli's disease) or intrinsic destructive cholangiopathy. In general, hepatic function is well preserved despite portal hypertension or bouts of cholangitis, although some patients experience progressive hepatic failure in long-term follow-up.

Treatment

Variceal Hemorrhage

The first line of treatment for this complication is institution of beta-adrenergic blockade or endoscopic variceal eradication (either sclerotherapy or ligation treatment). In most cases, varices may be successfully obliterated by the endoscopic approach, thereby controlling this potentially life-threatening complication. Surgical shunts or transjugular intrahepatic portal-systemic shunt (TIPS) are reserved for patients who fail endoscopic therapy or who bleed from gastric varices or portal hypertensive gastropathy. Occasionally patients will experience progressive hepatic fibrosis and hepatic dysfunction after long-standing portal systemic shunt surgery; development of this complication may necessitate consideration for liver transplantation.

Cholangitis

Radiological imaging (ultrasonography, biliary radioscintigraphy, CT, or magnetic resonance imaging) may be required to determine whether the patient with congenital hepatic fibrosis has concomitant biliary cystic disease. If the latter is present, the treatment of cholangitis is centered around provision of adequate biliary drainage, relief of obstruction (papillotomy with stone extraction or stricture dilation), and control of infection with antibiotics. In the absence of biliary cystic disease or cholangiocarcinoma (said to occur in as many as 6 percent of cases of congenital hepatic fibrosis), cholestasis may be related to idiopathic inflammatory destructive cholangiopathy and respond to ursodeoxycholate therapy.

Liver Transplantation

In general, patients with congenital hepatic fibrosis lack evidence of significant hepatic dysfunction or hepatic failure and respond to the management of complications, as noted above. Indications for hepatic transplantation include:

1. Variceal hemorrhage or hemorrhage from portal hypertensive gastropathy not responsive to endoscopic treatment of amenable to portal-systemic shunt surgery or TIPS
2. Recurrent cholangitis not amenable to medical, endoscopic, radiological, or surgical therapy
3. Hepatic failure (development of coagulopathy, biochemical deterioration, ascites, or portal-systemic encephalopathy)

Since patients with congenital hepatic fibrosis often have autosomal recessive polycystic kidney disease, one may need to consider combined liver-kidney transplantation in suitable candidates.

CHOLEDOCHAL CYST

Background

Choledochal cysts are cystic dilatations that may occur throughout the macroscopic intra- and extra-hepatic biliary tree. Although the term *choledochal cyst* has been used for any cystic dilatation of the biliary tree, isolated choledochal cysts are usually restricted to the common hepatic or bile duct only. Despite the uncommon occurrence of choledochal cysts there are hundreds of reports in the literature encompassing over three thousands cases. The first report was in 1723 by Vatano. Choledochal cyst is a rare condition in the western hemisphere; however, it is relatively more common among Japanese and other Oriental populations. Several classifications of choledochal cysts have been proposed, but the most commonly cited in the medical literature is by Todani (Fig. 8). The pattern of inheritance is unclear, and there have been no definitive studies of either the genetic markers or the molecular biology of choledochal cysts.

The pathogenesis of choledochal cyst is unknown. Several theories have been proposed. The most favored one is that congenital weakness of the common bile duct and relative distal obstruction, due to congenital pancreatobiliary malformation, facilitate ascending infection of the bile duct (cholangitis) or chronic reflux of pancreatic enzymes. Support for this theory is found in experimental models, where choledochal cysts have been produced by removing epithelium, ligating the distal portion of the bile duct, and anastomosing the pancreatic duct directly to the biliary system. Histologically, the cyst walls are made up of fibrous tissue representing a chronic inflammatory process, and the epithelial lining is either partially or completely absent.

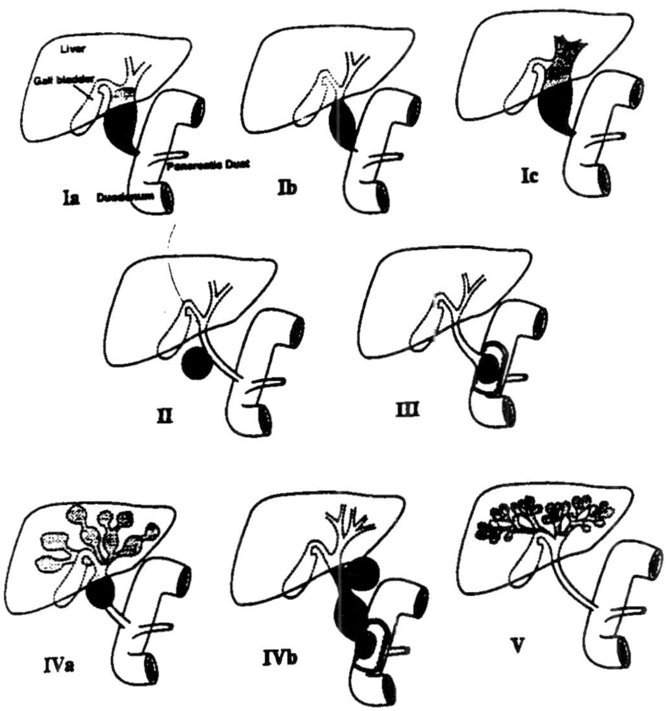

Figure 8 This figure shows the various anatomic types of choledochal cysts: type Ia, choledochal cyst; type Ib, segmental choledochal dilatation; type Ic, diffuse or cylindrical duct dilatation; type II, extrahepatic duct diverticulum; type III, choledochocele; type IVa, multiple intra- and extrahepatic duct cyst; type IVb, multiple extrahepatic duct cyst; type V, intrahepatic duct cyst (Caroli's disease). (From Todani et al., 1995.)

Clinical Features

The most common clinical presentation of choledochal cyst is a relatively young patient (child or adolescent) with pain, mass in the right upper quadrant or epigastrium, and jaundice. In one series of 740 cases, jaundice was the most common and consistent presenting feature. In infants, jaundice is often the only sign, and the disorder may be difficult to distinguish from biliary atresia. The majority of the patients have been diagnosed before age 30 and the male-to-female ratio in most series is about 1:4.

Reported complications include spontaneous and traumatic rupture, rupture during pregnancy, liver abscess, cirrhosis, and complications related to portal hypertension, including gastroesophageal varices and development of cholangiocarcinoma. The incidence of cholangiocarcinoma ranges from 2.5–17.5%, which is 5–35 times greater than among the population at large. The incidence of carcinoma increases throughout life and approaches 50% by age 50. Internal drainage procedures without cyst excision appear to accelerate the development of cholangiocarcinoma. Bacterial overgrowth and increased levels of secondary bile acids may contribute to cyst metaplasia and carcinoma. The tumors may originate in different parts of the pancreatobiliary system, including liver, gallbladder, intrahepatic ducts, pancreatic ducts, and pancreas.

Diagnosis

The diagnosis of a choledochal cyst should always be suspected in a child presenting with recurrent abdominal pain, jaundice, and raised serum amylase. Initial imaging of the biliary tree by ultrasonography or radioscintigraphy (HIDA scans) is usually diagnostic. Confirmation and anatomic definition may require CT, endoscopic retrograde cholangiopancreatogram (ERCP), or percutaneous transhepatic cholangiogram (PTC).

Patients with extrahepatic choledochal cysts have an increased incidence of anomalous pancreaticobiliary junction, which requires ERCP when excision of the cyst is planned. In recent years endoscopic ultrasonography (EUS) has been a useful imaging method for patients with suspected anomalous pancreaticobiliary junction. Prenatal ultrasonography can detect choledochal cysts in utero, which may help antenatal counseling, since early excision of the neonatal cyst and duct revision may be required.

Treatment

It is generally agreed that choledochal cysts require surgical treatment. The preferred surgical treatment is complete cyst excision with Roux-en-Y hepaticojejunostomy. This eliminates any opportunity for stasis, infection, stone formation, and possible development of cholangiocarcinoma. The procedure provides excellent long-term results with low morbidity and mortality, but lifelong follow-up may be necessary to avoid potential problems, such as biliary cirrhosis. Internal cyst drainage procedures (cystoduodenostomy, cystojejunostomy) have often been unsatisfactory, with a complication rate as high as 50%; this procedure may actually accelerate the development of cholangiocarcinoma. Unilobar intrahepatic cystic disease is usually treated by resection of the affected lobe of the liver. Radiological and endoscopic drainage procedures are used to stabilize patients with acute or recurrent cholangitis. However, recurrent symptoms are common and the risk of development of cholangiocarcinoma is not eliminated. When features of end-stage liver disease develop due to long-standing, progressive biliary obstruction or when endoscopic, radiological, or surgical therapy have failed to resolve the biliary infectious complications orthotopic liver transplantation may be considered.

CAROLI'S DISEASE

Background

In 1957, Caroli described a syndrome of congenital malformation of intrahepatic bile ducts characterized by segmental cystic dilatation of the intrahepatic ducts, increased incidence of biliary lithiasis, cholangitis and liver abscesses, absence of cirrhosis and portal hypertension, and association of renal cystic disease. Subsequent to Caroli's initial report, two distinct disease entities associated with Caroli's disease have been recognized: (1) a simple type, which is associated with medullary sponge kidney in 60–80% of cases, and (2) a periportal fibrosis type, which is associated with congenital hepatic fibrosis, cirrhosis, portal hypertension, and esophageal varices.

Clinical Features

The most common presenting symptoms of Caroli's disease are recurrent episodes of fever, chills, and abdominal pain due to cholangitis, with peak incidence in early adult life. Males and females are equally affected, in contrast to the female predominance of polycystic disease, simple hepatic cysts, and choledochal cysts. More than 80% present with symptoms before the age of 30 years. Rarely, the disease presents later in life with evidence of portal hypertension and its complications, most commonly bleeding esophageal varices. The risk of development of cholangiocarcinoma in Caroli's disease is about 7%. Biliary lithiasis is found in one-third of patients and predisposes them to recurrent episodes of cholangitis due to obstruction and ascending infections. Occasional patients also experience multiple liver abscesses. The genetics are unclear, with both autosomal dominant and autosomal recessive patterns of inheritance proposed. There have been no molecular biological studies of Caroli's disease.

Diagnosis

Caroli's disease is typically discovered by ultrasonography performed during evaluation of biliary obstruction or cholangitis. Communication of the intrahepatic cysts with the biliary tree is usually confirmed by scintigraphy, CT scan after biliary contrast, ERCP, or PTC. Some studies have suggested that CT is superior to ultrasonography in the initial evaluation of adult patients. Ultrasonography is preferred in children. PTC and ERCP provide detailed examination of the biliary tree and may aid in therapy.

Treatment Options

Biliary Drainage

Adequate biliary drainage is the primary approach in the management of Caroli's disease. Endoscopic therapy with ERCP is effective in removing sludge or stones from the common bile duct but is of limited utility in providing adequate drainage of intrahepatic cysts. In contrast, PTC is more effective in draining these cysts and avoids recurrent episodes of

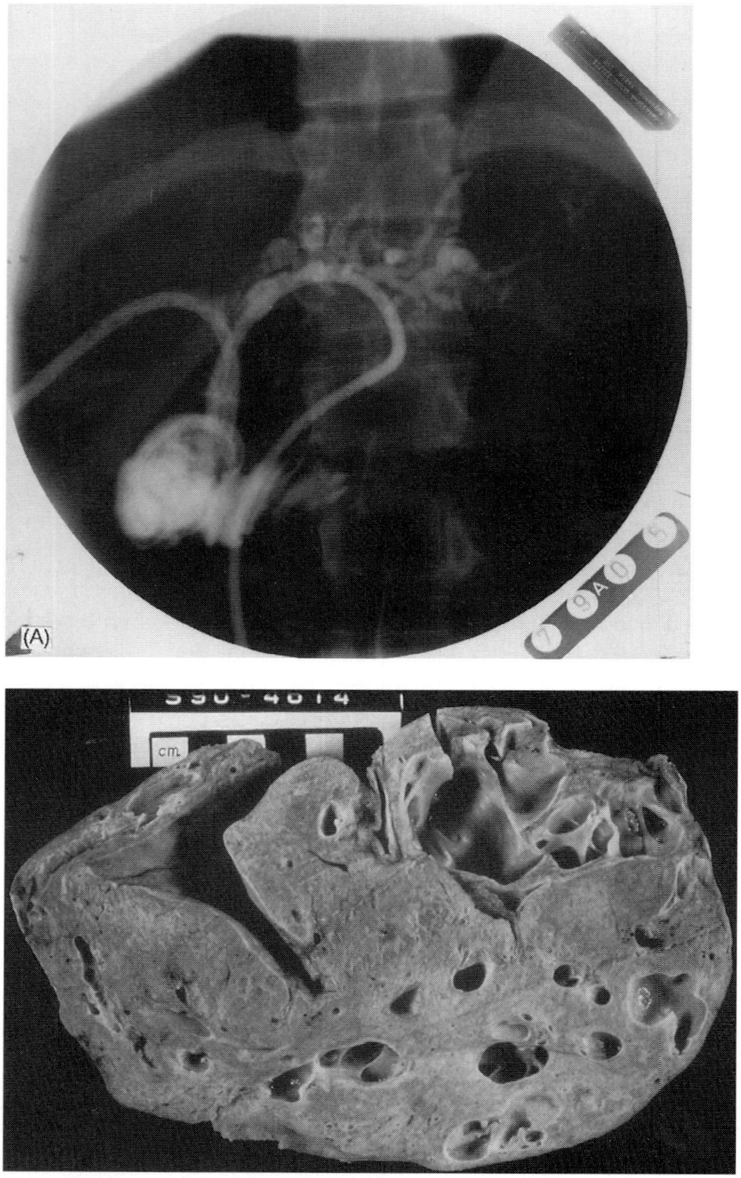

Figure 9 (A) This PTC radiograph demonstrates the typical intrahepatic biliary cysts of Caroli's disease and percutaneously placed pigtail drainage catheters. (B) Gross anatomic view of same patient's explanted liver posttransplantation.

cholangitis, especially if patients comply with periodic flushing and changing of drainage catheters (Fig. 9A and B).

Rarely, the cystic disease is confined to one hepatic lobe; in this circumstance, hepatic lobectomy is often curative. Although some have advocated hepaticojejunostomy after partial hepatectomy as primary therapy, the long-term efficacy of this procedure is uncertain, and the extensive surgery could compromise the outcome from hepatic transplantation.

Liver Transplantation

There are two main indications for hepatic transplantation in Caroli's disease: hepatic decompensation and recurrent cholangitis unresponsive to endoscopic or radiological interventions. Most patients with Caroli's disease have preserved hepatic function, but some have associated congenital hepatic fibrosis and portal hypertension. Bleeding from esophageal varices is usually controlled by endoscopic sclerotherapy or band ligation. TIPS placement to decompress portal hypertension is relatively contraindicated due to the extensive cystic disease, similar to polycystic liver disease. If, however, variceal bleeding recurs despite the maximum endoscopic therapy or if the patient develops cirrhosis (biliary type) and experiences decompensation with the development of ascites or encephalopathy, then transplantation is preferred. The most common indication for transplantation is recurrent cholangitis despite prior interventions. Transplantation should be considered if patients experience two or more bouts of cholangitis despite maximum radiological or endoscopic therapy.

BIBLIOGRAPHY

D'Agata ID, Jonas MM, Perez-Atayde AR, Guay-Woodford LM. Combined cystic disease of the liver and kidney. Semin Liver Dis 1994; 14:215–228.

Everson GT. Hepatic cysts in autosomal dominant polycystic kidney disease. Am J Kidney Dis 1993; 22:520–525.

Everson GT. Hepatic cysts in autosomal dominant polycystic kidney disease. Mayo Clin Proc 1990; 65:1020–1025.

Fabiani P, Mazza D, Toouli J, Bartels AM, Gugenheim J, Mouiel J. Laparoscopic fenestration of symptomatic non-parasitic cysts of the liver. Br J Surg 1997; 84:321–322.

Gigot JF, Jadoul P, Que F, Van Beers BE, Etienne J, Horsmans Y, Collard A, Geubel A, Pringot J, Kestens PJ. Adult polycystic liver disease: is fenestration the most adequate operation for long-term management? Ann Surg 1997; 225:286–294.

Huang JF, Chen SC, Lu SN, Lin ZY, Chuang WL, Hsieh MY, Wang LT, Tasi JF, Chang WY, Chen CJ. Prevalence and size of simple hepatic cysts in Taiwan: community- and hospital-based sonographic surveys: Kao-Hsiung i Hsueh Ko Hsueh Tsa Chih [Kao-Hsiung J Med Sci] 1995; 11:564–567.

Harris RA, Gray DW, Britton BJ, Toogood GJ, Morris PJ. Hepatic cystic disease in an adult polycystic kidney disease transplant population. Aust NZ J Surg 1996; 66(3):166–168.

Kabbej M, Sauvanet A, Chauveau D, Farges O, Belghiti J. Laparoscopic fenestration in polycystic liver disease. Br J Surg 1996; 83:1697–1701.

Klingler PJ, Gadenstatter M, Schmid T, Bodner E, Schwelberger HG. Treatment of hepatic cysts in the era of laparoscopic surgery. Br J Surg 1997; 84:438–444.

Klupp J, Bechstein WO, Lobeck H, Neuhaus P. Orthotopic liver transplantation in therapy of advanced polycystic liver disease. Chirurgie 1996; 67:515–521.

Madariaga JR, Iwatsuki S, Starzl TE, Todo S, Selby R, Zetti G. Hepatic resection for cystic lesions of the liver. Ann Surg 1993; 218:610–614.

Miller WJ, Sechtin AG, Campbell WL, Pieters PC. Imaging findings in Caroli's disease. AJR 1995; 165:333–327.

Miyano T, Yamataka A, Kato Y, et al. Hepaticoenterostomy after excision of choledochal cyst in children: a 30-year experience with 180 cases. J Pediatr Surg 1996; 31:1417–1421.

Pirson Y, Lannoy N, Peters D, Geubel A, Gigot J, Breunig M, Verellen-Dumoulin C. Isolated polycystic liver disease as a distinct genetic disease, unlinked to polycystic kidney disease 1 and polycystic kidney disease 2. Hepatology 1996; 23:249–252.

Sans M, Rimola A, Navasa M, et al. Liver transplantation in patients with Caroli's disease and recurrent cholangitis. Transplant Int 1997; 10:241–244.

Shrestha R, Mckinley C, Russ P, Scherzinger A, Bonner T, Showalter R, Everson GT. Postmenopausal estrogen therapy selectively stimulates hepatic enlargement in women with autosomal dominant polycystic kidney disease. Hepatology 1997; 26:1282–1286.

Tikkakoski T, Makela JT, Leinonen S, Paivansalo M, Merikanto J, Karttunen A, Siniluoto T, Kairaluoma MI. Treatment of symptomatic congenital hepatic cysts with single-session percutaneous drainage and ethanol sclerosis; technique and outcome. J Vasc Intervent Radiol 1996; 7:235–239.

Todani T, Watanabe Y, Urushihara N, Noda T, Morotomi Y. Biliary complications after excisional procedure for choledochal cyst. J Pediatr Surg 1995; 30:478–481.

vanSonnenberg E, Wroblicka JT, D'Agostino HB, Mathieson JR, Casola G, O'Laoide R, Cooperberg PL. Symptomatic hepatic cysts: percutaneous drainage and sclerosis. Radiology 1994; 190: 387–392.

Ward CJ, Turley H, Ong ACM, Comley M, Biddolph S, Chetty R, Ratcliffe PJ, Gatter K, Harris PC. Polycystin, the polycystic kidney disease 1 protein, is expressed by epithelial cells in fetal, adult, and polycystic kidney. Proc Natl Acad Sci USA 1996; 93:1524–1528.

33
Management of Liver Disease in Pregnancy

Vinod K. Rustgi
Georgetown University School of Medicine, Washington, D.C.

INTRODUCTION

The evaluation of liver disease in pregnant women is no different than it is in the general population. There are liver diseases specifically associated with pregnancy, liver diseases that may arise during the course of pregnancy, and, of course, those that may predate pregnancy. Pregnancy itself does not confer any special predisposition to liver disease, though there may be different manifestations.

The gross appearance of the liver is the same during pregnancy as during nonpregnancy. Histological changes may be nonspecific. The hepatocytes of pregnant women may show proliferation of the smooth and rough endoplasmic reticulum and increased numbers of peroxisomes. Other histological changes can include variability in the size and shape of hepatocytes, more frequent cytoplasmic fat vacuoles and centrilobular hepatocytes, and hypertrophy of the Kupffer cells.

To understand the physiological changes in the liver during pregnancy, it is helpful to remember that blood and plasma volume increase during pregnancy, with plasma volume expanding at a greater rate than total blood volume. Consequently, anemia normally develops and cardiac output increases, while hepatic blood flow remains unchanged. During pregnancy, 20% less of the cardiac output per unit time may reach the liver. High-clearance drugs that are cleared by the liver in a manner that is blood flow–dependent have a reduced clearance during pregnancy due to the larger volume of distribution.

EFFECT OF PREGNANCY ON MEASURES OF HEPATIC FUNCTION USED CLINICALLY

Occasionally, increased fat may be seen in the liver biopsies of some pregnant women. This may be due to the progressive increases in cholesterol (25–60%), phospholipids, and/or in plasma triglycerides (up to 300%) that may be seen.

Table 1 Effect of Pregnancy on Liver Parameters

Parameter	Effect
Excretory function	
BSP	122% increased storage capacity; 27% reduction in transport maximum
Bilirubin	Increase in unconjugated fraction, no change in total level
Bile acids	Slight increase in unconjugated levels
Synthetic function	
Albumin	20–25% reduction due to hemodilution
α_1-Globulins	50% increase
α_2-Globulins	50% increase
β-Globulins	50% increase
γ-Globulins	No change
Prothrombin time	No change
Metabolic function	Reduced clearance of high-extraction xenobiotics
	Variable changes (both an increase and a reduction) in low-extraction xenobiotics
Liver injury parameters	
Alkaline phosphatase	Increased total activity; no change in the level of the hepatobiliary fraction
Transaminases	Mild to moderate reductions due to hemodilution
γ-Glutamyl transferase	No change
Histology	Slightly enlarged hepatocyte size
	Slight increase in volume of the endoplasmic reticulum

While $alpha_1$, $alpha_2$, and betaglobulins tend to increase, gamma globulins remain within the normal range during pregnancy, given that they are the products of plasma cells rather than the liver. The conjugated fraction of bilirubin increases. Albumin levels decrease by almost 40% by term; transaminase levels also tend to decrease minimally, all probably as a consequence of dilution (see Table 1). Other proteins such as $alpha_1$ and $alpha_2$ globulins, like ceruloplasmin, tend to increase.

VIRAL HEPATITIS

The diagnosis of acute viral hepatitis during pregnancy is aided by serological testing. The main questions that need to be addressed when viral hepatitis occurs in pregnancy are the effects on the unborn fetus, the effect on the newborn infant, and whether the disease manifestations are different during pregnancy.

Management

Management during pregnancy is meant to be conservative. All extraneous medications are to be avoided. Aggressive evaluation and diagnostic tests are not usually necessary. In the pregnancy patient with hepatitis, amniocentesis is inadvisable, since it can provide an avenue for the spread of infection to the fetus. Furthermore, viral hepatitis is not an indication for cesarean section, either as a means of protecting the mother or preventing spread of the disease to the newborn. Finally, the patient with hepatitis can usually benefit from education about the disease. Mothers do not need to avoid contact with their babies. Breast-feeding need not be discouraged, because it has not been shown to be a way of spreading this disease. Prevention of spread should be achieved by immunoprophylaxis and not by isolation or restriction of activities.

EFFECTS OF VIRAL HEPATITIS ON PREGNANCY

Mortality and morbidity during pregnancy seem to be functions of nutritional status as well as the particular viral agents involved. In the western world, pregnant women seem to be no more adversely affected by viral hepatitis than is the nonpregnant population. Historical data show that poor socioeconomic conditions are associated with remarkably higher complication rates among pregnant women. This was shown in Israel during the years 1967–1977 and in Saudi Arabia as well. In the latter country, the mortality rate of viral hepatitis in third-trimester pregnant women fell from 70.8% in the years 1953–1962 to 14.3% for the period 1963–1975.

In other areas of the world, such as India and Africa, both the frequency and severity of hepatitis are far greater in pregnant women, particularly during the third trimester. A striking example of this phenomenon was reported during an epidemic of non-A, non-B hepatitis, probably hepatitis E, that occurred in Kashmir, India, in November 1978. In evaluating that outbreak, the attack rate was determined to be 2.8% among men, 2.1% among nonpregnant women, and 17.3% among pregnant women. A total of 22% of pregnant women developed fulminant hepatitis, all during the third trimester, and two-thirds of them died. Virtually none of the men or nonpregnant women suffered this complication.

Effect of Viral Hepatitis in Pregnancy on the Newborn

A common consequence of hepatitis during pregnancy does seem to be prematurity. Earlier concerns about a teratogenic effect have not been confirmed. Initially, Stoller and Collmann proposed the possibility that maternal exposure to viral hepatitis near the time of conception was associated with an increased frequency of births of infants with Down's syndrome. Similar observations were reported in Greece, though the theory was eventually disproven by larger series conducted in the United States and England.

Hepatitis A (HAV)

HAV is a small, 27-nm virus with a single-stranded RNA that belongs to the Picornaviridae family. It causes an acute self-limited disease; the incubation period averages 20–30 days (see Chap. 6). Though primarily transmitted via the fecal-oral route, hepatitis A can be transmitted by alternate paths, such as intravenous drug use and sexual contact. Some 80% of infected children and young adolescents are asymptomatic and anicteric, whereas jaundice occurs in more than 80% of adult patients.

Management of hepatitis A consists primarily of supportive measures. A diet adequate in protein (1 g/kg) and calories (30–35/kg) should be maintained. If the patient is unable to tolerate oral intake, hospitalization for intravenous alimentation may become necessary. Patients with evidence of fulminant hepatitis and those showing coagulopathy or encephalopathy require treatment in the setting of an intensive care unit. Most patients recover within 4–6 weeks.

Passive acquisition of antibodies by immune globulin offers effective protection from hepatitis A and was the mainstay until recently. The dose is 0.02 mL/kg, administered intramuscularly within 2 weeks of the onset of disease in the index case. Infants of mothers who may be infectious at or soon after delivery are candidates for immune globulin therapy. Its principal limitation is a relatively short period of efficacy lasting up to 6 months.

A formalin-inactivated hepatitis A vaccine is now available in the United States. This vaccine should be clinically useful in obstetric patients. Women who have children enrolled in day care or who live in endemic areas are certainly appropriate candidates for vaccination.

Hepatitis B

Hepatitis B is caused by a DNA virus. In the United States, more than 300,000 new cases of hepatitis B occur annually and more than 1 million Americans are chronic carriers (see Chap. 7).

If exposure to a patient with acute or chronic hepatitis B infection has occurred, a seronegative person should receive immunoprophylaxis with hepatitis B immune globulin, 0.06 mL/kg intramuscularly, followed by vaccination with recombinant hepatitis B vaccine.

Perinatal transmission occurs primarily as a result of the infant's exposure to infected blood and genital secretions during delivery; antenatal transmission is uncommon. The frequency of perinatal transmission increases to almost 90% in women who are seropositive for both hepatitis B surface antigen and hepatitis B e antigen. Women who become acutely infected in the third trimester of pregnancy are also more likely to transmit infection to their fetuses (80–90%) as compared with women who are infected in the first trimester. A combination of passive and active immunization is 85–95% effective in preventing neonatal hepatitis B infection. The Centers for Disease Control have recommended universal vaccination of all infants. Dosage recommendations vary depending upon the mother's serostatus (see Table 2). Therefore obstetricians must continue to screen all of their patients for hepatitis B (see Table 3). The number of births estimated to occur in HBsAg-positive women in the United States is approximately 16,500 per year, and perhaps only one-half would be identified by known risk factors.

Hepatitis C

This virus was identified in 1988 by scientists at the Chiron Corporation (see Chap. 9). There has been evidence that hepatitis C antibody is passively transferred to the infant, as is

Table 2 Recommended Doses and Schedules of Currently Licensed HBV Vaccines

	Recombivax HB (Merck Sharpe & Dohme)		Energix-B (SmithKline Beecham)
Age/status	Formulation/dose	Formulation/dose	Formulation/dose
Infants of HBsAg-negative mothers	2.5 μg	2.5 μg	10 μg
Infants of HBsAg-positive mothers	Adolescent/ high-risk infant 5.0 μg	5.0 μg	10 μg

Table 3 Prenatal Hepatitis B Virus Screening Recommendations

All gravidas should be screened routinely for HBsAg at the same time as other routine prenatal laboratory testing.
Women in high-risk groups should be screened again before delivery.
Women not tested prenatally should be tested as soon as possible after admission for delivery.
Infants born to HBsAg-positive mothers should receive appropriate immunization beginning within 12 h of birth.
Household and sexual contacts of HBsAg-positive women should be tested for susceptibility and considered for vaccination if appropriate.
Obstetric and pediatric hospital staff should be aware of HBsAg-positive mothers, so that babies receive timely vaccination.
Hospitals and health departments should establish programs for the education of patients and health professionals about perinatal transmission of hepatitis B virus and recommendations regarding screening.
In populations in which hepatitis B virus is highly endemic as well as in places where maternal screening is not logistically possible, vaccination of all neonates may be more effective than maternal screening.

Source: Immunization Practices Advisory Committee, 1988.

HCV-RNA when detected by polymerase chain reaction (PCR), but this rarely leads to chronic infection. The few cases where this does become chronic seem to have a complicating factor of simultaneous infection with human immunodeficiency virus (HIV). There have been suggestions of synergy between HIV and HCV.

Hepatitis Delta Virus

HDV is a defective virus that usually requires the presence of HBV for successful infection (see Chap. 8). It is rare to transmit HDV vertically. Prevention of vertical transmission of HBV is effective in preventing maternal-infant transmission of HDV.

Hepatitis E Virus

Hepatitis E is the agent of "epidemic" or water-borne hepatitis. An RNA virus, it is related to the caliciviruses. Its mean incubation period is 45 days, and it can cause severe disease in pregnant women.

Management again consists of supportive care. A chronic carrier state does not develop and perinatal transmission is not known to occur. Fetal outcome is not adversely affected. Administration of immune globulin produced in the United States and western Europe does not seem to be of benefit in preventing horizontal transmission of infection. If pregnant women must travel to areas at risk, the only option is to avoid potentially contaminated food or water, as recommended for the prevention of other enteric infections.

Herpes Simplex Hepatitis

Reported cases of herpes simplex hepatitis in pregnancy are limited. Manifestations include more common occurrence during the third trimester of pregnancy and generally an anicteric course. The characteristic liver lesions are usually a combination of microabscesses with or without hemorrhage and hepatocellular necrosis. Ground-glass nuclear viral inclusions are usually encountered more frequently than Cowdry type A inclusions. Clinicians should be alerted to the diagnosis by normal or mildly increased bilirubin and the presence of markedly elevated aminotransferases. Pregnant patients with this condition warrant close monitoring, particularly if a systemic viral syndrome is present. Initiation of acyclovir appears to result in a significant decrease in maternal and fetal morbidity, and preterm delivery may not be necessary. Rarely, the situation can deteriorate to fulminant hepatic failure and may have to be treated with orthotopic liver transplantation in conjunction with high-dose acyclovir.

Wilson's Disease

In women with Wilson's disease, concentrations of ceruloplasmin and copper in serum and urine increase during pregnancy or with use of estrogens. Treatment with D-penicillamine represents a problem, as it is potentially teratogenic. Trientine (triethylenetetraminedihydrochloride), a newer chelating agent, may be safer in pregnancy, though it has been reported to be teratogenic in rats. It is unclear whether the teratogenicity in rats was related to copper deficiency.

HEPATIC DISEASES UNIQUE TO PREGNANCY

Jaundice is unusual in pregnancy in normal women, with a reported prevalence of 1 in every 1500 pregnancies. From studying time courses, it is clear that all the unique and unusual hepatic diseases of pregnancy except for hyperemesis gravidarum usually occur in the third trimester or late in pregnancy (see Table 4).

Hyperemesis Gravidarum

Hyperemesis gravidarum is an unusual "syndrome" that can have its onset at any time in pregnancy but is most common in the first trimester. Transaminases are usually mildly elevated and hyperbilirubinemia may occur, but it rarely exceeds the level of 5 mg/dL. The etiology of the hyperbilirubinemia is uncertain, but it may be due to an exaggerating fasting-induced increase in heme-oxidase and the conversion of biliverdin to bilirubin.

Intractable vomiting may cause dehydration, electrolyte disturbances, or nutritional deficiencies. This occurs most often in women who are less than 25 years of age, who are

Table 4 Hepatic Diseases by Timing in Pregnancy

First trimester	Second trimester	Third trimester
Hyperemesis gravidarum Gallstones Viral hepatitis Drug-induced hepatitis	Intrahepatic cholestasis of pregnancy (uncommon) Gallstones Viral hepatitis Drug-induced hepatitis Preeclampsia/eclampsia (rare) HELLP syndrome (rare)	Intrahepatic cholestasis of pregnancy Preeclampsia/eclampsia Gallstones Viral hepatitis Drug-induced hepatitis HELLP syndrome Acute fatty liver of pregnancy Hepatic rupture

overweight, multiparous, and have had multiple births. Hyperthyroidism may occur in up to 50% of affected women.

Therapy consists of hospitalization, the initiation of intravenous fluids, and feeding in the form of total parenteral nutrition. If the symptoms are controlled, the dysfunction usually resolves, though it may recur in subsequent pregnancies.

Intrahepatic Cholestasis of Pregnancy

Intrahepatic cholestasis of pregnancy (IHCP) is a rare heritable disease of uncertain specific etiology; it probably represents an increased sensitivity to estrogen-induced cholestasis. It is characterized by pruritus and biochemical cholestasis, which appear late during a pregnancy, persist until delivery, and disappear after parturition. IHCP seems to be inherited in a Mendelian-dominant pattern. Some 50% of patients have a family history of jaundice in other members who have either been pregnant or have used oral contraceptive medications.

The geographic distribution is remarkably uneven. It is seen most commonly in Scandinavia; in Araucanian Indians in Chile, an incidence of 15–20% has been reported.

Classically, pruritus precedes clinical jaundice by 2–4 weeks. It generally starts in the palms and soles and then may extend to the trunk and extremities. Importantly, it recurs with subsequent pregnancy and tends to recur earlier.

Maternal health and prognosis are excellent with this condition. All abnormalities including minimal transaminase elevations, mildly abnormal prothrombin times, and pruritus and jaundice dissipate completely within 1 or 2 weeks of delivery. When liver biopsies have been obtained, only intrahepatic cholestasis has been demonstrated. The histology returns to normal within 2 weeks of delivery.

Unfortunately, the prognosis for the fetus can be quite poor. Fetal monitoring has shown high rates of fetal distress during labor. These findings have prompted suggestions of routine monitoring of these patients during the third trimester and to opt for cesarean section if any signs of fetal distress are found. In the absence of exogenous maternal vitamin K administration, fetal prothrombin activity can be negligible to absent, and such an infant may be subject to a great risk of intracranial hemorrhage during the delivery process. Maternal intrahepatic cholestasis has been associated with an increased incidence of prematurity, perinatal deaths, fetal distress, and meconium staining of amniotic fluid.

Therapy is directed to helping ameliorate pruritus and correct the biochemical parameters of cholestasis but to also improve the prognosis of the fetus and the newborn.

Cholestyramine has been used to alleviate pruritus but poses the problem of increasing steatorrhea and malabsorption of vitamin K and other fat-soluble vitamins. Phenobarbital has been used but does not improve pruritus or biochemical abnormalities substantially. Its use in pregnancy may be considered dangerous in the late stages due to the potential risk of inducing respiratory depression in the newborn.

S-adenosyl-L-methionine has also been tried. This is the principal endogenous methyl donor in several methyltransferase reactions and is also a key intermediary in the synthesis of glutathione. It appears to antagonize some of the cholestatic effects of estrogens in humans and to significantly improve pruritus. However, in a double-blind, placebo-controlled study, the drug was ineffective in Chilean patients with moderate to severe IHCP.

Ursodeoxycholic acid is widely used in the treatment of cholesterol cholelithiasis in various liver diseases, many of which affect women of childbearing age. It has been shown to be helpful in IHCP and in small trials has been safe, with no deleterious effects to the newborn.

Acute Fatty Liver of Pregnancy

Acute fatty liver of pregnancy (AFLP) was first recognized in the 1930s. The incidence in a largely Hispanic population was reported to be 1 per 13,328 deliveries. There seems to be an increased incidence in primiparas, particularly those carrying twins or male fetuses. AFLP occurs almost exclusively after the 35th week of pregnancy, although it has been noted as early as the 30th week.

Clinically, the disease consists of rapid onset of hyperemesis and right-upper-quadrant or midabdominal discomfort, followed by rapidly progressive encephalopathy that may progress to coma and death. Ammonia levels are increased, usually markedly.

The hematocrit is usually normal unless there is accompanying gastrointestinal bleeding. The peripheral blood smear demonstrates thrombocytopenia and normoblasts. There is usually evidence of diffuse intravascular coagulopathy with a low platelet count and presence of fibrin split products. Signs of preeclampsia, hypertension, and peripheral edema are common in AFLP and unusual in fulminant hepatitis. Liver biopsy using oil-red-O stain is very helpful but may not be possible when coagulopathy develops.

It is difficult to predict the clinical course in patients with AFLP. Recent studies have reported a patient survival rate of up to 90%. This improved prognosis has been ascribed, at least in part, to early recognition of disease and early termination of pregnancy. On gross examination, the liver is pale and small. Unlike the situation in macrovesicular fatty infiltration, the nuclei are centrally located rather than pushed to the periphery. There may be patchy hepatocellular necrosis, lobular inflammation, and reticular condensation. Electron microscopy may demonstrate subtle differences between the hepatic mitochondrial changes seen in Reye's syndrome and AFLP.

The cause of AFLP is not known in all cases. A metabolic disorder seems likely. Subsequent pregnancies have been normal in those who have survived. In the mother, improvement occurs in 2 or 3 days after delivery, although is some cases a transient worsening is noted, especially in the degree of encephalopathy. There is a subgroup of patients who exhibit a rapidly progressive downhill course. It is in these patients that liver transplantation may become necessary and may play a lifesaving role.

AFLP has been associated with LCHAD (long-chain 3-hydroxyacyl-coenzyme dehydrogenase) deficiency. The abnormality in many families may be a single guanosine-to-cytosine mutation of the alpha subunit of the trifunctional protein that metabolizes the last three steps of beta oxidation. LCHAD deficiency in many of these infants may be the cause of later problems, including hypoglycemia, hypotonia, acute or chronic skeletal and cardiac muscle dysfunction, developmental delay, and sudden infant death syndrome.

Preeclampsia/Eclampsia and HELLP Syndrome

Preeclampsia is the triad of hypertension, proteinuria, and edema. It occurs most frequently during the second half of gestation and usually during the third trimester. Eclampsia includes the signs and symptoms of preeclampsia as well as convulsions or coma.

Preeclampsia may often cause mild disturbances in liver function and histology if patients are carefully evaluated. Fortunately for most eclamptic patients, hepatic complications are relatively minor, present little threat to the mother and fetus, and resolve entirely and without sequelae after delivery. Therefore, for this majority of instances, management can be directed to control of blood pressure, edema, and salt retention with little concern for liver involvement.

The precise mechanism of preeclampsia/eclampsia is not understood, though vasospasm and activation of coagulation may be important factors. The risks to the fetus of preeclampsia/eclampsia include prematurity, fetal growth retardation, and low birth weight.

Clinical features do not differ greatly in patients with HELLP syndrome (hemolysis, elevated liver enzymes, low platelet count). These entities may represent a continuum of multisystem disorders that may involve the liver. Laboratory tests in HELLP syndrome are usually indicative of microangiopathic hemolysis. Elevated transaminases, thrombocytopenia, and moderate proteinuria are common. These laboratory abnormalities usually normalize within 5 days postpartum and the hypertension and proteinuria by 3 months. A neonatal thrombocytopenia and neutropenia may be noted.

The principles of therapy include supportive care and a prompt decision regarding timing and mode of delivery. Glucocorticoids may be helpful in hastening fetal lung maturity. Expansion of plasma volume, bed rest, magnesium sulfate, plasma exchange therapy, and antithrombin II all have been used in some patients. Most investigators recommend prompt delivery. There does not seem to be a recurrence in subsequent pregnancies, and oral contraceptives also seem to be safe.

Hepatic Rupture

Spontaneous rupture of the liver is a rare complication of pregnancy. In the nonpregnant individual, rupture of the liver is encountered in the setting of hemangioma, adenoma, amebic abscess, echinococcus cysts, and blunt trauma. Preeclampsia/eclampsia occurs in 85% of patients with spontaneous hepatic rupture of pregnancy; of these, 70% are multiparas. Preeclampsia in previous pregnancies is speculated to impair hepatic mechanisms for removing fibrin deposits. Subsequent preeclampsia leaves larger fibrin deposits, more vascular occlusion, larger hemorrhages, and ultimately sizable subcapsular hematomas. These hematomas may enlarge, and if Glisson's capsule weakens by ischemia, spontaneous hepatic rupture may result. Both maternal mortality and fetal death are reported to be greater than 50%.

A high clinical index of suspicion in the setting of acute abdominal pain, nausea, and vomiting in the last trimester may allow for early intervention. Abdominal computed tomography (CT) scans are currently the most helpful diagnostic tool.

When a hepatic hemorrhage is recognized, careful monitoring is essential. Indications for laparotomy include a continued need for transfusion or deterioration of vital signs; worsening pain or peritoneal signs; progressive expansion of the hematoma; and, finally, a septic hematoma.

Surgical methods of treatment include evacuation and drainage, oversewing of the damaged liver bed, application of a topical hemostatic agent, hepatic artery ligation, and possibly hepatic artery embolization or even hepatic lobectomy. Liver transplantation has also been done successfully.

Porphyria

Porphyrias are classified on the basis of the major site of expression of the enzymatic defect as either erythropoietic or hepatic. It is possible to have more than one enzymatic defect concurrently in the heme synthetic pathway. Clinical manifestations are more common in women, suggesting the importance of hormonal influences. Normal pregnancy is associated with an increase in urinary excretion of aminolevulinic acid (ALA) and coproporphyrin. The magnitude of these changes remains much smaller than that seen during porphyric attacks.

Neilson and Neilson reported 76 pregnancies in 40 patients with porphyria. The vast majority had a flare during pregnancy, and only 60% of these pregnancies progressed to the state of viability. The maternal death rate was high, with 17 maternal deaths due to attacks of porphyria, 14 of which were among primigravidas.

Management consists of hospitalization for supportive care with intravenous administration of glucose, correction of electrolyte imbalances, pain control, and the use of phenothiazines for nausea and vomiting. When tolerated, a high-carbohydrate diet of 300–500 g daily is instituted.

Porphyria cutanea tarda (PCT) is the most common disorder of porphyrin metabolism in Europe and North America. Due to its high association with hepatitis C in particular, hepatitis C antibody testing and measurement of circulating hepatitis C virus is recommended in pregnant women with this disorder. PCT is also associated with positive tests for antinuclear antibody in 30–40% of patients, which may have important implications for the gestation period. Testing for lupus anticoagulant and anticardiolipin antibodies is also recommended. During pregnancy, avoidance of alcohol, iron, and exposure to sunlight, especially during the first trimester, is recommended. The clinical manifestations of PCT improve as the pregnancy advances, perhaps due to the relative iron deficiency that develops. It is also important to assess the newborn in the immediate postpartum period and to screen for the presence of PCT, both for genetic purposes and avoidance of inducing factors in the child.

BIBLIOGRAPHY

Anita FP, Bharadwaja TT, Watsa MC, et al. Liver in normal pregnancy, pre-eclampsia and eclampsia. Lancet 1958; 2:776–778.

De Mola JRL, Muise KL, Duchon MA. Obstet Gynecol Surv 1996; 51:493–497.

Gelpi AP. Viral hepatitis complicating pregnancy: mortality trends in Saudi Arabia. Int J Gynecol Obstet 1979; 17:73–81.

Hunt CM, Carson KL, Sharara I. Hepatitis C in pregnancy. Obstet Gynecol 1997; 89:883–890.

Immunization Practices Advisory Committee. Prevention of perinatal transmission of hepatitis B virus: prenatal screening of all pregnant women for hepatitis B surface antigen. MMWR 1988; 37:341–346.

Khuroo MS, Teli MR, Skidmoor S, et al. Incidence and severity of viral hepatitis in pregnancy. Am J Med 1981; 70:252–255.

McNair RD, Jaynes RV. Alterations in liver function during normal pregnancy. Am J Obstet Gynecol 1960; 80:500–503.

Neilson DR, Neilson RP. Porphyria complicated by pregnancy. W J Surg Obstet Gynecol 1985; 66:134–138.

Perez V, Gorodisch S, Casavilo AF, et al. Ultrastructure of human liver and the end of normal pregnancy. Am J Obstet Gynecol 1971; 110:428–431.

Pockros PJ, Peters RL, Reynolds TP. Idiopathic fatty liver of pregnancy: findings in ten cases. Medicine 1984; 663:1–11.

Ribalta J, Reyes H, Gonzalez MC, et al. S-adenosyl-l-methionine and the treatment of patients with intrahepatic cholestasis of pregnancy: a randomized, double-blind, placebo-controlled study with negative results. Hepatology 1991; 13:1084–1089.

Rovinsky JJ, Jaffin H. Cardiovascular hemodynamics of pregnancy: III. Cardiac grade, stroke volume, total peripheral resistance and central blood volume in multiple pregnancy. Synthesis of results. Am J Obstet Gynecol 1966 95:787–794.

Rustgi VK, Hoofnagle JH. Viral hepatitis during pregnancy. Semin Liver Dis 1987; 7:40–46.

Shanley CJ, Braun DK, Braun K, et al. Fulminant hepatic failure secondary to herpes simplex virus hepatitis. Transplantation 1995; 59(1):145–149.

Sims HF, Brackett JC, Powell CK, et al. The molecular basis of pediatric long-chain 3-hydroxyacyl-coenzyme dehydrogenase deficiency associated with maternal acute fatty liver of pregnancy. PNAS 1995; 92:841–844.

Smithwick EM, Pascual E, Go SC. Hepatitis-associated antigen: possible relationship to premature delivery. J Pediatr 1972; 81:537–540.

Stoller A, Collmann RD. Incidence of infective hepatitis followed by Down's syndrome nine months later. Lancet 1965; 2:1221–1223.

Thaler MM, Park CK, Landers DV, et al. Vertical transmission of hepatitis C virus. Lancet 1991; 2:17–18

34
Management of Pruritus

Christine M. Hunt and Kelly L. Carson
Duke University Medical Center, Durham, North Carolina

INTRODUCTION

The pruritus of cholestasis can be severely debilitating, resulting in loss of productivity, sleep deprivation, and suicidal depression. Many therapies have been used in the treatment of the pruritus of cholestasis, including antihistamines, cholestyramine, rifampicin, metronidazole, ursodeoxycholate, phenobarbital, flumecinol, charcoal hemoperfusion, and anion resin exchange plasmapheresis. These therapies have largely proved ineffective in the amelioration of intractable pruritus associated with cholestatic liver disease. The broad range of therapies employed attests to the enormous difficulties encountered in discovering effective treatments. Many trials have been small and uncontrolled, leading to the use of multiple empiric regimens in the clinic.

Recently, important insights into the pathogenesis of the pruritus of cholestasis were revealed in a series of elegant experiments exploring the role of endogenous opioids in pruritus. Opioids have long been known to cause pruritus. Elevations in plasma opioids have been noted in animal models of cholestasis. A seminal observation was made in 1979; a patient with primary biliary cirrhosis (PBC) complicated by severe pruritus exhibited marked and rapid improvement of pruritus following administration of intravenous naloxone, an opioid antagonist. A subsequent unblinded trial of nalmefene in the treatment of severe pruritus associated with cholestatic liver disease confirmed the benefit of opioid antagonists in the amelioration of intractable pruritus. Administration of oral nalmefene 5 mg daily yielded marked and rapid improvement in pruritus, as well as in fatigue. Subsequent double-blind, placebo-controlled trials have confirmed the benefit of intravenous naloxone in the treatment of severe pruritus associated with cholestasis. Although opioid antagonists provide significant benefit to most patients with severe pruritus of cholestasis, not all patients experience relief. This suggests that while opioids are important in the pathogenesis of pruritus, additional pathogenic mechanisms are likely.

Investigators have explored the role of other mediators of nociception in an attempt to find novel agents to ameliorate intractable pruritus. The central nervous system (CNS) sedative propofol, and the serotonin antagonist ondansetron have been successfully employed in the treatment of severe pruritus of cholestasis.

CLINICAL PRESENTATION

The onset of pruritus secondary to cholestasis typically parallels the underlying liver disease, occurring either gradually or abruptly. PBC is associated with the insidious appearance of pruritus, a symptom frequently worsened prior to the menstrual cycle. Pruritus may predate the onset of jaundice in this disease. In contrast, drug-related cholestatic syndromes can rapidly result in both jaundice and pruritus.

Pruritis may be focal (e.g., involving the palms and soles) or generalized. Severe pruritis may be only minimally relieved by scratching; patients may employ instruments in a futile attempt to relieve the pruritus. Not infrequently, a dermatologist will initially be consulted for treatment of the pruritus of cholestasis; however, primary skin lesions are not present. Secondary skin lesions, including severe excoriations and lichenification, may result from self-induced damage.

Laboratory abnormalities associated with the pruritus of cholestasis include elevations in the alkaline phosphatase, 5′ nucleotidase, or gamma glutamyltranspeptidase and/or total and direct bilirubin and transaminases.

PATHOGENESIS

It was long held that the pruritus of cholestasis resulted from bile acids binding to nerve endings in the dermis; however, multiple lines of evidence have disproved this hypothesis. Serum and tissue concentrations of bile acids vary markedly in patients with cholestasis and are not predictive of pruritus. In addition, dermal concentrations of bile acids are not universally increased in patients with severe pruritus.

Substantive evidence supports the role of endogenous opioids in the pruritus of cholestatic liver disease. Pruritus, a well-recognized side effect of morphine administration, can be alleviated with opioid antagonists, and total endogenous opioid levels are elevated in patients with cholestatic liver disease.

The administration of the potent opioid antagonist nalmefene to patients with severe pruritus of cholestatic liver disease precipitates an opioid withdrawal syndrome, suggesting that elevated endogenous opioids are present. Further experiments have demonstrated that the pruritus of cholestasis can be lessened with opioid antagonists. When injected into the

Table 1 Therapeutic Agents for Amelioration of Mild to Moderate Pruritis of Cholestasis

Medication	Mode of action	Suggested dose
Cholestyramine/Colestipol	Intestinal anionic resin sequestrant	8 g PO prior to breakfast
Ursodeoxycholate	Hydrophilic bile acid that may inhibit hepatocellular membrane injury by toxic bile acids; modulates hepatic immune function, and stimulates choleresis	15–20 mg/kg PO daily
Rifampin	Postulated to decrease potentially toxic bile acids and/or improve intrahepatic sulfation	10 mg/kg PO daily

Table 2 Therapeutic Agents for Amelioration of Severe Pruritis of Cholestasis

Medication	Mode of action	Suggested dose
Naloxone	Opioid antagonist	0.4 mg IV bolus, followed by 0.2 μg/kg/min IV infusion
Naltrexone	Opioid antagonist	12.5–25 mg PO qd as starting dose; titrate to higher dose as needed. With prolonged therapy and diminished efficacy secondary to tachyphylaxis, a "drug holiday" of 2 days weekly may be required
Propofol	CNS sedative	2–3 mg/kg/h IV
Ondansetron	Serotonin antagonist	4–8 mg IV qd–bid

medullary dorsal horn of monkeys, plasma from cholestatic patients with pruritus induced facial scratching. Naloxone administration abolished this effect, suggesting that a pruritogenic substance with opioid agonist properties is produced in patients with the pruritus of cholestasis.

TREATMENT ALGORITHMS

Recommended treatments are subdivided into those that improve mild to moderate pruritus (Table 1) and those that are useful in severe refractory pruritus (Table 2). Alternative, less efficacious therapies are also discussed below.

MILD TO MODERATE PRURITUS

Cholestyramine and Colestipol

These insoluble sequestering agents have been widely used in the treatment of pruritus of cholestasis. Cholestyramine may successfully manage mild pruritus of cholestasis (Table 1), as proven in a placebo-controlled, double-blind, crossover-design trial. As anion-exchange resins, these compounds decrease the enterohepatic circulation of bile acids, cholesterol, etc., by intestinal binding and excretion. Cholestyramine is also a choleretic agent.

These sequestering agents are typically administered before breakfast to maximize binding of the overnight "store" of gallbladder contents (and potentially "trap" pruritogenic compounds in the bile). Some investigators recommend dosing both before and after breakfast. As anion-exchange resins, these compounds can also bind a variety of medications; therefore, medication administration must be carefully reviewed with the patient. If this "first-line" drug fails in more severe pruritus, the clinician is advised to pursue the more effective therapies outlined below.

Antihistamines

A small placebo-controlled, double-blind, crossover-design trial found the nonsedating antihistamine terfenadine to be efficacious in the treatment of pruritus (with a mean reduction of pruritus score from 20.3–15.8), yet found chlorpheniramine to be no better than placebo.

Phototherapy

Small, uncontrolled studies have suggested transient benefits from phototherapy. In a pilot study in PBC, pruritus recurred within 2 weeks of completion of 10-day phototherapy sessions.

MODERATE PRURITUS

Antibiotic Use

Rifampicin

The cytochrome P-450 inducer rifampicin has been found effective in the amelioration of pruritus in two double-blind, placebo-controlled trials. Pruritus visual analogue scores were improved 50% in comparison with placebo following 7-day treatment with rifampin. However, subsequent studies have revealed variable results with this drug.

Rifampicin impedes hepatocellular uptake of bilirubin and may thereby stabilize hepatocellular membranes. However, its antipruritic mechanism remains unproven. Potential risks of rifampicin include its hepatotoxicity (most frequently seen with coadministration of antituberculous therapy), lithogenicity (secondary to increasing the biliary cholesterol saturation index), and reduction in 25-hydroxycholecalciferol (hence contributing to bone disease in PBC).

Metronidazole

Metronidazole has been shown to improve pruritus in primary biliary cirrhosis. Its antipruritic effect has been attributed to its ability to alter gut flora (thereby potentially altering the production of the toxic secondary bile acid lithocholate), however, this remains unproven. A randomized trial of metronidazole used in the prevention of cholestasis in patients with Crohn's disease receiving total parenteral nutrition revealed significant improvement in cholestasis in the patients who were randomized to metronidazole therapy.

Ursodeoxycholate

Ursodeoxycholate has been reported to improve pruritus in PBC patients in a 2-year, multicenter, double-blind, placebo-controlled study by Poupon et al. In this trial, the patients had their pruritis graded as absent, occasional, or permanent. In the cohort who completed the study, the prevalence of pruritus decreased significantly from 53–23% in the ursodeoxycholate-treated group, in comparison to a 48–28% decrease in the placebo-treated group.

Ursodeoxycholate is reported to stabilize hepatocellular membranes against perturbation by toxic hydrophobic bile acids, to modulate hepatic immunological function, and to increase choleresis. Ursodeoxycholate has not been efficacious in improving pruritus in all cholestatic patients; however, its minimal side effects make it an attractive agent for initial therapy.

S-Adenosyl-L-Methionine

S-adenosyl-L-methionine (SAM) administered intravenously was beneficial in reducing pruritus in some trials in cholestatic liver disease. Oral SAM was then examined for the amelioration of pruritus and fatigue in patients with cholestasis in a large, multicenter, prospective, double-blind, placebo-controlled trial in Italy. Patients with stable cholestasis (greater than twofold elevations in bilirubin and alkaline phosphatase) were given oral SAM 1600 mg daily or placebo for 2 weeks. Pruritus and fatigue were quantified with visual analogue scales; global well-being was quantified by the "Face Scale." Serum bilirubin and alkaline phosphatase significantly improved in greater than half of the patients receiving SAM.

Notably, 77% (30/39) of SAM vs. 33% (14/42) of placebo-treated patients experienced a > 50% improvement in pruritus; 57% (39/68) of SAM vs. 12% (7/60) of placebo-treated patients noted a > 50% improvement in fatigue. However, the small subgroup of patients with PBC treated with SAM ($n = 6$) did not differ significantly from the placebo-treated group ($n = 8$). The benefits of SAM therapy were noted during therapy and quickly reversed with therapy discontinuation. The side effects of SAM were minimal (with transient insomnia noted in < 3%); no patients withdrew from the study because of side effects.

The efficacy of SAM is believed to be secondary to enhanced membrane fluidity (with SAM-dependent methylation of hepatic membrane phospholipids) or sulfation of hydrophobic bile acids. SAM has also proved efficacious in the treatment of depression. In summary, SAM has proved of some benefit in patients with mild to moderate pruritus of cholestasis.

Methotrexate

Pruritus occurring in conjunction with PBC has been reported to improve several months following the initiation of oral methotrexate therapy. However, the use of methotrexate in PBC remains controversial (see Chap. 12).

Phenobarbital

In controlled trials comparing the use of phenobarbital and rifampicin in the pruritus of cholestasis, phenobarbital did not significantly alter pruritus. This cytochrome P-450 inducer is both a choleretic and sedative agent; however, its use in the pruritus of cholestasis cannot be recommended.

Flumecinol

Flumecinol is a benzhydrol derivative and cytochrome P-450 inducer that has been used in the treatment of jaundice in Gilbert's syndrome. This agent has been assessed in randomized, double-blind, placebo-controlled trials and found to be efficacious and safe in the amelioration of pruritus in oral doses of 300 mg daily. Flumecinol decreased the mean pruritus score only slightly, from 45/100 to 32/100, after 3 weeks of therapy. No change in quality-of-life score was noted during flumecinol therapy. The minimal benefit of this therapy precludes its use in patients with significant pruritus.

SEVERE PRURITUS

Opioid Antagonists

A double-blind, placebo-controlled crossover design trial of intravenous naloxone treatment of severe pruritus of cholestatic liver disease confirmed the efficacy of opioid antagonists. Significant improvements in pruritus after naloxone administration were noted in both scratching activity (measured with a vibration transducer) and scores on visual analogue scales. Naloxone administration resulted in an opioid withdrawal syndrome in 3% (1 of 29) patients. Unfortunately, naloxone is limited by its lack of oral bioavailability, need for parenteral administration, and short half life (Table 2).

Pilot studies in Britain and a double-blind placebo-controlled trial in the United States reveal significantly improved pruritus in patients with cholestasis treated with nalmefene, a potent oral opioid antagonist. However, intravenous nalmefene is the only form available in the United States. Due to its potency as an opioid antagonist, nalmefene can precipitate an opioid withdrawal reaction, nausea, hallucinations, or insomnia in patients with cholestasis, necessitating careful monitoring and gradual increases in dosage over time.

Naltrexone, another oral opioid antagonist, was initially approved for use in the treatment of narcotic and alcohol dependence. A pilot single-blind trial of naltrexone 50 mg PO per day in the treatment of severe pruritus associated with cholestatic liver disease found it highly effective; however, 40% of patients developed nausea and/or emesis. To avoid these side effects, an initial naltrexone dose of 25 mg would be prudent with subsequent dose escalation. High-dose naltrexone (300 mg/day) when administered to obese subjects have been noted to produce mild, asymptomatic, reversible abnormalities in aminotransferases. No cases of hepatic failure have been reported with naltrexone. In the described pilot study, no significant change in aminotransferases was observed with naltrexone treatment.

Tachyphylaxis to the antipruritic effects of naltrexone may develop after several weeks of use. In patients requiring long-term naltrexone for continuing pruritus, this effect can be circumvented by the institution of "drug holidays" (where the drug is stopped for 2 days weekly).

Propofol

Propofol has been effective in the control of severe pruritus of cholestasis in a double-blind, placebo-controlled crossover study. In addition to global CNS depression, propofol is postulated to depress the posterior horn, a region associated with opioid-induced pruritus. The clinical utility of propofol is limited by its hypnotic properties and need for intravenous administration.

Ondansetron

Ondansetron, a potent serotonin antagonist, has been shown to significantly improve pruritus in cholestatic liver disease in a single-blind, placebo-controlled, crossover-design study. Studies to date have examined the use of intravenous ondansetron; however, an oral preparation is now available. Ondansetron is cleared through phase I hepatic metabolism, therefore, the dose should be decreased to once daily in patients with severe hepatic insufficiency.

Serotonin plays a central role in neurotransmission of nociceptive stimuli in the peripheral and CNS. Both pain and itch are transmitted through C fibers of polymodal nociceptors; serotonin excites C fibers, which also stimulate itching.

Orthotopic Liver Transplantation

Patients with severe pruritus refractory to the measures outlined above merit evaluation for orthotopic liver transplantation. However, hepatitis C, which may appear posttransplantation, has been associated with severe pruritus.

Charcoal Hemoperfusion/Plasmapheresis/Anionic Resin Plasmapheresis

Multiple uncontrolled trials suggest a temporary benefit from these modalities; however, the inconvenience, cost, and morbidity of these therapies markedly limit their utility.

Partial External Diversion of Bile

An uncontrolled pediatric trial suggested improvement of intractable pruritus from partial diversion of bile to an external stoma (approximately 50% of bile flow is diverted). Pruritus was reportedly markedly improved in four of six children with progressive intrahepatic cholestasis; children with arteriohepatic dysplasia exhibited amelioration but not cessation of pruritus. In view of the paucity of data, partial external diversion cannot be routinely recommended.

SUMMARY

The pruritus of cholestasis remains an often unbearable problem for the patient and a challenge for the physician. Multiple regimens have been employed often with disappointing results. The use of narcotics and serotonin antagonists in the treatment of the pruritus of cholestasis appears most promising. Further research is needed to improve our understanding and treatment of this disorder.

BIBLIOGRAPHY

Bergasa NV. The pruritus of cholestasis. Semin Dermatol 1995; 14:302–312.

Bergasa NV, Jones EA. The pruritis of cholestasis: potential pathogenic and therapeutic implications of opioids. Gastroenterology 1995; 108:1582–1588.

Bergasa NV, Alling DW, Talbot TL, Swain MG, Yurdaydin C, Turner ML, Schmitt JM, Walker EC, Jones EA. Effects of naloxone infusions in patients with the pruritus of cholestasis. Ann Intern Med 1995; 123:161–167.

Borgeat AI, Savioz D, Mentha G, Giostra E, Suter PM. Intractable cholestatic pruritus after liver transplantation-management with propofol. Transplantation 1994; 58(6):727–729.

Borgeat A, Wilder-Smith D, Mentha G, Huber O. Propofol and cholestatic pruritus. Am J Gastroenterol 1992; 87:672–674.

Carson KL, Tran T, Sharara AI, Hunt CM. Naltrexone in the treatment of severe pruritus of cholestatic liver disease. Am J Gastroenterology 1996; 91(5):1–2.

Cynamon HA, Andres JM, Iafrate RP. Rifampin relieves pruritus in children with cholestatic liver disease. Gastroenterology 1990; 98:1013–1016.

Frezza M, Surrentia C, Manzillo G, Fiaccadori F, Bortolini M, De Padova C. Oral S-adenosylmethionine in the symptomatic treatment of intrahepatic cholestasis. Gastroenterology 1990; 99:211–215.

Poupon RE, Balkau B, Eschwige E, Iglesias J, Gonzalez MC, Hernandez I, Alvarez C, Molina C, Danitz AM. A multicenter, controlled trial of ursodiol for the treatment of primary biliary cirrhosis. N Engl J Med 1991; 324:1548–1554.

Schworer H, Hartmann H, Ramadori G. Relief of cholestatic pruritus by a novel class of drugs: 5-hydroxytryptamine type 3 (5-HT3) receptor antagonists: effectiveness of ondansetron. Pain 1995; 61:33–37.

Turner IB, Rawlins MD, Wood P, James OFW. Flumecinol for the treatment of pruritus associated with primary biliary cirrhosis. Aliment Pharmacol Ther 1994; 8:337–342.

Wolfhagen FHS, Sternieri E, Hop WCJ, Vitale G, Bertolotti M, Van Buuren HR. Oral naltrexone treatment for cholestatic pruritus: A double-blind, placebo-controlled study. Gastroenterology 1997; 113:1264–1269.

35

Management of Upper Gastrointestinal Bleeding Secondary to Portal Hypertension

Arun J. Sanyal and Mitchell L. Shiffman
Medical College of Virginia–Virginia Commonwealth University, Richmond, Virginia

Portal hypertension is defined as an increase in portal venous pressure over 5 mmHg. Portal hypertension causes variceal hemorrhage, a principal complication of cirrhosis, and contributes substantially to the 32,000 deaths and over 20 million days of work loss due to cirrhosis annually. Therefore, control of portal hypertension and treatment of its complications are cornerstones of management of cirrhosis. The optimal management of portal hypertension requires a clear understanding of its anatomic and physiological basis, natural history, and the utility of specific therapies at specific stages in the natural history of portal hypertension.

GASTROESOPHAGEAL VARICES: ANATOMY AND CLASSIFICATION

The portal vein normally drains blood from the stomach, intestines, spleen, and pancreatic bed via the superior mesenteric, splenic, and left gastric veins (Fig. 1). The tributaries of the portal vein also communicate with veins draining into the systemic venous circulation. Such portasystemic communications exist primarily in five locations: (1) at the cardia via the intrinsic and extrinsic veins of the region, (2) in the anal canal via anastomoses between the superior and middle hemorrhoidal veins, (3) in the falciform ligament via recanalization of the paraumbilical veins and direction of flow to the veins draining the abdominal wall, (4) in the splenic venous bed and the left renal vein, and (5) in the retroperitoneum. Of these, the gastroesophageal collaterals are of the greatest clinical significance.

The veins draining the esophagus may be classified as intrinsic, extrinsic, and venae comitantes of the vagus nerve. The intrinsic veins comprise a subepithelial and submucosal plexus running along the length of the esophagus. These drain via perforating veins into an extrinsic plexus of veins, which drain into the inferior thyroid and brachiocephalic veins in

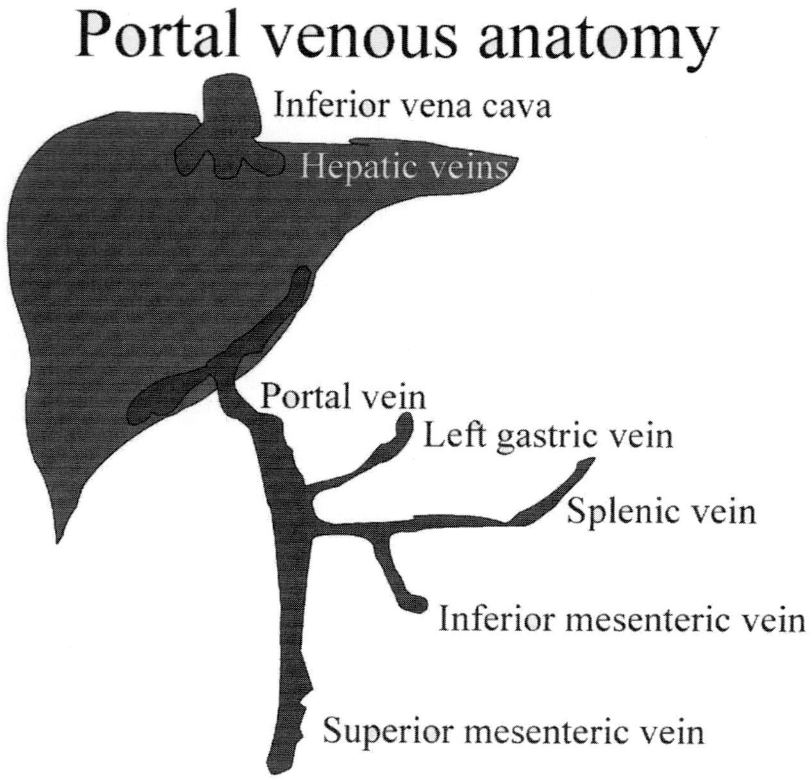

Figure 1 Anatomy of the portal venous system.

the neck, azygous veins in the thorax, and left gastric vein in the abdominal part of the esophagus.

The intrinsic veins of the gastroesophageal junction are divided into four well-defined zones (Fig. 2): (1) Gastric: this is a 2- to 3-cm zone with its upper border at the gastroesophageal junction and is composed of a radial band of veins in the submucosa and lamina propria. (2) Palisade zone: this commences at the gastroesophageal junction and extends cranially for 2–3 cm and is a direct extension of the veins of the gastric zone, which run in "palisades" or packs of longitudinally arrayed veins in the lamina propria. These veins are the primary site of communication between the portal bed and azygous bed. (3) Perforating zone: The intrinsic veins drain into the extrinsic veins primarily in this region via valved perforating veins, which only allow unidirectional flow normally. It extends 2–3 cm cranially from the palisade zone. (4) Truncal zone: A 8- to 10-cm zone extending upward from the perforating zone. The intrinsic veins are composed of three or four large venous trunks in the submucosa, which communicate with an irregular polygonal venous plexus in the submucosa. Blood in these veins flows from a cranial to caudal direction and drains via the perforating veins into the extrinsic veins.

When portal hypertension occurs, an adaptive increase in flow through the porta-systemic communications occurs to return blood to the heart. The vessels involved, especially the intrinsic veins around the gastroesophageal (GE) junction dilate and become

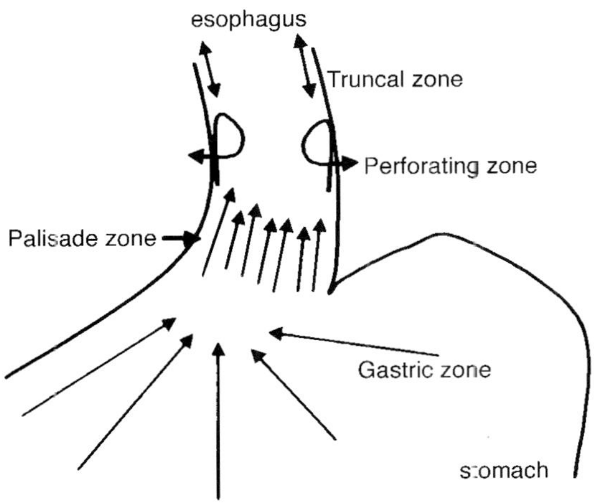

Figure 2 Illustration showing the venous drainage of the intrinsic veins of the gastroesophageal junction. Four zones are identified: (1) gastric, (2) palisade, (3) perforating, and (4) truncal. In patients with portal hypertension, blood flows from the gastric to the esophageal region via veins in the palisade region which dilate and enlarge to form varices.

tortuous forming varicose veins. GE varices occur in four basic patterns: (1) varices in the fundus of the stomach, (2) gastric and palisade-zone varices, (3) varices in the perforating zones, and (4) paraesophageal varices, which involve the extrinsic esophageal veins. In contrast to normal individuals, the valves in the perforating veins become incompetent, thereby permitting reverse flow into the intrinsic plexus from the extrinsic veins.

Clinically, varices are classified by location into esophageal and gastric varices. Esophageal varices are often graded by size (Fig. 3). A common system:

F1: Small, straight varices
F2: Enlarged, tortuous varices, occupying less than one-third of the lumen
F3: large, coil-shaped varices, occupying more than one-third of the lumen

Gastric varices are classified primarily by location. As agreed upon at the Baveno consensus conference, they are described as follows:

Gastroesophageal varices (GOV): Gastric varices in continuity with esophageal varices
Type I (GOV1): along the lesser curve (usually 2–5 cm in length)
Type II (GOV2): along the greater curve extending towards the fundus of the stomach
Isolated gastric varices (IGV):
Type I (IGV1): isolated cluster of varices in the fundus of the stomach
Type II (IGV2): isolated gastric varices in other parts of the stomach.

GOV1 varices form when a branch of the left gastric vein penetrates the gastric wall (cardiac vein) and joins the deep submucosal veins in the gastric zone; they are in direct continuity with those in the palisade zone and are usually associated with large esophageal varices. In contrast, large esophageal varices are present in only 50% of GOV2 varices. IGV1 are often associated with either segmental portal hypertension (splenic vein thrombosis) or the presence of spontaneous collaterals from the splenic vein to the renal vein,

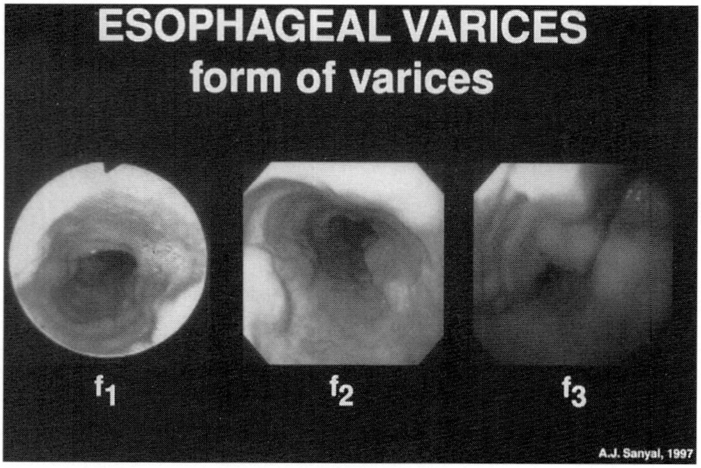

Figure 3 Endoscopic grading of esophageal varices.

which feed these varices (Fig. 4). About 50% of cases of ectopic varices including IGV2 are associated with portal vein thrombosis. The mechanisms responsible for this phenomenon are unknown.

PATHOPHYSIOLOGY OF PORTAL HYPERTENSION

The portal pressure is directly related to portal inflow and outflow resistance

$$\text{Portal pressure} = \text{portal venous inflow} \times \text{outflow resistance} \quad (1)$$

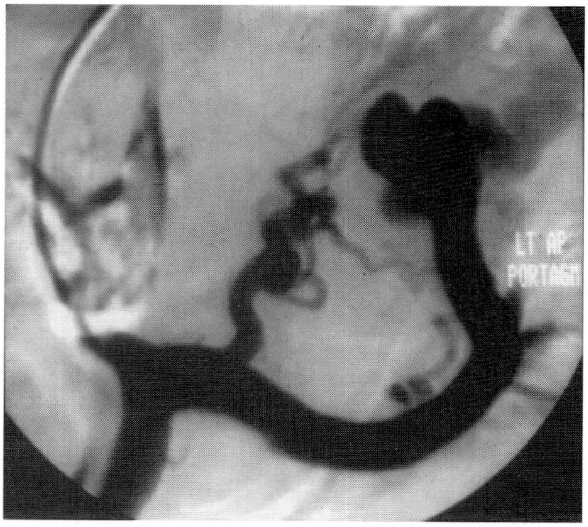

Figure 4 Angiographic study of a spontaneous splenorenal collateral feeding a gastric varix in the fundus of the stomach (IGV1).

Portal pressure is usually determined by hepatic venous catheterization and measurement of the free hepatic venous (FHV) and wedged hepatic venous pressures (WHVP) and calculation of the hepatic venous pressure gradient (HVPG):

$$\text{HVPG} = \text{WHVP} - \text{FHV} \tag{2}$$

Wedged hepatic pressures reflect sinusoidal pressures, while the free hepatic venous pressure corrects for the effects of intraabdominal pressures. Portal hypertension is initiated by an increase in outflow resistance from the portal venous bed. Table 1 lists the sites and common causes of portal hypertension. In cirrhosis, the portal hypertension is further worsened by splanchnic arteriolar dilation, which increases portal venous inflow.

Once portal hypertension occurs, a collateral circulation develops to return blood to the systemic circulation. For a given varix, the transmural pressure gradient is the product of flow and resistance:

$$P_1 - P_2 = Q \times R \tag{3}$$

where P_1 and P_2 are the pressures within and outside the varix respectively, Q is the blood flow per unit time, and R is the resistance to flow through the varix. Also Poiseuille's formula states that resistance to flow may be expressed as:

$$R = nl/\pi r^4 \tag{4}$$

where n is blood viscosity and r and l are the radius and length of the vessel. Variceal wall tension is determined by the transmural pressure, radius, and wall thickness (w) (Laplace's law):

$$\text{Wall tension} = [Q \times (nl/\pi r^4)] \times r/w \tag{5}$$

Variceal wall tension determines the probability of rupture. Based upon Eq. (5) above, along, large varices with high flow rates and thin walls are most likely to rupture and bleed. Conversely, by decreasing collateral flow, resistance to flow, or increasing wall thickness, the risk of variceal rupture should also be decreased. Most pharmacological treatments are directed at decreasing collateral flow, which is usually achieved by decreasing portal pressure and/or increasing collateral resistance. However, the latter has complex effects on collateral flow by directly increasing wall tension and indirectly decreasing it by reducing collateral flow. This may explain some of the interindividual variability in hemodynamic response to pharmacological treatment.

Table 1 Sites and Common Causes of Portal Hypertension

Presinusoidal portal hypertension	Sinusoidal portal hypertension	Postsinusoidal portal hypertension
Portal vein thrombosis	Cirrhosis	Venoocclusive disease
Extrinsic compression of portal vein	Vitamin A toxicity	Budd-Chiari syndrome
Sarcoidosis	Alcoholic hepatitis	Severe congestive heart failure
Noncirrhotic portal fibrosis		
Schistosomiasis		

NATURAL HISTORY OF GASTRIC AND ESOPHAGEAL VARICES:

Esophageal Varices

Approximately 5–15% of patients with cirrhosis without varices develop varices de novo each year. It is estimated that the majority of cirrhotic individuals will develop varices during their lifetimes. However, only about a third of all patients with esophageal varices will ever experience variceal hemorrhage. Considering the approximately 20–30% mortality from each episode of variceal hemorrhage, it is important to be able to target those at greatest risk of bleeding. Several factors predict the risk of bleeding from esophageal varices. These include:

Portal pressures: It has been clearly shown that varices do not develop and therefore cannot bleed when the HVPG is under 12 mmHg. Varices are invariably associated with an HVPG > 12 mmHg, but the risk of bleeding is not predicted by the absolute value of the HVPG above 12 mmHg.

Varix size and location: The likelihood of variceal rupture is directly related to variceal diameter due to the effects of the radius on wall tension (see above). Varices at the GE junction and palisade zone lie in the lamina propria and thus have a thinner coat and are most likely to bleed.

Variceal features on endoscopy: Several endoscopic features of esophageal varices have been shown to predict the risk of hemorrhage. Together, these are often referred to as "red signs," due to their color. These findings include:

- Red wale marks: These are longitudinal red streaks on varices which resemble red corduroy wales.
- Cherry red spots: These are discrete cherry-colored spots that are flat and overlie varices.
- Hematocystic spots: These are raised, discrete red spots overlying varices; they resemble "blood blisters."
- Diffuse erythema: as self-evident, this denotes the diffuse red color of the varix.

Degree of liver failure: Patients with more advanced liver failure are more likely to experience variceal hemorrhage. Thus, with increasing bilirubin and prothrombin time and decreasing albumin levels, the risk of bleeding increases.

Presence of ascites: Tense ascites is also an important risk factor for variceal hemorrhage.

All of these risk factors have been used to estimate the probability of variceal hemorrhage with relative precision (Table 2). Thus, in a patient with Child's class C cirrhosis, large varices, and red signs, the risk of hemorrhage is over 76% within 1 year, while another patient with Child's class A cirrhosis and small varices has a less than 10% likelihood of bleeding. The risk of bleeding also decreases over time from the time that varices are identified; most bleeding episodes occur within the first 2 years after identification of varices.

Once bleeding occurs, spontaneous cessation of hemorrhage occurs in only 50% of individuals. Those with Child's class C cirrhosis and actively spurting varices are particularly prone to continue to bleed without active intervention. Following cessation of active bleeding, there is a high risk of rebleeding for approximately 6 weeks. The risk of such early rebleeding is greatest within the first 48 h and about 50% of all early rebleeding episodes occur during this period. The risk factors for early rebleeding include large varices, age > 60 years, renal failure, and severe initial bleeding as defined by a hemo-

Table 2 Estimated 1-Year Percentage Probability of Bleeding as a Function of All Possible Combinations of the Endoscopic Variables Form (F) and Red Wale Markings in a Child's Class A, B, and C Patients

	Child's class								
	A			B			C		
Red wale markings	F1	F2	F3	F1	F2	F3	F1	F2	F3
−	6	10	15	10	16	26	20	30	42
+	8	12	19	15	23	33	28	38	54
++	12	16	24	20	30	42	36	48	64
+++	16	23	34	28	40	52	44	60	76

Source: Adapted from North Italian Endoscopic Club for the Study and Treatment of Esophageal Varices: Prediction of the first variceal hemorrhage in patients with cirrhosis of the liver and esophageal varices. N Engl J Med 319:983, 1988; with permission.

globin < 8 g/dL at admission. Also, overly aggressive volume replacement may cause rebound portal hypertension and precipitate early rebleeding. Survival during this acute phase depends not only on the control of active hemorrhage but also on the recurrence of bleeding. The long-term course after an index bleed is characterized by recurrent variceal hemorrhage, liver failure, and death. The risk of recurrent bleeding is related to the degree of liver failure, continued alcoholism, variceal size, renal failure, and the presence of a hepatoma. Overall, about 70% of untreated individuals rebleed and die within a year of their index bleed.

Gastric Varices

The likelihood of bleeding from gastric varices depend on their location. Although GOV1 constitute over 70% of gastric varices, only 11% of GOV1 ever bleed. In contrast, about 80% of IGV1 experience hemorrhage even though they represent only 8% of all gastric varices. Bleeding from IGV1 is often associated with lower portal pressures than in nonbleeding subjects with esophageal varices. Furthermore, bleeding from such varices is more severe and the risk of encephalopathy is higher than in patients with bleeding esophageal varices. Overall, gastric varices bleed less frequently but more severely than esophageal varices. Esophageal variceal sclerotherapy causes spontaneous obliteration of 60% of GOV1. In those in whom GOV1 persists for more than 6 months after esophageal variceal obliteration, the risk for rebleeding is substantially greater than in those whose varices disappear (28 vs. 2%). GOV2 are not affected by esophageal sclerotherapy. Recently, the risk of bleeding from IGV1 was shown to correlate with the size of the varices (> 10 mm), Child's class, and the presence of red spots on the varices. Based on these findings, the following prognostic index was calculated:

Prognostic index = (0.53)(Child's class + 0.78) (Varix size + 0.72)(Red spot)

where Child's class A = 0, B = 1, C = 2; the varix size is scored as small (< 5 mm) = 0, medium (5–10 mm) = 1, and large (> 10 mm) = 2; and red spot is scored as absent = 0 or present = 1. The risk of bleeding correlated directly with the prognostic index (Fig. 5).

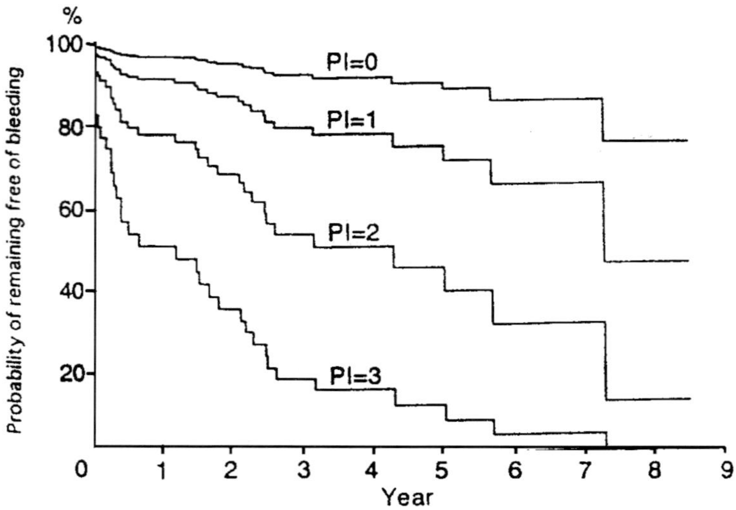

Figure 5 Risk of bleeding from gastric varices in the fundus based on a prognostic index derived by Kim et al. Reproduced with permission from T. Kim et al. Hepatol 1997; 25:307–312.

PRIMARY PROPHYLAXIS OF VARICEAL HEMORRHAGE

A key objective in managing the cirrhotic subject is the primary prevention of variceal hemorrhage. The importance of primary prevention is underscored by the continuing high mortality from active hemorrhage as well as the progressive decline in survival following the index bleed. Currently, despite the multitude of available treatments, only pharmacological treatment with nonselective beta blockers is recommended for primary prevention of variceal hemorrhage.

Pharmacological Treatment

Nonselective Beta Blockers

An important determinant of portal pressure is the portal venous inflow, which is dependent on mesenteric arteriolar resistance. Alpha-adrenergic agents constrict mesenteric arterioles, while beta-adrenergic agents dilate these vessels. Conversely, beta-adrenergic antagonists block the dilatory effects mediated via the beta receptors and allow unopposed alpha-adrenergic effects, resulting in mesenteric arteriolar constriction. Propranolol and nadolol are the two most studied beta-adrenergic antagonists.

Pharmacodynamic Effects. Following either an oral or intravenous dose of propranolol, the hepatic venous pressure gradient decreases by 9–31%. This decrease is primarily due to a decrease in hepatic wedge pressures, with a much lesser contribution from increased systemic venous pressures. In addition, decreases in heart rate and cardiac output contribute, to a lesser degree, to the portal hypotensive effects of these agents at higher doses.

Up to 50% of patients have failed to show a greater than 10% decrease in HVPG upon propranolol administration. This may be due to the following: (1) a concomitant increase in collateral and/or hepatic sinusoidal resistance may negate the hypotensive effects of decreased portal inflow and (2) a compensatory increase in hepatic arterial flow may maintain sinusoidal perfusion and maintain the increased wedge pressures. The site of portal obstruction, cause of cirrhosis, plasma propranolol levels, severity of liver failure, presence of ascites, or basal hemodynamic values and heart rate response to propranolol do not correlate with the portal hypotensive effects of propranolol.

In the long term, the portal hypotensive effects are maintained in most subjects. Tachyphylaxis does occur in some patients and is clinically important because only those with a sustained decrease in portal pressures may benefit from β blockade.

Pharmacokinetic Considerations. Propranolol is highly lipophilic and is almost completely absorbed after oral administration. It undergoes first-pass elimination to a variable degree, causing plasma levels to vary by up to 20-fold. With increasing doses, the relative hepatic extraction decreases, allowing plasma levels to rise. A sustained-release form of propranolol has also been developed which allows once-daily dosing. The clinical effects often do not correlate well with the plasma levels because of the formation of active metabolites, especially the (−) enantiomer, which are taken up by sympathetic nerve endings and then released slowly.

In contrast, nadolol is water-soluble and only incompletely absorbed orally. Also, its interindividual pharmacokinetic variability is much less than that of propranolol. Due to its hydrophilic nature, it does not cross the blood-brain barrier well. However, clinical trials have not shown a significant decrease in the incidence of CNS side effects compared to those of propranolol. Nadolol is excreted via the kidneys and its dose must be modified in response to renal insufficiency.

Adverse Effects. Beta blockade is associated with numerous side effects and multiple drug interactions that have been described in great detail in the literature. The most clinically important side effects involve bronchoconstriction, development of heart failure, and impotence in cirrhotics. Despite the increase in renin activity and decrease in renal blood flow, renal dysfunction occurs only occasionally after propranolol administration. The administration of beta blockers has not been shown to impair the hemodynamic response to acute blood loss.

Clinical Trials of Beta Blockers for Primary Prevention of Variceal Hemorrhage. A total of 10 placebo-controlled clinical trials of propranolol or nadolol have been reported and reviewed. Alcoholic liver disease was the most common etiology of cirrhosis across all trials. Analysis of the data is, however, complicated by the considerable heterogeneity among the patients studied and the treatment regimens used. With a single exception, only patients with esophageal varices were enrolled. Most patients enrolled had Child's class A cirrhosis, although one study excluded those with Child's class C cirrhosis. Only those with large varices were enrolled in four studies, while two studies only enrolled only those with an HVPG > 10–12 mmHg. Doses of 10–480 mg/day of short-acting propranolol or 40–320 mg/day of long-acting propranolol were used. Nadolol was used in two studies. The dose was titrated in these studies by measurement of heart rate, with a 25% decrease in the resting heart rate as the desired endpoint. In addition, a resting heart rate of 55 beats per minute was considered adequate in one trial.

Despite the heterogeneity among trials, several general observations were made across the studies. During the first year of follow-up (the period of greatest risk of bleeding), those treated with beta blockers had a lower risk of variceal hemorrhage than those treated with placebo (0–18% vs. 12–30%) (Fig. 6). These effects were even more pro-

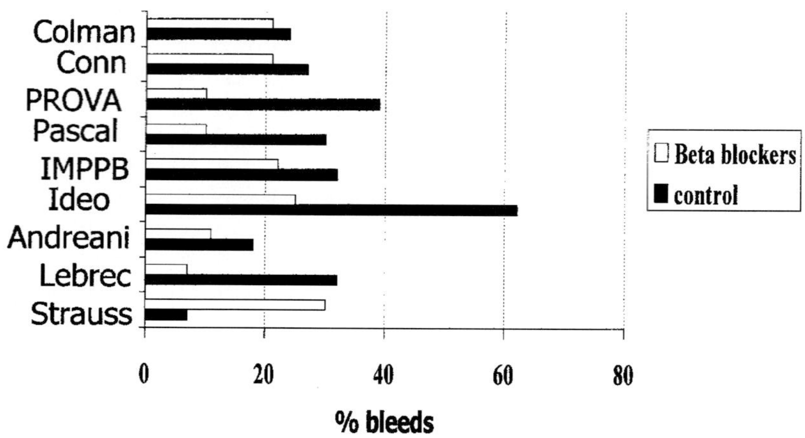

Figure 6 Effects of beta blockers on index bleeding from varices. (From A.J. Sanyal, P.P. Purdum, III, V.A. Luketic, and M.L. Shiffman. Bleeding gastroesophageal varices. Semin Liver Dis 1993; 13:328–342.)

nounced after 2 years of follow up. Although four studies showed a significant decrease in bleeding risk, only one found a survival advantage for those treated with beta blockers. However, variceal hemorrhage–related deaths were less likely among those receiving beta blockers. Metanalyses of the data suggest that nonselective beta blockade reduced the risks of initial variceal hemorrhage by 45% and bleeding-related deaths by 50%. Compliance with treatment was an important predictor of a good outcome, while failure of therapy was associated with younger age, large variceal size, advanced liver failure, and lower propranolol doses.

Nitrosovasodilators

Pharmacodynamics. Nitric oxide is a potent vasodilator and an important mediator of the vasodilated state seen in cirrhosis. The "nitrosovasodilator" group of drugs act via the nitric oxide pathway, producing vasodilation in their target vascular beds. At usual pharmacological doses, these agents are primarily venodilators and decrease cardiac output by decreasing venous return in those with normal myocardial length-tension relationships. Systemic venodilation decreases postsinusoidal resistance and decreases portal pressure. At high doses of drug, arterial dilation and systemic hypotension occur, causing reflex splanchnic vasoconstriction and further decreases in portal pressures. Also, nitrate-mediated baroreceptor reflexes in the pulmonary capillary bed trigger splanchnic vasoconstriction and contribute to the drugs' portal hypotensive action.

Effects on Portal Hemodynamics. Acute administration of either isosorbide mononitrate (ISMN) or dinitrate (ISDN) may cause up to a 40% decrease in HVPG, a 30% decrease in portal flow, and a 15% decrease in azygous flow. Plasma norepinephrine and renin activity increase, indicating increased sympathetic activity and enhanced tendency to retain Na. In the long term, the degree of portal decompression is variable and the systemic hemodynamic effects become less pronounced. The effects of ISDN are less predictable than ISMN presumably due to their variable hepatic extraction in cirrhotic subjects. Therefore, ISMN is the long-acting nitrate of choice for the treatment of portal hypertension.

Clinical Trials of Nitrates for Primary Prevention of Variceal Hemorrhage. An important study prospectively randomized 118 patients to receive either ISMN (20 mg thrice daily) or propranolol (to the maximum tolerated dose). After a median follow up of 29 months, no significant differences were noted in either bleeding rates (18 vs. 14%) or mortality (18 vs. 15%). However, after 7 years, an increased mortality especially in those > 51 years of age (72 vs. 48%) were noted in those receiving ISMN.

It is unclear whether the above findings reflect a beneficial effect of propranolol or an adverse effect of nitrates. Interpretation of the data is further confounded by the fact that about 50% of patients enrolled in each arm withdrew from the study. Nitrates are known to increase sodium retention and to cause tissue hypoxia and increased lactate levels in cirrhotic individuals. At this time, the data do not support a role for nitrates as monotherapy for the primary prophylaxis of variceal hemorrhage. Similarly, the role of combination therapy (beta blockers plus nitrates) has not been validated in clinical trials and its use is considered experimental.

Surgical Portal Decompression

Four prospective randomized trials comparing surgical portacaval shunts with medical therapy were carried out over twenty-five years ago. They demonstrated that while surgery could effectively prevent variceal hemorrhage, the benefit was offset by severe encephalopathy, which ensured in 30–60% of patients. Moreover, medically treated patients survived longer. Thus, the modality has been eliminated as an option for the primary prevention of variceal hemorrhage.

Transjugular Intrahepatic Portasystemic Shunts (TIPS)

In this procedure, a pathway is created between the hepatic vein and the intrahepatic portion of the portal vein by angiographic techniques using a transjugular approach. This pathway is then dilated and kept patent by deployment of an expandable metal stent, thereby creating a low-resistance track for blood from the hypertensive portal vein to return to the heart. Currently, no data exist to support a role for TIPS for primary prevention of variceal hemorrhage. In addition, TIPS does not improve the outcome of liver transplantation and in some cases may render the operation technically more difficult. TIPS is thus not recommended for the primary prevention of variceal hemorrhage.

Endoscopic Sclerotherapy

Injection of sclerosant substances into varices may be used to obliterate varices and treat variceal hemorrhage. The clinical trials of sclerotherapy for primary prevention of variceal hemorrhage are difficult to compare because fo the variability in patient populations and the use of sclerotherapy during episodes of active bleeding. Although three studies found sclerotherapy to be beneficial, a large multicenter study found a significantly higher mortality in those treated with sclerotherapy despite a decrease in variceal hemorrhage in these patients. Beta blockers alone are superior to sclerotherapy and equivalent to beta blocker plus sclerotherapy for this indication. Thus, sclerotherapy should not be used either alone or with beta blockers for the primary prevention of variceal hemorrhage.

Endoscopic Band Ligation

A recent study evaluated the role of endoscopic band ligation for the primary prevention of variceal hemorrhage. It demonstrated a decrease in rates of variceal hemorrhage and also a survival advantage for treated patients. These exciting data now await validation in cirrhotic populations in the United States.

Clinical Recommendations for Primary Prevention of Variceal Hemorrhage

Nonselective beta blockers are the only recommended treatment for the primary prevention of variceal hemorrhage in cirrhotic patients. They are clearly effective and have also been shown to be cost-effective. However, every patient with cirrhosis does not necessarily benefit from these drugs. It is therefore customary to target those at greatest risk of bleeding and therefore most likely to benefit.

All patients with cirrhosis should undergo an endoscopic examination as part of their evaluation. Patients with Child's class B or C cirrhosis with esophageal varices of any grade and those with Child's class A cirrhosis and large varices, especially with red signs, should be targeted for treatment. In those where varices are not present, endoscopy should be repeated at 2- to 3-year intervals. No evaluable data currently exist for the clinical utility of beta blockers for the various types of gastric varices, although it appears to make intuitive sense to treat those especially at high risk for bleeding.

It has been shown that those who experience a 25% or greater drop in HVPG or HVPG to values < 12 mmHg and maintain these changes over time are most likely to remain free of bleeding. It has therefore been recommended that the HVPG be measured prior to initiation of therapy and after 1–3 months of treatment and that the dosage of the drug be changed appropriately to achieve the desired endpoints. However, the cost-effectiveness of this approach remains to be demonstrated. Moreover, HVPG measurement is not possible at many medical centers. Where such facilities are unavailable, the dose should be titrated to achieve a decrease in resting heart rate to values of 55–60 beats per minute.

MANAGEMENT OF ACTIVE HEMORRHAGE

Active variceal hemorrhage accounts for about one-third of all deaths related to cirrhosis. Review of the literature on the management of active hemorrhage is confounded by the variable use of terminology across studies. Recently, several definitions were agreed upon that simplify evaluation of published studies and render new studies more comparable. These include:

Time zero: is the time of admission to a medical care facility.

Clinically significant bleeding: is defined by a transfusion requirement of two units of blood or more within 24 h of time zero together with a systolic blood pressure < 100 mmHg, a postural change of > 20 mmHg, and/or a pulse rate > 100/min at time zero.

Acute bleeding episode: represents the events in the interval of 48 h from time zero. Bleeding during this time is considered to represent failure of therapy.

Failure of therapy: is defined within two time frames: (1) < 6 h from time zero: a transfusion requirement of more than four units, inability to increase systolic blood pressure by 20 mmHg or to 70 mmHg, and/or a pulse rate < 100 per minute; (2) > 6 h from time zero: occurrence of hematemesis with a drop in systolic BP > 20 mmHg, increase in pulse rate by 20 beats per minute from the 6-h time point and need for two units or more of blood to keep the hemoglobin around 9 g/dL. Any bleeding occurring after initial hemostasis and more than 48 h from time zero but less than 6 weeks is considered to represent early rebleeding.

There are three primary goals of management during the active bleeding episode. These include hemodynamic resuscitation, prevention and treatment of complications, and treatment of bleeding. All three need to be pursued simultaneously and often require coordinated critical care.

Hemodynamic Resuscitation. This should be aggressively managed with large-bore peripheral intravenous lines or a central line. Lost blood should be replaced by packed cells and clotting factors should be replaced as needed. Platelet counts often drop within the first 48 h after bleeding and may necessitate transfusions if they fall below 50,000/mL in an actively bleeding patient. Care should be taken to avoid overtransfusion with volume overload because of the risk of rebound portal hypertension and inducing rebleeding. Also, in those receiving large volumes of blood products, the ionized [Ca^{2+}] and platelet counts must be monitored and corrected as necessary.

Prevention and Management of Complications (Table 3). Complications related to bleeding as well as the treatment of bleeding contribute substantially to mortality from active hemorrhage. An important complication with a frequently fatal outcome is aspiration pneumonia. All patients with altered mental status and active bleeding or those with massive hematemesis should be intubated for airway protection. Renal function must be monitored and fluid administered to maintain an urine output of at least 50 mL/h. If renal failure develops, it must be evaluated quickly and managed appropriately. Lactulose should be given orally once bleeding is controlled to wash the blood from the GI tract and also to prevent encephalopathy. In patients with ascites, oral antibiotics (e.g., norfloxacin) should be administered to prevent spontaneous bacterial peritonitis. Finally, a close watch for signs of infection must be kept and treatment started quickly and aggressively when infection is found. Aminoglycosides should be avoided (owing to their high incidence of nephrotox-

Table 3 Supportive Management of Active Variceal Hemorrhage

Hemodynamic resuscitation
Packed cell transfusion
Correction of coagulopathy
Correction of thrombocytopenia
Monitor for side effects of blood product administration
Airway protection
Renal support
Maintain urine output > 50 mL/h
Avoid aminoglycosides
Avoids NSAIDS for fever
Sepsis
Prophylaxis for spontaneous bacterial peritonitis in high-risk subjects
Neurological support
Monitor mental status
Avoid sedation
Metabolic
Thiamine when indicated
Monitor and treat delirium tremens
Monitor and treat acidosis or alkalosis
Monitor phosphate levels, treat hypophosphatemia
Monitor blood sugar

icity in patients with advanced cirrhosis) unless documented sepsis with bacteria sensitive only to aminoglycosides is found.

Treatment of Active Hemorrhage. All of the modalities discussed above for primary prevention are also available for active bleeding. The choice of treatment depends on its relative efficacy and safety, the expediency with which it can be implemented, and cost considerations. These are discussed below.

Pharmacological Treatment

Vasopressin and Its Analogues

Vasopressin directly constricts mesenteric arterioles and decreases portal venous inflow, thereby decreasing portal pressures. A large number of studies have evaluated the role of vasopressin in the management of active hemorrhage. Vasopressin can achieve initial hemostasis in 60–80% of individuals (Table 4) but has only marginal effects on early rebleeding episodes. Also, it does not improve survival from active variceal hemorrhage. In fact, it may contribute to mortality owing to its coronary vasoconstrictive properties and the resultant myocardial, cerebral, and bowel ischemia. Vasopressin has also been shown to induce a fibrinolytic state and, theoretically, can worsen the bleeding diathesis. Finally, recent studies have shown that the portal hypotensive effect of vasopressin in nonbleeding cirrhotics is attenuated when variceal hemorrhage occurs. These considerations have decreased the use of this drug for the management of variceal hemorrhage. Glypressin in an analogue of vasopressin in which a triglycyl group is attached to the N-terminal of lysine-

Table 4 Summary of Published Trials of Sclerotherapy for Control of Acute Variceal Hemorrhage

Reference	Study design	Control bleeding[a] (%)	Early rebleeding[a] (%)	Deaths[a] (%)	Comments
Barsoum et al[20]	Medical vs EST	42 vs 74	58 vs 26	42 vs 26	Rigid scope, 76% schistosomiasis
Larson et al[39]	BT[b] bs BT + EST	?	53 vs 23	13 vs 4	
Moreto et al[40]	BT vs EST	80 vs 100	43 vs 17	30 vs 30	Emphasizes high rebleeding rate of BT
Paquet and Feussner[41]	BT vs EST	73 vs 95	44 vs 20	27 vs 10	Survival advantage with EST
Soderlung and Ihre[42]	BT + VP[b] vs EST	84 vs 95	34 vs 30	36 vs 28	Total number of rebleeding rates by EST
Copenhagen Sclerotherapy Project[43]	Medical vs EST	?	54 vs 48	78 vs 65	EST improved survival after 30 days
Westaby et al[44]	VP + NTG[b] vs EST	65 vs 88	31 vs 31	39 vs 27	

[a]Control versus sclerotherapy.
[b]BT, balloon tamponade; NTG, nitroglycerin; VP, vasopressin.
Source: From A.J. Sanyal and M.L. Shiffman, Pharmacologic treatment of portal hypertension. In: J.H. Lewis et al., eds. Current Clinical Topics in Gastrointestinal Pharmacology. London: Blackwell Scientific, 1997:242–275.

vasopressin. Cleavage of this residue releases the drug in a slow and sustained manner at the vascular smooth muscle. Several clinical trials have shown equivalence to somatostatin and greater efficacy than placebo. Sufficient clinical experience with this agent does not exist to warrant its large-scale use.

Somatostatin and Its Analogues

Somatostatin is a 14–amino acid peptide named for its growth hormone–inhibiting properties. It inhibits release of vasodilator hormones (e.g., glucagon) and thereby indirectly causes splanchnic vasoconstriction and decreased portal inflow. Somatostatin has a very short half-life and disappears within minutes of a bolus infusion. Octreotide is a long-acting analogue of somatostatin.

Pharmacodynamics. Following a bolus injection of either agent, portal venous inflow, portal pressures, azygous flow, and intravariceal pressures decrease within seconds. Of these effects, the changes in portal pressures, as measured by wedged hepatic pressures, are most variable and the decrease in collateral flow (azygous flow) are those most consistently observed. The overall effects of a 250-μg bolus of somatostatin followed by an infusion at 250 μg/h has the same effects as a 500-μg bolus. Bolus doses are more likely to decrease cardiac output than continuous infusions. Octreotide has been reported to improve renal function, while somatostatin worsened renal function in one study. It must be noted, however, that neither drug causes clinically significant renal toxicity.

Clinical Trials. A number of clinical trials have compared somatostatin or octreotide to either vasopressin or placebo in the management of active bleeding. Although an initial placebo-controlled trial failed to demonstrate a benefit for somatostatin, several subsequent studies have shown it to be significantly superior to placebo with respect to the achievement of hemostasis as well as prevention of early rebleeding. It is also superior to vasopressin and balloon tamponade because of the virtual absence of side effects associated with somatostatin or octreotide therapy (Table 5). However, it must be noted that these beneficial effects on bleeding have not been shown to improve survival.

In one study, somatostatin was compared with sclerotherapy for the treatment of active variceal hemorrhage. Somatostatin was noted to be comparable to sclerotherapy in terms of both cessation of active hemorrhage as well as the incidence of early rebleeding and overall survival. In a similar paper, Sung et al. found octreotide to be comparable to sclerotherapy for the management of active variceal hemorrhage. Also, the use of either somatostatin or octreotide infusion for 5 days in addition to sclerotherapy have both been

Table 5 Comparison of Somatostatin or Octreotide to Vasopressin or Placebo in the Management of Active Variceal Hemorrhage

Author	Initial hemostasis Vp vs ss (%)	Mortality Vp vs ss (%)	Adverse effects Vp vs ss (%)
Kravetz	74 vs 87	45 vs 47	26 vs 0
Jenkins	33 vs 100	33 vs 20	17 vs 0
Bagarini	28 vs 68	28 vs 4	0 vs 0
Saari	57 vs 84	36 vs 34	14 vs 0
Hwang	54 vs 88	50 vs 46	0 vs 0
Huang	62 vs 75	43 vs 25	0 vs 0

shown in one study each to be superior to sclerotherapy alone for prevention of early rebleeding and improving survival. However, two other large studies using similar protocols did not demonstrate any additional benefit for octreotide over sclerotherapy alone.

As summarized in a recent consensus conference, somatostatin appears to be more effective than placebo or vasopressin and has fewer side effects than vasopressin. It has therefore replaced vasopressin as the pharmacological treatment of choice in the actively bleeding patient. Although the role of octreotide is less well established, it is the current drug of choice in the United States because of its easy availability as compared with somatostatin.

Endoscopic Treatment

Endoscopic treatment is currently the definitive treatment of choice for active variceal hemorrhage. It can be performed at the same time as diagnostic endoscopy at the bedside by virtually any trained gastroenterologist. Two forms of endoscopic treatment are available: endoscopic sclerotherapy and endoscopic variceal band ligation.

Clinical Trials. Both esophageal as well as GOV types I and II are amenable to treatment by sclerotherapy or band ligation. However, IGVs do not lend themselves to these modalities of treatment. Clinical trials have shown sclerotherapy to be superior to balloon tamponade alone, vasopressin alone, and a combination of vasopressin and balloon tamponade for control of active hemorrhage, prevention of early rebleeding, reduction of complication rates, and improved survival (Table 4). Both intravariceal and paravariceal injections are effective. In controlled clinical trials, band ligation has been shown to be as effective as sclerotherapy for achieving hemostasis and preventing early rebleeding. It is therefore reasonable to use either modality in the setting of active hemorrhage.

Complications. These may be categorized as local, regional, and systemic (Table 6). Local complications include ulceration, bleeding, dysmotility, and stricture formation; regional complications include esophageal perforation and mediastinitis. Systemic complications include sepsis, aspiration, and ventilation/perfusion mismatch with hypoxemia. All

Table 6 Complications of Sclerotherapy

Local complications	Regional	Systemic	Complications to physician
Ulcers	Esophageal perforation	Sepsis	Sclerotherapist's eye
Bleeding	Mediastinitis	Aspiration	
Stricture	Pleural effusions	Spontaneous bacterial peritonitis and candidemia	
Esophageal dysmotility	Acute gastric dilation	Ventilation-perfusion mismatch (hypoxia)	
Pain		Adult respiratory distress syndrome	
Odynophagia		Portal vein thrombosis	
Laceration			

Source: From A.J. Sanyal and M.L. Shiffman, Pharmacologic treatment of portal hypertension. In: J.H. Lewis et al., eds. Current Clinical Topics in Gastrointestinal Pharmacology. London: Blackwell Scientific, 1997: 242–275.

of these complications occur more frequently when endoscopy is performed emergently rather than electively.

What To Do When Endoscopic Treatment Fails?

Emergent endoscopic treatment fails to control bleeding in 10–20% of patients. These patients are at high risk for exsanguination as well as all of the complications related to active bleeding. Usually by the time a diagnosis of failed endoscopic treatment is established, patients have already received a trial of pharmacological treatment as well. In such patients, second attempts at endoscopic hemostasis may be made. However, if bleeding is not quickly and effectively stopped, more definitive therapy must be instituted immediately.

Balloon Tamponade. This is an effective way to achieve short-term hemostasis. However, following deflation of the balloon, there is a high risk of rebleeding. Also, the airway must be protected in all patients receiving such treatment owing to their failure to clear oral secretions and the high risk of aspiration. The only role of such treatment is to temporarily stabilize the patient so that more definitive treatment can be instituted.

Surgery. Both portal decompressive surgery (Table 7) and esophageal transection have been shown to be highly effective in achieving hemostasis. Emergency portacaval shunts are more likely to thrombose than elective shunts. Also, portacaval shunts alter vascular anatomy and may complicate future liver transplant surgery. Finally, portacaval shunts have been associated with an approximately 40–50% incidence of encephalopathy. Clinically, emergent endoscopic sclerotherapy has been shown to be as efficaceous as portacaval shunts when used as first-line treatment. These considerations have led to a decline in the use of surgery as first-line treatment of variceal hemorrhage. Nevertheless, surgical portal decompression remains an effective way to arrest variceal hemorrhage and prevent rebleeding. Similarly, esophageal transection has been shown to be as effective as sclerotherapy, although troublesome bleeding may occur from suture lines. The ideal patient for surgical therapy is one with well-preserved liver function who fails emergent endoscopic treatment and has no complications from the bleeding or endoscopy. The choice of surgery is usually dependent on the training and expertise of the surgeon.

Transjugular Intrahepatic Portosystemic Shunts (TIPS). TIPS function as side-to-side surgical portacaval shunts without exposing the patient to the risks of general anesthesia or major surgery. This has led to a resurgence of interest in portal decompression as a treatment for variceal hemorrhage. In initial studies, hemostasis was achieved in the vast

Table 7 Studies of Portacaval Shunt for the Emergent Treatment of Variceal Hemorrhage

Author	*N*	% Child's class C	30-day mortality
Cello	32	100	56
Villeneuve	36	0	19
Souttar	100	46	31
Levine	55	38	38
Orloff	94	100	20
Rikkers	22	64	41

majority of patients with refractory variceal hemorrhage despite endoscopic treatment. While the patient populations studied were heterogeneous, these studies demonstrated that TIPS could be performed in a reasonable period of time in most patients with low procedure-related morbidity or mortality.

Clinical Trials. In an important trial, patients who were actively bleeding and considered to be at high risk of dying from emergent surgery (defined by the presence of sepsis or deep coma, pneumonia, multiorgan failure, renal failure, severe comorbid conditions) despite emergent endoscopic treatment within the previous 72 h were stabilized by balloon tamponade and TIPS performed within 12 h. Hemostasis was achieved in over 90% of patients and the 30-day survival was 63%. In those without pulmonary compromise, a greater than 90% survival was noted at 30 days (Fig. 7). These data are far superior to those obtained with conventional treatment (i.e., surgery for this subset, where a 10–20% survival would have been expected). Thus, TIPS is the procedure of choice in patients with active hemorrhage despite endoscopic treatment who are at high risk for surgery.

A second study compared TIPS to a surgical small-diameter H graft in 70 patients with active hemorrhage regardless of their risk status. Of patients who received TIPS 57% rebled, as compared with only 26% of those who underwent surgery. These data underscore that surgical treatment is a viable and suitable option for active hemorrhage, especially in those who are not at high risk of dying from the procedure. It must be noted that the risk of failure of TIPS in this study was higher than that reported by any other center and the data are not therefore easily generalizable. Indeed, a nonrandomized trial of TIPS found it to be superior to esophageal transection. Clearly, more large-scale, randomized, prospective trials are needed to establish the roles of surgery vs. TIPS in average-risk subjects with active hemorrhage who have failed endoscopic treatment.

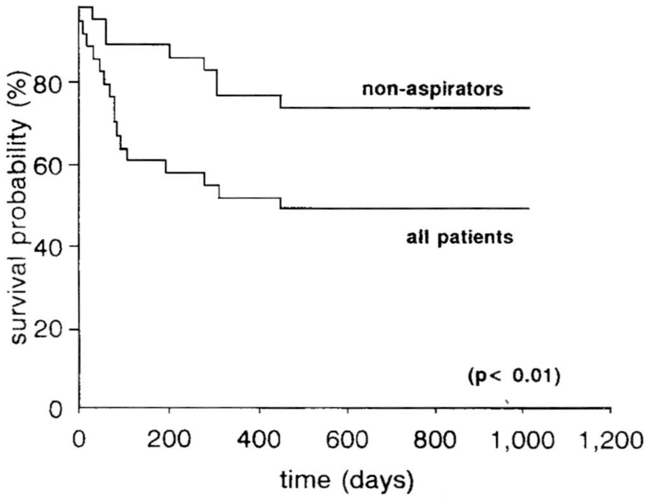

Figure 7 Effects of TIPS on survival in patients with active hemorrhage despite emergent sclerotherapy who were considered at high-risk of dying after emergent surgery. (From A.J. Sanyal, A.M. Freedman, V.A. Luketic, P.P. Purdem, M.L. Shiffman, J. Tisnado, and P.E. Cole. Transjugular intrahepatic portosystemic shunts for patients with active variceal hemorrhage unresponsive to sclerotherapy. Gastroenterology 1996; 111:138–146.)

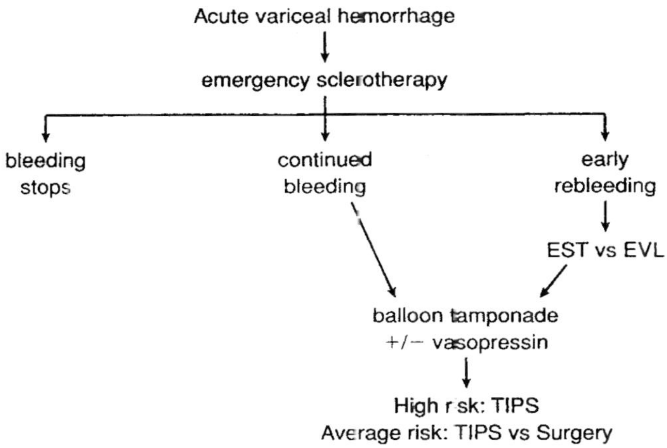

Figure 8 An algorithm for the management of acute variceal hemorrhage. (From A.J. Sanyal, A.M. Freedman, V.A. Luketic, P.P. Purdem, M.L. Shiffman, J. Tisnado, and P.E. Cole. Transjugular intrahepatic portosystemic shunts for patients with active variceal hemorrhage unresponsive to sclerotherapy. Gastroenterology 1996; 111:138–146.)

An Algorithm for the Management of Active Variceal Hemorrhage

The initial treatment of active hemorrhage must include hemodynamic resuscitation, prevention of complications and early endoscopy to establish the diagnosis and initiate specific treatment. Somatostatin or octreotide (50-μg bolus followed by 50-μg/h by intravenous infusion) may be started in the emergency room in those at high risk for variceal hemorrhage (Fig. 8). At endoscopy, bleeding esophageal varices are treated by either sclerotherapy or band ligation. If active bleeding persists or recurs within 48 h, it may be controlled by surgery or TIPS. The choice of the definitive procedure depends on the patient's clinical condition and the expertise available. When bleeding occurs more than 48 h after initial endoscopic treatment, a second attempt at controlling hemorrhage by endoscopy is reasonable before proceeding to salvage therapy.

Several caveats are of great importance in the management of actively bleeding patients to ensure a favorable outcome. First, repeated attempts to control bleeding by endoscopic, pharmacological, or mechanical means despite continued active hemorrhage only led to severe deterioration in the patient's condition and an increased risk of complications. At that stage, even if hemostasis is achieved, the patient often dies from liver failure, sepsis, and/or multiorgan dysfunction. Thus, the decision to proceed to salvage therapy should not be delayed once a patient fails initial endoscopic/pharmacological treatment. Next, many studies have demonstrated that pulmonary compromise is associated with a very high mortality and that the airway must be protected in all patients with severe active hemorrhage, especially if they are to be sedated or their mental state is altered. Finally, the need for balloon tamponade prior to TIPS is important. Most radiology suites are not equipped to manage actively bleeding or unstable patients. Temporarily stabilizing the patient by balloon tamponade allows the procedure to be performed under more controlled circumstances without detracting the attention of the angiography personnel from the procedure.

PREVENTION OF RECURRENT VARICEAL HEMORRHAGE

The natural history of the untreated patient who has survived an episode of variceal hemorrhage is characterized by recurrent hemorrhage with consequent liver failure, hepatic encephalopathy, and eventually death. It is therefore imperative to prevent such rebleeding. All of the modalities discussed above are also available for prevention for recurrent variceal hemorrhage.

Endoscopic Treatment

Endoscopic sclerotherapy has been extensively evaluated for the long-term prevention of recurrent variceal hemorrhage (Table 8). It has been shown to decrease both the risk of rebleeding (40–50% vs. 70%) and death (30–60% vs. 50–75%) as compared with placebo. It is controversial whether these effects represent the benefits of repeated episodes of sclerotherapy or the beneficial effects of sclerotherapy for episodes of active hemorrhage in these studies. The clinical outcome is similar whether intravariceal or paravariceal injections are made. Similarly, the nature of the sclerosant, its volume, or the frequency of sessions do not affect outcome. Most episodes of recurrent variceal hemorrhage occur before the varices are completely obliterated. Following obliteration, varices tend to recur over time, and surveillance endoscopy must be performed at 6-month intervals for 1 year and annually thereafter. All of the side effects of sclerotherapy described above during emergent sclerotherapy may also occur during repeated sessions.

Endoscopic band ligation has been developed as an alternate endoscopic treatment over the last 10 years. Many studies have evaluated the relative efficacy of band ligation with sclerotherapy. They demonstrate that band ligation is associated with earlier variceal obliteration, less complications, and less rebleeding as well as improved survival as compared with sclerotherapy (Figs. 9 and 10). Because of this, band ligation has replaced

Table 8 Effects of Sclerotherapy on the Prevention of Recurrent Variceal Hemorrhage

Reference	Design	Duration of follow-up (months)	Rebleeding[a] (%)	Number rebleeding[a]	Deaths[a] (%)
MacDougall et al.	No Rx[b] vs EST[c]	24	75 vs 43	100 vs 54	38 vs 21
Terblanche et al.	No Rx vs EST[d]	60	77 vs 58	73 vs 43	63 vs 62
Westaby et al.	No Rx vs EST	36	80 vs 55	125 vs 66	53 vs 32
Korula et al.	No Rx vs EST[c]	38	84 vs 49	98 vs 48	33 vs 33
Soderlund and Ihre	No Rx vs EST[c]	28	64 vs 58	99 vs 50	70 vs 62
Copenhagen Sclerotherapy Project	No Rx vs EST	? 9–52	54 vs 48	138 vs 64	78 vs 65
Burroughs et al. (abstract)	No Rx vs EST[d]	??	59 vs 55	183 vs 130	54 vs 47
Gregory et al. (abstract)	No Rx vs EST	60 vs 52	180 vs 116	56 vs 63	

[a]Control versus sclerotherapy.
[b]Rx: treatment
[c]Rebleeding in controls treated by shunt, vasopressin, Linton tubes.
[d]Acute episodes of bleeding in controls were treated with EST also.
Source: From A.J. Sanyal and M.L. Shiffman, Pharmacologic treatment of portal hypertension. In: J.H. Lewis et al., eds. Current Clinical Topics in Gastrointestinal Pharmacology. London: Blackwell Scientific, 1997:242–275.

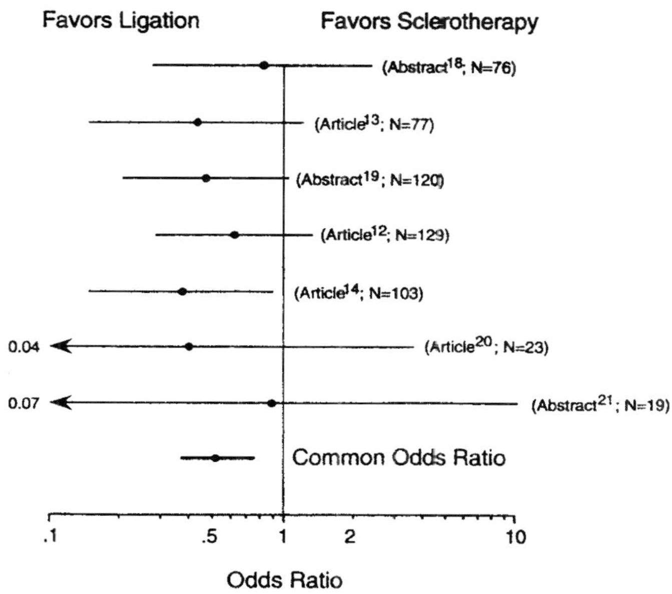

Figure 9 A metanalysis of endoscopic band ligation versus sclerotherapy for the prevention of recurrent variceal hemorrhage. Band ligation is superior to sclerotherapy for prevention of recurrent bleeding. (From Laine and Cook, 1995, with permission.)

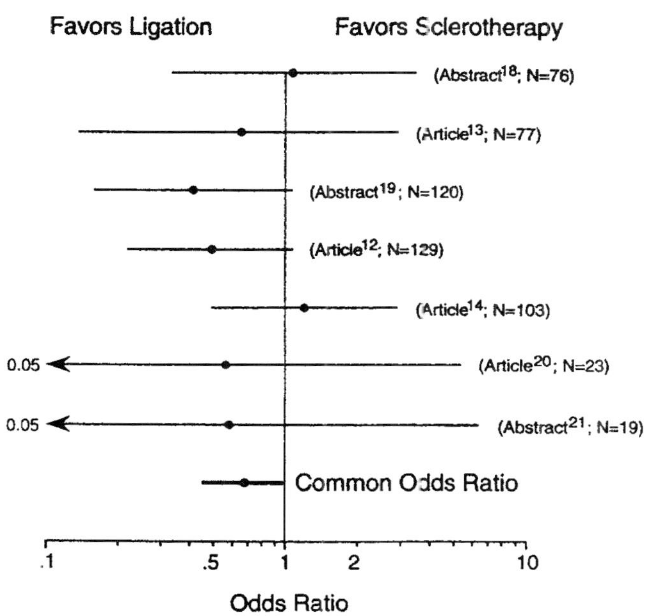

Figure 10 A metanalysis of endoscopic band ligation versus sclerotherapy for the prevention of recurrent variceal hemorrhage. Band ligation is superior to sclerotherapy with respect to survival. (From Laine and Cook, 1995, with permission.)

sclerotherapy as the first-line treatment for prevention of recurrent hemorrhage. However, band ligation is associated with a greater risk of variceal recurrence and is technically difficult when varices are very small. In such patients, sclerotherapy may be used.

Pharmacological Treatment

A large number of controlled clinical trials have examined the role of beta blockers for prevention of recurrent variceal hemorrhage in patients who have already bled at least once from esophageal varices. Over 428 patients received beta blockers while 400 patients received placebo. In these studies also, most patients had Child's class A alcoholic cirrhosis and the most important interstudy variable was the timing of entry into the study from the index bleeding episode (1 day to 1 month). Doses, varying to the same degree as in the primary prophylaxis trials, or propranolol or nadolol were used. Beta blocker doses were titrated to achieve a 25% decrease in resting heart rates. An improvement in rebleeding rates was noted in most studies, although a survival advantage was shown in only a single trial. Metanalyses of these data have been performed and suggest that the risk of bleeding is decreased by approximately 40%, while the risk of death is decreased by 20%.

A total of 10 controlled trials comparing beta blocker therapy to sclerotherapy have been published (Fig. 11). One trial showed a benefit in favor of beta blockers, while two showed a benefit in favor of sclerotherapy. Seven studies failed to show any significant differences in rebleeding rates. Importantly, with the exception of a single study, a survival advantage for beta blockers was not seen. A combination of sclerotherapy and beta blockade has also not been shown to be more efficacious than sclerotherapy alone (Table 9). Along the same lines, addition of transhepatic sclerotherapy to beta blockers does not add to the effects of beta blockade alone.

Transjugular Intrahepatic Portasystemic Shunts

Six clinical trials have evaluated the efficacy of TIPS vs. endoscopic treatment for the prevention of recurrent variceal hemorrhage; one study used band ligation while the others

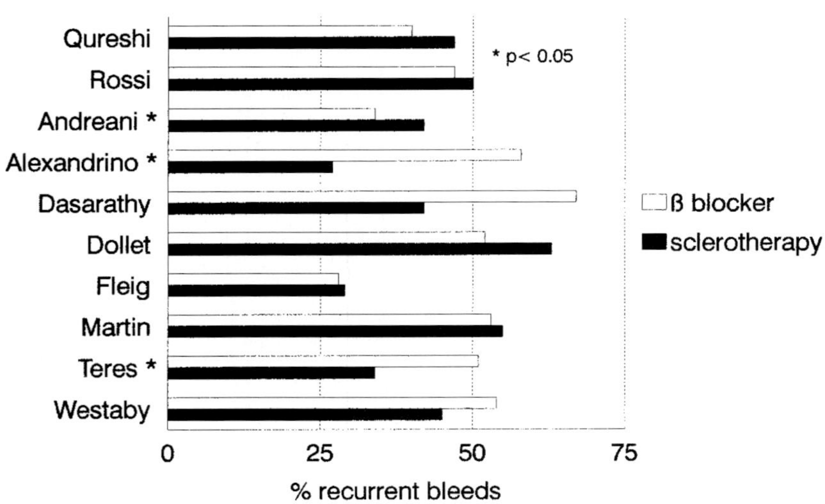

Figure 11 Comparison of beta blockers and sclerotherapy for the prevention of recurrent variceal hemorrhage. (From Sanyal et al., 1996, with permission.)

Table 9 Comparison of Beta Blockade plus Sclerotherapy vs. Sclerotherapy Alone for the Prevention of Recurrent Variceal Hemorrhage[a]

	% Rebleed (combination vs. EST)	% Survival (combination vs. EST)
Acharya	17/21	91/88
Avgerinos	31/52	82/78
Bertoni	7/28	93/79
Gerunda	20/23	97/90
Jensen	54/75	93/93
Lundell	10/9	95/77
Vickers	45/39	62/74
Vinel	18/39	87/86
Westaby	27/30	65/74

[a]No study demonstrated a survival advantage for combination therapy.

used sclerotherapy. The sclerotherapy protocols were also quite variable. While most studies randomized patients within 24 h of admission, one study focused primarily on long-term rebleeding and randomized patients after a mean of 7–8 days. Also, the severity of liver failure varied from study to study. Thus, these studies were too heterogeneous to be comparable.

All but one study demonstrated a significant decrease in the risk of rebleeding in patients undergoing TIPS (Fig. 12). The differences across studies were, however, due to the variable rebleeding rates after endoscopic treatment rather than after TIPS (approx 20%). Despite the beneficial effects on bleeding, TIPS was associated with either no survival advantage or actually poorer survival (Fig. 13), which reached significance by univariate analysis but not multivariate analysis in one study. TIPS is therefore used primarily as a salvage therapy for those with recurrent bleeding despite an adequate trial of endoscopic treatment.

The principal cause of rebleeding after TIPS is the recurrence of portal hypertension (Table 10). This may result from TIPS thrombosis, stent retraction and kinking, stent

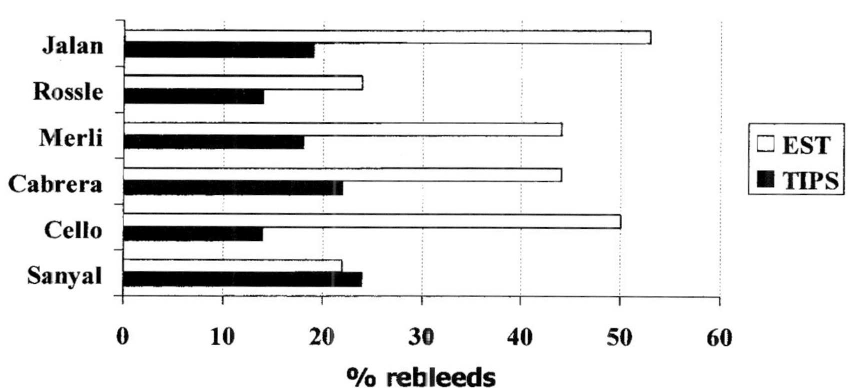

Figure 12 Comparison of TIPS vs. endoscopic treatment with respect to the rates of rebleeding when used for prevention of recurrent variceal hemorrhage.

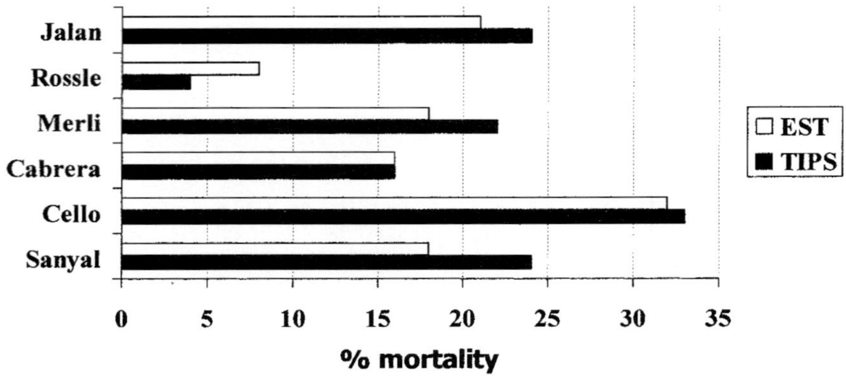

Figure 13 Comparison of TIPS vs. endoscopic treatment with respect to survival when used for the secondary prevention of variceal hemorrhage.

stenosis, and development of right heat failure. TIPS thrombosis usually occurs within the first month and is more likely to occur in moribund individuals. Its development has been associated with the presence of a biliary-TIPS fistula. It has been proposed that systemic anticoagulation can prevent TIPS thrombosis but carries the risk of inducing hemorrhage. It is rarely routinely used in North America. Stent retraction into the parenchymal tissue tract and stent kinking can be avoided by careful attention to technique. Quantitatively, the most common cause of recurrent portal hypertension is the ingrowth of tissue from the surrounding liver into the stent lumen, with eventual occlusion. Such pseudointimal hyperplasia results from the proliferation and migration of mesenchymal cells of smooth muscle phenotype into the lumen, where they synthesize and secrete collagen. Virtually all long-term survivors after TIPS experience TIPS stenosis within the first 2 years, necessitating surveillance by either Doppler sonography or angiography. Doppler sonography is specific but somewhat insensitive, depending on the specific cutoffs used for the diagnosis of stent stenosis (Table 11). Angiography is the gold standard for the detection of stent stenosis and is required for its treatment. A commonly used regimen is angiography at 6 and 12 months after TIPS and annually thereafter for the first 3 years. The propensity for development of stent stenosis decreases after 4 years.

Table 10 Causes of Upper-GI Bleeding after TIPS

Continued variceal hemorrhage
Stent dysfunction
Thrombosis
Retraction
Kinking
Displacement
Stenosis
Hemobilia
Persistent gastric varices
Associated with spontaneous splenorenal collaterals
Associated with massive splenomegaly

Table 11 Value of Doppler Ultrasound in the Detection of TIPS Stenosis

Author	Diagnotic criteria used	Shunt stenosis Sensitivity (%)	Specificity (%)
Dodd et al.	No flow in stent, Δ peak stent flow velocity >50 cm/s, hepatic venous flow reversal	93	77
Foshager et al.	Flow velocity in entire stent <60 cm/s, low velocity in stent with focal jet lesion	98	100[a]
Lafortune et al.	Change in stent flow volume, direction of flow in intrahepatic portal vein branches	84	89
Kanterman et al.	Peak shunt velocity <90 cm/s, Δ peak velocity >40 cm/s, main portal vein velocity <30 cm/s, flow in intrahepatic portal vein branches	92	72
Kimura et al.	Mean flow velocity <60 cm/s, drop in peak flow	92	89[b]
Feldstein	Direction of flow in intrahepatic portal vein branches, peak velocity in stent <50 cm/s	78	92
Lind et al.	Peak flow velocity in stent <30 cm/s	100	98
Sanyal et al.	Direction of flow in intrahepatic portal vein branches, reversed flow in hepatic vein, jet lesion in stent, stent flow volume <1 L/min, main portal vein flow velocity <10 cm/s	70	93

[a]Majority of patients had sonography after angiography in an "unblinded" study.
[b]Data interpretable only for stent occlusion, also recalculated predictive values less than published value.
Source: From A.J. Sanyal. The management of the cirrhotic patient after tranjugular intrahepatic portosystemic shunt. Semin Gastrointest Dis 1997; 8:188–199.

While hepatic blood flow (ICG clearance) and flow-dependent quantitative liver function (lidocaine metabolite formation) decrease after TIPS, this rarely has clinical significance. In some patients, liver function actually improves. This is invariably associated with resolution of associated ascites and improvement in oral intake and nutritional indices. Rarely, a syndrome of progressive jaundice occurs after TIPS placement (personal observation). Typically, this occurs in those with preexisting advanced liver failure. In these patients, progressive conjugated hyperbilirububinemia occurs and eventually multiorgan dysfunction follows. The treatment of this complication is orthotopic liver transplantation.

The adverse effects of TIPS are listed in Table 12. Hepatic encephalopathy occurs in about 30% of individuals after TIPS. It manifests itself as altered mental status and usually appears about 2–3 weeks after TIPS placement. It is often precipitated by dietary indiscretion, constipation, urinary tract infections, or electrolyte imbalances. Beyond 6 weeks after TIPS, most episodes are related to recurrent GI bleeding. Advanced age (> 60 years), Child's class C, and prior history of encephalopathy, and shunt diameter are risk factors for encephalopathy.

Hemolytic anemia (Sanyal's syndrome) occurs in about 10% of patients after TIPS. It is usually asymptomatic, although it may occasionally be severe enough to cause high-output heart failure. It is diagnosed by an increase in unconjugated bilirubin and reticulocytosis after TIPS. Hemolysis usually subsides within 8 weeks, although rarely it may be unremitting and require liver transplantation or shunt occlusion.

Table 12 Adverse Effects of TIPS

Technique related	Complications related to portosystemic shunting	Unique complications
Neck hematoma	Hepatic encephalopathy	TIPS-associated hemolysis
Cardiac arrhythmias	?Increased susceptibility to bacteremia	Infection of the stents
Perihepatic hematoma		
Rupture of liver capsule	Liver failure	
Extrahepatic puncture of portal vein		

Note: The question mark indicates a hypothetical possibility as yet unproven that TIPS increases susceptibility to sepsis.

Surgery and Orthotopic Liver Transplantation

A vast body of literature about the value of surgical treatment for prevention of recurrent variceal hemorrhage exists. In general, surgical treatment may be considered to either achieve portal decompression or mechanically disconnect the varices. The former include operations that behave as complete shunts (e.g., portacaval shunts and incomplete shunts, such as distal splenorenal shunts). The former decompress both the portal vein and hepatic sinusoids and convert the portal vein into an outflow tract. The latter preserve some sinusoidal perfusion while decompressing the portal veins. Each particular operation has its proponents, but their data are not easily generalizable due to the failure of others to obtain similar data. Virtually all of the operations described are effective in arresting hemorrhage and preventing rebleeding. However, they often do not provide any survival advantage over endoscopic treatment. They are therefore primarily used as salvage treatment for those who have failed endoscopic treatment. Theoretically, patients with Child's class A cirrhosis may benefit from surgery (compared to TIPS) if they fail endoscopic treatment. The non-decompressive operations do not treat the portal hypertension and are generally not recommended.

Orthotopic liver transplantation is the only treatment that not only effectively corrects the portal hypertension but also removes the cirrhotic liver and corrects liver failure. It is the only treatment that substantially improves the long-term outcome after variceal hemorrhage and must be considered in all patients who have survived in episode of variceal bleeding unless a contraindication exists.

An Algorithm for the Prevention of Recurrent Variceal Hemorrhage

The goal of long-term treatment is prevention of rebleeding, hepatic decompensation, and death (Fig. 14). Orthotopic liver transplantation is the only treatment that reliably achieves all three objectives. Thus, all survivors of a variceal bleed should be evaluated for liver transplant. While those with Child's class B or C should be listed right away unless a contraindication exists, listing for those with Child's class A cirrhosis should be individualized. While patients are waiting for transplant, endoscopic band ligation is the initial treatment of choice in most cases. Some patients with Child's class A cirrhosis who are compliant with therapy may be treated with propranolol or nadolol. Selected patients with Child's class A cirrhosis may benefit from surgical portal decompression.

If bleeding recurs, the acute bleeding is managed by endoscopic treatment. Those who continue to bleed or have bled despite adequate endoscopic treatment should be considered for salvage treatment with either TIPS or surgery. The choice of procedure

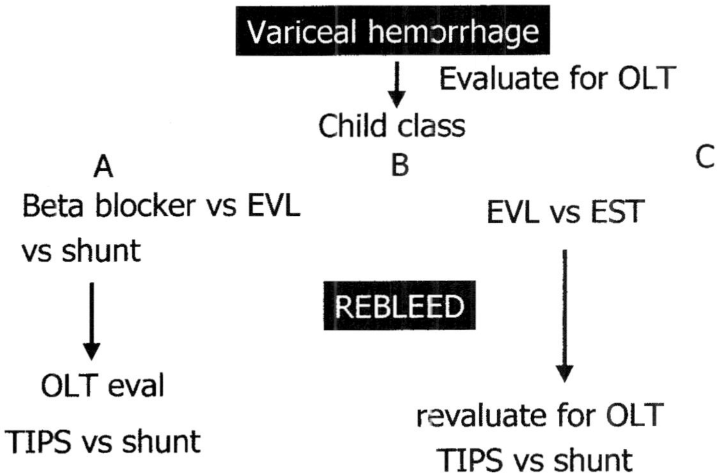

Figure 14 An algorithm for the prevention of recurrent variceal hemorrhage.

should be individualized based on the patient's condition and operator expertise. Bleeding occurring after surgery or TIPS should lead to a workup for shunt thrombosis or stenosis. Angiography is the procedure of choice in such a patient because a patent Doppler sonogram does not exclude the possibility of TIPS stenosis.

CONCLUSIONS

Many advances in the management of portal hypertension and variceal hemorrhage have occurred over the last 10 years. Effective therapy for primary prevention of variceal hemorrhage is now available in the form of nonselective beta blockers. Active bleeding should be managed with somatostatin or octreotide and endoscopic sclerotherapy; TIPS and surgery are reserved as salvage therapy for those who fail endoscopic treatment. Survivors of a variceal bleed should be evaluated for liver transplant. Specific treatment with endoscopic band ligation may be provided while they wait for transplant. Those who fail endoscopic treatment may be treated by TIPS or surgery.

BIBLIOGRAPHY

Angelico M, Carli L, Piat C, Gentile S, Capocaccia L. Effects of isisorbide 5 mononitrate compared to propranolol on first bleeding and long-term survival in cirrhosis. Gastroenterology 1997; 113: 1632–1639.

Freedman AM, Sanyal AJ. The spectrum of complications following transjugular intrahepatic porta-systemic shunts (TIPS). Semin Intervent Radiol 1994; 11:161–177.

Kim T, Shijo H, Tokumitsu H, et al. Risk factors for hemorrhage from gastric fundal varices. Hepatology 1997; 25:307–312.

Laine L, Cook DJ. Endoscopic ligation compared with sclerotherapy for treatment of esophageal variceal bleeding. Ann Intern Med 1995; 123:280–287.

Lay CS, Tsai YT, Teg CY, Doe J. Endoscopic variceal ligation in prophylaxis of first variceal bleeding in cirrhotic patients with high-risk esophageal varices. Hepatology 1997; 25:1347–1352.

Planas R, Quer JC, Boix J, et al. A prospective randomized trial comparing somatostatin and sclerotherapy in the treatment of acute variceal bleeding. Hepatology 1994; 20:370–375.

Poynard T, Cales P, Pasta L, et al. Beta-adrenergic antagonist drugs in the prevention of gastrointestinal bleeding in patients with cirrhosis and esophageal varices, an analysis of data and prognostic factors in 589 patients from four randomized clinical trials. N Engl J Med 1991; 324:1532–1538.

Rossle M, Haag K, Ochs A, et al. The transjugular intrahepatic portosystemic stent-shunt procedure for variceal hemorrhage. N Engl J Med 1994; 330:165–171.

Sanyal AJ, Freedman AM, Luketic VA, et al. Transjugular intrahepatic portosystemic shunts for patients with active variceal hemorrhage unresponsive to sclerotherapy. Gastroenterology 1996; 111:138–146.

Sarin SK, Lahoti D, Saxena SP, Murthi NS, Makwane UK. Prevalence, classification and natural history of gastric varices: long-term follow up study in 568 patients with portal hypertension. Hepatology 1992; 95:434–440.

36
Management of Hepatic Encephalopathy

Kevin D. Mullen, Annette Kyprianou, and Steedman A. Sarbah
MetroHealth Medical Center, Cleveland, Ohio

INTRODUCTION

As the term implies, hepatic encephalopathy (HE), encompasses a wide range of neuropsychiatric abnormalities occurring in patients with significant liver dysfunction. In the broadest of terms, one can classify HE into three main types: acute liver failure–associated (ALFA) HE, portosystemic shunt or bypass-associated HE, and HE seen in patients with chronic liver disease, usually cirrhosis (Table 1).

Acute liver failure–associated HE or fulminant hepatic failure is discussed in Chap. 25. It is mentioned only briefly in this chapter. Even though HE associated with portosystemic bypass and apparently normal liver function is not very common, it deserves some attention because it poses particular diagnostic difficulties. The vast majority of HE seen by clinicians occurs in patients with well-established cirrhosis. This is the focus of the majority of the discussion.

CLINICAL PRESENTATION

In addition to florid or clinically evident HE, there is a well-accepted entity of subclinical HE. This is defined as substandard performance on one or more psychometric tests (e.g., Digit Symbol, Trail Test, Perdue Peg Board, etc.) in a cirrhotic patient with a normal routine neurological examination. There is a great deal of interest in subclinical HE from the research perspective. However, from the practical point of view of patient management, clinicians need not concern themselves with attempts to diagnose this problem. The reason for this fairly strong statement is simple. It has not yet been established that subclinical HE has any meaningful effect on the patient's quality of life. Until this occurs, clinicians can ignore subclinical HE. Nonetheless, it is quite possible that study of this type of patient may lead to a better understanding of the pathogenesis of HE. Also, techniques to detect and measure the degree of cerebral dysfunction in subclinical HE may eventually have applications in the more overt variety of this disorder.

Table 1 Main Types of Hepatic Encephalopathy

Acute liver failure associated (ALFA) encephalopathy.
Massive loss of parenchymal liver function
Encephalopathy associated with portal-systemic bypass.
Classic historical cases of HE with pure shunting
Encephalopathy assoicated with chronic liver disease cirrhosis.
Combination of loss in parenchymal function plus bypass

In its clinically evident form, HE essentially consists of two elements: (1) alterations in consciousness and (2) a generalized motor disturbance. All clinicians are aware of the classic presentation of confusion and asterixis. Indeed, merely seeing a change in mental status in a patient with known or strongly suspected liver disease should immediately raise the possibility that HE is present. Problems arise when liver disease or portosystemic shunting is not obvious. Also, dramatic psychiatric presentations tend to lead the physician away from the consideration of HE even when liver disease is known to be present. Even more diagnostic difficulties arise when patients with advanced liver disease have multiple concurrent potential causes of encephalopathy existing simultaneously. Despite these difficult situations, the approach to the management of HE is highly standardized, which is rather remarkable, since we have no "gold standard" for the diagnosis of this disorder. Preceding a detailed discussion of management, some diagnostic difficulties are outlined below.

Occult Cirrhosis or Portosystemic Shunts

The diagnosis of *hepatic* encephalopathy requires appreciation that the patient has underlying *hepatic* dysfunction. Generally, this is obvious based on history, physical examination, and laboratory testing. However, because of the hepatitis C "epidemic" in the United States, we are now seeing many patients with normal or nearly normal liver tests who have fully established cirrhosis and portosystemic shunts. While it is still true that most of these patients will not frequently develop overt HE until advanced liver failure occurs, some patients will exhibit HE at an earlier stage of their liver disease. The diagnosis of HE is often missed in these patients. Noncirrhotic portal hypertension with portosystemic shunting is less common in the United States but can also lead to HE, which may be difficult to diagnose.

Clues to a possible underlying cirrhosis and/or portosystemic shunt can be uncovered by the patient's history. Two good examples are a past history of very heavy alcohol intake and blood transfuction prior to availability of hepatitis C testing. Change in mental status in patients with histories of this type should lead to the consideration of HE even if the liver tests are normal. Physical findings of spider nevi, hepatomegaly, or splenomegaly in a patient with mental status changes should also bring HE into the differential diagnosis. In relation to laboratory testing, one of the more reliable indications of possible underlying portal hypertension is mild to moderate thrombocytopenia. Elevated serum globulins can be seen in patients with portosystemic shunting in the absence of any other laboratory abnormalities. The role of blood ammonia testing is discussed later.

Patients not suspected to have significant liver disease are increasingly being uncovered because of incidental findings on computed tomography (CT) or ultrasound imaging of

Table 2 Motor Disturbances in Hepatic Encephalopathy

Hyperreflexia
Babinski sign
Cogwheel rigidity/parkinsonian features
Gegenhalten
Asterixis
Monotone speech
Loss of fine motor coordination
Fine tremor
Sluggish pupillary response
Ocular saccades
Immobile facies

the abdomen (see Chap. 2). Prominent venous collateral vessels, splenomegaly, or a very irregular liver may be noted. Occasionally, these findings are ignored or not followed up because liver tests are normal. Subsequent symptoms or signs of HE may be misdiagnosed by physicians unaware of the radiological findings. Two incidental findings on brain imaging may, for the first time, indicate the possible presence of an underlying liver problem. These are evidence of cortical atrophy; this, however, is nonspecific. More dramatic is hyperintensity of the basal ganglia on T1-weighted magnetic resonance imaging (MRI). This finding should immediately raise the possibility of an underlying portosystemic shunt.

Classic Presentations of HE

The most familiar presentation of HE occurs in patients with advanced decompensated cirrhosis. Patients will, over hours to days, develop a gradual onset of change in mental status with or without the generalized motor abnormalities listed in Table 2. Asterixis, when observed, is a useful indication of possible HE but is not specific for the syndrome (Table 3). Vivid visual hallucinations and extreme agitation are more likely to represent delirium tremens than HE. At times it is difficult to differentiate these two syndromes, especially in septic patients. Until total end-stage liver disease is reached, most HE episodes are precipitated by discrete identifiable events. Correcting these is one of the cornerstones of treating HE. Unfortunately many patients with advanced liver disease develop other conditions that can also lead to encephalopathy (Table 4). Distinguishing between HE and other causes of encephalopathy is impossible at times, hence an empirical approach to

Table 3 Causes of Asterixis

Hypercapnia
Salicylate poisening
Brainstem lesion
Polycythemia
Drug intoxication

Table 4 Other Causes of Encephalopathy in Liver Patients

Hypoxia
Hyperglycemia
Hypoglycemia
Metabolic acidosis
Sepsis
Intracranial hemorrhage
Intracranial hypertension
Electrolyte disturbances
Drug overdose/excessive effect
Delirium tremens

treatment is outlined below. Patients can have single or multiple episodes of HE and return to an apparently normal baseline between attacks, especially if effective therapy is employed.

A less common presentation is persistent HE which never returns to a normal neurological state. Some cases are mild enough that patients can continue to function with, for example, persistent clumsiness of fine hand movement. Rarer are patients who continually have a clouded sensorium and fluctuating neurological status. Within this group one encounters the now rare cases of non-Wilsonian hepatolenticular degeneration. This form of hepatocerebral degeneration was associated with surgically created shunts but can arise in patients with long-standing spontaneous shunts. Spastic paraparesis has also been described as a complication of long-standing portosystemic shunts.

Blood Ammonia Testing

The role of measurement of blood (usually plasma) ammonia concentration in the diagnosis of HE is debatable. Patients with clear-cut decompensated liver disease and signs and symptoms of HE have HE even if ammonia levels are normal. Indeed, this is a common phenomenon when venous blood samples are assayed. Arterial ammonia levels tend to be elevated more frequently but add nothing in terms of diagnosis to typical cases. Subjecting patients to arterial puncture is unwarranted if one has already formulated a clinical diagnosis of HE. If it is done and happens to be normal, the inexperienced clinician will hesitate to initiate therapy. Given that poor correlation between blood ammonia concentrations and the severity of HE is well described, it is hard to understand why such emphasis has been placed on obtaining this measurement in some centers. We feel very strongly that measurement of blood ammonia should be undertaken only in research settings or when there is considerable doubt about the clinical diagnosis.

An elevated blood ammonia, assuming that the assay has been performed properly, can be helpful in indicating that underlying liver disease and/or portosystemic shunting of blood is present in a patient with a change in mental status. Occasionally a congenital or acquired urea-cycle enzyme defect can be discovered from the unexpected finding of a significantly elevated blood ammonia level. If poor assay techniques are used (Table 5), blood ammonia levels will be elevated, leading to a great deal of confusion.

Table 5 Proper Ammonia Assay

Arterial blood ... taken onto ice
Prompt assay
Right clinical context

Another misuse of ammonia measurements is to determine improvement. This should be judged on clinical grounds and never based on ammonia levels. The lack of correlation of ammonia concentrations and the clinical severity of HE is even more striking during treatment in our experience. Hence, we totally discourage the use of ammonia measurements to gauge the improvement of HE. Its only place may be in research studies.

Management of Hepatic Encephalopathy

Once the diagnosis of HE is considered to be possibly present in a patient, an empirical but effective treatment plan is instigated. In patients with severe HE, this management process should be initiated in an intensive care unit, since so many things have to be done simultaneously. In all patients the following should occur:

1. Other causes of "encephalopathy" should be sought and treated.
2. Precipitating factors for the development of HE should be identified and corrected.
3. Gut cleansing by nasogastric (NG) lavage and enemas should commence.
4. Lactulose should be delivered into the small intestine if possible.

Other Causes of Encephalopathy

Perhaps one of the most difficult aspects of the diagnosis and treatment of HE in patients with advanced liver disease is the susceptibility of these patients to other serious medical problems. Cirrhotics appear to be immunocompromised and often develop severe infection. Bronchopneumonia, urinary tract infections, and spontaneous bacterial peritonitis can be lethal. The ill-defined but well-recognized "septic" encephalopathy may be present in infected cirrhotic patients mixed with a sepsis-induced hepatic encephalopathy. Hypotension, hypovolemia, respiratory failure, uremia, and nosocomial infections can all play a role in altering the mental status of cirrhotic patients. As one searches for the site of sepsis and tries to correct the many other concurrent problems, treatment for HE has to be started. There is no way to distinguish hepatic encephalopathy from all of these other potential causes of change in mental status. As noted in Table 4, factors such as untoward responses to CNS-active drugs taken on prescription or by more surreptitious means should be screened for in most cases. Early consideration should be given to performing a CT scan of the head, particularly in patients with lateralizing neurological signs. No degree of coagulopathy precludes a diagnostic aspiration of ascitic fluid to check for spontaneous bacterial peritonitis.

In patients with less severe HE or who are repeatedly admitted with HE, the intensity of the workup can be reduced, especially if there is an immediately recognized precipitating factor that can be corrected.

Precipitating Factors

It is impossible to overemphasize the importance of identifying and correcting precipitating factors in the management of HE. Successful achievement of this goal alone corrects HE in the vast majority of patients with chronic liver disease. Paradoxically, this fact makes it exceptionally difficult to conduct controlled treatment trials to test the efficacy of new treatments for this syndrome. Comparison of treatment consisting of lactulose and correction of precipitating factors is very likely to show no difference in efficacy unless the patient's numbers are very high. In other words, even if the drug being tested against lactulose is ineffective, it may still appear to have a positive action, because correction of precipitating factors is the dominant mechanism of benefit. This problem can be solved by only studying patients with "spontaneous" bouts of HE, but such patients are difficult to find in significant numbers.

Detailing the clinical problems in identifying and treating precipitating factors (Table 6) could be the subject of a chapter on its own. A selection of some of the more common difficulties will illustrate the issues. Sepsis is a particular problem. As noted earlier, patients with advanced chronic liver disease develop severe sepsis syndromes, which lead to multiple independent causes of encephalopathy. Worse still, absence of the usual signs of sepsis can occur; in comatose patients, a history of illness may not be available. One must operate on the principle that cirrhotic patients with a major change in mental status are infected until proven otherwise. This, in addition to the simultaneous empiric diagnosis of HE, leads to commencing a large amount of aggressive treatment with uncertainty as to what is occurring in the patient. Nonetheless, treatment has to be instigated immediately to ensure that survival is optimized.

Precipitation of HE by major gastrointestinal hemorrhage is generally easily recognized. However, increasing abdominal distention attributed to worsening ascites or an ileus sometimes turns out to be due to an unrecognized hemorrhage. This becomes evident when gut cleansing is commenced. Experienced clinicians know the importance of not overtransfusing these patients, which would result in even more episodes of brisk hemorrhage from varices.

Table 6 Precipitating Factors of Hepatic Encephalopathy

Hypokalemia
Alkalosis
Sepsis
GI hemorrhage
Uremia
Sedatives/analgesics
Constipation
Dehydration
Lactulose noncompliance
Excessive oral proteins
Ileus or bowel obstruction
Superimposed liver injury
Ketanserin

One issue, about which we have learned from our clinical studies of the potential role of "endogenous" benzodiazepines in the pathogenesis of HE, is the extraordinary availability of prescription benzodiazepines to patients for whom these drugs have never been prescribed. Relatives or friends provide these for insomnia, sometimes in deliberately mislabeled bottles.

Dehydration without electrolyte changes or with "normal" serum sodium levels can occur in cirrhotic patients due to multiple causes. Diuretics are the most common culprits, but excessive free water loss from lactulose-induced diarrhea can also be responsible. Patients with dehydration-precipitated HE respond very rapidly to volume restitution. Having a chart of the patient's best-functioning body weight can be helpful in identifying this precipitating factor. Patients with advanced cirrhosis and serum sodium concentrations in the normal range should be viewed as potentially dehydrated, since these patients usually have concentrations in the 125–130 mEq/mL range.

Gut Cleansing

The main cause for hesitation in commencing active gut cleansing in severe HE is the unwarranted fear of inducing variceal bleeding with nasogastric tube insertion. Variceal bleeding is felt to be a volcano-like explosion from within rather than erosion of the surface of varices by gastric acid or nasogastric tubes. Placement of nasogastric tube is an essential aspect of the initial management of a comatose, cirrhotic patient for a number of reasons. First, it often reveals that gastrointestinal hemorrhage is a precipitating factor for the episode of HE. Second, it potentially allows aspiration of a certain amount of the blood from the stomach, which reduces the nitrogenous load to the gut in those patients and, when functioning properly, can be a guide to the existence of ongoing bleeding. Third, this is the route whereby laxatives and fluids can be safely delivered into the gastrointestinal tract. The sooner these measures are commenced, the better, since no number of enemas can really cleanse the intestinal tract. Nonetheless, if firm stool is palpable on rectal examination, a few enemas can accelerate the gut-cleansing process. Only in the case of bowel obstruction or ileus should enema treatment exclusively be used. It is worth emphasizing that patients already on lactulose may have air/fluid levels on abdominal x-ray without actually having bowel obstruction or ileus. If bowel sounds are present and stool is being passed, then ileus is not present and gut cleansing from above can usually be continued safely. At times, abdominal x-rays will demonstrate large quantities of fecal material in the right colon. Finding this in an HE patient who is not improving on treatment can be helpful in management. Strenuous efforts should be made to clear stool, a process that is usually successful only with laxatives (usually lactulose but potentially other agents) delivered into the upper gastrointestinal tract.

In patients with severe ileus due to spontaneous or postoperative bacterial peritonitis, major difficulty may be encountered in treatment. Limited parenteral therapy is available for HE, which at best is of uncertain efficacy. Supportive treatment until the ileus resolves is all that can usually be employed.

Lactulose Delivery

It used to be common practice to initiate purgation with traditional agents such as magnesium citrate. In theory, proprietary bowel preparations could also be utilized, but the volume of fluid required may exceed gastric emptying capacity in some patients. Today, lactulose is generally instilled via a nasogastric tube in 30- to 60-mL amounts every few hours until bowel movements are induced; it is then titrated to keep the bowel movements loose but not voluminous. The induction of a similar appearance of the rectal effluent to the instilled lactulose is undesirable, since dehydration or electrolyte abnormalities can occur as a result of an overly aggressive purgation.

Lactulose enemas are often mentioned as an alternative treatment if nasogastric deliver of lactulose is not advisable. We find this to be ineffective and advise against it. In theory, lactose enemas can be substituted with a great reduction in cost.

Hepatic Encephalopathy "Resistant" to Therapy

The vast majority of patients should be clearly responding to empirical HE therapy by 72 h. Reasons for failure to improve are listed in Table 7. The commoner reasons for failure to respond are inadequate gut cleansing, missed sepsis, or an uncorrectable precipitating factor. Hesitation to place a nasogastric tube in a comatose patient because of fear of precipitating variceal bleeding is common. Enema therapy is often inadequate, so upper intestinal delivery of lactulose via a nasogastric tube is strongly recommended if the patient is unable to take anything by mouth. We emphasize again that variceal bleeding is usually caused by eruption rather than surface erosion; accordingly, one should not hesitate to place a well-lubricated nasogastric tube, even in a patient with known esophageal varices. Overvigorous aspiration via the nasogastric tube is, of course, discouraged. One problem in managing severe HE around the time of variceal bleeding is the banding technique. When multiple ligations are done, it is unwise to place a nasogastric tube, since the bands can be dislodged by tube placement. Perhaps after 24 h a fine-bore (e.g., Dubhoff) tube can be used more safely, but little is published on this issue.

As mentioned earlier overuse of lactulose can induce dehydration, which may independently cause HE. This is an example where resistant HE may be due to a complication of empirical treatment.

The most difficult issue with encephalopathy in cirrhotic patients is sepsis. Almost like to neonatal patients, cirrhotic patients need to be thoroughly checked for sepsis whenever there is a change in their status. Peritoneal, pleural, and cerebrospinal fluids need to be checked for infection. Urine cultures and careful scrutiny for septic phlebitis and cellulitis are mandatory. The lungs represent the most common site of sepsis. However, diverticulitis, pyelophlebitis, cholecystitis, and cholangitis can arise without helpful signs of their presence. Failure to identify a septic focus should always be a consideration in patients with unresponsive HE.

The presence of intestinal ileus or mechanical bowel obstruction in cirrhotic patients with severe HE is a major problem. Deciding if ileus is present is very important since, as

Table 7 Causes of Failure of Empiric Therapy

Failure to deliver lactulose into intestines
Failure to identify and treat precipitating factors
Other causes of encephalopathy missed
Empirical treatment has induced a new problem
True resistant hepatic encephalopathy

noted, lactulose treatment can produce a picture on abdominal x-rays of air/fluid levels even when bowel function is normal. Audible bowel sounds are helpful in this decision. One hopes not to encounter cirrhotic patients with HE who need surgery for mechanical bowel obstruction. Treatment of severe HE when intestinal cleansing is not feasible is not very effective.

The three known parenteral therapies for HE are (1) branched-chain amino acid–enriched intravenous formulations, (2) ornithine aspartate, and (3) sodium benzoate. The efficacy of intravenous "hepatic" formulations is uncertain, but they may have a role to play in certain cases. Ornithine aspartate and sodium benzoate promote the excretion of waste nitrogen and therefore should be helpful. However, ornithine aspartate is available only in Europe and has not yet been used to treat severe HE. Oral sodium benzoate is effective, but no parenteral study has been performed. In reality, with ileus we treat everything we can and hope that intestinal function will return, at which time resistant HE may improve.

There is a subset of patients who just seem to be difficult to awaken. Formerly, neomycin was started on these patients. There is some evidence for synergism with lactulose in resistant HE. However, oral metronidazole or even broad-spectrum penicillins can awaken many resistant cases. Likewise, some success has been reported with oral vancomycin. Metronidazole must be used with caution, since it is cleared by the liver. We start 250 mg PO and titrate the dose within days to the minimum effective level. This works so well that we have to remind our house staff that it is second-line therapy. In our limited experience, parenteral metronidazole is ineffective.

Issues with Outpatient Management of HE

Lack of compliance with oral lactulose is so prevalent that one should operate on the principle that no one is taking it. Its very sweet taste causes aversion in many patients, and patients may not want to tell their doctors that they are not taking it; thus, lack of compliance is often missed. The simple maneuver of advising patients to take their lactulose in iced tea greatly enhanced compliance.

Many patients with clear HE drive to their clinic appointments. Convincing them to do otherwise is not usually successful. Likewise when one phones patients and suspects HE by hearing a remarkably monotonous voice pattern, transport may be a problem, since patients are disinclined to have someone else drive them to be seen. Talking to a family member in this situation can be helpful.

One severely underutilized management strategy for patients with persistent or recurrent HE is the vegetable protein diet. More patients these days are interested in their

Table 8 Treatment Options with Resistant Hepatic Encephalopathy

Addition of metronidazole/vancomycin/neomycin PO or via nasogastric tube
Reduction in diameter of/occlusion of stent oral or parenteral administration of branched-chain amino acid–enriched formulations
Sodium benzoate
Flumazenil...(short-acting)
Orthotopic liver transplantation

diet and are, therefore, willing to eat a vegetable-based protein diet. Making this more palatable would enhance its more frequent use.

Periodically we find that zinc repletion, branched chain amino acid supplement by mouth, and elimination of analgesics and tranquilizers from "helpful" friends improves HE control. Rarer still, reduction in shunt diameter in patients with a transjugular infrahepatic portosystemic shunt (TIPS) and occlusion of shunts can improve the intractable cases. However, in many patients with intractable or recurrent HE, liver transplantation becomes the main treatment option.

Liver Transplantation and HE

Ideally, physicians should refer patients for transplant assessment long before intractable HE is present. When this is not done, an interesting array of problems arise. The first is trying to get patients through a detoxification program, which, in many states, is a mandatory prerequisite for liver transplantation in alcoholics. Patients may be too encephalopathic to go through the program or will literally not be able to remember to go to treatment sessions. Frequent hospital admissions for HE and other problems often punctuate their detoxification program. Likewise, cardiac and pulmonary testing may be difficult because of HE, and the entire assessment process suffers as a result.

In the patient with truly chronic, severe HE, candidacy for liver transplantation can be compromised by the concern of irreversible brain injury (e.g., hepatocerebral degeneration). The concerned transplant team needs to see at least an evanescent glimpse of normal brain function to proceed with liver transplantation comfortably. The frequency of frontoparietal brain atrophy and hyperintense basal ganglia on brain imaging even in patients with normal mentation needs to be remembered in confronting with this situation. Occasionally, intravenous flumazenil can temporarily arouse patients with intractable HE, which can assist in transplant assessment. However, a recent well-described report of improvement in so-called hepatocerebral degeneration after liver transplantation suggests that we should be cautious in excluding patients from liver transplantation on the basis of hepatocerebral degeneration.

One final issue in relation to liver transplantation is the occasional case wherein mild HE episodes continue after an otherwise successful transplant. Patients recognize the "fuzziness" and "clouding" that went with their more frequent and severe HE episodes

Table 9 Therapies Used to Treat Hepatic Encephalopathy

Gut detoxification	Ammonia elimination	Dietary manipulations	Therapeutic potpourri
Lactulose	Sodium benzoate	Branched chain amino acids	L-dopa
Lactose	Branched chain ketoacids	Vegetable supplementation	Bromocriptine
Neomycin	Ornithine aspartate	Zinc supplementation	Flumazenil
Kanamycin	Arginine	*Lactobacillus*	Naloxone
Vancomycin	Glutamate	*Enterococcus faecium* tablets	
Rifaximin	Sodium phenylacetate		
Sorbitol			
Paramomycin			

pretransplant. These milder episodes of HE may be due to persistent portosystemic shunts, which eventually close many months after transplantation.

ACKNOWLEDGMENT

This work is supported in part by NIH Grant RO1AA10410.

BIBLIOGORAPHY

Blei AT, Cordoba J. Subclinical encephalopathy. Dig Dis 1996; 14(suppl 1):2–11.

Bresci G, Parisi G, Banti S. Management of hepatic encephalopathy with oral zinc supplementation: a long-term treatment. Eur J Med 1993, 2:414–416.

Kircheis G, Quack G, Erbler H. L-ornithine, L-aspartate in the treatment of hyperammonemia and hepatic encephalopathy. In: Cohn HO, Bircher J, eds. Hepatic Encephalopathy. Syndromes and therapies. Bloomington, IN: Medi-Ed Press, 1994: 373–383.

Krieger S, Jaub M, Jansen O, Theilmann L, Geibler M, Krieger D. Neuropsychiatric profile and hyperintense globus pallidus on T1-weighted magnetic resonance images in liver cirrhosis. Gastroenterology 1996; 111:147–155.

Marchesini G, Dioguardi FS, Bianchi GP, et al. Long term oral branched chain amino acid treatment in chronic hepatic encephalopathy: a randomized double-blind case-controlled trial. J Hepatol 1990; 11:92–101.

Mendoza G, Marti-Fàbregas J, Kulisevsky J, Escartin A. Hepatic Myelopathy: a rare complication of portacaval shunt. Eur Neurol 1994; 34:209–212.

Morgan MY, Read AE, Speller DC. Treatment of hepatic encephalopathy with metronidazole. Gut 1992; 23:1–7.

Mullen KD, Szauter KM, Kaminsky-Ross K. "Endogenous" benzodiazepine activity in body fluids of patients with hepatic encephalopathy. Lancet 336:81–83.

Powell EE, Pender MP, Chalk JB, Parkin PJ, et al. Improvement in chronic hepatocerebral degeneration following liver transplantation. Gastroenterology 1990; 98:1079–1082.

Sushma S, Dasrathy S, Tandon RK, et al. Sodium benzoate in the treatment of acute hepatic encephalopathy: a double blind randomized trial. Hepatology 1992; 16:138–144.

37
Management of Ascites

Enrique J. Martinez
LifeLink Transplant Institute, Tampa General Hospital, Tampa, Florida

Lennox Jeffers
University of Miami and Veterans Affairs Medical Center, Miami, Florida

INTRODUCTION

The detection of ascites in any patient heralds the beginning of a significant decline in function and should prompt a thorough evaluation of the patient to ascertain its etiology and help direct appropriate therapy. While massive ascites is easily appreciated, mild to moderate ascites can be missed in up to 50% of cases, even when examined by experienced gastroenterologists. Flank dullness is a sensitive finding seen in up to 90% of cases, whereas shifting dullness is more specific but less sensitive. Amounts of fluid as small as 120 mL have been purported to be demonstrated by the puddle sign, which requires the patient to be in a knee-hand position. Imaging studies, such as ultrasound, are much more sensitive and specific than the physical examination and can detect amounts as small as 100 mL. Parenchymal liver disease will be inculpated in about 80% of the ascites cases, whereas etiologies such as malignancy (12%), heart failure (5%), tuberculosis (2%), pancreatic ascites (1%), and other miscellaneous etiologies need to be considered as part of the differential.

DIAGNOSIS

Diagnostic paracentesis, which can generally be performed safely in most patients, serves an invaluable role in helping to delineate etiologies through the calculation of the gradient from serum to ascites albumin. If one subtracts the amount of ascites albumin from the amount of serum albumin, the resultant gradient can be used to differentiate among the ascites etiologies. A high gradient (greater than or equal to 1.1 g/dL) is associated with cirrhosis, alcoholic hepatitis, fatty liver of pregnancy, massive liver metastases, fulminant liver failure, portal vein thrombosis, Budd-Chiari syndrome, veno-occlusive disease, cardiac ascites, or myxedema. A low gradient (less than 1.1 g/dL) is associated with peritoneal carcinomatosis, tuberculous peritonitis, biliary or pancreatic ascites, nephrotic syndrome, or serositis due to collagen vascular disease.

PROGNOSIS

In general, the development of ascites marks a decline in liver function and foretells an overall decrease in survival. Earlier reports suggested that the development of ascites in a cirrhotic patient is associated with a 50% 2-year survival rate. Other studies in alcoholic patients who developed ascites have likewise shown a diminished 5-year survival rate, from 89–52%, with an even further worsening of survival to 32% if patients continued to drink. Prospective data would suggest that the development of ascites in cirrhotic patients can reduce 5-year survival rates from 14 to 9%.

When one considers causes of death, ascites has been implicated in 50% of cases. Spontaneous bacterial peritonitis has been attributed to a mortality rate as high as 70%, with this accounting for 5–10% of all deaths in cirrhotics (see Chap. 38). Some 10% of deaths in cirrhotic patients are due to hepatorenal syndrome (see Chap. 39). Iatrogenic complications of the management of ascites account for up to 10% of deaths in cirrhotic patients. These factors alone can account for the significant decline in survival that is seen in cirrhotic patients with ascites.

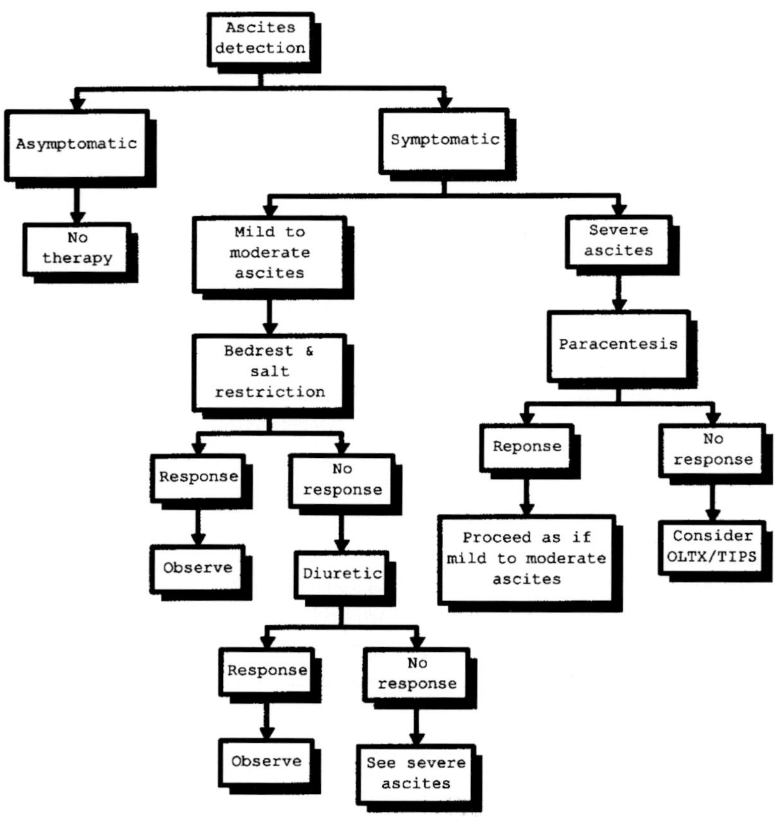

Figure 1 Approach to therapy of ascites.

PATHOGENESIS

A variety of theories have been presented to account for the known abnormalities seen in the cirrhotic patient with ascites. The overflow theory supports renal sodium retention as an initiating event triggered by liver disease or portal hypertension and resulting in plasma volume expansion and subsequent ascites. The underfill theory proposes an imbalance between the hepatic sinusoidal hydrostatic and oncotic forces, which leads to excess peritoneal lymph accumulation, decreasing plasma volume. It triggers renal sodium retention, leading to the fluid overload state. The arterial vasodilation theory attempts to bring these two theories together by suggesting that cirrhotic patients have a circulating humoral factor that causes peripheral vasodilation and leads to renal sodium retention via a variety of other factors, including increased sympathetic tone, altered intrarenal blood flow, and altered balance of renin, angiotensin, and aldosterone.

THERAPY

The decision to treat a patient with ascites should be based upon the clinical course. Anywhere between 5 and 10% of patients will form an equilibrium between ascites production and the ability to function; this group should merely be monitored. For the remaining 90%, a stepwise approach to the management of ascites should be considered.

Bed Rest

The use of bed rest to help with ascites stems from its potential to help restore the central venous circulating volume and reduce activation of the renin-angiotensin system, thereby improving renal perfusion and deceasing sodium retention. This therapy is of limited use because of its significant impact on the patient's lifestyle.

Dietary Restriction

It is known that limiting salt intake will help influence fluid accumulation in cirrhotic patients, who tend to excrete a very low sodium urine; thus, any effective reversal of this process will require that the dietary sodium intake be limited. Every gram of sodium (23 mEq) ingested over sodium excretion is estimated to lead to 200–300 mL of fluid retention. Extreme dietary reduction of sodium to < 500 mg/day does result in fluid loss but is impractical owing to poor out-of-hospital compliance. A 2-g sodium restriction results in a more practical dietary manipulation that can be tolerated by most patients. Actual fluid restriction should not be recommended unless hyponatremia (serum sodium < 125 mEq/L) ensues. It is vitally important to stress that maintenance of appropriate dietary sodium restriction will help minimize further use of medication, as medications taken by cirrhotic patients are associated with significant complications. It is also important to note that recommendations for good nutrition and abstinence from alcohol should be recommended to patients to help stabilize the patient's synthetic functioning.

Diuretics

Only 10% of patients will be managed by the use of bed rest and dietary salt restriction, thus leaving a much larger proportion of patients who will be exposed to the risks of diuretics. The ultimate goal of diuretic use would be to produce an effective diuresis without giving rise to any significant side effects. The rate of diuresis should be limited to 700–900 mL/day if no peripheral edema is present and to 3 lb/day if peripheral edema is present.

Spironolactone is the standard for therapy in cirrhotic ascites. Its mechanism of action is through direct antagonism of aldosterone at the level of the collecting duct, thus blocking sodium reabsorption and potassium excretion. By comparison with a loop diuretic such as furosemide, spironolactone has been shown to be more effective as a single agent in 65% of patients. Given its 1-week half-life in cirrhotic patients, spironolactone should initially be given at 50–100 mg/day; increases can be made every week thereafter to a maximum dose of 400 mg/day. Doses up to 200 mg/day may be given at a single administration. Development of gynecomastia and breast tenderness may prompt a change to another potassium-sparing diuretic such as amiloride or triamterene. Caution must be exercised with the use of triamterene as it may act in a synergistic fashion with nonsteroidal anti-inflammatory agents in producing renal failure. Detection of severe hyperkalemia may prompt either a dose reduction of spironolactone or concomitant administration of a loop diuretic to counterbalance potassium retention.

If diuresis is not sufficient with aldactone, the addition of a loop diuretic such as furosemide may lead to effective diuresis in an additional 20% of patients. Furosemide may be started at 20–40 mg/day and increased progressively, if tolerated, to a maximum dose of 160 mg/day. Careful evaluation for hypokalemia as well as renal function is indicated whenever any diuretics are used. Other loop-acting agents such as ethacrinic acid, bumetanide, or torasemide may be substituted, and each has slightly different pharmacological effects. Torasemide has been purported to have a potential benefit due to its longer half-life, increased bioavailability, and greater natiuretic effect.

Metolazone may help some patients who are otherwise refractory to spironolactone and a loop diuretic. It acts on the cortical diluting segment and can cause massive diuresis in some patients. Its use must be tempered by the significant risk of secondary electrolyte and renal dysfunction; its administration calls for very close observation.

Potassium-canrenoate is a European aldosterone antagonist that has less anti-andrenergic side effects and may be more effective than amiloride.

Surgical Management of Ascites

Approximately 10–20% of patients will be refractory to medical management of ascites. The ultimate surgical management of ascites would be liver transplantation, which is associated with a 2-year survival of over 70%. But given the donor shortage, this is not a practical immediate option. Other surgical therapies must therefore be used to stabilize the patient or help manage the ascites.

Paracentesis

Paracentesis provides the patient with an almost immediate improvement in the volume of ascites but does pose the risk of potentially serious side effects. Studies have found that up to 75% of all patients with ascites have had large-volume paracentesis performed and that it has been performed in 93% of refractory ascites patients. Study trials comparing large-volume paracentesis with albumin infusion versus spironolactone and furosemide have demonstrated that paracentesis is more effective than medical therapy in eliminating ascites (96–72%) and in decreasing the length of hospitalization (11.5 vs. 31 days); it is also associated with a decreased incidence of encephalopathy, renal dysfunction, and electrolyte problems (16 vs. 60%).

The issue of exactly when to give plasma volume expanders has led to extended research. Most studies suggest that when 5 L or less of ascites is removed, there are no significant changes in plasma volume, renin activity, or aldosterone levels. Paracentesis exceeding 5 L should be accompanied by some type of plasma volume expansion, as there can be up to a 20% incidence of hyponatremia or renal impairment with these patients. It appears that the decrease in intravascular problems tends to occur 12–24 h after the paracentesis; therefore, agents that have a longer duration should be used. Currently, studies favor the use of three plasma expanders. Albumin has a 21-day half life; it is extremely expensive and sometimes in short supply. Hemaccel has a 16-h half-life. Dextran 70 has a 24-h half-life. Albumin is by far the most commonly used plasma expander and is administered intravenously at 6–8 g/mL of ascites removed during the large-volume paracentesis.

Reinfusion of Ascites

Reinfusion of ascites offers the advantage of volume expansion with prevention of protein loss and decreased cost. Larger studies are still required before this process can become streamlined and be made less cumbersome for the practicing physician.

Peritoneovenous Shunting

A variety of peritoneovenous shunts have been introduced, including the Leveen, Denver, and Minnesota shunts. They all act as an artificial thoracic duct by draining the ascitic fluid directly into the central venous system, with the valve requiring only 3 cm of water pressure to open. The main problem of these shunts has been the high rate of postprocedure complications. The use of peritoneovenous shunts has been shown to be superior to medical management in relieving tense ascites more rapidly and decreasing the length of hospital stay. The nutritional status of patients with long-standing peritoneovenous shunts may also be improved long term, most likely related to the cessation of protein loss with paracentesis.

Postshunt coagulopathy has been reported in 10–60% of patients, with a higher subclinical than clinical rate of overt coagulopathy. Peritoneal cell production of tissue plasminogen activator and postoperative platelet decreases due to intravascular coagulation are felt to be causative. There appears to be a reduction in the coagulopathy if the majority of the ascitic fluid is removed at the time of surgery. Likewise, the intraoperative administration of aspirin or heparin may help to decrease the intravascular coagulation.

Other complications related to technical problems created by the shunt placement are common. Shunt failure can be seen in 30–40% of patients within the first year for a variety of technical reasons including tip thrombosis, kinking, or clogging of the valve. Infection due to ascitic leakage can be seen in up to 26% of patients. Late peritonitis, due to probable transient bacteremia, can be seen in 10%, with all shunt patients requiring antibiotics before undergoing any invasive procedures. Thrombosis of the superior vena cava can be noted in 2–23%, with 8% developing pulmonary emboli over 5 years. It is also postulated that peritoneovenous shunting may increase the risk of variceal bleeding by increasing intravascular volume.

Transjugular Intrahepatic Portosystemic Shunting (TIPS)

A growing body of evidence appears to support the conception of TIPS for refractory ascites. Summarizing data from these studies, there appears to be a 77–100% technical success in placement of the TIPS, with a 50–92% response of ascites to treatment. The lowest response rate was seen in one series in which pre-TIPS encephalopathy, elevated total bilirubin > 5 mg/dL, and early death may have prevented any observation of improvement in ascites. Ochs et al., in one of the larger TIPS series, found that TIPS decreased portosystemic venous pressure gradients in 63%, with complete remission of ascites seen in 74% and partial remission in 18%. TIPS occlusion by thrombus occurred in 10%, with late shunt malfunctions characterized by ascites being noted in 32% and most malfunctions being corrected by dilation or revision of the stents. A hospital mortality rate of 4% was noted, with a 58% cumulative 9-month mortality. Trends for predicting a worse outcome were suggested by rising bilirubin level post-TIPS and age > 60 years at the time of procedure. Encephalopathy increased from 40–50% post-TIPS, being debilitating in one-third of these patients. Interestingly, encephalopathy improved in 6% and appeared de novo in 16%.

Ongoing clinical trials are being prepared to try to address further the efficacy of TIPS for ascites and also to try to compare it with total-volume paracentesis.

CONCLUSIONS

The development of ascites is a poor prognostic indicator in any patient with liver disease. Whenever it occurs, a thorough evaluation needs to be performed to elucidate the cause. A variety of noninvasive and invasive options are available for ameliorating symptoms in patients with ascites, but the only proven therapy that has had any positive impact on survival is liver transplantation. Organ shortages and prolonged waiting times dictate that we manage these patients carefully with other means while they await transplantation if they are indeed candidates for this procedure.

BIBLIOGRAPHY

Angelli P, Dalla Pria M, De Bei E, Albino G, Caregaro L, Merkel C, Ceolotto G, Gatta A. Randomized clinical study of the efficacy of amiloride and potassium canrenoate in non-azotemic cirrhotic patients with ascites. Hepatology 1994; 19:72–79.

Burroughs AK. Paracentesis for ascites in cirrhotic patients. Gastroenterol Int 1990; 2:120–123.

Dunn CJ, Fitton A, Brogden RN. Torasemide: an update of its pharmacological properties and therapeutic efficacy. Drugs 1995; 49:121–142.

Garcia-Villareal L, Zozaya JM, Betes M, Herrero JI, Prieto J. Transjugular intrahepatic portal-systemic shunt in the treatment of refractory ascites: effect on clinical, renal, humoral, and hemodynamic parameters. Hepatology 1995; 21:986–994.

Gines P, Arroyo V. Paracentesis in the management of cirrhotic ascites. J Hepatol 1993; 12:S14–18.

Longmire-Cook SJ. Pathophysiologic factors and management of ascites. Surg Gynecol Obstet 1993; 176:191–202.

Ochs A, Rossle M, Haag K, Hauenstein KKH, Deibert P, Siegerstetter V, Huonker M, Langer M, Blum HE. The transjugular intrahepatic portosystemic stent shunt procedure for refractory ascites. N Engl J Med 1995; 332:1192–1197.

Somberg K, Lake JR, Tomlanovich SJ, LaBerge JM, Feldstein V, Bass NM. Transjugular intrahepatic portal-systemic shunt in the treatment of refractory ascites: effect on clinical and hormonal response and renal function. Hepatology 1995; 21:709–716.

38

Management of Spontaneous Bacterial Peritonitis

John C. Hoefs, Victoria Alagiozian-Angelova, and Afshin Khatibi
University of California, Irvine Medical Center, Orange, California

INTRODUCTION

Spontaneous bacterial peritonitis (SBP) is an infectious process within the peritoneal cavity, mostly occurring in cirrhotic patients with ascites in whom a contiguous local source of infection is not present. The incidence of SBP in cirrhotic patients admitted to hospital with ascites has been estimated at 7–23%. The diagnosis is established on the basis of a polymorphonuclear (PMN) cell count in ascitic fluid higher than 250/mm^3, a positive ascitic fluid culture (70–80% of cases), and absence of an intraabdominal source of infection. Clinical signs and symptoms are often not present. SBP can also develop in patients with ascites, as a result of acute liver failure, nephrotic syndrome, or massive hepatic metastasis when the ascitic protein concentration is < 1 g/dL. It is uncommon in patients with cardiac ascites and extremely rare in patients with disease causing ascites with high protein levels—e.g., peritoneal carcinomatosis.

TYPES OF ASCITIC FLUID INFECTION

Based on the characteristics of ascitic fluid analysis [polymorphonuclear (PMN) cell count and culture], different variants of ascitic fluid infection have been identified as SBP, culture-negative neutrocytic ascites (CNNA), monomicrobial nonneutrocytic bacterascites, and polymicrobial bacterascites. These variants behave almost identically; they appear to occur in the same population of patients and have similar outcome.

SBP is defined as an ascitic fluid PMN cell count of $\geqslant$ 250/mm^3 with a positive ascitic fluid culture, usually for a single organism, with no evidence of an intraabdominal source of infection. A recent study observed that 15% of culture-positive SBP cases become negative spontaneously before the initiation of therapy, whereas 85% of cases remain culture-positive for the same organism.

CNNA is defined as an ascitic fluid PMN cell count of $\geqslant$ 250/mm^3 with a negative ascitic fluid culture. Other causes of neutrocytic ascites should be carefully excluded, such as previous antibiotic therapy, peritoneal carcinomatosis, tuberculosis, systemic lupus erythematosus, penetrating duodenal ulcer, pancreatitis, hepatocellular carcinoma, or bleeding into the peritoneum. Patients with SBP who are placed on antibiotic therapy prior to paracentesis and the 15% of SBP patients who spontaneously become culture-negative are included in this group. These patients are clinically identical to patients with SBP regarding symptomatology, laboratory findings, response to antibiotics and mortality rate.

Approximately one-third of blood cultures in CNNA are positive for organisms characteristic of SBP. Approximately one-quarter of survivors have either had a previously documented episode of SBP or will develop such in the future. These findings suggest that there may be several reasons for culture negativity, such as SBP that resolved spontaneously or clinical laboratory techniques that are inadequate to detect all infected patients.

Bacterascites is a culture-positive ascites with an ascitic fluid PMN cell count of < 250/mm^3. When there is evidence of a host response to the presence of bacteria, the implications of the infection and, therefore, the diagnosis changes. Bacterascites becomes spontaneous bacterial peritonitis when the neutrophil count rises in response to the infection. Presumably, at an early stage, the organisms in the ascitic fluid can be eradicated by host defenses by means of specific and nonspecific opsonins and macrophages, without an influx of neutrophils. In some instances however, infection persists and chemotactic factors are released, initiating a polymorphonuclear response.

Monomicrobial nonneutrocytic bacterascites (MMNA) is defined as an ascitic fluid PMN cell count of < 250/mm^3 with a positive ascitic fluid culture for a single organism. Spontaneous resolution of bacterascites occurs in 62–86% of cases. It is suggested that the underlying liver disease is usually less severe in patients with monomicrobial bacterascites than in those with SBP. In other words, monomicrobial bacterascites involves the process of colonization of ascites without a host response. It may represent either an early stage of infection, prior to the inflammatory response, or just a poor host response to infection. Patients with bacterascites have the same mortality rate as those with SBP.

Polymicrobial bacterascites is infrequent and usually results from a needle perforation of the gut during a diagnostic or therapeutic paracentesis. It rarely progresses to peritonitis unless the ascitic protein concentration is < 1 g/dL.

Secondary bacterial peritonitis is an infection of the peritoneal cavity with positive ascitic fluid bacterial cultures, ascitic fluid PMN cell count of > 250/mm^3, and evidence of an intraabdominal source of infection. It is very important to differentiate spontaneous from secondary peritonitis, because treatment of secondary peritonitis is mostly surgical. Secondary infection of ascites may result from a nearby "contained" infection, such as an abscess, or penetration of a colonized hollow viscus (e.g., the colon). A contained infection may initially be similar to SBP but evolves more rapidly to severe infection and does not respond well to antibiotics. Bowel perforation evolves even more rapidly (due to the large number of organisms initially entering the peritoneal cavity) and can be distinguished from SBP by the number and type of infecting organisms as determined by Gram staining for multiple organisms and cultures positive for multiple organisms, ascitic fluid analysis [lactic dehydrogenase (LDH) and glucose levels compared to serum], presence of a contiguous source of infection, air under the diaphragm, and poor response to antibiotic therapy. Ascitic fluid analysis in SBP meets two or more of the following criteria: total protein > 1 g/dL, glucose < 50 mg/dL, and LDH > 225 mU/mL or higher than the upper limit of normal for serum. Secondary peritonitis represents < 10% of ascitic fluid infections in cirrhotic patients.

Table 1 Bacteria Isolated from the Ascitic Fluid in 267 Episodes of Spontaneous Bacterial Peritonitis in 246 Patients

Bacteria	No. of Isolates	%
Escherichia coli	131	43
Klebsiella pneumoniae	26	8
Streptococcus pneumoniae	24	8
Alpha-hemolytic streptococcus	17	5
Group D streptococcus	17	5
Unclassified streptococcus	13	4
Beta-hemolytic streptococcus	12	4
Enterobacteriaceae	8	3
Pseudomonas	6	2
Staphylococcus aureus	5	2
Miscellaneous	48	16
Total	307	100

Source: Courtesy of Hoefs JC, Runyon BA: Disease-a-Month 31, September 1985.

ETIOLOGY OF SBP

Table 1 shows the most common organisms isolated in patients with SBP. *Streptococcus* represents 26% of all isolates from spontaneously infected ascitic fluid. *Escherichia*, *Streptococcus*, and *Klebsiella* represent 77% of the isolates. Despite the fact that gut flora cause the majority of SBP, anaerobes are cultured in approximately 6% of cases. This may be due to the relatively high PO_2 of ascitic fluid and the inability of anaerobes to survive under these circumstances. The polymicrobial infections (10% of cases) usually include one or more isolates typical for SBP plus one or more peculiar organisms, such as *Staphylococcus aureus*, *Candida* species, or anaerobes.

PATHOGENESIS

SBP is a consequence of multiple alterations in the immune defense of patients with cirrhosis. The most accepted hypothesis in the pathogenesis of SBP explains it as the colonization of the ascitic fluid from an episode of bacteremia. Although the passage of microorganisms from bloodstream to ascites has never been documented, it can be assumed that bacteria present in the circulation may easily reach the ascites because of the constant fluid exchange between these two compartments. Once ascites is colonized by microorganisms, the development of SBP would depend on the defensive capacity of the ascitic fluid (Fig. 1). Decreased antimicrobial activity of ascitic fluid would predispose to development of SBP.

Another option is the passage of enteric organisms from the intestinal wall. Evidence in favor of a transintestinal wall route includes the presence of mucosal edema and the demonstration of transfer from lumen to peritoneal cavity of both live and dead C-14–labeled *E. coli*.

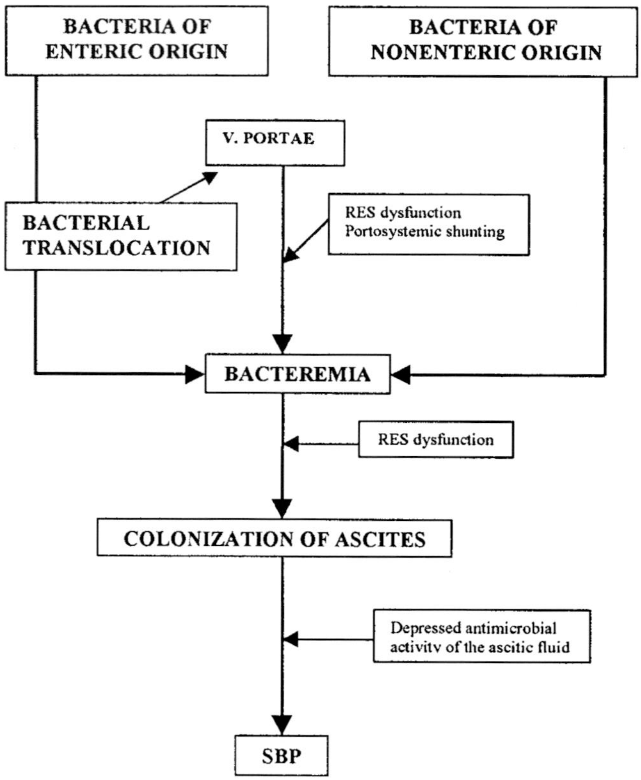

Figure 1 Bacteremia is a necessary precursor for SBP from either enteric or nonenteric organisms. Enteric organisms initially translocate across the gut wall from the intestinal lumen to the submucosal space. The organisms in the intestinal interstitial space may enter the central blood stream from: (1) *lymph* via the intestinal lymphatic chain to the left thoracic duct or (2) the small *portal venous* radicals to bypass the liver through intra- or extrahepatic shunts. The major route of movement of bacteria from the blood compartment to ascites is across the surface of the liver during bacteremia resulting in the small number that eventually contaminate ascites. An ascites protein concentration < 1 g/dL indicates low opsonic activity that allows growth of these organisms.

Since SBP is caused predominantly by enteric organisms, the most accepted pathogenic mechanisms, explaining passage of enteric organisms from the lumen of the bowel to the systemic circulation are:

- The depression of the hepatic reticuloendothelial system (RES), causing failure of the liver to "filter" these bacteria and allowing them to pass through the wall of the bowel to the systematic circulation via the portal vein.
- The relative increase of aerobic gram-negative bacilli in the jejunal flora in cirrhosis and the possible alteration in the intestinal barrier caused by circumstances decreasing mucosal blood flow (e.g., acute hypovolemia or splanchnic vasoconstrictor drugs).
- Bacterial translocation, or the process by which enteric bacteria normally present in the gastrointestinal tract, cross the mucosa, infect the mesenteric lymph nodes,

and reach the bloodstream through the intestinal lymphatic circulation. Bacterial translocation to mesenteric lymph nodes has been observed in an experimental model of cirrhosis in rats as well as in some other conditions associated with a high incidence of gram-negative bacterial infections, like obstructive jaundice or hemorrhagic shock.

Recent studies have demonstrated a genetic identity of different bacteria, cultured simultaneously from intestinal lumen, mesenteric lymph nodes, and ascitic fluid in cirrhotic patients. Bacterial translocation has been documented in patients with intestinal obstruction and cirrhosis undergoing laparotomy.

In order to explain the mechanism of SBP caused by nonenteric bacteria, one can assume that they enter the circulation from the skin or upper respiratory tract, penetrating the mucocutaneous barriers naturally present. Dental abscesses, periodontal disease, and pneumonic infections are common sources.

Whatever the source of bacteria reaching the bloodstream, a bacteremic event can be more prolonged and therefore can more easily become clinically significant in cirrhotic than in noncirrhotic patients. This is generally explained by the depressed RES function in cirrhotics. Once ascitic fluid has been colonized by microorganisms, the development of SBP would depend only on the defense capacity of the ascitic fluid.

PREDISPOSING FACTORS

Predisposing factors can be divided into iatrogenic and noniatrogenic groups, the latter including intestinal barrier changes, altered activity of the reticuloendothelial system, decreased opsonic activity of the ascitic fluid, and neutrophil dysfunction.

Iatrogenic Factors

Cirrhotic patients are frequently subjected to different diagnostic and therapeutic maneuvers that may alter their normal defense barriers and thus increase the risk of bacterial infections. Endoscopic sclerotherapy for variceal bleeding in emergency settings was estimated to be associated with bacteremia in 5–30%. The placement of a transjugular intrahepatic portosystemic stent for the treatment of bleeding esophageal varices has not been documented to be associated with bacterial infections. A peritoneovenous shunt (Le Veen shunt) was reported to be associated with a 20% of incidence of bacterial infections. The most common invasive techniques, such as diagnostic or therapeutic paracentesis and endoscopy, are associated with a very low risk for the development of bacterial infections. Despite the frequency of procedures in cirrhotic patients, the vast majority of episodes of SBP are unrelated to procedures.

Noniatrogenic Factors

Major alterations in the normal intestinal flora of cirrhotic patients occur. The aerobic (facultative) gram-negative bacilli are present in low numbers in the small bowel of normal subjects. Their number is significantly increased in the jejunum of cirrhotic patients. This phenomenon is called *intestinal bacterial overgrowth.* This may increase the chances of aerobic gram-negative bacilli invading the bloodstream (bacterial translocation) and causing infection of enteric origin in these patients. Additionally, it has been documented in animal models that there is increased passage of bacteria from the intestinal lumen to extraintestinal sites. Bacterial translocation can be caused by a disruption of the intestinal permeability barrier, bacterial overgrowth, and/or a decrease in host immune defense. Some patients with cirrhosis have intestinal mucosal congestion and edema attributed to portal hypertension, which may cause increased intestinal permeability and facilitate bacterial translocation. Endotoxin is associated with bacterial translocation by increasing gut permeability and altering host immune defense. Changes in permeability of the intestinal mucosa have also been observed in hemorrhagic shock, sepsis, and injury.

The reticuloendothelial system (RES) is widely distributed throughout the body, but approximately 90% of the defensive system is in the liver, where Kupffer cells and endothelial sinusoidal cells are the major components. The special location of the RES is thus considered the main defensive mechanism against bacteria and other infections acquired through a hematogenous route, such as SBP. There are studies showing marked depression of the RES, especially its hepatic fraction, in patients with cirrhosis. It has been shown that the risk of acquiring bacteremia and SBP in cirrhosis is directly related to the degree of RES dysfunction in these patients. The exact pathogenesis of the depression of phagocytic activity of the RES is not clear. However, the most accepted theory suggests that it is the result of intrahepatic shunting of blood, which escapes the phagocytic action of the RES cells located in the sinusoids. A significant amount of hepatic blood flow circulates through anatomic or functional intrahepatic shunts and therefore is not available for blood-tissue exchange. Other mechanisms may also be involved, like reduction in the phagocytic capacity of monocytes, considered as Kupffer cell precursors, as well as impaired function of macrophage Fc-gamma receptors in alcoholic cirrhosis. Serum opsonic activity has been found to be reduced in most cirrhotic patients, probably as a consequence of a decreased serum concentration of complement and fibronectin, substances that normally stimulate phagocytosis by enhancing the adhesiveness of microorganisms to the reticuloendothelial cell surface.

It has been demonstrated that the nonspecific antimicrobial capacity of ascitic fluid in cirrhosis, which varies greatly in different patients, may be involved in the pathogenesis of SBP. There is an inverse and highly significant correlation between the opsonic activity of the ascitic fluid and the risk of developing peritonitis in patients with ascites admitted to hospital. Opsonic activity of ascitic fluid in cirrhosis is directly correlated with the concentration of defensive substances, such as immunoglobulins, complement, and fibronectin as well as with the concentration of total protein in ascites. Several investigators have found that the concentration of total protein in ascitic fluid correlates well with the risk of SBP. It has been demonstrated that patients with protein concentration in ascitic fluid below 1 g/dL develop peritonitis during their hospital stay with a significantly higher frequency than those with a greater protein concentration (15 vs. 2% respectively), and the cumulative probability of developing peritonitis during long-term follow-up is significantly greater in cirrhotic patients with ascites whose ascitic protein concentration is below 1 g/dL compared with others (20 vs 2% respectively, after 1 year). The probability of the first episode of SBP in cirrhotic patients with ascites is significantly influenced by the antimicrobial capacity of the ascitic fluid and by hepatic function, ascitic fluid protein levels, and serum bilirubin levels. Since iron is an essential growth factor for microorganisms, a recent preliminary study has suggested that ascitic fluid transferrin levels also could play an important role in the predisposition for SBP development in cirrhosis. The authors suggest that cirrhotic patients with low ascitic fluid transferrin concentration would have high free iron levels in ascitic fluid that could facilitate SBP.

A high proportion of cirrhotic patients show altered PMN cell function at different

Table 2 Factors Predisposing to Spontaneous Bacteria Peritonitis in Cirrhotic Patients with Ascites

Confirmed factors
End-stage liver disease
GI bleeding
Ascitic fluid total protein $\leqslant$ 1 g/dL
History of SBP
Suspected but not confirmed factors
Urinary tract infection
Indwelling catheters (bladder and intravascular)
High free iron levels in ascitic fluid
Factors not likely to predispose
Diagnostic paracentesis
Large-volume therapeutic paracentesis
Endoscopy
Sclerotherapy
Hepatocellular carcinoma

levels. The most frequent disturbance is a marked reduction of chemotaxis, probably caused by the presence of substances in serum that are capable of inhibiting granulocyte migration. The nature of these chemotactic inhibitory substances has not been determined. The phagocytic and bactericidal capacity of PMNs has been found to be reduced in many cirrhotic patients. PMN dysfunction has not been adequately investigated in relation to the risk of acquiring bacterial infections in cirrhotic patients. However, as the types of infection frequently developed by patients with congenital or acquired PMN function abnormalities (chronic granulomatous diseases and recurrent staphylococcal and fungal infections) are very different from the infections developed by cirrhotic patients, it seems unlikely that PMN dysfunction plays a major role in the susceptibility of patients with cirrhosis to bacterial infections.

Another way of interpreting predisposing factors for SBP can be seen in Table 2.

CLINICAL PRESENTATION

SBP usually presents on a background of cirrhosis with voluminous ascites. Clinical features may be variable depending on the stage at which SBP is diagnosed.

Abdominal pain and fever are the most characteristic symptoms. However, nonspecific symptoms and signs—such as hepatic encephalopathy, vomiting, diarrhea, jaundice, GI bleeding, shock, or hypovolemia—may also be present. Some patients may present with only mild deterioration in mental status or progressive kidney failure. SBP can also be totally asymptomatic in about 9% of cases.

Analysis of blood usually shows peripheral leukocytosis and evidence of marked liver failure. Acidosis can also be present, and kidney failure occurs in about one-third of cases.

Approximately half of the cases with SBP are community-acquired. Frequently patients are diagnosed with SBP on admission to hospital. Between 40 and 55% are diagnosed within 2–7 days of admission.

Since the clinical picture of SBP is frequently insidious, careful evaluation for the disease in cirrhotic patients with ascites is required. Diagnostic paracentesis is extremely helpful and is highly recommended not only in patients presenting with the clinical features of SBP but also in cases where there is marked deterioration of the previous clinical status.

DIAGNOSIS

The variability in presentation of SBP necessitates a high clinical suspicion for this diagnosis, which should generally be considered in cirrhotic patients with advanced disease and new onset of ascites, those with ascites admitted to hospital, those suspected of having a bacterial infection, and those with clinical deterioration or a complication such as gastrointestinal hemorrhage, hepatic encephalopathy, or renal insufficiency.

Ultimately, the diagnosis of SBP rests on ascitic fluid analysis and culture. An absolute ascitic fluid PMN count greater than 250/mm^3 is diagnostic of ascitic fluid infection. Virtually 99.9% of patients with SBP have absolute neutrophil counts of 250/mm^3 or higher. In comparison, the mean number of PMNs in uninfected ascites is 60/mm^3. Differentiation of neutrophil-predominant ascitic fluid also helps to distinguish bacterial infection of ascitic fluid from other causes of elevated white blood cell count in the ascitic fluid. For instance, in peritoneal carcinomatosis, an elevated white blood cell count with mononuclear predominance is seen, whereas with tuberculous peritonitis, a lymphocyte predominance is generally observed.

Ascitic fluid analysis should also include comparison of serum and ascitic levels of total protein, albumin, glucose, and LDH. Serum levels should be obtained at the time of paracentesis. Patients with SBP generally have total protein concentrations less than 1.5 g/100 mL. There is an inverse correlation with the level of serum total protein and risk of SBP. Cardiac ascites is the only condition in which SBP may be observed, albeit extremely rarely, in the presence of a normal total protein concentration. Determination of the serum-ascites albumin gradient also potentiates the diagnosis of SBP. A serum-ascites albumin concentration of 1.1 g/dL or greater was correlated closely with presence of portal hypertension. Virtually all patients with SBP have portal hypertension. The only exception is patients with nephrotic syndrome, in whom the serum-ascites albumin gradient is less than 1.1 g/dL and in whom SBP has been reported. Interestingly, in both, a low ascitic total protein concentration is observed, which, as mentioned, is a risk factor for SBP.

Comparison of ascites-serum glucose and LDH levels can yield important information about the cellular metabolic activity in the ascitic fluid. With SBP, the ascitic glucose concentration does not decrease; however, the ascites/serum glucose ratio may decrease. Additionally, the ascitic concentration of LDH will usually increase. These changes are observed in approximately 30% of SBP cases. The low concentration of bacteria usually observed in SBP will result in smaller changes in these two measurements and hence a lower metabolic activity in the ascitic fluid. Conversely, high concentration of bacteria is often seen in secondary bacterial peritonitis. This results in higher cellular metabolic activity in ascitic fluid with lower ascites/serum glucose ratios and higher LDH levels. These parameters can, therefore, be useful in differentiating between spontaneous bacterial peritonitis and secondary bacterial peritonitis. Gut perforation may result in secondary bacterial peritonitis. In a study by Runyon and Hoefs, all six patients with gut perforation met at least two of the following criteria; ascitic fluid total protein concentration greater than 1 g/dL, glucose concentration less than 50 mg/dL, and LDH concentration greater than

225 mU/mL (or greater than the upper limit of normal for serum). Only 2 out of 33 patients with spontaneous bacterial peritonitis met two of these criteria.

Gram stain of ascitic fluid in SBP frequently fails to demonstrate an organism. It is usually positive in 30% of cases. If ascitic fluid is centrifuged, the yield may increase to 55%. Finding multiple and different organisms should prompt a search for gut perforation with abdominal x-rays and contrast studies, as appropriate.

Bacterial culture will ultimately result in the identification of the causative organism for SBP. The low concentration of bacteria in ascitic fluid (often less than one organism per milliliter) requires other than conventional culture methods. It is recommended that 10 mL of ascitic fluid immediately be inoculated into each of two bacterial blood culture bottles at the bedside. The yield with this method for positive cultures reaches 80–90%. In comparison, the conventional culture technique yields positive cultures in only 50%. BacT/Alert is a new system that may detect bacteremia sooner than the conventional blood culture bottles. In a study by Ortiz and colleagues, ascitic fluid cultures were positive at a mean time of 13.3 h compared to 43.0 h with conventional blood culture bottles. Further studies are needed to assess the efficacy of the BacT/Alert system.

In cases of bacterascites and MMNA, it is recommended that a second paracentesis be performed in 24 to 48 h to reevaluate the ascitic fluid prior to institution of antibiotic therapy. Up to 40% of symptomatic patients with MMNA will develop SBP; this population of patients should be promptly treated.

Currently the routine testing of ascitic fluid for lactate, pH or various cytokines (i.e., tumor necrosis factor alpha, $alpha_1$ antitrypsin, C-reactive protein) is not recommended. Though cytokines concentrations are elevated in infected ascitic fluid, the delay in their measurement and uncertainty regarding their exact role limits their utility in diagnosis of SBP.

MANAGEMENT

Empiric antibiotic treatment should be initiated immediately in cases where SBP is suspected or if ascitic fluid analysis reveals a PMN count of 250/mm^3 or greater. Symptomatic patients with bacterascites (MMNA) should also be treated or the decision based on repeat paracentesis when the positive culture is reported.

In empiric therapy of SBP, the antibiotic of choice has been cefotaxime, a third-generation cephalosporin. Cefotaxime covers the flora most commonly responsible for SBP. Its low toxicity and adequate penetration of ascitic fluid makes it a suitable choice. It has been shown to be superior to ampicillin plus tobramycin in efficacy, with lower hospital mortality in treatment of SBP.

Studies with regard to dosing regimens have shown treatment with cefotaxime at 2.0 g every 8–12 h to be as effective as every 6 h. The length of therapy has also been evaluated, and it appears that a 5-day course is as effective as a 10-day one.

Following a single dose of cefotaxime, nearly complete sterilization of ascitic fluid culture occurs, with subsequent negative cultures. The absolute PMN count in ascitic fluid also falls predictably to less than 50% of the initial concentration within 48 h. A second paracentesis in 48 h is therefore recommended to assess successful control of infection. In cases of secondary bacterial peritonitis, repeat paracentesis in 48 h often yields a higher absolute neutrophil count than at baseline and can be used in differential diagnosis. Ascitic fluid cultures also remain positive. If secondary bacterial peritonitis is suspected based on the latter findings, radiological studies are necessary to localize a source of infection (i.e., gut perforation or abscess) and surgical consultation should be obtained.

Aminoglycosides are generally associated with a poor resolution of SBP and a high incidence of nephrotoxicity in cirrhotic patients despite controlled serum levels. In a study by Hoefs, all cirrhotic patients being treated for SBP who developed a serum creatinine level greater than 2.1 g/dL, expired; these included six patients treated with gentamicin. Aminoglycosides *should therefore be avoided* in this population of patients.

Aztreonam use in treatment of SBP has resulted in *poor resolution* of the infection, with considerable incidence of suprainfection. It also lacks gram-positive coverage, and generally *should not be used* as initial treatment of SBP.

Amoxicillin-clavulanic acid is similar to cefotaxime with regard to initial treatment of SBP. A cure rate of 85% has been observed, with no significant side effects. It has an excellent cost/benefit ratio. It is, however, not available in its parenteral form in the United States. Studies are also needed to assess its efficacy comparatively with third-generation cephalosporins.

Ofloxacin, an oral quinolone, has good ascitic fluid penetration with excellent coverage of gram-negative bacilli and some coverage of gram-positive cocci. In a recent randomized trial, ofloxacin at a dose of 400 mg every 12 h was compared with intravenous cefotaxime in treatment of cirrhotic patients with uncomplicated SBP. Infection resolution rate and hospital survival rate were similar in both groups. Ofloxacin may therefore be a suitable substitute in the treatment of uncomplicated SBP as initial therapy. It may, however, be utilized in cirrhotic patients with uncomplicated SBP who have favorably responded to 2 or 3 days of inpatient parenteral cefotaxime and may then complete their treatment with an outpatient course of oral ofloxacin.

PROGNOSIS

Survival of an episode of SBP is clearly dependent on timely and appropriate antibiotic therapy. This results in a 93% success rate compared with a 25% success rate in patients receiving inappropriate therapy. Overall, there appear to be two distinct populations with different outcomes following an episode of SBP. A series by Hoefs observed one population with a rapid death rate (less than 7 days from onset of SBP) and one with a slower death rate. Rapid death was associated with lack of a previous hospitalization for liver disease, hepatomegaly, elevated serum bilirubin levels, abnormal levels of creatinine, and peripheral leukocytosis. The majority of these patients had acute alcoholic hepatitis. The second population are patients with advanced quiescent liver disease. This group has a slower death rate and overall better prognosis.

Prognostic factors have been sought in order to determine short and long-term survival following SBP. A study by Runyon and Hoefs found peripheral leukocytosis, jaundice, and absence of chills to predict a poor outcome for the specified episode of SBP, while peripheral leukocytosis, jaundice, and an elevated serum creatinine level predicted a poor outcome for the hospitalization. Serum bilirubin concentrations greater than 8 mg/dL and/or a serum creatinine concentration greater than 2.1 g/dL resulted in a 90% mortality, while the absence of both parameters yielded a 50% mortality. A study by Llovet et al. has also demonstrated renal and liver insufficiency to serve as independent risk factors of short-term survival following SBP. A recent large trial by Toledo also found serum BUN level at time of SBP diagnosis to be the best independent predictor of survival.

The probability of SBP recurrence is 69% at 1 year. Serum bilirubin grater than 4 mg/dL, prothrombin time greater than 4 s prolonged above control, and ascitic fluid protein concentration less than 1 g/dL correlate with an increased risk of recurrent SBP.

Long-term survival in cirrhotic patients following an episode of SBP is poor. Hoefs reported 1-year survival following discharge from the hospital at approximately 38%. Death was attributed to liver failure and recurrent SBP. Cirrhotic patients who survive an episode of SBP should, therefore, be referred for liver transplantation.

PROPHYLAXIS

Predisposition to the development of SBP appears to be related to decreased bactericidal and opsonic activity of ascitic fluid. Specifically, an ascitic fluid protein < 1 g/dL, C3 < 15 μg/mL, and low opsonophagocytic activity pose risks for the development and recurrence of SBP. Some efforts have been allocated to nonantibiotic strategies to prevent SBP. These have included elimination of ascites and increasing the ascitic fluid protein concentration.

Therapeutic paracentesis, though it may, theoretically, deplete ascitic fluid protein, has been shown not to increase the risk of SBP development in cirrhotic patients with tense ascites. On the other hand, therapeutic paracentesis may not decrease the risk of SBP either. Diuresis will serve to remove fluid and hence increase the concentration of protein in ascitic fluid, yet it also has not been shown to reduce the incidence of SBP.

Antibiotic prophylaxis strategies are aimed at reducing the potential pathogens of SBP. It is well established that the bulk of the pathogens responsible for SBP reside in the gut. Up to 80% of the pathogens are aerobic gram-negative bacteria. Efforts have therefore been centered on identification of an agent capable of selective decontamination of the gut (SDG), with reduction of gram-negative aerobes. The preservation of the remaining flora, particularly the anaerobes, is important in preventing intestinal colonization by pathogenic and resistant bacteria. The ideal agent must also have minimal toxicity even in the presence of liver failure, must be able to prevent SBP, should be cost-effective, and ought to be more efficacious than the current means of detection and treatment of SBP.

Norfloxacin is an oral quinolone with excellent activity against aerobic gram-negative bacteria, with preservation of anaerobic flora and infrequent emergence of resistant bacterial strains. It is also poorly absorbed from the intestinal tract and has a low incidence of side effects. It is therefore an ideal agent for SDG. In experimental studies by Runyon, prophylactic norfloxacin was associated with a 60% reduction in the overall rate of bacterial peritonitis.

Short-term antibiotic prophylaxis may reduce the incidence of SBP in cirrhotic patients with low ascitic fluid total protein concentration at time of admission to hospital and at presentation with gastrointestinal hemorrhage. Soriano studied norfloxacin prophylaxis in preventing nosocomial SBP in hospitalized cirrhotic patients with low ascitic fluid total protein concentration. He found a lower incidence of SBP in treated patients than in placebo-treated patients during the course of hospitalization. Mortality however was not significantly changed. In another study, Soriano also found that norfloxacin prophylaxis significantly decreased the incidence of SBP in cirrhotic patients admitted with gastrointestinal hemorrhage. A significant change in mortality was not observed.

Long-term prophylaxis may be necessary in particular subgroups of cirrhotic patients with ascites. Cirrhotic patients with low ascites fluid protein levels (less than 1 g/dL) or high serum bilirubin (greater than 2.5 mg/dL) have a greater than 50% probability of developing an initial episode of SBP during a 1-year follow-up. Novella studied the effect of norfloxacin prophylaxis in this particular population of patients in preventing an initial episode of SBP. He observed a lower incidence of SBP in patients given long-term (daily, continuous) norfloxacin prophylaxis as compared with short-term (daily, hospitalization period only) prophylaxis. However, more norfloxacin-resistant *Escherichia coli* organisms were isolated from infections in the long-term-treatment group.

An economic analysis by Younossi et al. found norfloxacin prophylaxis in high-risk patients with cirrhosis (previous history of SBP) to be cost-effective. Similarly, a cost-analysis study by Inadomi also found norfloxacin prophylaxis to be cost-effective in cirrhotic patients with a prior history of SBP and in those with an ascitic fluid protein concentration < 1 g/dL.

SBP may occur in cirrhotic patients on norfloxacin for selective gut decontamination. Llovet studied the characteristics of 229 episodes of SBP in cirrhotic patients with or without norfloxacin prophylaxis and did not find any difference in clinical features, response to treatment, or prognosis. However, a significantly higher proportion of SBP cases in patients on prophylaxis was caused by gram-positive bacteria (30 vs. 79%).

Ciprofloxacin and trimethoprim-sulfamethoxazole have been used as alternatives to norfloxacin for SBP prophylaxis. These agents have higher systemic absorption and broader bacterial coverage that may result in a higher incidence of resistant strains. A study by Rolachon showed that a weekly dose of ciprofloxacin 750 mg significantly lowered the incidence of recurrent or initial episodes of SBP in cirrhotic patients with low ascitic fluid protein concentrations in comparison with control. Mortality, however, was not significantly changed. A study by Singh randomized cirrhotic patients to receive either no prophylaxis or one double-strength trimethoprim-sulfamethoxazole five times a week as prophylaxis for SBP. The treated group had a lower incidence of SBP compared with the "no prophylaxis" group. Mortality was again not significantly changed.

At the present time, our recommendations regarding SBP prophylaxis in cirrhotic patients are as follows:

1. While awaiting liver transplantation, cirrhotic patients with a prior episode of SBP should be placed on oral norfloxacin 400 mg daily on a continuous basis.
2. Cirrhotic patients with an ascitic fluid total protein concentration below 1 g/dL who require admission to the hospital should be placed on oral norfloxacin 400 mg daily for the duration of their hospitalization.
3. Cirrhotic patients with ascites who present with variceal hemorrhage should be placed on a 7-day course of oral norfloxacin 400 mg daily.
4. Though promising, further studies with trimethoprim-sulfamethoxazole and ciprofloxacin are needed before they can be recommended as alternatives to norfloxacin prophylaxis.

BIBLIOGRAPHY

Garcia-Tsao G. Treatment of spontaneous bacterial peritonitis with oral ofloxacin: inpatient or outpatient therapy. Gastroenterology 1996; 111:1147–1150.

Gomez F, Ruiz P, Schreiber AD. Impaired function of macrophage Fc gamma receptors and bacterial infection in alcoholic cirrhosis. N Engl J Med 1994; 331:1122–1128.

Guarner C, Runyon BA. Macrophage function in cirrhosis and the risk of bacterial infection. Hepatology 1995; 22:367–369.

Llovet JM, Rodrigues-Iglesias P, Moitinho E, et al. Spontaneous bacterial peritonitis in patients with cirrhosis undergoing selective intestinal decontamination. J Hepatol 1997; 26:88–95.

Navasa M, Follo A, Llovet JM, et al. Randomized, comparative study of oral ofloxacin versus intravenous cefotaxime in spontaneous bacterial peritonitis. Gastroenterology 1996; 111:1011–1017.

Navasa M, Rimola A, Rodes J. Bacterial infections in liver disease. Semin Liver Dis 1997; 17:323–333.

Novella M, Sola R, Soriano G, et al. Continuous versus inpatient prophylaxis of the first episode of spontaneous bacterial peritonitis with norfloxacin. Hepatology 1997; 25:532–536.

Rimola A, Salmeron JM, Clemente G, et al. Two different dosages of cefotaxime in the treatment of spontaneous bacterial peritonitis in cirrhosis: Results of a prospective, randomized, multicenter study. Hepatology 1995; 21:674–679.

Ortiz J, Soriano G, Coll P, et al. Early microbiologic diagnosis of spontaneous bacterial peritonitis with BacT/Alert. J Hepatol 1997; 26:839–844.

Rolachon A, Cordier L, Bacq Y, et al. Cirpofloxacin and long-term prevention of spontaneous bacterial peritonitis: results of a prospective controlled trial. Hepatology 1995; 22:1171–1174.

Runyon BA, McHutchison JG, Antillon MR, et al. Short course versus long-course antibiotic treatment of spontaneous bacterial peritonitis: a randomized controlled study of 100 patients. Gastroenterology 1991 100:1737–1742.

Singh N, Gayowski T, Yu VL, Wagener MM. Trimethoprim-sulfamethoxazole for the prevention of spontaneous bacterial peritonitis in cirrhosis: a randomized trial. Ann Intern Med 1995; 122: 595–598.

Soriano G, Guarner C, Tomas A, et al. Norfloxacin prevents bacterial infection in cirrhotics with gastrointestinal hemorrhage. Gastroenterology 1992; 103:1267–1272.

39
Management of Functional Renal Failure (Hepatorenal Syndrome)

Robert D.J. Henihan and Lawrence S. Friedman
Harvard Medical School and Massachusetts General Hospital, Boston, Massachusetts

INTRODUCTION

The hepatorenal syndrome (HRS) is the clinical association of liver disease and functional renal failure (that is, renal failure without demonstrable intrinsic renal pathology). This clinical picture has been recognized for well over a century. In 1863, Austin Flint noted that in patients with cirrhosis and renal failure, the histology of the kidney at autopsy appeared normal. Not until 1956, however, did Hecker rekindle interest in the topic by observing that cirrhotic patients with renal failure had no proteinuria and a low urinary sodium concentration. Evidence for the reversible nature of HRS came when the kidney of a patient with the syndrome was transplanted into a recipient and functioned normally. The reversibility of the syndrome was confirmed when a patient with HRS underwent liver transplantation and recovered renal function. These findings suggest that the cause of renal failure in affected patients is liver disease rather than a primary renal process.

In this chapter we first review the pathophysiology underlying HRS. Because treatment of this condition is limited and the prognosis grim, the importance of avoiding potential precipitants and excluding other potentially reversible causes of renal dysfunction are emphasized. Last, we review current therapeutic options for the syndrome and suggest an approach to the evaluation of patients with cirrhosis in whom renal failure develops.

PATHOPHYSIOLOGY

Renal Abnormalities in Cirrhosis

The earliest change in renal function seen in patients with cirrhosis is renal sodium retention, which can be found when cirrhosis is entirely compensated. Renal sodium retention becomes clinically significant when the patient is unable to excrete a daily sodium load and develops ascites. The primary defect is increased absorption of sodium in the proximal and distal renal tubules, usually in the presence of a normal glomerular filtration rate (GFR). The mechanisms responsible for increased sodium absorption include activation of the renin-angiotensin-aldosterone system (RAAS), resulting in increased serum levels of renin and aldosterone, and stimulation of the sympathetic nervous system (SNS), resulting in increased serum levels of norepinephrine. However, a substantial number of patients with ascites have a normal RAAS and SNS, implying that other antinatriuretic mechanisms play a role.

Many patients with ascites are unable to excrete free water and may develop dilutional hyponatremia. Water retention occurs after sodium retention is established. However, in patients with compensated cirrhosis and even in some patients with ascites, renal water excretion is normal. The presumed mechanisms responsible for reduced water excretion in patients with cirrhosis are multiple. Among the abnormalities that have been described in patients with ascites are elevated levels of antidiuretic hormone (ADH); reduced synthesis of renal prostaglandins (PGs), particularly PGE_2; and reduced delivery of filtrate to the ascending limb of Henle (the diluting segment of the nephron). The relative contributions of these three factors varies; alterations in ADH and renal PGs appear to be more important in patients without renal failure, whereas reduced delivery of filtrate to the distal nephron is more important in those with HRS.

The final alteration in kidney function in patients with cirrhosis is renal vasoconstriction, which causes a decrease in both renal blood flow (RBF) and GFR. The effect of renal vasoconstriction on renal function can vary from reduced clearance of an exogenously administered solute (e.g., inulin) to full-blown HRS. HRS occurs in the setting of marked stimulation of both the RAAS and SNS in addition to elevated serum levels of both ADH and endothelin, all of which contribute to potent vasoconstriction. In addition, there is a reduction in the synthesis of local vasodilators (e.g., PGE, PGF, and kallikrein) in the kidney.

Mechanisms of Renal Vasoconstriction

As described previously, the pathophysiological basis of HRS is intense vasoconstriction affecting the renal vasculature. Activation of RAAS, with resultant elevations in the levels of renin, angiotensin II, and aldosterone, has both an antinatriuretic and direct renal vasoconstrictive effect and is thought to be a response to the profound systemic vasodilatation seen in patients with cirrhosis. Raised serum norepinephrine levels indicate an activated SNS, and lumbar sympathetic blocks have been shown to improve RBF in HRS. Serum levels of ADH are also increased in cirrhosis and cause predominantly medullary vasoconstriction in the kidneys. However, the principal effect of ADH is to reduce water excretion in an attempt to maintain systemic circulatory volume.

A number of natriuretic peptides have been found to be elevated in patients with HRS, including atrial (ANP), brain, and C-type natriuretic peptide. The effect of ANP is mediated by dilation of afferent arterioles and constriction of the efferent arterioles in renal glomeruli, with a resulting increase in GFR. ANP also has a direct inhibitory effect on sodium reabsorption at the inner medullary collecting tubules. Patients with ascites typically exhibit renal resistance to the natriuretic effects of ANP, however, presumably because of activation of the antinatriuretic systems (RAAS and SNS).

Serum levels of nitric oxide have been demonstrated to be increased in patients with cirrhosis and may be responsible for systemic vasodilatation. Although inhibition of nitric oxide synthesis alone has no direct effect on the renal circulation in rat models of cirrhosis, inhibition of both renal PG and nitric oxide synthesis results in marked renal vasoconstric-

Table 1 Vasoactive Mediators That Are Altered in Patients with Varying Degrees of Hepatic Dysfunction

	Compensated cirrhosis	Cirrhosis with ascites and normal glomerular filtration rate	Hepatorenal syndrome
		Plasma levels	
Renin activity	↔ or ↓	↑	↑↑
Norepinephrine	↔ or ↓	↑	↑↑
Antidiuretic hormone	↔	↑	↑↑
Atrial natriuretic peptide	↔	↑	↑↑
Glucagon	↑	↑	↑↑
Platelet activating factor	↔	↑	↑↑
Endothelin	↔	↑	↑↑
		Urine levels	
Prostaglandin E_2	↔	↑	↓
6-K-$PGF_1\alpha$	↔	↑	↓
PGI-M	↑	↑	↑
Thromboxane B_2	↔	↑	?
Kallikrein	↔	↑	↓
Cysteinyl leukotrienes	↔	↑	↑

Key: 6-K-$PGF_1\alpha$, 6-keto prostaglandin F-1 alpha ($PDF_1\alpha$) (a stable metabolite of renal prostacyclin); PGI-M, 2,3-dinor-6-keto-$PDF_1\alpha$ (a stable urinary metabolite of systemic prostacyclin); thromboxane B_2, a stable metabolite of thromboxane A_2
Source: Badalamenti et al., 1993.

tion. The precise role of nitric oxide in the renal circulatory changes seen in cirrhosis is under active investigation.

In the past decade, levels of numerous intrarenal substances have been shown to be altered in patients with HRS. Production of vasodilatory peptides, including kallikrein-kinin, PGE_2, and PGI_2, is reduced in patients with functional renal failure, whereas levels of vasoconstrictors like thromboxane A_2, endothelin, and platelet activating factor are elevated. An overview of the changes in various humoral mediators in HRS is shown in Table 1.

Overall, it appears that systemic vasoactive factors are activated to maintain arterial blood pressure in the presence of increased vascular capacitance in cirrhosis. At the same time, intrarenal processes attempt to protect RBF by producing locally acting vasodilatory molecules. When the renal protective effect begins to fail, renal dysfunction can occur and ascites may develop. If this process continues unabated, extreme renal vasoconstriction and HRS may ensue. The specific mechanisms responsible for renal dysfunction in cirrhosis remain to be elucidated. Which factors are primary and which are secondary, or compensatory, still needs to be clarified. What is clear is that HRS is one end of a spectrum of renal changes seen in cirrhosis. Figure 1 provides an overview of the cascade of hemodynamic alterations that may result from cirrhosis.

Hypotheses to Explain the Development of Renal Dysfunction and HRS

A number of theories have been proposed to explain the development of ascites and renal dysfunction in cirrhosis (see also Chap. 37). The original explanation proposed in the

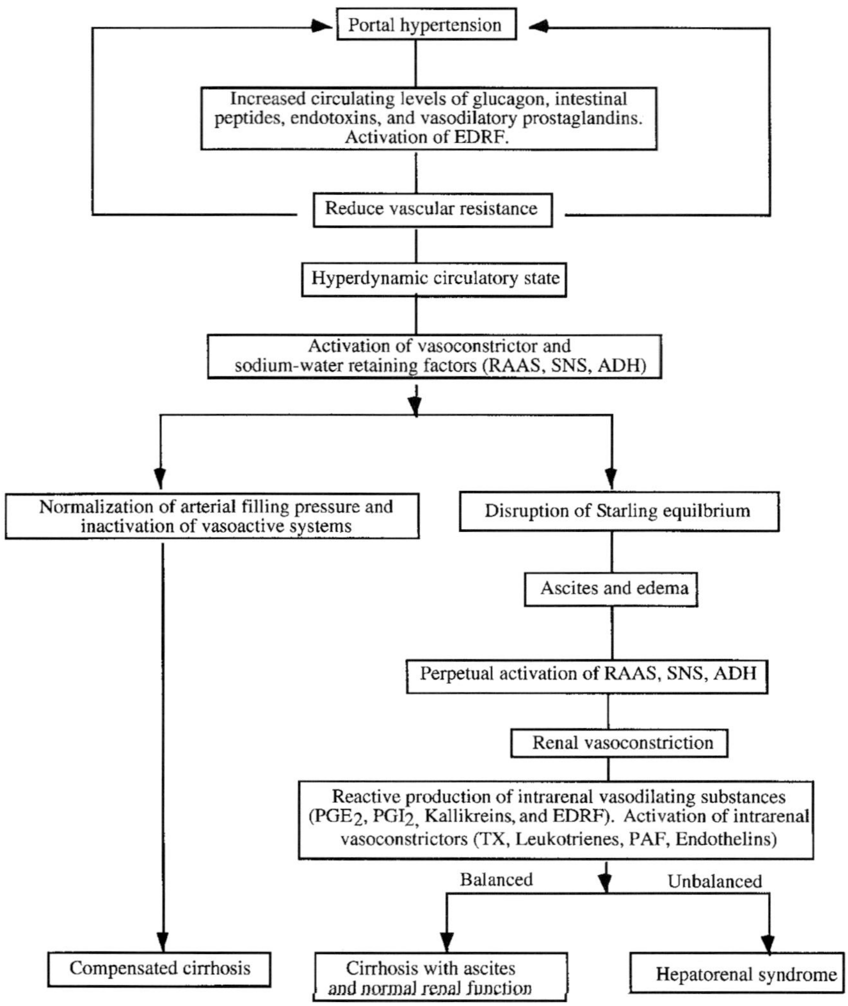

Figure 1 Factors thought to be involved in the development of circulatory changes seen in cirrhosis.

underfill hypothesis advocates that excess production of interstitial fluid in the liver results from portal hypertension, overwhelms the lymphatic drainage of the liver, and leads to accumulation of ascites in the peritoneal cavity. The consequence is intravascular hypovolemia, which triggers compensatory mechanisms (RAAS, SNS, and ADH) that cause sodium and water retention by the kidney. According to this theory, cardiac output and plasma volume should be low in patients with cirrhosis, but in fact the opposite is true.

To account for the hypervolemia that is typically found in patients with cirrhosis, the *overflow hypothesis* was proposed in 1970. This theory suggests that the primary event is a hepatorenal reflex (possibly mediated by the autonomic nervous system) that results in primary sodium retention by the kidney, leading, in turn, to hypervolemia and ascites. However, this theory fails to account for activation of the RAAS and SNS, which according to this hypothesis, should be depressed in the presence of an expanded plasma volume.

The peripheral vasodilatation hypothesis was put forward in 1988 in an attempt to reconcile the underfill and overflow hypotheses and account for the limitations of each. This theory suggests that portal hypertension directly causes splanchnic arterial vasodilatation, which leads to underfilling of the vascular compartment and a diminished effective arterial blood volume. Vasopressor mechanisms are then stimulated and result in renal compensation, including increased renal sodium absorption. When renal sodium absorption leads to effective replacement of arterial volume, cirrhosis remains compensated. On the other hand, if effective arterial filling remains low, vasoactive compensation leads to continuing renal sodium and water retention and eventually to ascites, reflecting a decompensated state. If equilibrium is not ultimately achieved, the final consequence of this attempt at compensation is unrelenting renal vasoconstriction and progression to HRS (Fig. 1).

CLINICAL FEATURES

Functional renal failure, or HRS, is a common complication of end-stage liver disease. In a prospective study, HRS developed in 18% of patients with cirrhosis and ascites after 1 year and 39% after 5 years. Typically, HRS develops in patients with advanced liver disease and ascites, although it can be seen in patients with acute liver failure as well. Invariable findings in HRS are profound renal vasoconstriction, with marked reductions in RBF and GFR and normal-appearing kidneys on histology.

Two clinical forms of HRS are recognized. Type 1 HRS is characterized by a rapid reduction in renal function, defined as a twofold increase in serum creatinine levels to greater than 2.5 mg/dL or a 50% drop in the creatinine clearance to less than 20 mL/min in less than 2 weeks. This type of HRS typically occurs in patients with advanced liver failure (often due to alcohol), jaundice, ascites, encephalopathy, and coagulopathy. In half of these patients, a precipitant such as surgery, gastrointestinal bleeding, infection, or recent paracentesis may be recognized. The patient develops progressive oliguria, dilutional hyponatremia, and hyperkalemia. The serum blood urea nitrogen (BUN) level typically reaches 60–120 mg/dL, and the serum creatinine level reaches 3–8 mg/dL. The prognosis is grim, with a median survival of only 2 weeks, far worse than that seen with other causes of acute renal failure in cirrhosis.

In Type 2 HRS the onset is more gradual, with a slow decline in GFR over weeks to months. Affected individuals often have well-preserved hepatic function and typically present with diuretic-resistant ascites. Usually the BUN is less than 50 mg/dL and serum creatinine less than 2 mg/dL. Although the short-term outlook of these patients is better than that of patients with type 1 HRS, they ultimately progress to a type 1 picture.

DIAGNOSIS

It is important to distinguish HRS from other causes of acute renal failure (ARF) that may develop in patients with cirrhosis, because the prognosis varies considerably depending on the etiology. The main challenge is to exclude prerenal azotemia and acute tubular necrosis, from which patients may be expected to recover. Unfortunately, there is no definitive test to confirm a diagnosis of HRS. Table 2 summarizes the characteristic laboratory and clinical findings that may help differentiate the three most common causes of ARF in a patient with cirrhosis.

Table 2 Urinary Findings in the Three Common Causes of Renal Failure in Patients with Liver Disease

	Hepatorenal syndrome	Prerenal azotemia	Acute tubular necrosis
Urine output (mL/24 h)	<500	<500	May be nonoliguric
Urine sodium (mEq/L)	<10 (often <5)	<20	>20–30
Urine:plasma creatinine ratio	>30	>30	<30
Urine:plasma urea ratio	>20	>20	<5
Fractional excretion of sodium (%)[a]	<1	<1	>1.5
Urine osmolality (mOsm/kg water)	>400	>400	Similar to plasma
Sediment	Normal or granular casts	Normal or granular casts	Renal tubular cells or muddy brown casts
Response to plasma expansion	None	Increase in urine output	None

[a]Fractional excretion of sodium = 100 × (urine/plasma sodium)/(urine/plasma creatinine)
Source: Badalamenti et al., 1993.

Patients with acute tubular necrosis (ATN) have an elevated urine sodium concentration, usually over 30 mEq/L, and urine that is nearly isosmolar with plasma. The findings reflect a loss of renal tubular function. Other markers of renal concentrating ability are deranged, including a urine-to-plasma creatinine ratio of less than 30:1 and a fractional excretion of sodium of greater than 1.5%. Cellular casts in the urinary sediment, when present, can help confirm a diagnosis of ATN.

As can be seen in Table 2, distinguishing prerenal azotemia from HRS can be difficult on the basis of urinary findings alone. Therefore, an intravenous fluid challenge is essential. In patients with prerenal azotemia, fluid administration is followed by a significant and prolonged improvement in urine output and serum markers of renal function. In contrast, in patients with HRS, the response to plasma expansion is limited and short-lived. Which fluid to administer is a matter of preference. In the criteria of the International Ascites Club described below, a challenge with 1.5 L of normal saline is recommended. However, normal saline can worsen the ascites typically present in patients with HRS, and others recommend use of salt-poor albumin, which remains in the vascular compartment longer than saline. Occasionally, measurements of central venous or capillary wedge pressure may be needed to exclude hypovolemia and titrate volume expansion.

In an attempt to standardize the nomenclature and definitions of syndromes associated with ascites, the International Ascites Club has recommended criteria for the diagnosis of HRS (Table 3). Five major criteria must be present for a diagnosis of HRS. In addition, five minor criteria are supportive of but not required for the diagnosis.

The first major criterion is that the patient have significant liver dysfunction and portal hypertension. The second criterion is renal dysfunction. Since synthesis of creatinine may be diminished in patients with cirrhosis and protein malnutrition, the serum creatinine can underestimate GFR. In addition, an elevated serum bilirubin level can interfere with the measurement of creatinine. Therefore, it is important to be aware that significant renal dysfunction may be present in patients with serum creatinine levels in the upper range of normal. Determination of the 24-h creatinine clearance may be helpful in borderline cases.

Table 3 Criteria of the International Ascites Club for Diagnosing the Hepatorenal Syndrome

Major criteria (all criteria must be met)
1. Chronic or acute liver disease with advanced hepatic failure and portal hypertension.
2. Low glomerular filtration rate, as indicated by a serum creatinine of >1.5 mg/dL or 24-h creatinine clearance <40 mL/min.
3. Absence of shock, ongoing bacterial infection, and current or recent treatment with nephrotoxic drugs. Absence of gastrointestinal fluid losses (e.g., vomiting or diarrhea) or renal fluid losses (e.g., overaggressive diuresis).
4. No sustained improvement of renal function (i.e., a decrease of serum creatinine < 1.5 mg/dL or increase in creatinine clearance to >40 mL/min) following the removal of diuretic therapy and volume expansion with 1.5 L of normal saline intravenously.
5. Proteinuria <500 mg/dL and no ultrasound evidence of either obstructive uropathy or parenchymal renal disease.

Additional criteria (usually present)
1. Urine volume <500 mL/day.
2. Urine sodium <10 mEq/L.
3. Urine osmolality greater than plasma osmolality.
4. Urine red blood cells <50 per high-power field.
5. Serum sodium concentration <130 mEq/L.

Source: Arroyo et al., 1996.

The other major criteria for HRS represent an attempt to exclude other causes of ARF. Acute tubular necrosis (ATN) is a frequent occurrence in patients with hypotension and low-flow states as a result of gastrointestinal bleeding, rapid fluid losses (e.g., diarrhea, vomiting, diuresis), or infection. ATN can even occasionally complicate HRS, but usually not in the early stages. The presence of β_2-microglobulin in urine may be used as a marker of tubular damage, and its absence can be helpful in excluding ATN. It is important to keep in mind that renal impairment develops in one-third of patients with spontaneous bacterial peritonitis (SBP), of whom one-third will recover renal function with antibiotic therapy. Cirrhotic patients with acute renal failure should therefore undergo a diagnostic paracentesis, as should any patient with decompensated cirrhosis, to exclude SBP.

The fact that some medications can precipitate renal failure should be considered. The main offenders include aminoglycosides, which can cause ATN, nonsteroidal anti-inflammatory drugs (NSAIDs), which inhibit renal vasodilatory prostaglandins synthesis, and diuretics, which may cause prerenal azotemia through volume depletion.

The last of the major criteria for HRS is the absence of significant proteinuria, which is a marker of glomerular disease. A renal ultrasound is recommended to exclude both parenchymal renal disease and postrenal obstruction as the cause of renal failure. Certain glomerulonephropathies may be associated with liver disease. For example, membranous or membranoproliferative glomerulonephritis has long been recognized as a complication of hepatitis B infection. Polyarteritis nodosa is also well described in hepatitis B surface antigen–positive patients, some of whom also have cryoglobulinemia or a serum sickness-like illness. Similarly, patients with hepatitis C infection can develop type II cryoglobulinemia and membranoproliferative glomerulonephritis. Membranous glomerulonephriphritis is an important complication of autoimmune hepatitis, since it is usually responsive to therapy with corticosteroids. Last, IgA nephropathy can be seen in patients with alcoholic cirrhosis.

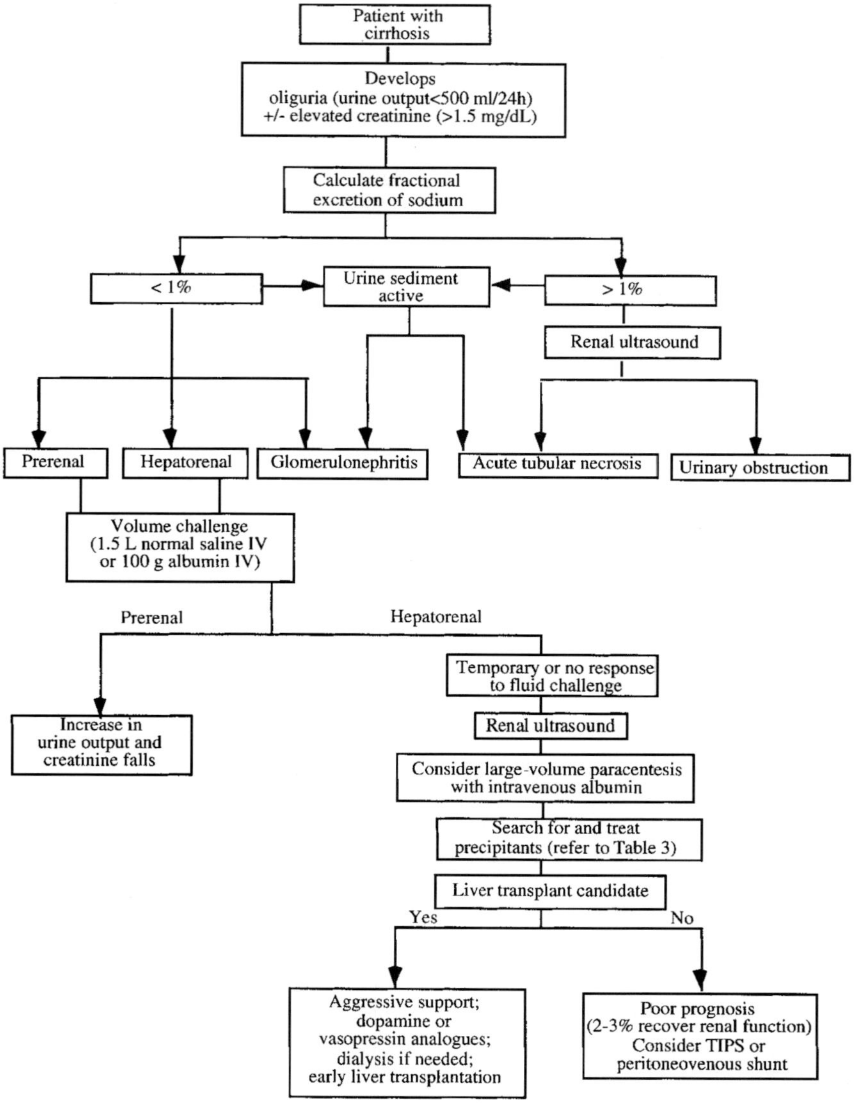

Figure 2 A suggested approach to evaluating the patient with advanced liver disease in whom renal failure develops.

The minor criteria for HRS consist mainly of the urinary findings described above. One should be cautious in making a diagnosis of HRS in the absence of these findings, but well-documented cases of HRS without oliguria or a urine sodium concentration below 10 mEq/L have been reported.

Figure 2 presents an overall approach to the evaluation of patients with cirrhosis in whom renal failure develops (see below).

PROGNOSTIC FACTORS

In view of the poor outcome of patients with HRS, the question arises as to whether there is any way to predict the risk of developing the syndrome. In 1993, Ginès et al. reported that neither the Child-Pugh score nor etiology of cirrhosis was helpful in predicting the risk of HRS. However, among cirrhotic patients hospitalized with ascites, the following findings were associated with an increased risk of HRS: hepatomegaly, serum sodium concentration < 134 mEq/L, and plasma renin level > 3.5 ng/mL/h.

More recently, Platt et al. described the use of Doppler ultrasound of the renal arteries at the corticomedullary junction or the interlobular arteries to calculate a resistive index (RI) as a measure of renal vasoconstriction. Among patients with an elevated RI (i.e., $>$ 0.7), renal dysfunction developed in 42% and frank HRS developed in 26% over a mean follow-up of 263 days. In contrast, only 6% of patients with a normal RI (i.e., $<$ 0.7) developed renal dysfunction, and only 1% developed HRS. An elevated RI was predictive of the risk of developing HRS in this study. If this finding is reproducible, it may allow high-risk patients to be identified prior to the development of HRS so that preventive treatment can be initiated.

THERAPEUTIC APPROACHES

Unfortunately, treatment of HRS is limited. The only effective long-term treatments are those that reverse hepatic dysfunction, such as liver transplantation. In fact, following liver transplantation, patients with HRS have the same long-term survival rate as those without functional renal failure. Therefore, patients with HRS should be considered for liver transplantation as early as possible if they are otherwise eligible.

In addition to supportive care and a search for treatable precipitants, a number of pharmaceutical approaches have been attempted in patients with HRS. Intravenous administration of low "renal" dose dopamine (1–3 μg/kg/min) may improve renal function in some cases by increasing RBF. However, GFR may not improve, and when the infusion of dopamine is discontinued, oliguria usually recurs. Other dopaminergic agonists such as ibopamine and fenoldopam have not proved helpful.

In an attempt to correct systemic hypotension, alpha and beta sympathomimetic agents such as phenoxybenzamine, isoproternol, and metaraminol have been tried without success. Other vasoactive medications, including calcium-channel blockers, angiotensin converting enzyme inhibitors, alpha-adrenergic receptor blockers, and clonidine (to reduce central sympathetic outflow) have also failed to show a benefit. Use of prostaglandins in patients with HRS has also been disappointing. In one report of four patients with HRS in whom the PGE_1 agonist misoprostil was used in association with volume expansion with albumin, only transient improvement in renal function was demonstrated, and all four patients died within 1 month. Subsequent studies using misoprostil have failed to confirm a beneficial effect. Use of endothelin-receptor antagonists or adenosine to improve renal circulation has been suggested as a therapeutic approach but has not been studied.

Analogues of vasopressin have been reported to be of some benefit in HRS. Ornipressin, administered in a dose of 6 IU/h, causes splanchic and mesenteric vasoconstriction without increasing intrarenal resistance. Lenz et al. have shown that ornipressin increases renal sodium excretion and inulin clearance and reverses the hyperdynamic circulation nearly to normal. Unfortunately, the drug has to be given as a continuous intravenous infusion, and the observed changes reverse on discontinuation of the medication. Terlipressin, a vasopressin analogue that can be given intravenously in a dose of 1–3 mg twice daily, has been used as an alternative to ornipressin to maintain renal function in a patient with HRS for 2 months until a liver became available for transplantation, but experience with this approach is limited. More recently, aprotinin (an inhibitor of the kallikrein-kinin system) has been shown to increase systemic vascular resistance in patients with cirrhosis complicated by ascites, with resulting increases in RBF, GFR, and natriuresis. These findings require confirmation in larger studies.

Surgical portacaval shunts have occasionally been reported to improve renal function in patients with HRS, presumably by increasing effective blood volume. However, others have not confirmed these results, and in view of the high operative mortality rates associated with this approach, surgery in patients with advanced liver disease has fallen out of favor. Although the use of peritoneovenous shunts has been successful in the treatment of refractory ascites, results are less impressive in HRS, although occasional successes have been described. The high complication rate—with disseminated intravascular coagulation, vascular thrombosis, and infection—argues against the use of peritoneovenous shunts in most patients.

Insertion of a transjugular intrahepatic portosystemic shunt (TIPS) has been tried in a number of patients with HRS. In an abstract, Brensing et al. described eight patients with well-documented HRS (two on dialysis) in whom urine output and sodium excretion improved over the 2 weeks following placement of a TIPS. BUN and serum creatinine levels fell, and dialysis was withdrawn. Seven of the patients were discharged from the hospital, and only one patient died 4 weeks later (of liver failure). A number of case reports have also described dramatic improvement in renal function following TIPS placement in patients with HRS. Although promising, these initial reports have been limited to abstracts and case reports. Controlled studies will be needed before TIPS can be generally recommended. It is important to remember that in patients with refractory ascites in whom TIPS is performed, initiation of natriuresis may take 2 weeks, and negative sodium balance may not be achieved for 4 weeks. Also, patients over age 70 may respond less favorably and are at greater risk of complications from the procedure than younger patients. Nevertheless, TIPS looks like a promising approach for the future, especially in patients who are not eligible for liver transplantation.

Dialysis may be considered in patients with HRS who are awaiting liver transplantation until a donor organ becomes available. Otherwise, patients with HRS obtain no survival benefit and should not undergo dialysis. Patients with nonfunctional renal failure due to other causes may benefit from dialysis.

OVERALL APPROACH TO THE CIRRHOTIC PATIENT WITH RENAL FAILURE

It is essential that physicians caring for patients with liver disease be aware of risk factors for HRS. Both physicians and patients should be alert to early signs of clinical deterioration, such as weight gain or diuretic resistance, or overt complications like gastrointestinal bleeding or infection. These should be treated promptly to avoid a further decline in liver or renal function. In patients with ascites, diuresis should be initiated, and weight loss should not exceed 0.5 kg/day, or 1 kg/day if peripheral edema is present. If large-volume paracentesis is attempted, intravascular volume repletion with salt-poor albumin should occur simultaneously or be completed within 6 h of the paracentesis (5–10 g of salt-poor albumin per liter of ascites removed). In addition, patients should be advised to avoid use of over-the-counter medications such as NSAIDs. Nevertheless, despite close monitoring and avoidance of precipitants, HRS may still develop. Figure 2 offers an approach to the evaluation of a cirrhotic patient in whom renal failure develops.

When renal failure develops in a patient with cirrhosis, the first step in management is to exclude causes of renal failure other than HRS. The urine should be examined for findings suggestive of ATN (Table 2). If the clinical and urinary pictures are consistent with prerenal azotemia, volume expansion should be initiated with normal saline or with albumin if the serum albumin is < 2.5 g/L. Failure of urine output to increase after a suitable challenge (e.g., at least 1.5 L of saline) confirms the diagnosis of HRS (Table 3). Some authorities advocate performance of a large-volume paracentesis (4–6L over 1 h) with intravenous administration of albumin (100 g in 500 mL normal saline). Large-volume paracentesis increases cardiac output by improving venous return and reduces renal venous congestion, thereby improving renal circulation. If there is concern about the adequacy of volume expansion, a central venous catheter may be placed to exclude hypovolemia and guide fluid resuscitation. Last, a renal ultrasound should be obtained to exclude postrenal obstruction.

In the patient with functional renal failure, a search for aggravating factors should be conducted; if identified, there should be treated appropriately (see Table 3). All patients should have a diagnostic paracentesis to exclude spontaneous bacterial peritonitis. This can be carried out even in the presence of coagulopathy, using a 20-gauge needle. Patients with acute liver failure should be evaluated promptly for liver transplantation, and those who are candidates should be supported aggressively until a donor organ becomes available. Patients with chronic liver disease may already be on a transplant waiting list, and their priority status can be increased. Unfortunately, due to the shortage of donor organs, patients with HRS often succumb to advanced liver disease before transplantation can be performed.

In patients with HRS awaiting liver transplantation, a number of pharmacological therapies may be considered, as discussed above. Intravenous infusion of low-dose dopamine (1–3 μg/kg/min) or the vasopressin analogues ornipressin (2–6 IU/h) or terlipressin (2–6 mg/day) can help stabilize renal function. Dialysis can also be used to support a patient. However, these measures provide only temporary improvement and should be reserved for cases in which liver transplantation is anticipated or deterioration in liver function is potentially reversible.

Therapeutic options are limited in patients with HRS who are not candidates for liver transplantation. The aforementioned therapies (other than liver transplantation) do not alter the natural history of HRS and, in general, should not be pursued in this group of patients. However, in these patients with a uniformly bleak outlook, novel therapies have been tried, as mentioned above. Early reports suggest that TIPS may successfully reverse renal failure associated with HRS, at least in some cases. In patients unsuitable for transplantation and aware of the significant morbidity involved (including the risk of developing encephalopathy, bleeding, and worsening liver function), TIPS may offer a chance for prolonged survival and should be considered, preferably in a study setting. Another option that can be considered is a peritoneovenous (e.g., LeVeen) shunt, for which limited success has been described.

SUMMARY

Although our understanding of the pathophysiology of HRS has advanced in the past decade, the precise mechanisms and mediators involved still need to be clarified. Optimal management is based on early recognition of HRS and exclusion of other forms of renal failure. In addition, avoidance of precipitating events and early treatment of complications are critical. Unfortunately, therapeutic options for HRS remain limited; in fact, liver transplantation is the only long-term treatment of proven efficacy. Recently, TIPS has been reported to reverse progressive renal failure in some patients with HRS, but controlled studies are needed to confirm these findings and to help identify patients who may benefit from this intervention. In the future, improved understanding of the humoral derangements seen in HRS may allow new pharmacological approaches to be explored. For now, HRS remains a significant cause of mortality in patients with liver disease.

BIBLIOGRAPHY

Arroyo V, Ginès P, Gerbes AL, Dudley FJ, Gentilini P, Laffi G, Reynolds TB, Ring-Larsen H, Scholmerich J. Definition and diagnostic criteria of refractory ascites and hepatorenal syndrome in cirrhosis. Hepatology 1996; 23:164–176.

Badalamenti S, Graziani G, Salerno F, Ponticelli C. Hepatorenal syndrome: new perspectives in pathogenesis and treatment. Arch Intern Med 1993; 153:1957–1967.

Brensing KA, Textor J, Raab P, Schiedermaier P, Strunk H, Falkenhausen MV, Perz J, Gorich J, Klehr HU, Schild H, Sauerbruch T. Sustained improvement of hepatorenal syndrome after TIPS insertion in patients with terminal liver cirrhosis not eligible for transplantation. Gastroenterology 1996; 110:A1158.

Forrest EH, Jalan R, Hayes PC. Review article: renal circulatory changes in cirrhosis—pathogenesis and therapeutic prospects. Aliment Pharmacol Ther 1996; 10:219–231.

Ginès A, Escorell A, Ginès P, Salo J, Jimenez W, Inglada L, Navasa M, Caria J, Rimola A, Arroyo V, Rodes J. Incidence, predictive factors, and prognosis of the hepatorenal syndrome in cirrhosis with ascites. Gastroenterology 1993; 105:229–236.

Lenz K, Hortnagel H, Drum W, Reither H, Schmid R, Schneeweiss B, Laggner A, Grimm G, Gerbes AL. Ornipressin in the treatment of functional renal failure in decompensated liver cirrhosis. Gastroenterology 1991; 101:1060–1067.

Platt JF, Ellis JH, Rubin JM, Merion RM, Lucey MR. Renal duplex Doppler ultrasound: a noninvasive predictor of kidney dysfunction and hepatorenal failure in liver disease. Hepatology 1994; 20:362–369.

Roberts LR, Kamath PS. Ascites and hepatorenal syndrome: pathophysiology and management. Mayo Clin Proc 1996; 71:874–881.

40

Management of the Hematological Complications of Liver Disease

Richard F. Branda
University of Vermont College of Medicine, Burlington, Vermont

Hematological abnormalities are diverse and frequent in patients with liver disease (Table 1). For the most part, the magnitude of the hematological changes parallels the severity of the liver disease. Clinically the most important hematological complication of liver disease is the highly complex coagulopathy that affects virtually every aspect of the clotting system. It has been estimated that 85% of patients with liver disease have at least one hemostatic abnormality and that 15% have a clinical bleeding tendency. In general, clotting test abnormalities are more predictive of clinical bleeding in patients with acute hepatitis than in patients with cirrhosis. For example, among 104 patients with acute infectious hepatitis, the coagulation defect was mild and not associated with bleeding in those without liver failure, while patients with liver failure had severe coagulopathies and nearly 60% had significant bleeding. In contrast, the relationship between coagulation abnormalities and clinical, particularly variceal, bleeding is less clear in patients with chronic hepatocellular disease, perhaps because the bleeding is due to the interaction of multiple factors. In patients with severe or advanced liver disease, anemia, leukopenia, and thrombocytopenia may be prominent. Effective management of the hematological complications of liver disease utilizes systematic evaluation and judicious treatment based upon an understanding of the underlying pathophysiology.

PATHOPHYSIOLOGY OF COAGULATION FACTOR ABNORMALITIES

Several mechanisms have been identified in liver disease that eventuate in a coagulopathy. These include a fall in clotting factor and natural protease inhibitor production, increased consumption of clotting factors, decreased clearance of activated clotting factors, and production of functionally abnormal clotting proteins.

Vitamin K deficiency is the most easily correctible hemostatic abnormality due to decreased clotting factor production. This fat-soluble vitamin is malabsorbed by patients with intra- or extrahepatic biliary obstruction and by patients being treated with bile acid

Table 1 Hematological Abnormalities in Patients with Liver Disease

- I. Erythrocytes
  - A. Decreased number
    - 1. Impaired production
      - a. Folic acid deficiency
      - b. Vitamin B_{12} deficiency
      - c. Iron deficiency
      - d. Anemia of chronic disease
      - e. Ethanol toxicity
    - 2. Increased destruction
      - a. Hypersplenism
      - b. Spur cell hemolytic anemia
      - c. Zieve's syndrome
      - d. Stomatocytosis
  - B. Relative anemia secondary to increased plasma volume
  - C. Morphological changes
    - 1. Acanthocytes
    - 2. Target cells
    - 3. Macrocytes
    - 4. Spherocytes
- II. Granulocytes
  - A. Decreased number
    - 1. Drug toxicity
    - 2. Folic acid deficiency
    - 3. Vitamin B_{12} deficiency
    - 4. Ethanol toxicity
    - 5. Infection
  - B. Abnormal distribution due to splenic sequestration
- III. Platelets
  - A. Decreased number
    - 1. Splenic sequestration
    - 2. Folic acid deficiency
    - 3. Vitamin B_{12} deficiency
    - 4. Ethanol toxicity
    - 5. Immune-mediated
    - 6. Disseminated intravascular coagulation
    - 7. Drug toxicity
  - B. Impaired platelet function
    - 1. Abnormal platelet aggregation in vitro
    - 2. Prolonged bleeding time
- IV. Clotting factor abnormality
  - A. Decreased clotting factor and natural protease inhibitor production
  - B. Increased consumption of clotting factors
  - C. Decreased clearance of activated clotting factors
  - D. Production of functionally abnormal clotting proteins
- V. Aplastic anemia

binders such as cholestyramine. Vitamin K is also synthesized by intestinal bacteria. Therefore patients receiving antibiotics are particularly susceptible to vitamin K deficiency. Since body stores of this vitamin are limited, frank deficiency can develop within a few weeks of reduced bile salt availability or from the combination of poor dietary intake and antibiotics. Characteristically, vitamin K deficiency results in a dissociation of clotting factor antigen levels and the procoagulant activities of these factors: antigen levels are normal while coagulant activities are low due to decreased availability of vitamin K for postribosomyl carboxylation and hypocarboxylated factors. In contrast, when liver synthetic function is impaired, both antigen and coagulant levels are low. The vitamin K–dependent factors are II, VII, IX, and X and proteins C and S. These factor deficiencies are usually detected by a prolonged prothrombin time (PT), but the activated partial thromboplastin time (PTT) may also be abnormally long because deficiencies of factors II, IX, and X also affect this test.

Failure of Clotting Factor Production by the Diseased Liver

Damage to liver parenchymal cells leads to a decrease in the level of most plasma clotting factors due to impaired synthesis. The factor deficiencies that are of greatest clinical relevance are factors VII, X and II. Factor IX is affected to a lesser extent by hepatocellular disease. Factor V is regularly decreased in chronic liver disease but variably reduced in acute hepatitis. Since the bleeding abnormality associated with factor V deficiency is relatively mild, the likely contribution of a decrease in factor V to the hemostatic defect in liver disease is probably modest. Likewise, the decrease in plasma levels of prekallikrein, high-molecular-weight kininogen, and factors XIII, XII, and XI associated with liver disease appear to contribute little to the bleeding diathesis. Fibrinogen levels are usually normal or high in patients with liver disease because fibrinogen is an acute-phase reactant. However, patients with advanced cirrhosis or severe acute hepatitis may develop hypofibrinogenemia. Fibrinogen levels under 100 mg/dL are associated with abnormal clotting tests [the thrombin time (TT) is most sensitive, but the PT and PTT may also be prolonged] and a bleeding tendency. Liver disease also can eventuate in reduced synthesis of plasma anticoagulants: deficiencies of antithrombin III, protein C, and heparin cofactor II have been reported. The clinical significance of these changes in anticoagulant levels is uncertain at present but it's probably modest, since abnormalities of protein C are usually not associated with an increased thrombotic risk in patients with liver disease.

In contrast to the deficiencies in clotting proteins associated with liver disease, levels of factor VIII:C and von Willebrand antigen and activity are typically mildly to moderately increased because they are synthesized in extrahepatic sites. This observation can be used to distinguish between those patients with liver disease who have predominantly decreased synthesis of clotting factors from patients with superimposed disseminated intravascular coagulation (DIC), since in the former group the factor VIII level will be high, while in the latter group it will be low due to consumption. Thus, the typical clotting test profile in patients with liver disease and decreased synthesis of clotting factors is a prolonged PT that correlates with the severity of the hepatocellular damage, normal to variable lengthening of the PTT, a TT that is usually normal unless hypofibrinogenemia develops, and elevated levels of factor VIII.

Increased Consumption of Clotting Factors

Coagulation factors equilibrate into ascitic or edema fluid, thereby reducing intravascular levels of these proteins. The extent to which chronic low grade DIC contributes to the coagulopathy of liver disease is controversial. DIC could be initiated by hepatocellular necrosis or by entry of endotoxin into the circulation from the intestine in patients with portal hypertension and sustained by decreased clearance of activated clotting factors. Observations favoring the presence of DIC in liver disease include shortened fibrinogen survival, increased thrombin/antithrombin III complex formation, elevated levels of fibrinopeptide A (FPA), increased levels of D-dimers and other fibrin degradation products (FDP), and decreased levels of factor VIII. Thus both increased thrombin generation and elevated plasmin formation have been found in patients with liver disease. However, these abnormalities are seen in many but not all patients with significant liver disease, and each might have other explanations (Fig. 1). Therefore, the diagnosis of DIC in the setting of liver disease is often difficult because of the multiple abnormalities of the coagulation system and the lack of specific tests for DIC. Since the extent of any chronic DIC is related to the severity of the underlying liver disease, there is little to be done to correct it short of improving liver function. In contrast, it is important to recognize superimposed DIC due to another, more treatable cause such as sepsis, shock, or pulmonary embolus. In these cases it is critical to identify and treat the precipitating factor so as to correct the additional coagulopathy leading to decompensated DIC. Laboratory tests indicative of new DIC are a dropping platelet count, red cell fragments, a decrease in levels of fibrinogen and factor

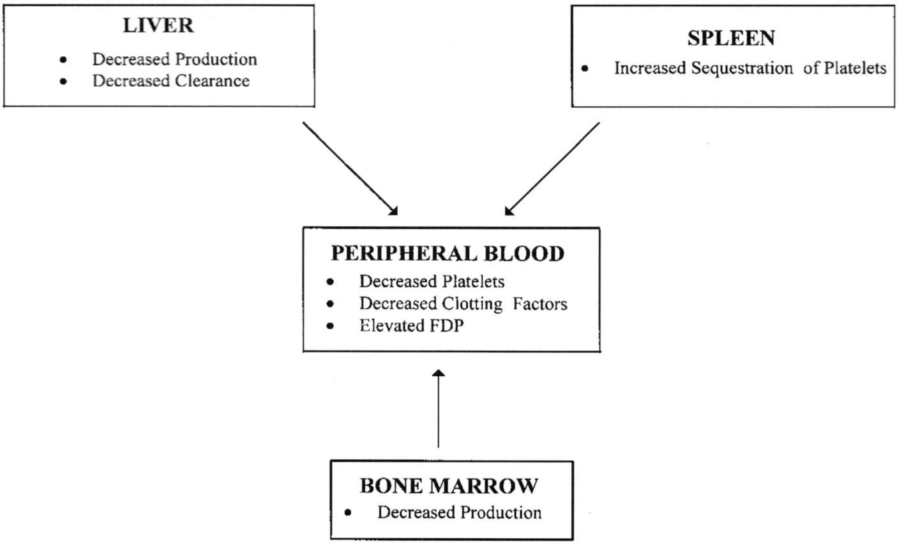

Figure 1 Net effect in blood compartment can mimic DIC. Decreased clotting factor and blood cell production, decreased activated factor clearance, and increased sequestration of platelets in liver disease can mimic the laboratory abnormalities of DIC or exacerbate ongoing DIC.

VIII, and rising FDPs. The fibrinogen level is a particularly robust assay for this purpose, since fibrinogen levels usually remain adequate in the face of all but the most advanced liver disease. Therefore, a fibrinogen level of less than 120 mg/dL should raise a suspicion of DIC.

Another cause of increased clotting factor consumption in patients with liver disease is accelerated fibrinolysis. This may be secondary to DIC or to alterations in the plasminogen/plasmin system. Elevated levels of plasminogen activators such as TPA—together with reduced synthesis of plasminogen and impaired clearance of plasminogen activators by the reticuloendothelial system—result in increased fibrinolytic activity. A relationship between the extent of increased fibrinolysis and clinical bleeding in patients with liver disease has been postulated. The presence of hyperfibrinolysis is suggested by a shortened euglobulin lysis time and elevated fibrin degradation products. Unfortunately, the former test is not widely available and the latter is nonspecific. Thus, like DIC, increased fibrinolysis is difficult to identify accurately in patients with liver disease.

Decreased Clearance of Activated Clotting Factors

The reticuloendothelial system of the liver is involved in clearance of activated clotting factors (IXa, Xa, and XIa), plasminogen activators, and fibrin degradation products. The resulting abnormalities in the regulation of coagulation in patients with liver disease contribute to the development of primary fibrinolysis and DIC.

Synthesis of Abnormal Clotting Proteins

Reduced carboxylation of clotting factors due to vitamin K deficiency leads to the production of nonfunctioning molecules. Synthesis of fibrinogen containing excess negatively charged sialic acid residues can result in dysfibrinogenemia. This abnormal protein has a decreased capacity for fibrin polymerization due to the increased net negative charge. Dysfibrinogenemia is identified by a prolonged TT in the presence of normal levels of fibrinogen and fibrin degradation products. Abnormal prothrombin (des-gamma-carboxy prothrombin) and protein C molecules have been described in patients with hepatocellular carcinoma. Abnormal prothrombin can be identified by the native II enzyme-linked immunosorbent assay (ELISA).

PATHOPHYSIOLOGY OF PLATELET ABNORMALITIES

Mild to moderate thrombocytopenia is common in liver disease. It has been estimated that 16% of patients with acute hepatitis without liver failure, 52% with liver failure, and one-third of cirrhotic patients will have thrombocytopenia. In most cases this is due to *splenic sequestration* from congestive splenomegaly. In these patients, platelet survival is reduced, but platelet production is nearly doubled. The platelet count is typically between 50–100,000/μL and rarely drops below 20,000/μL. Consequently, thrombocytopenia secondary to hypersplenism usually does not produce a bleeding diathesis by itself.

Folic acid deficiency is an easily treatable cause of thrombocytopenia. Patients with alcoholic liver disease are particularly susceptible to folate deficiency. In one study, megaloblastic hemopoiesis developed 5–10 weeks following initiation of a low-folate diet in chronic alcoholics as compared with 19 weeks in normal subjects. Moreover, ethanol per se accelerated the development of megaloblastic anemia by 2 weeks in the same subjects. This acceleration probably reflects the direct toxic effect of alcohol on hematopoiesis and on folate metabolism. Decreased absorption of folate, impaired intracellular folate metabolism, and increased urinary folate excretion have been described in alcohol abusers.

Patients with chronic liver disease of diverse origin can develop *immune-mediated thrombocytopenia*; this complication is particularly common in autoimmune hepatitis and is also seen in patients with chronic hepatitis C, sometimes only after interferon-alpha treatment. Platelet-associated IgG and serum immune complex levels are elevated and thrombocytopenia has resolved following splenectomy. A second mechanism causing shortened platelet survival in liver disease is *DIC* (Table 1). Rapid DIC can accompany fulminant hepatitis with severe hepatocellular damage, while features of chronic, low-grade DIC have been observed in cirrhotic patients. In any patient with thrombocytopenia, *drugs* should be considered as a possible cause. Usually the thrombocytopenia is due to immune-mediated platelet destruction except in the case of thiazide derivatives, which impair platelet production. All nonessential drugs should be discontinued and, if possible, essential drugs should be replaced by chemically unrelated compounds with similar clinical effects. In general, the thrombocytopenia will improve within 1–2 weeks of stopping the offending drug. The drugs most frequently associated with thrombocytopenia include heparin, valproic acid, thiazide derivatives, antibiotics (sulfas, penicillins, and cephalosporins) and gold salts, although many others have been implicated. *Ethanol ingestion* has a direct toxic effect on the bone marrow and thereby decreases platelet production. The thrombocytopenia persists for several days following withdrawal of alcohol before rising to normal or supranormal levels.

Platelet function is usually normal, but abnormalities in some patients with liver disease have been described. These include impaired in vitro platelet aggregation, prolonged bleeding time out of proportion to the extent of thrombocytopenia, and reduced ATP and serotonin release by platelets. The degree of abnormal platelet function often parallels the severity of the underlying liver disease. Platelet aggregation in response to ADP and thrombin was consistently abnormal in patients with prolonged TTs but not in those with normal or only slightly prolonged (< 5 s) TTs. This abnormality in platelet aggregation has been attributed to FDPs. Abnormal platelet function in patients with advanced cirrhosis has been implicated in bleeding from esophageal varices and is considered by some investigators to be a poor prognostic sign.

EVALUATION OF HEMOSTATIC DEFECTS

The initial hematological evaluation of a patient with liver disease (Table 2) should include a personal and family history of bleeding tendency; a careful drug and dietary history; physical examination for evidence of bleeding and splenomegaly; an examination of the peripheral blood smear; measurement of hemoglobin, hematocrit, red cell indices, white blood cell count, and differential; and also platelet count, PT, PTT, and TT.

Prolonged PT and/or PTT

Perform a 50:50 mix. If the prolonged test corrects, a deficiency of one or more clotting factors is present. Incomplete correction suggests an inhibitor/inactivator. Appropriate studies, including an antiphospholipid antibody assay and a dilute Russell's viper venom test, should be considered.

Prolonged TT

This suggests the presence of fibrin split products, abnormal fibrinogen, or low fibrinogen level. Measure D-dimer or FDPs and fibrinogen. Elevated fibrin split products may indicate DIC or fibrinolysis. A precipitating cause of DIC such as infection should be sought. Measuring a factor VIII level can be helpful in identifying DIC, since it is usually normal or high in liver disease but low in DIC. The combination of low fibrinogen and increased fibrin split products can also be found in increased fibrinolysis. A shortened euglobulin lysis time would support this diagnosis if the test is available. Normal levels of fibrin split products and fibrinogen suggest dysfibrinogenemia.

Thrombocytopenia

Measure serum vitamin B_{12} and folate levels, since the latter vitamin is frequently deficient in patients with liver disease and both deficiencies are easily treatable. Assays of antiplatelet antibodies may be useful in selected patients. In patients who have extensive mucosal or cutaneous bleeding despite seemingly adequate platelet counts, a bleeding time or platelet function test may be of diagnostic value. It should be noted, however, that anemia alone can lengthen the bleeding time. All drugs the patient is receiving should be reviewed and any that are associated with thrombocytopenia discontinued. Bone marrow examination is helpful in assessing megakaryocyte number and morphology, cellularity, and the presence of other disease states that are contributing to the thrombocytopenia. However, a bone marrow examination is usually not necessary in most patients with thrombocytopenia and liver disease.

Table 2 Management of the Coagulopathy in Liver Disease

I. Initial evaluation
   A. Personal and family history of bleeding tendency
   B. Drug and dietary history
   C. Physical exam for evidence of bleeding and splenomegaly
   D. Examination of peripheral smear
   E. Measurement of hemoglobin level, hematocrit, red cell indices, and reticulocyte count
   F. White cell count and differential
   G. Platelet count
   H. PT, PTT, TT

II. If no clinical bleeding or need for invasive studies and laboratory abnormalities are stable:
   A. Prolonged PT and/or PTT: do 50:50 mix
      1. If corrects, administer vitamin K
      2. If does not correct, investigate for inhibitor/inactivator
   B. Prolonged TT
      1. Measure D-dimer or FDP; if elevated suggests DIC, fibrinolysis or decreased clearance of FDPs
         a. Low factor VIII suggests DIC
         b. Shortened euglobulin lysis time suggests fibrinolysis
      2. Measure fibrinogen
         a. Low fibrinogen and elevated D-dimer or FDP suggests DIC or fibrinolysis
         b. Normal or slightly decreased fibrinogen and normal or slightly increased D-dimer or FDP suggests dysfibrinogenemia
   C. Thrombocytopenia
      1. Measure serum vitamin B_{12} and folate levels and red cell folate level
      2. Stop any drug associated with thrombocytopenia
      3. Antiplatelet antibody test may be of some use
      4. Bone marrow aspirate and biopsy if a disease process in addition to liver disease is suspected
      5. Anemia may contribute to a bleeding tendency

III. If clinically significant bleeding is present or invasive procedure in needed:
   A. Administer vitamin K
   B. If vitamin K ineffective or rapid correction required
      1. Fresh frozen plasma
      2. Cryoprecipitate for fibrinogen <100 mg/dL
      3. Platelet transfusion if actively bleeding or for invasive procedure if platelet count $<50{,}000/\mu L$
      4. Desmopressin (DDAVP)

IV. Severe bleeding where patient cannot tolerate large fluid volumes
   A. Prothrombin complex concentrates
   B. Exchange transfusion

V. If laboratory abnormalities are progressive or evidence of DIC
   A. Investigate for initiating factor, particularly infection
   B. Replace clotting factors and platelets
   C. Therapeutic measures of unproven value
      1. Heparin
      2. Antithrombin III concentrates
      3. Antifibrinolytic agents (may be dangerous)
      4. Antiplatelet agents

MANAGEMENT OF HEMOSTATIC FAILURE IN LIVER DISEASE (Table 2)

Clotting Factor Deficiencies

A trial of vitamin K is worthwhile in patients with liver disease and a prolonged PT. *Vitamin K_1*, 10 mg daily for a maximum of 3 successive days, is given slowly intravenously to avoid hypotension. The subcutaneous route can be used but may be associated with unpredictable absorption. Intramuscular injections should be avoided because of hematoma formation. Correction of the PT should begin within 6–8 h and be totally correct within 3 days. Incomplete correction indicates the presence of another cause for the clotting factor deficiency.

If the patient is bleeding or requires an invasive procedure, the PT should be corrected to less than 3 s over control. Many experienced clinicians consider invasive procedures such as liver biopsies, thoracocentesis, paracentesis, and placement of central lines contraindicated if the PT is prolonged more than 3 s. *Fresh frozen plasma (FFP)* contains all of the clotting factors that are diminished in patients with liver disease, but total correction of the hemostatic defect with FFP is often difficult. The amount of FFP needed to provide adequate levels of coagulation factors is 25–30% of the total plasma volume, estimated from the formula:

$$\text{Plasma volume} = (70 \text{ mL/kg} \times \text{kg body weight})(1 - \text{hematocrit})$$

For example, for a 70-kg individual,

$$\text{PV} = 70 \text{ mL/kg} \times 70 \text{ kg} = 4900 \text{ mL} \times (1 - 0.4) = 2940 \text{ mL}$$

The clotting factor with the shortest half-life determines how often FFP must be given. Since factor VII has a half-life of 2–5 h, and a level of 20% or more is needed to provide adequate hemostasis, FFP may be required as often as every 6–12 h. Many patients, particularly those with cardiovascular disease, cannot tolerate the FFP volumes required to normalize the PT. These volumes are increased further in patients with added clotting factor consumption or with sequestration into ascitic fluid. Monitoring for evidence of bleeding and measuring the PT 4–6 h after transfusion provides a guide to further therapy.

Other blood products available for replacement are *cryoprecipitate* and *prothrombin complex concentrates*. Patients with fibrinogen levels below 100 mg/dL can be conveniently corrected with cryoprecipitate. Each unit of cryoprecipitate contains approximately 250 mg of fibrinogen. Generally 0.5–1.0 U/100 mL of plasma volume is adequate, but larger volumes may be required in patients with ascites. Prothrombin complex concentrates lack some clotting factors that are deficient in patients with liver disease and therefore must be given in conjunction with FFP. Prothrombin complex concentrates contain activated clotting factors that are cleared poorly by a diseased liver. Therefore their use should be avoided, if possible, because of the attendant risk of thromboembolic complications. In some cases, heparin has been used in conjunction with prothrombin complex concentrates to reduce the thrombotic risk, but heparin is particularly difficult to manage in patients with liver disease. Prothrombin complex concentrates or *exchange transfusion* may have a role in emergency situations where the patient cannot tolerate large volumes of FFP.

Platelet transfusions should be restricted to patients who are actively bleeding or who require an invasive procedure. Because of splenic sequestration, the rises in the platelet count following platelet transfusion will be less than in other thrombocytopenic patients. Most patients will tolerate invasive procedures with platelet counts $\geqslant$ 50,000/μL. Preferably the PT should be corrected as well, but one series reported only 3.4% bleeding complications in patients with platelet counts $\geq 50{,}000/\mu L$, even with PTs up to 4 s and PTTs up to 9 s prolonged. However, patients with malignancies had a higher risk of bleeding with similar hemostatic compromise. *Desmopressin (DDAVP)* may be helpful in patients with bleeding and abnormal platelet function. This drug has been shown to shorten the bleeding time and the PTT in patients with chronic liver disease. It is particularly helpful in patients with the additional complication of renal failure.

Heparin has been used in some patients with liver disease, particularly those with evidence of DIC. However, its use is of unproven value and may aggravate the hemostatic disorder. The roles of fibrinolytic inhibitors such as *ε-aminocaproic acid* and *tranexamic acid* are unclear at present. These drugs should be employed cautiously at best in patients with liver disease, since their use is contraindicated in the presence of DIC. Similarly, the role of *antithrombin III* concentrates in patients with liver disease requires further investigation.

RED CELL ABNORMALITIES

Changes in red cell number, shape, and size occur in patients with liver disease. *Anemia* is common and often the cause is multifactorial. Increased plasma volume causes a relative anemia. Underproduction of red cells can be due to folic acid or vitamin B_{12} deficiency, the anemia of chronic disease, iron deficiency following gastrointestinal bleeding, or, in alcohol abusers, the direct toxic effect of ethanol on the bone marrow. Hypersplenism with sequestration and premature destruction of red cells may contribute to anemia. Morphologically, *spherocytes* become more prominent in the blood film. The lipid abnormalities associated with severe liver disease induce dramatic morphological changes in the red cells and a hemolytic anemia. The red cells acquire cholesterol from the plasma, increase in surface area, and develop a scalloped cell contour. These cells are remodeled and sequestered in the spleen, after which they lose cell surface area and transform into a spiculated *acanthocyte* (Fig. 2, top). The hemolytic anemia is rapidly progressive, splenomegaly and jaundice become more prominent, and the majority of patients die within weeks to months. Splenectomy decreases the hemolytic rate but is attended by a high risk in these patients with advanced liver disease. Less ominous changes in red cell size and shape that accompany liver disease are *target cells* and *macrocytes* (Fig. 2, bottom). Both reflect excess red cell membrane cholesterol in patients with obstructive or hepatocellular liver disease. In patients with mild to moderate liver disease, these are of no clinical significance. On occasion, severe hemolysis, marked hypertriglyceridemia, and active fatty cirrhosis occur together; this has been called *Zieve's syndrome*. The cause of hemolysis in this syndrome is unclear. Finally, a transient hemolytic anemia with *stomatocytosis* has been described in patients with liver disease.

The *laboratory evaluation* of anemia should begin with examination of the peripheral smear and measurement of the reticulocyte count. A low reticulocyte count in conjunction with macrocytic red cell indices, macrocytes, hypersegmented neutrophils, and large platelets suggest vitamin B_{12} or folate deficiency. Measurement of serum and red cell folate and of serum vitamin B_{12} levels is then indicated. Other causes of decreased production should also be considered, with measurement of serum iron, iron-binding capacity, and serum ferritin. Usually the anemia of chronic disease can be distinguished from iron-deficiency anemia with the help of these iron studies. Identification of ethanol toxicity may

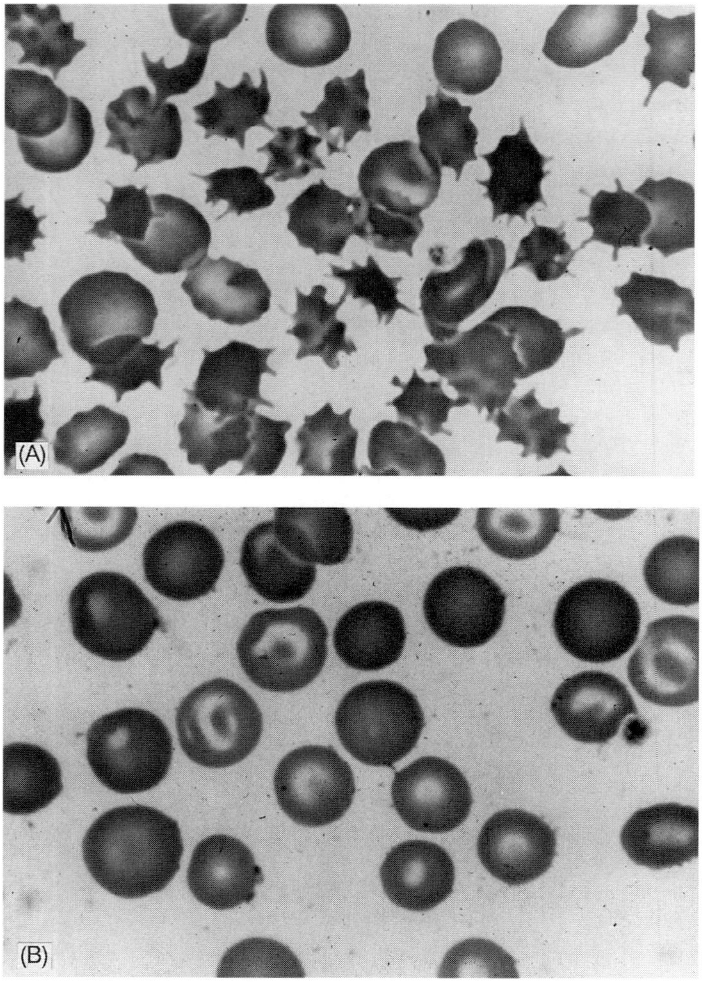

Figure 2 (A) Peripheral blood film from a patient with advanced liver disease showing spur-shaped red cells. (B) Peripheral blood film from a patient with chronic liver disease showing target cells and macrocytes.

require a bone marrow examination to demonstrate vacuolization of red cell precursors or ringed sideroblasts. An elevated reticulocyte count indicates bleeding or hemolysis. In this case the red cell indices will be macrocytic and the red cell morphology should be helpful. Sources of bleeding should be sought.

LEUKOPENIA

A decrease in white blood cells can be seen in patients with liver disease. The causes are similar to those for other cytopenias: splenic sequestration, drug toxicity, vitamin B_{12} or folate deficiencies, and ethanol toxicity. Decreased granulocyte survival has been reported in liver disease. Newly developed or more severe granulocytopenia should initiate a search for infection.

APLASTIC ANEMIA

Severe aplastic anemia can follow acute hepatitis and carries a poor prognosis. The disease usually develops in adolescent boys within 6 months of clinical hepatitis. The median survival is less than 6 months, with 90% mortality at 1 year. Hepatitis A, B, or C cannot be implicated in most cases of hepatitis-associated aplastic anemia. Several features of the disease suggest that it is mediated by immunopathological mechanisms.

BIBLIOGRAPHY

Boks AL, Brommer EJP, Schalm SW, Van Vliet HHDM. Hemostasis and fibrinolysis in severe liver failure and their relation to hemorrhage. Hepatology 1986; 6:79–86.

Colon-Otero G, Menke D, Hook CC. A practical approach to the differential diagnosis and evaluation of the adult patient with macrocytic anemia. Med Clin North Am 1992; 3:581–597.

Gallus AS, Lucas CR, Hirsh J. Coagulation studies in patients with acute infectious hepatitis. Br J Haematol 1972; 22:761–771.

Joist JH. Hemostatic abnormalities in liver disease. In: Colman RW, Hirsh J, Marder VJ, Salzman R, eds. Hemostasis and Thrombosis: Basic Principles and Clinical Practice. 3rd ed. Philadelphia: Lippincott, 1994:906–920.

Mammen EF. Coagulation abnormalities in liver disease. Hematol/Oncol Clin North Am 1992; 6:1247–1257.

McVay PA, Toy PTCY. Lack of increased bleeding after liver biopsy in patients with mild hemostatic abnormalities. Am J Clin Pathol 1990; 94:747–753.

Shohet SB. Hemolysis and changes in erythrocyte membrane lipids. N Engl J Med 1972; 286:577–581, 638–644.

Stein SF, Harker LA. Kinetic and functional studies of platelets, fibrinogen, and plasminogen in patients with hepatic cirrhosis. J Lab Clin Med 1982; 99:217–230.

Violi F, Ferro D, Quintarelli C, Saliola M, Cordova C, Balsano F. Clotting abnormalities in chronic liver disease. Dig Dis 1992; 10:162–172.

41

Management of Pulmonary Complications of Liver Disease

Jason Kelley
University of Vermont College of Medicine, Burlington, Vermont

INTRODUCTION

Liver disease, as it advances, frequently brings with it secondary pulmonary disorders. At their mildest, the pulmonary complications of liver disease simply represent unusual or confusing physical, radiographic, or laboratory findings but cause little harm or disability. At the other end of the spectrum of pulmonary disorders are rapidly lethal disorders with cryptic presentations. An example of the former is the respiratory alkalosis of advanced hepatic encephalopathy; instances of the latter include such disorders as pulmonary veno-occlusive disease and primary pulmonary hypertension associated with biliary cirrhosis. In this chapter emphasis is placed primarily on the former syndromes; several case presentations show how the cases were managed.

The connection between hepatic disease and pulmonary complications has long been thought to be a consequence of metabolic communication via the vasculature. This notion is supported by a wealth of ongoing research implicating the pulmonary vasculature as a major target of injury or remodeling in advanced hepatic disease. The precise cells and mediators involved are the subject of intense research. Excess generation of nitric oxide has recently been seen as a key pathogenetic feature of the hepatopulmonary syndrome (HPS) that may soon lead to new therapies (Table 1).

HEPATOPULMONARY SYNDROME

Basic Features of the Hepatopulmonary Syndrome

The HPS is the combination of advanced liver disease, hypoxemia, and intrapulmonary vascular dilatations. To this triad can be added the presence of a hyperdynamic circulatory state and the failure of hypoxic pulmonary vasoconstriction. It has been estimated that HPS may occur in as many as one-third of subjects with advanced hepatic disease. Usually it goes unrecognized until the patient is hospitalized for fulminant hepatic failure. However,

Table 1 Pulmonary Syndromes Associated with Liver Disease

Hepatopulmonary syndrome
Typical causes: alcoholic cirrhosis
Presentation: incidental finding on arterial blood gas analysis
Pulmonary hypertension
Typical causes: biliary cirrhosis, alcoholic cirrhosis
Presentation: often cyptic

for the minority of patients who develop the syndrome, the severity of the hypoxemia can be debilitating. Growing interest in liver transplantation has renewed clinical interest in issues surrounding the HPS (Table 2).

A typical case presents some of the perplexing manifestations of the HPS.

Case 1A

A 53-year-old accountant had manifestations of alcohol-induced liver disease for 3 years. One year previously she had been admitted for the first of several episodes of variceal bleeding. Then she stopped drinking entirely and resumed work full time. Recently, however, she presented to her primary care physician because marked and progressive dyspnea troubled her at rest. Review of her history was initially unrewarding: she had smoked cigarettes (less than one pack per day) but only until the age of 27 and had had no employment involving exposure to industrial toxins. She denied a cough; a prior chest radiograph at the time of previous hospitalization had shown only a modest degree of atelectasis that resolved before discharge. A careful physical exam showed only the changes of her advancing liver disease, including spider nevi. On listening to the posterior chest, her doctor heard a few crackles in the lung bases posteriorly. There was only minimal ascites and her abdomen was not tense. Her skin was not cyanotic and there was only a small amount of edema about the ankles. The pH of arterial blood was 7.46, the Pa_{O_2} was only 53 mmHg, and the Pa_{CO_2} was 32 mmHg. While she was breathing pure oxygen, her arterial PA_{O_2} rose to 600 mmHg; her Pa_{CO_2} remained at 33 mmHg.

This case demonstrates key features of this often misunderstood and frequently overlooked syndrome. The patient presented the basic triad of the HPS: advancing liver disease, marked hypoxemia, and subtle but typical radiographic features. Despite ending the ongoing insult to her liver, she had developed marked hypoxemia and dyspnea. Her respiratory alkalosis, although chronic, was only partially compensated. The arterial oxygen level rose markedly when she breathed pure oxygen. Nevertheless, her Pa_{CO_2} was

Table 2 Key Features of Hepatopulmonary Syndrome

Basic triad	Additional features
Advanced hepatic failure	Hyperdyamic (systemic) circulatory state (high cardiac output, low vascular resistance)
Hypoxemia	
Intrapulmonary vascular dilatations	Blunted pulmonary vasoconstrictor response to hypoxia or vasoconstrictor

persistently low even when the arterial oxygen level was above the normal range. These changes were all present, although the physical exam was nearly normal.

> Management point: No single test establishes the diagnosis of HPS. It is important to rule out unusual causes of hypoxemia in patients likely to have HPS. The hypocapnia of this patient was not mediated by her hypoxemia as the Pa_{CO_2} did not rise when oxygen was administered.

Physical Findings in HPS

As noted above, although sings of advanced liver disease are usually present, no particular findings on the physical exam distinguish patients with HPS. Patients with cutaneous spider nevi may be more likely to have more systemic and pulmonary vasodilatation. They also have more profound gas exchange abnormalities and less hypoxic pulmonary vasoconstriction than subjects without nevi. Possibly both cutaneous and pulmonary vascular pathological anomalies of HPS (see below) are under the control of the same biochemical and cellular mediators. Pleural effusions and ascites may be present but are not essential parts of the HPS.

> Management point: Despite often marked respiratory alkalosis and increased minute ventilation, the patient with HPS may not appear to be hyperventilating.

Pulmonary Physiology in HPS

Case 1B

> Spirometry was carried out on the patient described above. It documented only mild restrictive ventilatory impairment: the forced vital capacity was reduced to 72% of the predicted value. Complete pulmonary function tests a week later added the following information: the diffusing capacity for carbon monoxide (DL_{CO}) was only half of the predicted value; the lung volumes were symmetrically reduced to 71–75% of the predicted values.

There is often a restrictive pattern of lung function with decreased total lung capacity. A restrictive ventilatory pattern is found in about 25% of patients. To a degree, this ventilatory pattern may also be due to airway obstruction, since cigarette smoking is frequent among alcoholics, but the pulmonary function manifestations of liver disease are not a direct consequence of smoking. Only a minority of patients with HPS have an obstructive pattern on spirometry (Table 3).

The most common pulmonary abnormality in advanced liver failure is a reduction in the diffusing capacity; one recent study suggested that the diffusion for carbon monoxide is reduced in 50% of such patients. Although patients with the HPS often have low values for diffusing capacity, their lung volumes and expiratory flow rates may remain normal.

> Management point: The vital capacity and FEV_1 (forced expiratory volume in 1 s) can be determined using an office or bedside spirometer. A pattern of airflow obstruction (proportionally greater reduction of the FEV_1 than of the forced vital capacity) suggests the presence of a primary airway disease coexisting with HPS. It does not rule out pulmonary manifestations of hepatic failure.

Although the HPS may not be associated with pathognomonic physical pulmonary findings, many patients with advancing liver diseases have a characteristic combination of

Table 3 Pulmonary Function in Hepatopulmonary Syndrome

Uncompensated respiratory alkalosis (low Pa_{CO_2})
Low diffusing capacity (DL_{CO})
Hypoxemia, sometimes significantly corrected by breathing pure oxygen
Orthodeoxia
Mild restrictive ventilatory impairment

pulmonary function tests. By the time a patient is placed on a liver transplant list, many abnormalities in pulmonary function tests are usually quite apparent.

Management point: Because airway obstruction is not a feature of HPS, bronchodilators are not effective therapy in patients with HPS. They should not be used unless the patient has coexisting chronic obstructive pulmonary disease or asthma.

Oxygen Uptake and Delivery in HPS

Impaired arterial oxygenation is a central feature of the HPS. Mild hypoxemia (Pa_{O_2} in the range of 60–75 mmHg) is a frequent feature of chronic liver disease and occurs in about one-third of all such patients. It can often be traced to pleural effusions or ascites with reduction in lung volume. Less commonly, it is the result of interstitial pulmonary edema. More severe cases of hypoxemia should suggest the possibility of the HPS. The special features that distinguish the hypoxemia of HPS include (1) orthodeoxia (see below) and (2) the dramatic correction of the abnormal gradient for oxygen that occurs when the patient breathes pure oxygen.

The alveolar-arterial oxygen gradient is a more specific index of gas exchange than the Pa_{O_2} by itself. This is because it takes into account the partial pressure of carbon dioxide (Pa_{CO_2}) as well as the inspired oxygen concentration. This is particularly true in advanced liver disease associated with significant hypocapnia. The mean alveolar-arterial oxygen gradient has been reported to be widened (35 and 45 mmHg) in series of patients awaiting portocaval shunt or liver transplantation; the normal gradient (while breathing room air) is no more than 5–10 mmHg when healthy subjects breathe room air. As many as two-thirds of the patients awaiting liver transplantation have an elevated alveolar-arterial oxygen gradient.

Moderate degrees of hypoxemia are quite common in liver disease. In one series of 100 patients with cirrhosis, 28% were found to have a resting room air Pa_{O_2} of less than 70 mmHg, but only 5% had a resting room air Pa_{O_2} of less than 60 mmHg (Naeije and colleagues, 1981). In a large but retrospective analysis of patients with the HPS, Krowka and colleagues found that 59% had a Pa_{O_2} below 60 mmHg (the mean Pa_{O_2} for this group was only 62 mmHg when arterial blood was drawn with the patient in the supine position).

Another basic feature of the HPS is the greater than expected increase in arterial oxygen levels that occurs when patients are given pure oxygen to breathe. This finding does not accord with the notion that true anatomic shunts are the sole cause of hypoxemia in HPS. An unusual pattern of local mismatching of gas diffusion and blood perfusion has therefore been invoked by Krowka and colleagues. The notion behind what they have termed a "diffusion-perfusion impairment" is that the affected pulmonary vessels are too dilated to allow proper geometry for optimal oxygen transfer. Oxygen molecules have too little time to traverse to the center of the dilated vessel to oxygenate erythrocytes. Unlike the behavior of a classic shunt, this mechanism (a diffusion-perfusion imbalance) can be overridden when pure oxygen is administered. Conversely, oxygenation could be expected to worsen when the patient exercises, and this is indeed the case. Reduction in the transit time through the focal dilatations of the pulmonary vascular bed decreases the time available for oxygen diffusion. Indeed, when exercising patients with cirrhosis breathe pure oxygen there is further impairment of oxygenation and development of a larger shunt fraction.

Case 2

> A disabled 51-year-old automobile mechanic with proven alcoholic cirrhosis complained of severe dyspnea. A basic evaluation including physical exam, chest radiograph, and simple spirometric tests was all normal except for signs of advanced hepatic insufficiency. However, during evaluation in the pulmonary function laboratory, an oximeter was used to evaluate his exercise tolerance. When he lay on an examining table at rest, his oxygen saturation was 0.92. When he stood, it fell to 0.87; with walking, it fell further to 0.84.

As demonstrated by this patient, two unusual physiological features of the dyspnea noted by patients with HPS are the related gravitational phenomena of platypnea and orthodeoxia. Platypnea is dyspnea that is induced by the upright position and relieved by recumbency. Orthodeoxia is its objective counterpart: arterial deoxygenation that is accentuated in the upright position. Orthodeoxia is caused by preferential perfusion through intrapulmonary vascular dilations in the lung bases such that shunting is increased when the patient stands up.

These positional changes in both signs and symptoms are seen in as many as 5% of patients with cirrhosis. Published series focusing on patients with more advanced liver disease suggest that an even higher proportion of patients eventually develop orthodeoxia. The Pa_{O_2} may fall to extremely low levels in patients with orthodeoxia. In one case series describing nine patients with cirrhosis, the mean Pa_{O_2} was less than 45 mmHg. The presence of orthodeoxia, although not pathognomonic of HPS, strongly suggests the diagnosis in patients with established liver insufficiency.

> Management point: Patients with advancing liver disease should be asked about the presence of dyspnea during screening. When pulmonary function tests are done, remember to carry out oximetry in both the supine and upright positions. The wide availability of pulse oximeters allows for rapid screening for orthodeoxia in the office or at the bedside.

Focal dilatations of the pulmonary microvasculature, primarily in the lower lung zones, are the pathological hallmarks of the HPS. These lesions, rather than hepatopulmonary venous shunts, are thought to be quantitatively the most important cause of the severe hypoxemia. They were first identified using injections of gelatin into postmortem samples. This technique illustrated dilatation of the fine peripheral branches of the pulmonary artery at both the precapillary and capillary levels; the same technique was also used to display spider nevi on the pleural surfaces.

Clinically available physiologically based studies can be used to demonstrate focal intrapulmonary vascular dilatations. Intravenously injected ^{99m}technetium-labeled macroaggregated albumin particles exceeding 25 μm in diameter, such as are routinely used in perfusion lung scans, are normally filtered out during passage through the pulmonary microvasculature. In HPS, they traverse the pulmonary circulation and enter the systemic circulation, where they can be detected in richly vascular tissues such as brain and kidneys. The intrapulmonary capillary and precapillary vascular dilatations of HPS, ranging in size from 15–500 μm in diameter, fail to trap these particles.

> Management point: In patients with liver disease and unexplained pulmonary complaints, radionuclide scanning may prove helpful. However, it is important to consult with the radiologist in advance and explain the goal of the study and why images of the kidneys, brain, or whole body are sought.

The degree to which intrapulmonary vascular dilatations affect hemodynamics and gas exchange among patients with the HPS can be quite variable. The fraction of cardiac output shunted through the lungs ranges from as little as 20% to as much as 70% of the total cardiac output. Moreover, the extent of intrapulmonary shunting is not closely correlated with the severity of the liver disease. Nor does it correlate with the presence or extent of ascites or portal hypertension. In general, though, gas exchange worsens over time, despite apparent stabilization of the patient's liver function.

Accompanying hypoxemia and orthodeoxia of HPS is a blunted hypoxic pulmonary vasoconstrictor response. This is an important cause of hypoxemia in patients with the HPS. It usually becomes important in management when the patient is stressed by coexisting disorders such as infections.

Pathophysiology of the HPS

The basic causes of the vascular abnormalities in HPS have only recently begun to be determined. Key features include chronic vasodilation with low pulmonary vascular resistance, failure of the pulmonary vasculature to constrict in response to pharmacological agents, the presence of multiple discrete vascular dilatations, and a high cardiac output state. Investigators have long hypothesized that the liver or the portal circulation synthesizes mediators that modulate vasoreactivity of the pulmonary circulation. Alternatively, the failing liver may not be able to clear or inactivate one or more mediators involved in pulmonary acute vasodilation and chronic remodeling. Whether the same mediators involved in acute vasodilator responses are also involved in the tissue remodeling that leads to the formation of focal vascular dilatations is unclear.

The list of candidate vasodilator substances includes prostaglandins (such as prostacyclin, prostaglandin E_1, and prostaglandin I_2), vasoactive intestinal peptide (VIP), calcitonin, substance P, glucagon, atrial natriuretic factor, and platelet-activating factor. Conversely, there might be inactivation of normally active vasoconstrictor substances including tyrosine, serotonin, or endothelin. Some experimental evidence points to impaired vascular responsiveness to angiotensin II as a common feature of cirrhosis.

Nitric oxide, a powerful local vasodilator of endothelial origin, is increased in animal models of cirrhosis. In one such study in rats, the attenuated vasoconstriction in response to angiotensin II could be reversed by inhibiting nitric oxide synthesis. This suggests that reduced vascular reactivity to angiotensin II in cirrhosis is mediated by nitric oxide. In a rat model of biliary cirrhosis, partial reversal of attenuated hypoxic pulmonary vasoconstriction can be affected by angiotensin II.

Recent basic investigations have implicated an unusual population of pulmonary vascular cells in the genesis of the HPS. Pulmonary intravascular macrophages are a cell population normally present in certain nonhuman species. However, chronic liver disease induces the development of this cell population in humans and other species in which they are normally not present. Through the local release of vasoactive mediators, these reticuloendothelial cells might participate in the vasodilatation and vascular remodeling that results in the formation of permanent pulmonary vascular anomalies. The ability of intravascular macrophages to generate high local levels of nitric oxide may account for the chronic vasodilation seen in patients with HPS.

These studies suggest that the liver plays an important role in regulating pulmonary vascular tone. A recent case report from Italy shows a clear role for nitric oxide in the hypoxemia of HPS. Investigators briefly infused methylene blue (a nitric oxide inhibitor) in a woman and markedly corrected the hypoxemia and orthodeoxia associated with her alcoholic cirrhosis. Clearly the roles of angiotensin and nitric oxide deserve further evaluation.

Acid-Base Disorders in HPS

As illustrated in Case 1, the typical blood gas result in the HPS shows an uncompensated or partially compensated respiratory alkalosis and variable degrees of hypoxemia. Various mediators of the hyperventilation have been postulated. These include ammonia and low albumin, but neither has been shown to induce respiratory alkalosis. Because of parallels with the hyperventilation of pregnancy, investigators have postulated that the respiratory alkalosis of cirrhosis is hormonally driven. Indeed, the combined effects of progesterone and estradiol seem to play a role in the hyperventilation of HPS. The actual levels of progesterone and estradiol found in patients with cirrhosis are several orders of magnitude lower than in pregnant women. However, there is a reasonable correlation between the plasma levels of these hormones in liver failure patients and the degree of their hyperventilation. The lack of a perfect correlation is not surprising, as the arterial Pa_{CO_2} level is an indirect measure of respiratory drive; it is the latter that is presumably directly affected by hormones. Moreover, it has been postulated that the levels of these hormones within the central nervous system would be the ones that more directly drive the hyperventilation.

Complicating the acid-base picture in patients with HPS is the frequent coexistence of metabolic alkalosis. Metabolic alkalosis can be induced by vomiting, hyperaldosteronism, and the inappropriately assertive use of diuretic drugs. When any of these occurs, the patient with HPS is unable to protect arterial pH. The appropriate respiratory compensation (reduced minute ventilation with a consequent rise in Pa_{CO_2}) is blocked.

Systemic Hemodynamic Complications of HPS

Patients with advanced liver disease have a hyperdynamic circulatory state characterized by inappropriate systemic vasodilatation and elevated cardiac output. Unexplained tachycardia is present and the systemic blood pressure is typically low. When measured with a right heart catheter, the systemic vascular resistance is low and the cardiac output high. The size of these hemodynamic changes generally correlates with the extent of impairment of liver function. For example, there is usually (but not always) evidence of portal hypertension. The high-output cardiac state is usually particularly obvious when the patient is admitted to a critical care unit for evaluation for bleeding, hypotension, or possible infection. As a consequence of the high cardiac output relative to the peripheral oxygen utilization, the difference between the arterial and the mixed venous oxygen content is narrow, as excess amounts of oxygenated blood pass through the systemic circulation (Table 4).

Table 4 Pulmonary Hemodynamics in the Hepatopulmonary Syndrome

Low pulmonary vascular resistance
Multiple discrete vascular dilations in lower lung zones and on pleural surfaces
Failure to vasoconstrict pulmonary vascular bed in response to hypoxia or pharmacological vasoconstrictors
Chronically low systemic blood pressure
Low systemic vascular resistance with high cardiac output
Limited capacity to respond to hypotensive events such as acute hemorrhage, sepsis syndrome, myocardial infarction

> Management point: Awareness of the hyperdynamic cardiovascular state in HPS is important, as it can be incorrectly assumed to represent a manifestation of the sepsis syndrome. Such misdiagnosis is common and leads to inappropriate hemodynamic management and overuse of broad-spectrum combinations of antibiotics. An important clue to the correct diagnosis is obtained when the high-output state does not resolve during empirical therapy for infection and shock.

Radiographic Evaluation of HPS

Chest radiographic abnormalities seen in patients with cirrhosis are generally nonspecific. Nearly half of such patients have small lung volumes. Other findings include pleural effusions (19%), increased interstitial markings (14%), and increased pulmonary vascular markings (4%). HPS is associated with characteristic increases of basilar interstitial and pulmonary vascular markings (Fig. 1).

A recent study by McAdams and colleagues reviewed the radiological manifestations of HPS. Chest radiographs showed bibasilar, medium-sized (1.5–3.0 mm) nodular or reticulonodular opacities in all 10 cases studied. The vascular basis for these opacities was

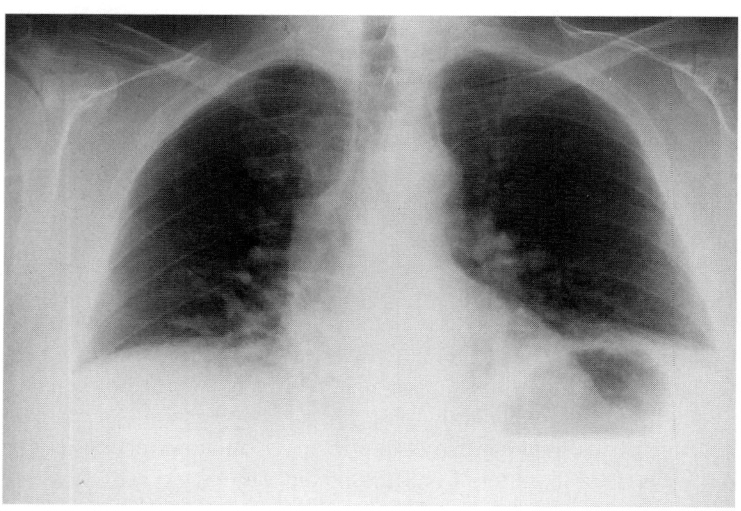

Figure 1

best appreciated on computed tomography (CT). Conventional (thick) CT cuts showed that these opacities represent dilated lung vessels. High-resolution CT images may also be helpful in excluding pulmonary fibrosis or emphysema as the cause of these opacities and of the accompanying hypoxemia.

> Management point: Once abnormalities on chest radiographs are securely identified as due to vascular dilatations further evaluation is not required each time a patient is admitted to hospital. CT scans of the chest are not a necessary component of the evaluation of patients suspected of having HPS.

Intrapulmonary Vascular Dilatations: Imaging Techniques

Three additional imaging modalities are available for confirming the presence of intrapulmonary vascular dilatations: contrast-enhanced echocardiography, ^{99m}technetium-labeled macroaggregated albumin injection followed by gamma-counter scanning of systemic vascular beds, and pulmonary angiography.

Contrast-Enhanced Echocardiography

This technique employs agitated saline, which provides a stream of microbubbles that normally opacify the vascular spaces during echocardiography. When the pulmonary vascular bed is normal, only the right heart becomes opacified. This is because the injected microbubbles are filtered in the pulmonary capillary bed and therefore cannot cross into the left side of the heart as an opaque bolus. Thus the presence of microbubbles in the left heart chambers shows the presence of an intrapulmonary or intracardiac right-to-left shunt. The distinction between intrapulmonary and intracardiac shunts is based on the rapidity of bubble appearance in the left heart.

Contrast-enhanced echocardiography is emerging as a particularly useful technique. It is rapid and can be carried out in hospitals without access to perfusion lung scanning or angiography. When an intrapulmonary shunt is present, contrast echocardiography cannot distinguish between precapillary, capillary, or pleural dilatations and direct arteriovenous anastomoses. It can be predicted that invasive transesophageal echocardiography may prove to offer additional advantages over surface echocardiography in localizing shunt to specific pulmonary veins and thereby determining the major site of intrapulmonary vascular dilatations.

Hopkins and colleagues studied 53 candidates for liver transplantation using contrast echocardiography. They found that nearly half of the patients studied had positive results on a contrast-enhanced echocardiogram, although none of their patients had overt hypoxemia (Pa_{O_2} less than 60 mmHg). Although patients with greater degrees of opacification had a lower Pa_{O_2} than those without shunt, the mean Pa_{O_2} did not differ between those with positive and negative echocardiographic results. Thus, echocardiography detects subclinical pulmonary vasodilatation before the development of overt hypoxemia.

Perfusion Scanning for Shunt Detection

Perfusion lung scanning with ^{99m}technetium-labeled macroaggregated albumin is an alternate method of detecting intrapulmonary vascular dilatations. Gamma-labeled macroaggregates greater than 15 μm in diameter are trapped in the normal pulmonary capillary bed. Therefore, a scan showing uptake of radionuclide over the brain or kidneys indicates transit through the lung caused by either an intrapulmonary or an intracardiac shunt. The magnitude of the shunt can be calculated from the ratio of systemic to total body activity of the radionuclide. Normally, no more than 6% of the macroaggregate bolus passes through the pulmonary vasculature. In contrast, as much as 70% has been shown to pass through the lungs of patients with severe hypoxemia of HPS. This technique is particularly useful in hospitals with a gamma camera but no pulmonary function laboratories or echocardiographic services. It appears to be about as sensitive as contrast echocardiography, although this point has not been rigorously tested.

Pulmonary Angiography

Before the availability of contrast-enhanced echocardiography and ^{99m}technetium-labeled macroaggregated albumin scanning, pulmonary angiography was the chief method of imaging pulmonary vascular lesions. Because of its more invasive nature, its utility is not limited to research studies. When angiography is used, it retains the advantage that direct measurements of intraluminal pressures can be made via the pulmonary artery catheter. These can be helpful in excluding associated pulmonary hypertension.

Pulmonary Infections and Injury

Whether patients with chronic liver disease have an increased risk of pulmonary infection remains a complex issue. In part this may be due to their frequent instrumentation and contact with the hospital environment and its attendant exposure to nosocomial pathogens. A recent study by Moss and colleagues indicated that patients with excessive chronic alcohol use have an increased risk of developing acute respiratory distress syndrome (ARDS). As with patients who do not suffer from chronic alcohol use, ARDS in the alcoholic occurs after a discrete event such as shock, infection, severe pancreatitis, or abdominal trauma. The risk for developing ARDS after such an insult was twice that found in control subjects; the risk of dying from ARDS once it developed was fourfold higher. Hence, there is double jeopardy for subjects with alcoholism.

It is somewhat puzzling that the multiple focal intrapulmonary vasodilatations of HPS do not result in paradoxic left-sided infections such as endocarditis or brain abscess. Possibly the presence of an activated pulmonary intravascular population prevents passage of viable organisms through the pulmonary circuit. In any case, such infections do not appear to be common in patients with HPS.

Evaluation for HPS

The basic evaluation for patients with advancing liver disease and suspected HPS should include screening spirometry and a blood gas to document Pa_{CO_2} and the level of hyperventilation. A chest radiograph may detect abnormalities requiring better definition by CT. If hypoxemia is present, oximetry or blood gases should be obtained in both the supine and standing positions to assess for orthodeoxia. Pulmonary function studies should include measurement of the diffusing capacity (DL_{CO}). Contrast echocardiography or perfusion scanning seem to be equally sensitive in defining intrapulmonary vascular dilatations. Angiography is not required for routine evaluation. Similarly, right heart catheterization is useful only when the patient is acutely hypotensive.

Differential Diagnosis of HPS

The diagnosis of HPS is based on the combination of characteristic pulmonary and systemic findings in patients with advanced liver disease rather than on a single pathognomonic feature or test. It, therefore, remains important to rule out other causes of primary or secondary pulmonary disease. Left ventricular failure with pulmonary edema typically presents with diffuse pulmonary shadows of edema, hypoxemia, and hypocapnic alkalosis.

Therapy for HPS

Therapy for the HPS is generally limited to supportive care until liver transplantation can be carried out. Supplemental oxygen is traditionally used in patients with debilitating hypoxemia but its efficacy has not been subjected to any analysis in clinical trials. It is important to continue to rule out ancillary causes of hypoxemia and systemic vasodilatation each time the patient presents with worsening of these findings. Recent evidence implicating local nitric oxide generation within the lung suggests the importance of this vasodilator in the nosology of HPS. This line of research is very likely to open up new approaches to therapy in the very near future.

Medical Therapy

HPS appears to result from the release of mediators from the hepatic axis that result in acute pulmonary physiological disorders and chronic remodeling. Therefore, appropriate medical therapy based on treatments to block this process carry a certain logic. Unfortunately, this approach has yet to produce significant therapeutic gains. Small trials have examined several drugs, including indomethacin and almitrine bismesylate. The latter drug has been tested in Europe for its ability to improve ventilation/perfusion matching in patients with chronic obstructive pulmonary disease. The somatostain analogue octreotide has been administered to a few patients with HPS in an attempt to improve ventilation/perfusion matching. Unfortunately, none of these therapies has been associated with significant improvement in the various manifestations of HPS. Plasma exchange has been equally disappointing. Even an extract of garlic (*Allium sativum*) has been put forward in one case report.

Occasionally, clinicians have an opportunity to correct the hepatic disorder resulting in HPS by means other than liver transplantation. For example, one recent case report recounts the course of a patient with transient noncirrhotic hepatocellular failure resulting from angioimmunoblastic lymphadenopathy. Appropriate antineoplastic treatment with cyclophosphamide and corticosteroids markedly reduced the defect in oxygen transfer. Such opportunities to correct underlying defects in liver function should not be overlooked.

Mechanical Obliteration of Vascular Malformations

Angiographic embolization of vascular malformations has been used successfully in patients with hereditary hemorrhagic telangiectasia and other disorders associated with discrete intrapulmonary shunts. Such an approach would seem ideally suited for patients with HPS. At least one group has reported on their attempt to correct the hypoxemia of the HPS by embolizing intrapulmonary vascular dilatations under angiographic guidance. However, the response to coil embolization in their case report was disappointing. The improvement in Pa_{O_2} ranged from 38–53 mmHg after multiple coil-spring devices were inserted; however, multiple angiographic sessions resulted in only minimal sustained improvement in overall oxygenation.

Transplantation

Liver transplantation (see Chaps. 43 and 44) is rapidly becoming the definitive treatment for HPS. The intrapulmonary gas exchange defects of the HPS are clearly reversible with liver transplantation. In early studies of patients with HPS who underwent transplantation, severe hypoxemia seemed to persist after transplantation, particularly in those patients with the most profound levels of preoperative hypoxemia. Recent publications, however, correct the older view that hypoxemia is a contraindication to liver transplantation. Hypoxemia and digital clubbing can be reversed whatever the etiology of the liver disease. Transplantation can also be expected to restore the increased cardiac index and elevated splanchnic blood flow in many but not all patients with HPS.

Although the reversibility of the HPS is now established, the effect of the severity of pretransplantation hypoxemia on perioperative morbidity and mortality remains controversial. Some reports suggest a high mortality when the preoperative Pa_{O_2} is less than 60 mmHg (on room air). In contrast, other surgical studies suggest that the only additional burden for patients undergoing transplantation for HPS is a prolonged postoperative ventilator time. The few studies published to date are based on relatively small series of patients. They indicate that at least half of those undergoing transplantation show improvement in oxygenation as determined by reduction in shunt fractions and improved oxygenation (mean alveolar-arterial oxygen gradient).

In summary, HPS can be reversed by successful liver transplantation. This observation challenges the older view of hypoxemia as a contraindication to liver transplantation. Nevertheless, the hypoxemia of HPS may progress despite stabilization of the hepatic dysfunction. Future guidelines for the management of patients with very severe HPS will have to be based on further clinical studies. Whether patients with the most severe hypoxemia (Pa_{O_2} below 50 mmHg) also benefit from transplant remains unclear.

Prognosis of HPS

It is difficult to predict which patients with liver disease will ultimately develop HPS, as no known hereditary factors or coexisting morbidities have been found. No reliable markers identify the patients with liver disease who are most likely to develop pulmonary vasodilations or hypoxemia. No consistent predictor has been identified among the severity of liver disease, the Child's severity index, or other scoring systems. Indeed, in some cases the derangements of gas exchange predate the recognition of hepatic disease.

The presence of large intrapulmonary vascular dilatations puts patients with HPS at risk for cerebral embolic events. It has been anticipated that patients with HPS are at particular risk of cerebral embolic events immediately following transplantation. During this time phase, the long-term coagulopathy is rapidly corrected but the large intrapulmonary shunts persist, putting the patient at particular risk.

PULMONARY HYPERTENSION ASSOCIATED WITH LIVER DISEASE

Pulmonary hypertension that occurs without left ventricular disorders or congenital heart disease is a rare disorder. It is called either primary pulmonary hypertension (PPH) to denote the absence of left ventricular causes or, alternatively, plexigenic pulmonary hypertension in reference to the characteristic pathological lesions. The association between advanced liver disease and PPH is well established. The clinical features of PPH are listed in Table 5. As can be seen, they are not at all specific and therefore the bedside diagnosis of PPH is often overlooked.

Physical findings of PPH are those of right heart strain and failure. There is often a prominent right ventricular heave, a loud second heart sound with a prominent second

Table 5 Clinical Feature of Primary Pulmonary Hypertension

Intense dyspnea (60–89%)
Syncope, near syncope, or dizziness (13–88%)
Chest pain (7–47%)
Peripheral edema (3–37%)
Palpitations (5–33%)

pulmonic sound, and a loud right ventricular gallop. A tricuspid murmur may accompany these findings. In addition, there are findings of chronic right heart failure (dependent edema), and the neck veins are elevated. Raynaud's phenomenon may be present.

The pulmonary vasculature exhibits a number of pathological features in cases of pulmonary hypertension. One common feature is medial hypertrophy of the muscular pulmonary arteries and extension of muscle cells to the (normally nonmuscular) arteriolar level. The pathognomonic pulmonary vascular lesion of PPH is the plexogenic malformation. These are dilation lesions found in small muscular arteries and arterioles; they consist of hyperplasia of the media and intima with resultant stenosis of the lumen. They have a characteristic onionskin appearance. Arterial thrombi are occasionally found but are considered a complication rather than a cause of plexogenic pulmonary arteriopathy. Aside from their dilation, large vessels are not affected and appear normal at postmortem exam.

Pulmonary function studies disclose mild or moderate restrictive impairment and a decreased diffusing capacity. Analysis of arterial blood may indicate an uncompensated respiratory alkalosis with hypoxemia. The chest film (or chest CT scan, if done) is often normal but may document the features of pulmonary hypertension: enlarged pulmonary arteries and right heart. Perfusion and ventilation lung scans, sometimes done when pulmonary embolism is being ruled out, show normal or near normal perfusion and ventilation without unmatched perfusion defects of pulmonary embolic disease. Lung biopsy, via either thoracotomy or bronchoscopy, is never a part of the evaluation. It would be particularly hazardous in the face of the extreme elevations of pulmonary artery pressures.

The electrocardiogram often shows right ventricular hypertrophy. Considerably more revealing are echocardiograms and right heart catheterization. Image and color flow–directed continuous-wave Doppler echocardiography allows noninvasive estimation of right heart performance. The pulmonary artery systolic pressure can be estimated from the tricuspid regurgitant jet if it can be imaged and measured. In skillful hands, estimates of right-sided filling pressures are quite accurate.

For greater precision, right heart catheterization can be used to specifically measure markedly elevated pulmonary artery pressures. Often in cases of PPH, the pulmonary artery pressures are elevated to the same range as in the systemic vessels. In contrast, the pulmonary capillary wedge pressure is low or normal, indicating the absence of left ventricular dysfunction. Cardiac output is usually low. In consequence, the oxygen tension or saturation of mixed venous blood is low.

PPH occurs in conjunction with cirrhosis of varying etiology, including alcoholic cirrhosis, chronic hepatitis, and primary biliary cirrhosis. Although epidemiological data are limited, PPH is considerably more common (five to tenfold) in patients with certain hepatic disorders than in the general population. It can occur in patients with cirrhotic and noncirrhotic portal hypertension. As many as 2% of patients with portal hypertension have occult or symptomatic PPH (Hadengue and colleagues, 1991). The risk of developing pulmonary hypertension seems to increase with the duration of portal hypertension.

Case 3

> A 57-year-old woman with primary biliary cirrhosis was referred for review of her pulmonary status during evaluation for liver transplantation. She had previously been hospitalized twice for respiratory failure thought to be due to pneumonias. She was severely dyspneic with the slightest exertion; hypoxemia was so severe as to warrant the use of continuous home oxygen. On exam, she had only mild ascites and Raynaud's phenomenon. There was significant digital clubbing and early bibasilar inspiratory crackles were heard in the chest. Screening pulmonary function tests were completely normal. However, when monitored during exercise with a pulse oximeter, she had a drop in her Sp_{O_2} from 0.93–0.88 and a rise in her heart rate from 88 to 125.

Management Point: manifestations of pulmonary hypertension are often overlooked or incorrectly diagnosed as chronic airway disease or pneumonia.

The prognosis for PPH, even without liver disease, is not good. Only one-third of patients survive for 5 years, with death usually a consequence of the progressive compromise of the right heart. Vasodilator therapy has been effective in many patients but requires hospitalization and cardiac catheterization to monitor the initial response to medications. Even under these circumstances, vasodilators can prove lethal.

Only a subset of patients, perhaps those with greater reactivity of their pulmonary vasculature, respond to vasodilators. Hydralazine, nifedipine, and continuously infused intravenous prostacyclin (Epoprostenol) have all been used with some success. In the absence of liver disease, lung transplantation is the only therapy that offers relief for patients who do not respond to vasodilator therapy. Multiple organ transplantation (liver and lung) may be required for patients with pulmonary hypertension and advanced liver disease.

BIBLIOGRAPHY

Caslin AW, Heath D, Madden B, Yacoub M, Gosney JR, Smith P. The histopathology of 36 cases of plexogenic pulmonary arteriopathy. Histopathology 1990; 16:9–19.

Hadengue A, Benhayoun MK, Lebrec D, Benhamou JP. Pulmonary hypertension complicating portal hypertension: prevalence and relation to splanchnic hemodynamics. Gastroenterology 1991; 100:520–528.

Hopkins WE, Waggoner AD, Barzilai B. Frequency and significance of intrapulmonary right-to-left shunting in end-stage hepatic disease. Am J Cardiol 1992; 70:516–519.

Krowka MJ, Porayko MK, Plevak DJ, Pappas SC, Steers JL, Krom RAF, Wiesner RH. Hepatopulmonary syndrome with progressive hypoxemia as an indication for liver transplantation: Case reports and literature review. Mayo Clin Proc 1997; 72:44–53.

McAdams HP, Erasmus J, Crockett R, Mitchell J, Godwin JD, McDermott VG. The hepatopulmonary syndrome: radiologic findings in 10 patients. AJR 1996; 166:1379–1385.

Moss M, Bucher B, Moore FA, Moore EE, Parsons PE. The role of chronic alcohol abuse in the development of the acute respiratory distress syndrome in adults. JAMA 1997; 275:50–54.

Naeije R, Hallemans R, Mols P, Melot C. Hypoxic pulmonary vasoconstriction in liver cirrhosis. Chest 1981; 80:570–574.

Rich S, Pietra GG, Kieras K, Hart K, Brundage BH. Primary pulmonary hypertension: radiographic and scintigraphic patterns of histologic subtypes. Ann Intern Med 1986; 105:499–502.

42
Management of Cirrhotic Cardiomyopathy

Zenghua Ma and Samuel S. Lee
University of Calgary, Calgary, Alberta, Canada

CLINICAL CHARACTERISTICS

Altered cardiovascular function in cirrhosis is manifest as decreased peripheral vascular resistance and blood pressure and increased cardiac output. Despite the baseline increase in cardiac output, the ventricular responses to physiological and pharmacological stimuli are blunted, a condition termed cirrhotic cardiomyopathy. A large body of evidence amassed over the past four decades has conclusively demonstrated the existence of cardiomyopathy in both cirrhotic patients and animal models of cirrhosis. However, in the absence of stimuli, impairment of cardiac contraction usually cannot be observed. This is probably because at baseline, the reduced peripheral vascular resistance masks any attenuation of cardiac contractility. Although several studies have attempted to explore the mechanisms of cirrhotic cardiomyopathy, there is, to date, a noticeable paucity of data on treatment of cirrhotic cardiomyopathy. Cirrhosis is also associated with pulmonary abnormalities including hypoxemia and occasionally pulmonary hypertension with right heart failure. These abnormalities have been collectively called "hepatopulmonary syndrome" and are discussed in Chap. 41. In this chapter we briefly discuss the pathogenesis underlying left ventricular cardiomyopathy and potential clinical management strategies.

PATHOGENESIS

Diminished β-Adrenergic Receptor Signal Transduction Function

β-Adrenoceptor function is the major determinant of ventricular contractility. The mechanism by which the β-adrenergic receptor regulates cardiac contraction has been clarified in recent years (Fig. 1).

Several previous studies have examined β-adrenergic receptor characteristics in cirrhosis. Patients with decompensated cirrhosis show decreased lymphocyte β-adrenoceptor density. Although β-adrenergic receptor status in cirrhotic human heart tissue

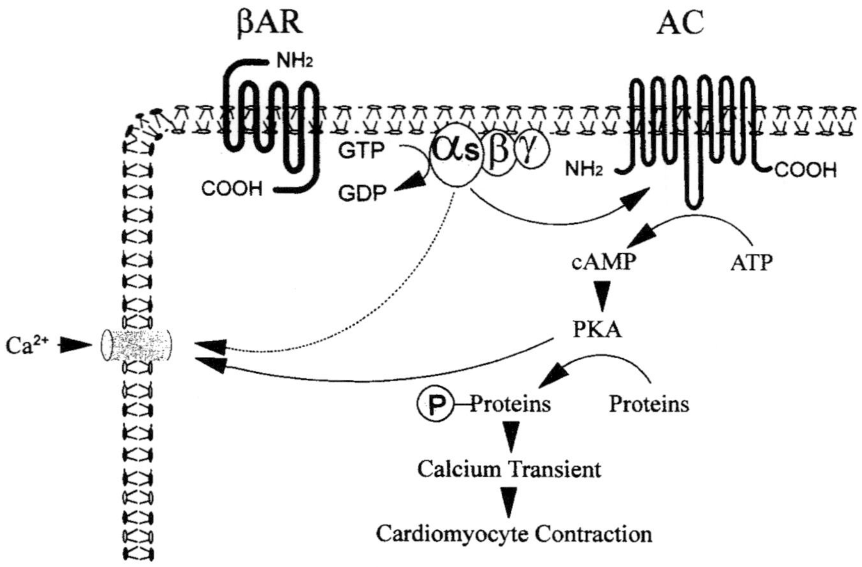

Figure 1 Schematic representation of the β-adrenergic receptor signal transduction pathway. βAR, β-adrenergic receptor; AC, adenylate cyclase; PKA, cAMP-dependent protein kinase. αs, β, and γ represent the heterotrimeric components of G protein. Receptor-ligand binding induces guanine nucleotide exchanges, with the subsequent dissociation of the stimulatory αs-GTP subunit, which activates adenylate cyclase to produce cAMP. cAMP stimulates PKA, which phosphorylates several proteins leading to a positive contractile response. These proteins include the membrane calcium channel, phospholamban on the sarcoplasmic reticulum and troponin I. The αs subunit can also directly activate the membrane L-type calcium channels, causing increased calcium influx. (From Ma and Lee, 1996, with permission.)

has not been directly examined, a good concordance between lymphocyte and myocardial β-adrenoceptor characteristics has previously been demonstrated. In a rat model of biliary cirrhosis, a reduced β-adrenergic receptor density in the ventricular sarcolemmal plasma membrane is found, and this is associated with blunted chronotropic and inotropic responses to the β-adrenergic agonist isoproterenol. In the heart, in contrast to other tissues, spare β-adrenergic receptors are rare. Moreover, maximum cardiac contractile responses generally require participation of all receptors. Therefore, a reduction in β-adrenoceptor density in the heart almost always leads to impairment of β-adrenergic signaling function.

In the β-adrenergic receptor signal transduction pathway, generation of cAMP as the second messenger is a central event, as shown in Fig. 1. In cirrhotic cardiomyopathy, it has been demonstrated that cAMP production is reduced in response to stimulation at the receptor, G protein, and adenylate cyclase levels. Moreover, the expression of Gsα, the stimulatory component of G protein, in cirrhotic rat hearts has been shown to be significantly reduced. The pathophysiological role of diminished β-adrenergic receptor function has recently been tested. It has been shown that β-adrenergic receptor–stimulated papillary muscle contractility is blunted in cirrhotic rats (Fig. 2). Thus, it can be concluded that diminished β-adrenergic receptor signaling function plays an important role in cirrhotic cardiomyopathy.

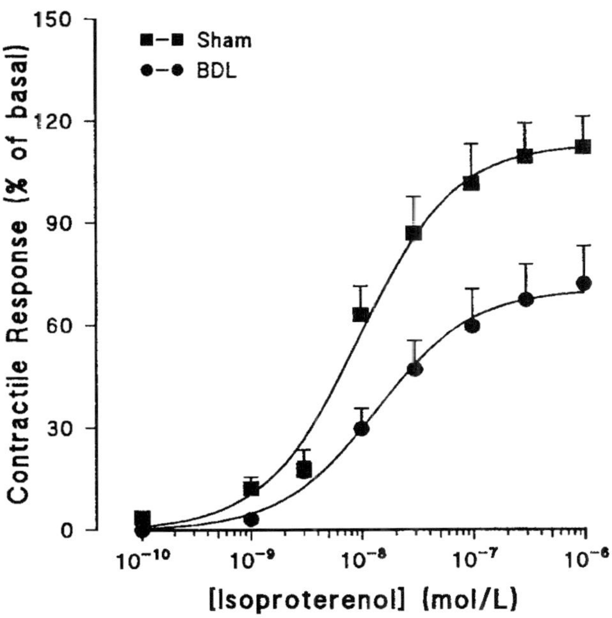

Figure 2 Left ventricular papillary muscle contractile responses under isoproterenol stimulation. The data were collected from 15 sham and 14 bile duct–ligated cirrhotic rats. Maximum contractile responses to β-adrenergic receptor stimulation in cirrhotic rats were significantly reduced, $p < 0.01$, compared with sham-operated rats. (From Ma et al., 1996, Ref. 5, with permission.)

β-Adrenergic Receptor Function and Plasma Membrane Physical Properties

The plasma membrane plays an important role in cardiomyocyte contractile function, since it forms the lipid environment for the β-adrenergic receptor and its second-messenger system. The plasma membrane's physical properties are determined by many factors, among which membrane cholesterol content is crucial. The sterol ring in the cholesterol molecule, which interacts with fatty acyl chains, is rigid, thus reducing the membrane fluidity—a parameter used to represent the membrane's physical properties. Ventricular membranes from cirrhotic rats have been demonstrated to have decreased membrane fluidity.

High serum cholesterol is often observed in cirrhosis. This is at least partly due to a decreased activity of serum lecithin-cholesterol acyltransferase (LCAT), which catalyzes esterification between free cholesterol and long-chain fatty acyl residues from lecithin. The functional impairment of LCAT leads to an increment of serum free cholesterol, which then facilitates incorporation of more cholesterol into cardiac plasma membranes.

It has been shown that in vitro fluidization of cirrhotic cardiac plasma membranes to restore fluidity to normal values also results in restoration of isoproterenol-stimulated cAMP generation to normal levels. However, when the β-adrenoceptor signal-transduction pathway is stimulated at the G-protein and adenylate-cyclase levels, fluidization of cardiac plasma membranes has no effect on cAMP production. Furthermore, effects of change in membrane fluidity on cAMP generation stimulated at the receptor level are not mediated through an increase in β-adrenergic receptor density, or through changes in the receptor binding affinity because these parameters were not found to be significantly different before and after membrane fluidization. These studies suggest that changes in the physical properties of the cardiac plasma membrane may interfere with the coupling process between the receptor and G protein and thereby lead to attenuated ventricular contractility.

Humoral Factors

Hepatic cirrhosis is a complex condition associated with many different pathological changes that can affect the cardiovascular system. First, in cirrhosis, because of hepatocellular insufficiency, toxic substances absorbed from the gut may not be inactivated. Furthermore, because of portal hypertension, portosystemic shunting develops, consequently permitting some toxic substances to bypass hepatic inactivation and shunt directly into the systemic circulation. Those toxic substances may exert inhibitory effects on the heart.

It is also well known that cirrhotic patients are more prone to suffer from bacterial infection and endotoxemia due to diminished immune function and possibly intestinal translocation. Endotoxins and cytokines stimulated by them, such as interleukins and tumor necrosis factor alpha (TNF-α), are known to inhibit ventricular contractility.

Second, it has been established that plasma norepinephrine levels are elevated in cirrhotic patients. Baseline norepinephrine levels are correlated with the severity of cirrhosis. Sustained increases in norepinephrine have been reported to cause myocardial injury and β-adrenergic receptor desensitization, a phenomenon known as catecholamine cardiomyopathy.

Third, an increase in plasma bile salt contents may lead to a reduction in cardiac contractility. It has been shown that ventricular contractility is diminished in jaundiced patients and animals. Previous research has also demonstrated in vitro that the contractile responses of ventricular papillary muscle are blunted when hydrophobic bile salts are added to the tissue bath. Since plasma bile salt levels are known to be increased in cirrhotic patients, such hypercholemia could be one of the pathogenic factors leading to cirrhotic cardiomyopathy.

CLINICAL MANAGEMENT

Monitoring Cardiac Function During Stressful Procedures

Since the characteristic feature of cirrhotic cardiomyopathy is the appearance of heart failure when the patient is exposed to physical stress, it is important to monitor cardiac function closely when patients undergo stressful procedures. It is recommended that routine cardiac function assessment—such as electrocardiography, nuclear imaging studies, or echocardiography—be performed to determine if patients can tolerate stressful procedures such as portocaval shunting and liver transplantation. If patients have obvious heart failure symptoms or severely abnormal cardiac functional assessment, as noted above, the surgery should be postponed, if possible, until ventricular function improves, because perioperative mortality is expected to be very high under these circumstances.

Supportive Measures

If the cirrhosis is caused by alcohol abuse, it is very important for patients to stop alcohol intake, since it is known that both hepatic and cardiac functional impairment due to alcohol may be improved by a period of abstinence. Furthermore, alcohol per se is a known direct cardiotoxin. If cirrhotic patients suffer from any bacterial infection, it should be vigorously treated as soon as possible to reduce the levels of endotoxins and associated inflammatory cytokines.

The general supportive measures for noncirrhotic cardiac failure also apply to cirrhotic heart failure. These include bed rest, sedation, dietary management, and correction of metabolic and electrolyte disorders. Bed rest interspersed with periods in a semirecumbent chair aids diuresis and decreases the cardiac workload. Such rest also helps to alleviate anxiety and stress, which thereby also decreases the workload. We prefer not to use tranquilizers to decrease anxiety because of the risk of precipitating or worsening hepatic encephalopathy with these drugs. In patients with cirrhosis, the "autoanticoagulation" due to hepatic insufficiency markedly diminishes the risk of developing venous thromboembolic disease, which is normally a complication of prolonged bed rest.

Dietary manipulation includes institution of a low-salt diet to aid in fluid mobilization. We prefer a no-added-salt diet (2–4 g of salt daily) for most situations because of the difficulties in compliance with more severe salt restriction. If further salt restriction becomes necessary, it may be more practical to start diuretic therapy rather than trying to enforce a severely salt-restricted and unpalatable diet. Many cirrhotic patients have protein-calorie malnutrition; therefore, we allow a relatively liberal protein intake up to 80 g/day unless encephalopathy supervenes (see Chap. 16).

Because many patients with cirrhotic cardiomyopathy tend to have advanced cirrhosis with renal dysfunction, serum electrolytes such as potassium, magnesium, and phosphate should be monitored and corrected if necessary. The cardiac contractile and electrophysiological dysfunction induced by disturbances in these ions are well known.

Diuretics

The use of diuretics should be considered among the mainstays of management for moderately severe heart failure in cirrhotic patients. Since patients with cirrhosis are known to have increased blood and plasma volume, it would seem relatively straightforward to remove some of this excess through the use of potassium-sparing and loop diuretics. Unfortunately, cirrhosis is also the most avidly salt- and water-retaining pathophysiological state known, and patients with advanced cirrhosis can elaborate a virtually sodium-free urine. The difficulties in promoting significant amounts of diuresis in this population are well known. Moreover, since many regional vascular beds behave as if tissue perfusion were inadequate, the "ineffective circulating volume," removing some of the excess extracellular fluid volume in cirrhotic patients may be deleterious to organs such as the kidney.

Despite these concerns, judicious use of diuretics such as spironolactone at doses starting at 100 mg/day, with increments of 50 mg to a maximum of 400–500 mg/day, and furosemide starting at 20 mg/day with increments of 20 mg to a maximum of 160 mg/day usually succeed in mobilizing fluid in up to 90% of cirrhotic patients. Serum electrolytes and renal function should be closely monitored during diuretic therapy.

Inotropic Drugs and Vasodilators

No published data are available at present regarding specific treatment for cirrhotic cardiomyopathy. It is recommended that routine heart failure therapy be followed should compromised ventricular function become overt. Because the β-adrenergic receptor is desensitized, it is unlikely that patients will benefit from inotropic drugs that act selectively on the β-adrenergic receptor, such as dobutamine, which is commonly used in low-output congestive failure. Instead, amrinone, a phosphodiesterase inhibitor that decreases cAMP degradation, may be a good choice, given that β-adrenergic receptor signaling function is attenuated, particularly cAMP production.

In addition, traditional inotropic agents such as cardiac glycosides may also be tried, although the evidence for a significant benefit from these agents is scant. The short-acting cardiac glycoside ouabain was found to be ineffective in improving contractility in a group of patients with alcoholic cirrhosis and relatively severe cardiomyopathy. However, it should be noted that most if not all of the patients in that study may have had alcoholic cardiomyopathy, which is generally more severe than nonalcoholic cirrhotic cardiomyopathy. It is important to emphasize that when cardiac glycosides such as digoxin are used, serum electrolytes, especially potassium, must be closely monitored, because these patients with cardiomyopathy tend to suffer from electrolyte imbalances, as noted above. As in patients with noncirrhotic heart failure, we generally avoid the use of glycosides if the heart size is normal. Also if high-output heart failure occurs, cardiac glycosides should be avoided, because these drugs sometimes exacerbate high-output congestive failure.

Angiotensin-converting enzyme (ACE) inhibitors such as captopril, which are currently the first-line drugs for noncirrhotic congestive heart failure, may not be effective in cirrhotic cardiomyopathy, because these drugs act by reducing peripheral vascular resistance, which is already low in cirrhotic patients. However, in urgent or emergent situations, vasodilators such as ACE inhibitors to reduce afterload and preload can be tried cautiously. Some patients with cirrhosis have marked activation of the renin-angiotensin system, and blockade with ACE inhibitors may result in dramatic acute arterial hypotension. Accordingly, therapy with ACE inhibitors should be started at low doses.

Antiarrhythmic Therapy

Recent studies have documented that some cirrhotic patients suffer from prolongation of the Q-T interval, which can lead to lethal arrythmias, especially ventricular arrythmia. Furthermore, prolongation of the Q-T interval appears to be correlated with the severity of cirrhosis. Therefore, for patients with these electrophysiological abnormalities, prevention of ventricular arrythmia may be of importance. Lidocaine, phenytoin, tocainide, mexiletine, and propranolol are the antiarrhythmic drugs that shorten the Q-T interval, especially when the Q-T interval is prolonged. Thus, these drugs could be used if profound Q-T interval prolongation is evident. Recently, we demonstrated that ventricular cardiomyocyte outward potassium currents are decreased, which may be responsible for the Q-T interval prolongation. Thus, any abnormalities in serum potassium should be corrected promptly. In addition, antiarrhythmic drugs that prolong the Q-T interval—such as quinidine, procainamide, and amiodarone—should be avoided in cirrhotic patients.

SUMMARY

It is clear that cardiomyopathy can be present in cirrhosis. Impairment of the cardiac β-adrenergic receptor signal transduction pathway, changes in membrane physical properties, and different humoral factors may play crucial roles in the pathogenesis of cirrhotic cardiomyopathy. Although therapeutic clinical studies are not available, supportive measures such as bed rest, dietary manipulation, and cessation of alcohol—in conjunction with more specific treatment such as careful diuretic therapy, positive inotropic agents, and, if necessary, antiarrhythmic drugs—should be beneficial.

BIBLIOGRAPHY

Gerbes AL, Remien J, Jungst D, Sauerbruch T, Paumgartner G. Evidence for down-regulation of β_2-adrenoceptors in cirrhotic patients with severe ascites. Lancet 1986; 1:1409–1410.

Grose RD, Nolan J, Dillon JF, Errington M, Hannan WJ, Bouchier IAD, Hayes PC. Exercise-induced left ventricular dysfunction in alcoholic and non-alcoholic cirrhosis. J Hepatol 1995; 26: 326–332.

Hausdorff WP, Caron MG, Lefkowitz RJ. Turning of the signal: desensitization of β-adrenergic receptor function. FASEB J 1990; 4:2881–2889.

Jacob G, Nassar N, Hayam G, Ben-Haim S, Edoute Y, Better OS, Bomzon A. Cardiac function and responsiveness to β-adrenoceptor agonists in rats with obstructive jaundice. Am J Physiol 1993; 265:G314–G320.

Kempler P, Szalay F, Varadi A, Keresztes K, Kadar E, Tanczos E, Petrik J. Prolongation of the QTc-interval reflects the severity of autonomic neuropathy in primary biliary cirrhosis and in other non-alcoholic liver diseases. Zeitschr Gatroenterol 1993; 31(suppl 2):96–98.

Lee SS. Cardiac abnormalities in liver cirrhosis. West J Med 1989; 151:530–535.

Lee SS, Marty J, Mantz J, Samain E, Braillon A, Lebrec D. Desensitization of myocardial β-adrenergic receptors in cirrhotic rats. Hepatology 1990; 12:481–485.

Lumlertgol D, Boonyaprapa S, Bunnacheck D, Thanachaikun N, Praisontarangkul OA, Phornphutkul K, Keoplung M. The jaundiced heart: evidence for blunted response to positive inotropic stimulation. Ren Fail 1991; 13:15–22.

Ma Z, Lee SS. Cirrhotic cardiomyopathy: getting to the heart of the matter. Hepatology 1996; 24: 451–459.

Ma Z, Miyamoto A, Lee SS. Role of altered β-adrenergic receptor signal transduction in the pathogenesis of cirrhotic cardiomyopathy in rats. Gastroenterology 1996; 110:1191–1198.

Ma Z, Meddings JB, Lee SS. Membrane physical properties determine β-adrenergic receptor function in cirrhotic rats. Am J Physiol 1994; 267:G87–G93.

Zavecz JH, Battarbee HD, O'Donnell JM Cardiac β-adrenoceptor-effector coupling in portal vein-stenosed rats. Am J Physiol 1995; 268:G410–G415.

43
Management of the Patient Awaiting Liver Transplantation

Fredric D. Gordon, Roger L. Jenkins, and W. David Lewis
Beth Israel Deaconess Medical Center and Harvard Medical School, Boston, Massachusetts

INTRODUCTION

The national shortage of donor organs has resulted in longer waiting times for patients awaiting liver transplantation. Patients experience more complications and may arrive at their transplant centers in severely debilitated states. The outcome of liver transplant surgery clearly depends upon the recipient's preoperative condition. For patients committed to a procedure as demanding as organ transplantation, an aggressive approach to pretransplant complications is appropriate. It is a challenge to both patients and physicians to avoid, limit, or treat these complications in order to increase the likelihood of successful transplantation.

MANAGEMENT OF COMPLICATIONS

Variceal Bleeding

Over 50% of patients awaiting liver transplantation will have variceal bleeding prior to transplantation. Frequently this is the initial event that will prompt the primary gastroenterologist to refer the patient to a transplant center. Variceal bleeding is a dramatic event that continues to have up to 30% mortality despite recent advances in therapy.

Endoscopic sclerotherapy is effective in controlling active variceal bleeding in over 90% of the cases. Unfortunately the rebleeding rate is quite high, with 60% of patients experiencing a second bleeding episode within 1 year. The complications of scleropathy include rupture of varices, esophageal stricture, esophageal perforation, chemical pericarditis, and pleuritis. Endoscopic variceal band ligation has reportedly yielded similar results; however, it is more difficult to perform during the acute bleeding episode. Band ligation has fewer complications and achieves earlier obliteration of varices. In order to offer the patient the least likelihood of rebleeding, varices must be treated repeatedly until obliteration is achieved. A typical program would include sclerotherapy or band ligation at the time of the initial bleed, 7 to 14 days later, and then monthly until obliteration. Varices should be

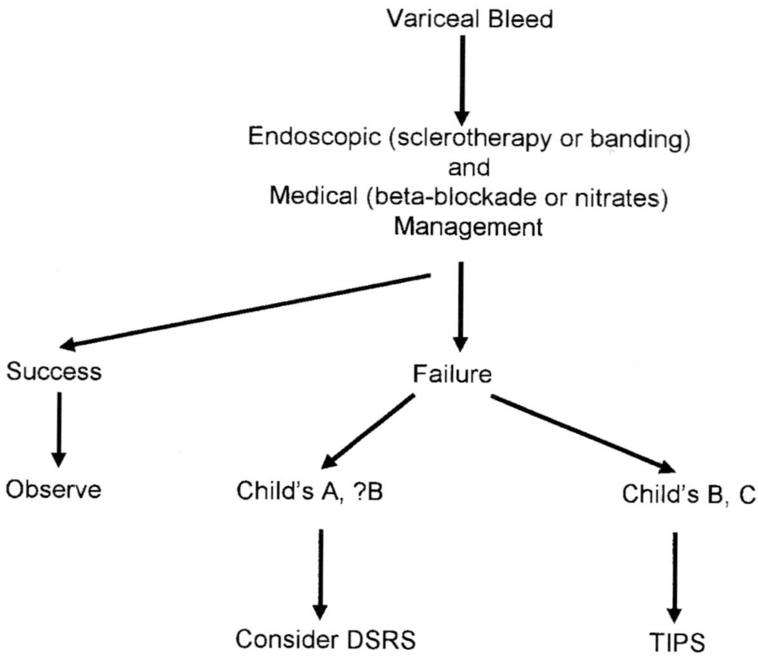

Figure 1 Management algorithm for patients with variceal bleeding. TIPS = transjugular intrahepatic portosystemic shunt; DSRS = distal splenorenal shunt.

endoscopically reevaluated every 3 to 6 months to be sure they have not recurred. Once varices have recurred, monthly therapy sessions should again be undertaken until obliteration.

In patients with refractory variceal bleeding despite adequate medical and endoscopic treatment, there are several options. In patients with relatively well-compensated liver disease (Child's Pugh class A), surgical distal splenorenal shunting offers long-term relief with an acceptable operative morbidity and mortality while not increasing the risks of transplantation, should it become necessary in the future. In patients with poor hepatic function or nutritional depletion, transjugular intrahepatic portosystemic shunting (TIPS) can be considered (see below). An algorithm for the management of patients with variceal bleeding is shown in Fig. 1 (also see Chap. 35).

When patients are diagnosed with cirrhosis, endoscopic evaluation is indicated to assess the esophagus for the presence of varices. Recent data clearly show that prophylactic treatment of varices with nonselective beta blockade will delay the first variceal bleed. Optimal results are seen when propranolol or nadolol is titrated to achieve a 25% reduction in baseline heart rate. Additionally, patients who have already had variceal bleeding may also benefit by reducing the risk of future bleeding. Similar data are available for orally administered nitrate therapy. There is no role for prophylactic sclerotherapy as morbidity and mortality may be increased.

Ascites

Ascites is among the most difficult pretransplant complications to manage. It requires patience and close attention by both the physician and the patient. The initial treatment of ascites is restriction of dietary sodium to less than 2000 mg/day and fluid restriction to 2 L/day. Diuretics can be added in a progressive, stepwise fashion until a maximum of 400 mg of spironolactone and 120 mg of furosemide is reached. Increments in diuretic dosing must be approached cautiously, as the risk of hyperkalemia, hyponatremia, and azotemia is great. Periodic large-volume paracentesis may also be employed, although the detrimental effects increase with more frequent taps. Specifically, proteins and nutrients are removed and discarded with each paracentesis, which, in patients with chronic liver disease, may result in severe emaciation, which can preclude successful transplantation (also see Chap. 37).

Refractory ascites is defined as persistent, tense peritoneal fluid despite adherence to treatment with dietary restrictions and diuretic therapy. In some instances the development of electrolyte abnormalities, azotemia, or portosystemic encephalopathy may preclude diuresis. In this circumstance, TIPS should also be considered. A growing body of literature suggests that TIPS is an effective treatment for refractory ascites in approximately 80% of cases. Typically, diuretic doses are reduced and their side effects are consequently minimized. Peritoneovenous shunting has no role in the patient awaiting liver transplantation. These shunts quickly become occluded and act as a nidus for infection in a nutrient-rich environment.

Portosystemic Encephalopathy

Portosystemic encephalopathy (PSE) is a frequent but intermittent occurrence in many patients awaiting liver transplantation (see Chap. 36). PSE is rarely spontaneous and usually has an inciting cause. This may include gastrointestinal bleeding, dietary noncompliance, electrolyte abnormalities, renal failure, infection, and omission of medication. In patients presenting with PSE, each of these entities must be considered and treatment should be directed at reversal.

For patients with ongoing or recurrent encephalopathy, the initial treatment should be lactulose. Lactulose is a minimally absorbed sugar that causes an osmotic diarrhea. This results in rapid transit of nitrogenous waste products through the gut, decreasing absorption into the bloodstream. Bacterial degradation of lactulose also acidifies the lumen, favoring retention of ammonia and other toxic products within the gut. Lactulose may be a substrate for the production of short-chain fatty acids.

The lactulose dose should be titrated to achieve three to five soft, controllable bowel movements per day. A reasonable starting dose is 30 mL twice daily, and patients can be taught how to self-titrate the dose to achieve maximal benefit. For patients who are intolerant of lactulose or ineffectively treated, Neomycin 500–1000 mg qid can be substituted or added. Neomycin, although minimally absorbed from the gastrointestinal tract, can cause nephrotoxicity and ototoxicity when used continuously over a long period of time. Other antibiotics such as metronidazole and ciprofloxacin have also been reported to be effective.

Limitation of protein intake should be reserved only for patients who have spontaneous encephalopathy refractory to all other medical therapies. Early limitation of protein results in emaciation, increasing the risk of infection and a poor outcome after transplantation. Protein intake of 1.0–1.2 mg/kg/day should be maintained if at all possible.

Role of Transjugular Intrahepatic Portosystemic Shunts

The success of TIPS has been well demonstrated in variceal bleeding. TIPS can be placed in patients whose initial variceal bleeding was not controlled with sclerotherapy or band ligation. In addition, patients who rebleed despite adequate endoscopic therapy can have a TIPS placed semielectively. TIPS is also gaining wide acceptance in the management of refractory ascites and hepatic hydrothorax. Although TIPS placement is associated with several side effects including portosystemic encephalopathy, peritoneal bleeding, and renal failure, its placement can be lifesaving in appropriately selected individuals.

Placement of the TIPS is critical and should be performed only by experienced individuals. Location of the TIPS either proximally into the superior mesenteric vein or distally into the inferior vena cava can preclude transplantation for technical reasons. Malpositioning of the TIPS increases the patient's risks in the operating room as well as putting the surgeon at risk of wire-stick injury. A team approach involving the hepatologist, transplant surgeon, and radiologist is preferred so that patient selection, TIPS placement, and transplantation can occur smoothly.

Because the TIPS is a foreign material in a low-flow vascular system, occlusion or stenosis is common. Approximately 5–10% of stents will occlude within 24 h of placement and up to 66% will stenose within 1 year resulting in clinical portal hypertension. A Doppler ultrasound performed 1 day after TIPS placement and then every 3–6 months will detect most critical occlusions or stenoses before the patient develops variceal bleeding or an increase in ascites. The occurrence of these signs should also alert the physician that the TIPS is stenosed, regardless of the Doppler findings. TIPS revision is often easily accomplished when Doppler ultrasound or clinical findings suggest the recurrence of portal hypertension.

The use of prophylactic TIPS in potential liver transplant recipients has not been well studied. Several retrospective analyses have indicated that intraoperative blood use is diminished; however, outcomes do not appear to be different. In our experience, TIPS can be detrimental, as decompressed varices—suddenly filled with blood when the patient is anhepatic with portal vein occlusion—often bleed profusely or the patient develops sudden massive bowel edema leading to difficulty in graft placement. Further study will be required to determine if TIPS should be considered routinely prior to transplantation.

Hepatorenal Syndrome

Hepatorenal syndrome (HRS) encompasses a spectrum of renal disease in patients with late-stage liver failure. It is characterized by a steadily rising creatinine, oliguria, and a urinary sodium concentration of less than 10. It is typically seen in patients who are hospitalized with severe jaundice and ascites. Hepatorenal syndrome can be induced by overzealous paracentesis and aggressive diuretic therapy. Differentiation between prerenal azotemia and HRS is critical, as the former can be easily treated with intravenous fluid. The latter condition is terminal unless treated by liver transplantation (see Chap. 39).

In addition to the criteria above, other causes of acute renal failure should be ruled out before making a diagnosis of HRS. These patients are particularly susceptible to intravascular volume depletion because of diuretic use, poor oral intake, and physicians' fear of worsening ascites. Treating physicians should be comfortable giving 1–2 L of saline per day in an effort to avoid dehydration. Any excesses resulting in symptomatic ascites can easily be removed with large-volume paracentesis, whereas prolonged dehydration can result in acute tubular necrosis and the need for hemodialysis. To be certain of intravascular volume status, pulmonary artery catheterization is often necessary before confirming a diagnosis of hepatorenal syndrome. In all cases, diuretics and other nephrotoxic drugs should be stopped. Hemodialysis can be performed in patients with HRS who remain candidates for liver transplantation.

Spontaneous Bacterial Peritonitis

Spontaneous bacterial peritonitis (SBP) affects up to 25% of cirrhotic patients with ascites and is a marker of advanced disease. The classic triad of fever, abdominal pain, and an elevated white blood cell count is rarely encountered and patients are usually asymptomatic. As a general rule, all hospitalized patients with ascites should undergo diagnostic paracentesis. Ascitic neutrophil counts above 250/mL indicate SBP. A lack of identification of an organism by culture is common and should not preclude treatment. For hemodynamically stable, nonseptic patients, therapy with an oral quinolone can be initiated; however, a low threshold for intravenous therapy should be maintained. Unless the responsible organism and its sensitivities are discovered, a repeat paracentesis and white cell count should be performed after 48 h to ensure that effective therapy has been chosen. There is now good evidence to suggest that recurrent SBP can be delayed or averted with the daily use of prophylactic antibiotics such as norfloxacin, ciprofloxacin, or trimethoprim-sulfamethoxazole (see Chap. 38).

Nutrition

Because of the national shortage of donor organs, it has become increasingly important to choose potential liver transplant recipients wisely. Malnutrition is a virtually universal finding in patients awaiting liver transplantation. Pretransplant nutritional status clearly affects posttransplant morbidity and mortality and is therefore one of the critical factors in determining transplant candidacy (Table 1).

Identification of patients who are poor risks for liver transplantation because of nutritional deficiencies is critical. Shaw et al. developed a formula to identify characteristics that would predict 6-month survival after liver transplantation. The total risk score included encephalopathy score, ascites score, malnutrition score (normal = 0, mild to moderate malnutrition = 1, severe muscle wasting and generalized malnutrition = 2), serum bilirubin score, transfusion score, and coagulopathy score. Of these, the nutrition score is the only variable that is reversible, emphasizing the important influence of nutritional status on outcome. More recently, a group from Germany found that among a large number of

Table 1 Potential Benefits of Improved Nutrition Before Transplantation

Reduced catabolism
Hepatic regeneration
Replete nutrient stores
Diminish portosystemic encephalopathy
Immune competence
Avoid deficiencies of essential nutrients
Tissue growth and repair
Decreased morbidity and mortality

Source: From Porayko et al., 1991.

variables known to be of prognostic significance in chronic liver disease, only the body cell mass and deviation in measured from predicted resting energy expenditure (ΔREE) separated high- from low-risk transplant recipients (see Chap. 16).

Aggressive nutritional intervention is indicated for those awaiting liver transplantation. The numerous benefits the patient may receive are listed in Table 1. The goal of nutritional therapy should be to decrease endogenous protein catabolism and provide enough amino acids and glucose to maintain or improve nitrogen balance. We feel that 1.0 g/kg/day of protein achieves this goal. Further protein restriction often worsens the patient's nutritional status and is appropriate in special circumstances only, such as severe PSE and uremia. Even in these situations, alternative forms of protein [casein, vegetable, and branched chained amino acids (BCCAs)] may be used.

Macro- and micronutrient deficiencies have been demonstrated to reduce immune function. This theoretically increases the patient's risk of sepsis, a major cause of both pre- and postoperative mortality. Protein malnutrition also influences intestinal mucosal barriers negatively, possibly increasing susceptibility to spontaneous bacterial peritonitis. This influence is greater when enteral nutrition is not maintained; therefore, enteral feeding is preferred to parenteral as long as the gut is intact. Total parenteral nutrition (TPN) can be useful when the patient is in hepatic coma and the risk of aspiration is high. TPN contains 18–50% BCCAs and can provide optimal support in patients with nitrogen-accumulating disorders (i.e., PSE and uremia).

DISEASE-SPECIFIC MANAGEMENT

Hepatitis C

Cirrhosis related to hepatitis C virus (HCV) is now the leading indication for liver transplantation in the United States. At present, it is estimated that approximately 4 million Americans have chronic hepatitis C. It is anticipated that 50% of these patients will have progressive histological disease and up to 20% will develop decompensated cirrhosis in the next 20 to 30 years. These estimates suggest that nearly 400,000 patients will have end-stage liver disease due to hepatitis C. Most of these patients will be symptomatic in some way and many will require liver transplantation. In addition to the complications of portal hypertension, discussed earlier in this chapter, there are several problems more commonly seen in patients with cirrhosis secondary to hepatitis C. Fatigue is an almost universal finding in these patients, although the cause remains unclear. The possibility of coexistent depression must always be considered and psychiatric evaluation is often warranted. Management of fatigue is quite difficult. Patients should be encouraged to maintain some degree of physical activity, and formal structured programs can be helpful. In addition, nutritional assessment should be performed and advice given. Last, subclinical portosystemic encephalopathy can be manifest by fatigue. If appropriate, a trial of lactulose may be indicated.

Cryoglobulinemia occurs in 1–2% of patients with HCV cirrhosis. This complication may be manifest by any combination of painful pruritic skin rash (pulpable purpura), renal failure, arthralgias, myalgias, and symptoms of peripheral neuropathy. Low-dose interferon has been found to be useful in managing several of these complications. Although cirrhotic patients are usually intolerant of standard-dose interferon therapy, 1–3 million units of interferon alpha two to three times weekly is often well tolerated and just enough to control the symptoms (see Chap. 9). Cessation of interferon often results in a return in symptoms.

Because hepatitis C viremia persists after liver transplantation in over 95% of patients, clearance of the virus prior to transplantation would be ideal. As stated earlier, interferon alone is not well tolerated and has a high side-effects profile, with poor efficacy. Clearance of the virus occurs on only 7–20% of patients treated for 6–12 months. Patients with cirrhosis have lower success rates than patients with precirrhotic diseases. Furthermore, the ability to use interferon in these patients is often limited by thrombocytopenia, leukopenia, and the impact of side effects on an already limited lifestyle.

The recent addition of ribavirin to interferon therapy offers more hope for viral clearance. It is not yet known what minimal dose of interferon is required in combination with ribavirin to eradicate the virus. Perhaps it will be low enough to be tolerated by patients with HCV cirrhosis. At present, combination therapy can be recommended only for selected individuals awaiting liver transplantation. The much anticipated HCV protease inhibitors will likely offer better opportunities for pretransplant viral clearance.

Vaccines

Vaccines to protect against hepatitis A and B are extremely effective in the general population, with immunity rates approaching 95%. The use of the hepatitis A vaccine has been studied in patients awaiting liver transplantation. Vento et al. recently reported several cases of fulminant hepatitis A in patients chronically infected with hepatitis C. They suggested that patients with HCV receive routine vaccination against hepatitis A. The efficacy of the hepatitis A vaccines in cirrhotic patients has not been evaluated.

A recent study by Chalasni et al. analyzed the efficacy of recombinant hepatitis B vaccine in patients with chronic liver disease awaiting liver transplantation. Fifty-seven patients without any positive markers for HBV were vaccinated with 1 mL of Engerix-B (SmithKline Beecham, Philadelphia, PA) at 0, 1, and 2 months. The response rate, as determined by the development of HBsAb, was a mere 16%. This likely indicates a failure of immune response in cirrhotic patients, although the degree of liver failure did not correlate with response. Further studies are needed to determine the optimal timing, dose, and schedule to achieve adequate response rates.

Hepatitis B

Despite infection control practices in blood banking and increasing safe sex practices, hepatitis B remains a rather common indication for liver transplantation. Because hepatitis B can manifest as both chronic and fulminant liver failure, the management strategies differ dramatically (see Chaps. 7 and 25).

The outcome after liver transplantation for fulminant hepatitis B is, perhaps surprisingly, quite good. Typically, viral replication has ceased by the time of presentation and patients are able to clear the virus without specific treatment. After transplantation, patients will commonly be positive or negative for hepatitis B surface antigen and negative for hepatitis B e antigen and HBV DNA. Superinfection with hepatitis delta (HDV) often confers even more protection from recurrent disease, with survival rates of 89%. Because of the fulminant nature of the disease, pretreatment of hepatitis B with antiviral agents is not practical. Many transplant programs use hepatitis B immune globulin (HBIg) intra- and postoperatively for patients with FHF due to HBV; however, this is not yet standard therapy in the United States.

Patients with chronic hepatitis B infection who undergo liver transplantation without immunoprophylaxis have a reinfection rate of 70–90%. In patients who are viremic at the time of transplantation, survival without the use of HBIg is 20% and with posttransplant HBIg, 50–70%; nonviremic patients have 45% and 60–70% survival rates, respectively.

Just as in hepatitis C, the ideal goal would be clearance of the virus prior to transplantation in order to avoid posttransplant recurrence. The pretransplant treatment of hepatitis B now offers several options that have not been available previously.

Interferon should be the first antiviral treatment considered in patients with chronic hepatitis B virus. Its use in this population will be limited by its marrow-suppressive effects, side effects, and degree of hepatic decompensation. Reduction in white blood cell and platelet counts of 30–50% can be expected. Side effects in unselected cirrhotic patients can also be devastating. These include a flu-like syndrome, anorexia, headaches, arthralgias, and myalgias. Patients with decompensated cirrhosis—that is, with uncontrolled ascites, encephalopathy, or variceal bleeding—should not be treated with interferon. Interferon-alpha dosing for hepatitis B is 30 million units per week given as either 10 million units three times a week or 5 million units six times a week. The duration of treatment is 4 months. In nondecompensated cirrhotic patients, the viral clearance rate ranges from 40–60% in several studies. As waiting times lengthen across the country, patients with hepatitis B will likely be placed on transplant waiting lists at a time when interferon therapy can be reasonably entertained. Hopefully, successful use of interferon will not only reduce the number of patients with hepatitis B requiring liver transplantation but also improve the posttransplant outcome in those who are ultimately transplanted. A study from Canada has shown that of eight patients with HBV DNA or hepatitis B e antigen positivity, all have seroconverted by 24 weeks of interferon therapy at 3 million units three times weekly. Seven of the eight, all treated with postoperative HBIg, are alive without evidence of recurrence after transplantation.

Lamivudine, or 3-TC, is an orally bioavailable nucleoside analogue. It has remarkable efficacy in reducing HBV DNA to undetectable levels in up to 100% of patients taking this medication. Early studies by Dienstag et al. demonstrated clearance of HBV DNA in all patients treated with 100 or 300 mg of lamivudine daily for 12 weeks. In 19% this response persisted for at least 24 weeks after withdrawal of therapy. Disappearance of hepatitis B e antigen was seen in 12%. The side-effects profile of lamivudine is nearly nil and it is extremely well tolerated by cirrhotic patients. Nevertheless, there is growing concern regarding the need for prolonged administration and the induction of resistance, even in patients who have undetectable HBV DNA levels. A recent study, however, demonstrated that HBV mutants, selected by lamivudine, had abnormal reverse transcriptase, resulting in impaired viral replication within the cell. This is particularly important, as lamivudine will likely have a role in the posttransplant management of recurrent hepatitis B.

Currently it seems most rational to use lamivudine in two specific settings. First, the medication can be used in patients who have a reasonable chance of avoiding liver transplantation if the progression of their disease can be halted at its present state. Before initiating lamivudine in this population, interferon should either have been tried unsuccessfully or considered but ruled out for other reasons. HBV DNA levels should be checked periodically as well as hepatitis B e antigen status. If the hepatitis B e antigen converts from positive to negative, the medication can be stopped and the patient observed with serologies and liver function tests checked periodically. The second group of potential lamivudine candidates are those in whom transplantation is a near certainty. It seems intuitive that the new liver would have a lower chance of reinfection if the viral load at the time of transplantation were diminished. Although this regimen has not been proven, we prefer to withhold lamivudine until approximately 6 months prior to anticipated transplantation. This will likely result in the patient undergoing transplantation with an undetectable circulating HBV DNA level and an extremely low likelihood that resistant virus might appear after 1 year of treatment.

Famciclovir, another nucleoside analogue, has been tested against hepatitis C in several small clinical trials. Dramatic reductions in HBV DNA level have been demonstrated, although clearance is rare. Seroconversion of hepatitis B e antigen to antibody has been reported and may be durable if it occurs. Larger studies are in progress to determine the efficacy of this drug prior to transplantation.

New antiviral agents with activity against hepatitis B are currently in development and will be undergoing clinical testing in the near future. It is likely that combination antiviral therapy with posttransplantation HBIg will be the standard in the near future.

Family members and other household contacts of patients with chronic hepatitis B should be tested for the presence of hepatitis B surface antigen (HBsAg), hepatitis B core antibody (HBcAb), and hepatitis B surface antibody (HBsAb). Vaccination should be administered to those who are negative for these markers. Those who are HBsAg-positive should be referred to a hepatologist for further evaluation (see Chap. 7).

Alcohol-Related Chronic Liver Disease

Very few patients awaiting liver transplantation will present as difficult and unique a challenge as the patient with cirrhosis due to alcohol. The ethics of transplantation for patients with alcoholic cirrhosis has been debated for many years. The current understanding of alcoholism suggests that it results from a combination of genetics and environment. Because of the genetic component and the ability to change learned behavior, liver transplantation is now an accepted method of treatment for alcoholic cirrhosis.

Population-based studies of alcoholics suggest that recidivism rates are as high as 80% in patients who have attempted to stop all alcohol intake. Alcoholics awaiting liver transplantation make up a subset of this population. In this group, recidivism rates are thought to be somewhat lower, possibly due to the gravity of disease, family support, and rigid medical follow-up, but data in this area are difficult to obtain and interpret. Nearly 20% of all alcoholics who have undergone liver transplantation return to drinking alcohol to some degree. One would expect a worse outcome in these patients, however, this has not been proven to occur in several studies.

Most transplant centers insist on at least 6 months of sobriety before listing a patient for liver transplantation. In fact, 6 months is an arbitrary duration of time but has very little basis in actual results. A patient's ability to maintain sobriety for 6 months does not necessarily correlate with the risk of recidivism, the likelihood of undergoing liver transplantation, nor the outcome after liver transplantation. Nonetheless, 6 months may be enough time to demonstrate both tangible and intangible effects of the cessation of alcohol. First, this seems to be an adequate amount of time to assess whether enough hepatic regeneration will occur that liver transplantation may be avoided. Second, it allows the patient to become involved in a rehabilitation program and/or Alcoholics Anonymous. This gives the transplant team a better long-term assessment of the risks of returning to alcohol abuse and addictive personality traits. Third, it may allow the resolution of interpersonal and family relationships so that the necessary support will be available at the time of transplantation.

Table 2 Stratification of Alcoholic Patients

High risk	Low risk
Undocumented or short period of abstinence (<1 month)	Long documented period of abstinence (>6 months)
Multiple failures to remain abstinent	No previous failure at rehabilitation
Poor or absent social support system	Good social support system
Absolute psychiatric contraindications	No psychiatric disorder

The physician caring for the alcoholic awaiting liver transplantation faces a seemingly dichotomous role, that of supporter and disciplinarian. In reality, however, this is a single role as the insistence of abstinence is a necessary part of support prior to liver transplantation. Therefore, it is incumbent upon the physician to detect signs of recidivism and report these to the transplant team. Most transplant centers will inactivate patients until they complete another period of sobriety with rehabilitation and documentation of abstinence. Overall care and detection of relapse must be individualized from patient to patient. Those patients who are found to be at high risk (see Table 2) may benefit from periodic, random, or weekly toxic screening. Low-risk patients may be managed with visits and discussion with family members. Missed appointments, noncompliance with medications, ongoing deterioration despite seemingly adequate and appropriate medical support, and a lack of support structure are potential markers of recidivistic behavior.

Alcoholic hepatitis is currently considered an absolute contraindication to liver transplantation as a definitive marker of ongoing alcohol abuse. Signs and symptoms suggesting alcoholic hepatitis include jaundice, fevers, leukocytosis, and an AST:ALT ratio of 2:1. Although hospitalization for acute alcoholic hepatitis carries a significant mortality, recovery is not unusual (see Chap. 15). These patients often recover without the need for transplantation as long as sobriety is maintained.

Primary Sclerosing Cholangitis

Primary sclerosing cholangitis (PSC) is a chronic progressive hepatobiliary disease often leading to significant complications related to cholestasis. Up to 20% of patients with PSC are referred for liver transplantation during the course of their disease. Outcomes after transplantation for PSC are similar to those of other noninfectious, nonmalignant liver diseases and approach a 5-year survival of 85%. It is therefore critical that the PSC patient be managed aggressively so that transplantation can occur safely and effectively.

Unfortunately, there are no proven therapies to control the progression of PSC. A variety of immunosuppressive, cupruretic, and antifibrogenic agents that have been analyzed in trials are ineffective (see Chap. 13). The treatment of patients with PSC awaiting liver transplantation therefore focuses on the management of complications.

The sudden onset of jaundice or fever raises the suspicion of a dominant biliary stricture, possibly causing bacterial cholangitis. In approximately 10% of patients, this will be evidence of cholangiocarcinoma. Therapeutic endoscopy or percutaneous cholangiography (if endoscopy is not feasible) should be performed to obtain cytological brushings and to dilate the stricture. If repeated attempts at dilation fail and the stricture is in the extrahepatic portion of the biliary tree, surgical biliary tract reconstruction can be performed.

The diagnosis of cholangiocarcinoma is important, as it is a contraindication to transplantation. The 5-year posttransplantation survival rate for patients with known cholangiocarcinoma is unacceptable at less than 20%. In patients with PSC, incidental cholangiocarcinoma is found in approximately 10% of explants. Several studies have shown that survival in these patients with small intrahepatic lesions is no different from that of the general transplant population (see Chap. 23).

Chronic nonspecific ulcerative colitis (CUC) coexists with PSC in nearly 70% of cases. Because CUC can be considered a premalignant lesion, yearly colonoscopy with biopsies is recommended for patients with pancolitis. This recommendation should be strictly adhered to in patients with PSC awaiting liver transplantation. Immunosuppression reduces natural surveillance for oncogenesis and can allow rapid growth of preexisting malignancy. Because the presentation of colon cancer in patients with CUC is typically a sessile lesion or malignant field defects rather than the usual adenomatous polyp progressing to carcinoma, pretransplant identification of malignancy is critical and can only be accomplished with colonoscopy.

Steatorrhea and deficiencies of fat-soluble vitamins can complicate PSC. Other concomitant causes of these conditions, including celiac sprue and pancreatitis, should be excluded. Pancreatic enzymes administration and supplementation of vitamins A, D, E, and K may be necessary. The management of pruritus and hepatic osteodystrophy is discussed below.

Primary Biliary Cirrhosis

Primary biliary cirrhosis (PBC) is another gradually progressive cholestatic liver disease. Many patients become symptomatic and signs of liver failure may develop. The posttransplant outcome, as in PSC, is good. Unlike PSC, however, ursodeoxycholate (UDCA) treatment is effective in delaying the progression of disease and the need for liver transplantation (see Chap. 12). Recently, data were combined from three large prospective, randomized, clinical trials comparing UDCA with placebo in patients with PBC. Transplant-free survival was significantly improved in patients, particularly those with a total bilirubin > 1.4 mg/dL or cirrhosis. Patients with PBC should, therefore, be placed on UDCA 12–15 mg/kg/day in divided doses. Recent evidence suggests that methotrexate may have a role in selected patients, and enrollment in clinical trials can be considered (see Chap. 12).

Hypercholesterolemia is commonly seen in patients with PBC, particularly early in the course of their disease. Typically the high-density lipoproteins are elevated in proportion to the total cholesterol. There does not seem to be an association between the hypercholesterolemia of PBC and coronary artery disease, and cholesterol-lowering agents are not indicated.

Pruritus

Patients with cholestatic liver diseases often develop severe pruritus, a symptom that can be as debilitating as chronic pain. Cholestyramine, 4 g given two to four times per day, offers effective control in many patients, possibly by binding bile salts. UDCA, thought to alter the type of bile salts produced, can also be used either alone or in combination with cholestyramine. When these agents are used together, doses must be separated by at least 2 h, as cholestyramine binds UDCA in the intestinal lumen. Refractory cases of pruritus can be treated with oral naloxone or nalmefene. Rifampin has been used but is potentially hepatotoxic in its own right. When oral therapy is ineffective, plasmapheresis can be considered (see Chap. 34).

Hepatic Osteodystrophy

Hepatic osteodystrophy is commonly seen in patients with primary biliary cirrhosis and primary sclerosing cholangitis. Lumbar bone density is below the fracture threshold in 35% of patients with cholestatic liver diseases. Many therapies—including calcium supplementation, vitamin D supplementation, sodium fluoride, estrogens, and calcitonin—have been studied but are ineffective in reliably increasing bone mineral density and decreasing fracture rates. Supportive care, pain management, and structural support, such as braces, may be indicated. The role of bisphosphonate therapy is unclear at this time.

Hereditary Hemochromatosis

Hereditary hemochromatosis (HH) is a homozygous disorder effecting approximately one in 250 people. It is a cause of progressive liver failure, adult onset diabetes, hypopituitarism, gonadal atrophy, and arthritis. If detected in the precirrhotic state, it is fully treatable with serial phlebotomy. Progression to liver failure can be halted and the patient can achieve a normal life expectancy.

Patients with cirrhosis caused by HH often require liver transplantation. If the patient maintains an adequate hematocrit, phlebotomy can be continued, as it affords symptomatic relief and improves the patient's general sense of well-being. Diabetes can be managed in standard fashion and generally requires insulin. The management of arthritis can be more problematic in the cirrhotic patient. Nonsteroidal anti-inflammatory agents, while effective in controlling arthritic symptoms, can induce hemorrhagic gastritis, which can be severe in the coagulopathic patient. Furthermore, patients with cirrhosis often have tenuous renal function because of azotemia or hepatorenal syndrome and these agents can exacerbate chronic renal insufficiency.

The incidence of hepatocellular carcinoma in patients with hemochromatosis is reportedly as high as 30%. Surveillance ultrasound and serum alpha-fetoprotein levels at 3- to 6-month intervals may be warranted in this population.

Children, siblings, and parents of patients diagnosed with HH should be screened for the disease. Serum ferritin, iron, and transferrin with calculation of transferrin saturation are good screening tests for Hh (see Chap. 27). Elevated levels may be evaluated either by biopsy with measurement of the hepatic iron index or genetic testing. The former test is invasive but is the gold standard of iron overload. If HH is present the biopsy also allows accurate staging of the disease. Genetic testing for HLA HFE (cys 282 tyr) is now commercially available but this trait is present in only about 85% of patients.

Familial Amyloidotic Polyneuropathy

Familial amyloidotic polyneuropathy (FAP) is a rare inherited disorder primarily seen among people of Mediterranean descent. This disorder is characterized by the hepatic production of abnormal transthyretin (TTR), which is deposited in a variety of organs including nerves, heart, kidneys, and the gastrointestinal tract. The liver is spared and patients, as a rule, do not develop portal hypertension or other complications of chronic liver disease. Liver transplantation halts the production of abnormal TTR and is the only known treatment for this disease. The pretransplant management of patients with FAP therefore focuses on maintaining adequate nutrition, renal function, and physical strength. Cardiac assessment is critical, as arrhythmia and cardiomyopathy are common and will often have a direct impact on the patient's transplant candidacy. Patients with FAP should be considered for transplantation when the diagnosis is confirmed and the first signs of organ dysfunction become evident.

Hepatocellular Carcinoma

The incidence of hepatocellular carcinoma (HCC) ranges from 2–50/100,000 persons per year. The primary risk factor for the development of HCC is cirrhosis; therefore, most patients awaiting liver transplantation are at risk. Three-year survival with HCC is rare. Although no studies have definitively shown that population-based screening for HCC is cost-effective, it is prudent to screen patients awaiting liver transplantation as there can be a significant impact on posttransplant survival. Common screening regimens include determination of serum alpha fetoprotein levels every 3 months and liver ultrasound every 3–6 months.

Tumors $>$ 5 cm in size, bilobar involvement, multifocal lesions, and vascular invasion of the portal vein portend a poor posttransplant outcome. The AJCC tumor stage is also a useful predictor of outcome. The 5-year survival rates of stage I and II disease are acceptable, being between 65 and 77%. Stages III, IVa, and IVb have poor 5-year survival rates, ranging from 0–25%. A variety of treatments have been demonstrated to control HCC to varying degrees, including transarterial chemoembolization, cryosurgery, percutaneous ethanol injection, hormonal therapy, immunotherapy, and standard chemotherapy. Transplantation for HCC should occur only in the setting of a formal protocol, which may involve any of the previously mentioned therapies (see Chap. 22).

Fulminant Hepatic Failure

A practical approach to the management of fulminant hepatic failure is discussed in Chap. 25. In cases of intentional toxic ingestion causing fulminant hepatic failure, there are several unique issues related to transplantation. Urgent psychiatric assessment, preferably before the patient becomes encephalopathic, should be obtained. It is critical to determine whether the patient is at high risk of repeated suicide attempts or has a psychiatric condition that would make compliance after liver transplantation unreliable. The patient's support system must also be carefully evaluated to ensure that adequate systems will be in place after transplantation. Although the assessment of candidates for transplantation must occur rapidly, a thorough transplant evaluation should be completed and standard inclusion/exclusion criteria applied.

Patients with fulminant hepatic failure have markedly elevated prothrombin times (PTs). The only reliable marker of hepatic recovery is the PT, and a falling PT is a clear indicator to the transplant team to inactivate the patient. Any tendency to give fresh frozen plasma (FFP) to correct the PT should be avoided unless the patient is actively bleeding or an invasive procedure is planned. This will eliminate falsely decreased PTs, which could result in inappropriate inactivation from the transplant list.

INTENSIVE CARE

Patients with chronic liver disease awaiting liver transplant are frequently hospitalized for a variety of problems, many of them detailed above. Life-threatening complications are not uncommon and intensive care is often indicated. The principles of management are similar to those in other patients in the intensive care unit, with a few notable exceptions. Patients with stage 4 hepatic encephalopathy or massive variceal bleeding should be intubated for airway protection. This may reduce the incidence of aspiration pneumonia. Because patients with liver failure are relatively immunocompromised, there should be a low threshold for initiation of empirical antibiotics. Active and uncontrolled infections are contraindications to liver transplantation; therefore prevention of infection may allow for timely transplantation.

THE WAITING LIST

In January 1998 the United Network on Organ Sharing (UNOS) mandated a sweeping change in the ranking criteria of the liver transplant waiting list. Primary emphasis was placed on the degree of illness as determined by the Child-Turcotte-Pugh (CTP) classification with secondary emphasis on time awaiting transplantation. The CTP score is calculated for each patient (see Table 3). Those candidates with 9 or fewer points are listed in status III by order of listing date. Those patients with 10 or more points are elevated to a higher tier (status IIB), again ranked by earliest to latest listing date. Status IIA, a tier above status IIB, is for patients with 10 or more CTP points who are ICU-bound with refractory bleeding, ascites, encephalopathy, or HRS and with a life expectancy of less than 7 days. Status I is reserved for patients with fulminant hepatic failure or primary graft nonfunction after liver transplantation. Clinical and laboratory assessment of the patient may be performed at any time deemed appropriate by the physician, and patients can be upgraded or downgraded based on their CTP scores. Computer modeling of this system suggests that there will be fewer deaths among patients awaiting transplantation, as "sicker" patients will have shorter waiting times. It is anticipated that in the near future a minimal listing criterion of 7 CTP points will be required before a patient is placed on the liver transplant waiting list. It is therefore imperative for referring physicians to maintain contact with the transplant center to inform them of any changes in the CTP criteria, as this may have a direct impact on ranking and waiting time. Further changes in the current allocation system are expected

Table 3 Child-Turcotte-Pugh Scoring System

	1	2	3
Ascites	None	Mild-moderate or controlled with diuretics	Severe
Encephalopathy	None	Mild	Moderate-severe
Albuin	>3.5	2.8–3.5	<2.8
Prothrombin time (INR)	<15 (<1.7)	15–17 (1.7–2.1)	>17 (>2.1)
Total bilirubin	<2	2–3	>3
(in cholestatic liver disease, substitute)	<4	4–10	>10

as the Department of Health and Human Services seeks government oversight regulations in place over the Organ Procurement and Transplantation Network.

Management of the patient awaiting liver transplantation is a challenging task; it requires recognition of current problems and especially anticipation of future complications. As waiting times increase nationwide, physicians will likely see more complications of chronic liver disease before transplantation occurs. An appropriately aggressive approach should be employed for these often critically ill patients. Portal hypertension continues to be the major cause of morbidity and mortality. Fortunately, new and successful treatments have been developed. An understanding of disease-specific complications is also essential. Liver transplantation remains a viable and cost-effective therapy for end-stage liver disease.

BIBLIOGRAPHY

Dienstag JL, Perillo RP, Schiff ER, Bartholomew M, Vicary C, Rubin M. A preliminary trial of lamivudine for chronic hepatitis B infection. N Engl J Med 1995; 333:1657–1661.

Edwards CQ, Kushner JP. Current concepts: Screening for hemochromatosis. N Engl J Med 1993; 328:1616–1620.

Jenkins RL. Defining the role of transjugular intrahepatic portosystemic shunts in the management of portal hypertension. Liver Transplant Surg 1995; 1:225–228.

Lucey MR, Merion RM, Henley KS, et al. Selection for and outcome of liver transplantation in alcoholic liver disease. Gastroenterology 1992; 102:1736–1741.

Petruff CA, Bedford A, Gordon FD, Chopra S. Hepatitis vaccines. Dig Dis 1997; 15:1–22.

Poupon RE, Lindor KD, Cauch-Dudek K, Dickson ER, Poupon R, Heathcote EJ. Combined analysis of randomized controlled trials of ursodeoxycholic acid in primary biliary cirrhosis. Gastroenterology 1997; 113:884–890.

Samuel D, Feray C, Bismuth H. Hepatitis viruses and liver transplantation. J Gastroenterol Hepatol 1997; 12:S335–S341.

Skinner M, Lewis WD, Jones LA, et al. Liver transplantation as a treatment for familial amyloidotic polyneuropathy. Ann Intern Med 1994; 120:133–134.

Wong RCK, Van Dam J. Endoscopic management of variceal hemorrhage. Practical Gastroenterol 1998; 22:13–25.

44
Management of the Patient After Liver Transplantation

Emmet B. Keeffe
Stanford University Medical Center, Stanford, California

The management of the posttransplant patient after discharge from the hospital and return to the referring physician is the focus of this review. The details of routine posttransplant management, evaluation of elevated liver chemistries, surveillance and treatment of the consequences of immunosuppression, diagnosis and treatment of late biliary tract complications, management of late infections, and the detection and treatment of recurrent disease after transplantation are all discussed.

ROUTINE POSTTRANSPLANT MANAGEMENT

Routine Monitoring

Patients are typically discharged from the hospital 1 to 2 weeks after liver transplantation and followed twice weekly initially and then weekly at the transplant center for several weeks. From 4–8 weeks after transplantation, recipients are discharged to the management of their local physicians in long-term consultation with the transplant center. Management of the complications that may occur after liver transplantation requires attention to detail and prompt evaluation of what may seem to be trivial complaints. The results of all laboratory tests are typically sent by fax and maintained on a master flow sheet at the transplant center, and local physicians should also maintain their own flow sheet. Even though referral physicians may become proficient with immunosuppressive medications, transplant center personnel will typically monitor and direct use of all immunosuppressive drugs and changes in dosage. Referral physicians should be prepared to communicate regularly with transplant nurse coordinators, who play a major role in communicating management plans to physicians and transplant recipients. General recommendations regarding when to call the transplant center are listed in Table 1.

After the patient returns home, routine monitoring consists of office visits with symptom survey and assessment of drug compliance; physical examination with attention to weight, blood pressure, abdominal wound, and new symptoms; and laboratory monitor-

Table 1 When to Contact the Transplant Center

Fever: Unexplained, sustained fever >38.5°C (101.5°F), with or without associated leukocytosis
Hypertension: Uncontrollable hypertension of persistently elevated blood pressures associated with severe symptoms or any change in antihypertensive regimen
Respiratory disorders: Any pneumonitis or complicated pneumonia
Gastrointestinal disorders: Vomiting for >24 h, diarrhea >24 h, gastrointestinal bleeding, or abdominal pain
Renal disorders: Acute or chronic increase in serum creatinine
Hematological disorders: Persistent leukopenia (<3000 mm^3) or unexplained leukocytosis with or without associated symptoms; acute or chronic unexplained lymph node enlargement or tonsillar enlargement
Neurological disorders: Any central nervous system infection (meningitis, encephalitis) or symptoms
Surgery: Before elective major surgery or as soon as possible (before or after) emergency surgery
Medications: Whenever discontinuing or starting any new medication

Source: Modified from Shaw et al., 1989.

ing with complete blood count (CBC), chemistry panel with a liver profile, and trough cyclosporine or tacrolimus levels. Visits are gradually reduced in frequency with stabilization of liver tests, immunosuppressive drug levels, and associated medical problems. By 6–12 months after transplantation, patients may be seen monthly or less frequently. Transplant centers advise long-term laboratory evaluation at intervals no less than monthly, with visits every 2–4 months after the first year according to need.

Daily Activities and Quality of Life

Most patients are able to return to their daily activities by 2–4 months after transplantation. Some reduced endurance appears to be related to poor cardiovascular fitness and lack of concentration. Most patients report significant improvement in both of these parameters over the course of the first posttransplant year. An active physical fitness program and sometimes psychotherapeutic support facilitate return to normal or near-normal daily activities. Regular physical exercise is encouraged for improvement in cardiovascular fitness, but contact sports are generally contraindicated.

The 10-year survival for patients who survive the first year after transplantation is greater than 80%. The quality of life is good as measured by self-assessment scales. Detailed assessment of quality of life by psychometric tests, however, has revealed that functional capacity does not return entirely to normal for all cognitive and psychomotor processes.

Diet

Most patients are able to resume and tolerate a regular diet. The early posttransplant nutritional program is aimed at correcting the malnutrition that occurred pretransplantation. The late posttransplant focus is to avoid the problem of weight gain with obesity. Some patients experience edema and occasionally ascites that require salt restriction and a brief period of diuretic therapy.

Immunosuppressive Drug Management

In general, the transplant center will take the primary responsibility for overseeing the immunosuppressive drug management. However, the referral physician should develop familiarity with drug dosage and the ranges of therapeutic trough levels for cyclosporine and tacrolimus. General guidelines for immunosuppressive drug dosages and blood level monitoring for tacrolimus, cyclosporine, and azathioprine are outlined in Tables 2 and 3.

Fever and Viral Syndromes

Liver transplant recipients experience common viral illnesses with the same frequency as the general population and do not experience more prolonged or severe courses. The primary differential diagnosis of importance is bacterial infection, which may progress rapidly from a self-limited infection to potentially lethal sepsis. A patient who experiences a body temperature above 38.5 °C for more than 24 h should be examined by a physician and evaluated by CBC, liver chemistries, chest x-ray, and urinalysis, with other tests as appropriate according to the nature of the symptoms. Suspected bacterial infections should be treated aggressively with broad-spectrum antibiotics, which can subsequently be mod-

Table 2 General Guidelines for Drug Dosage and Blood Level Monitoring for Tacrolimus, Cyclosporine, and Azathioprine

Weeks posttransplant	Daily dosage (mg/kg/day)	Target blood level
Tacrolimus (FK506, Prograf)	(Two divided doses)	(ng/mL)
0–2	0.30	10–15[a]
2–8	0.15	7–10
8–26	0.10	5–10[b]
26–52	0.05	5–10[b]
>52	0.05[c]	~5
Cyclosporine (Sandimmune or Neoral)	(Two divided doses)	(ng/mL)
0–2	20	300–400[d]
2–4	15	300–400
4–12	8–12	300–400
12–26	6–10	300–400
26–52	4–6	200–300
>52	2–4	100–200[e]
Azathioprine (Imuran)	(Single daily dose)	
0–1	2	
>1	1[f]	

[a]Target therapeutic blood level by IMX.
[b]During posttransplant weeks 8–26, target blood levels should be closer to 10 ng/mL; from weeks 26–52, target levels should be closer to 5 ng/mL.
[c]After weeks 52, dosage should be tapered to achieve target drug levels of approximately 5 nm/mL as long as liver tests remain stable.
[d]Target blood level by whole blood assay
[e]Target blood levels for cyclosporine should not fall below 100 ng/mL long-term.
[f]For treatment of recurrent rejection, azathioprine is usually discontinued after 3 months of therapy if liver tests are normal. When initiated for nephrotoxicity associated with tacrolimus or cyclosporine therapy, azathioprine is administered long-term at a typical dosage of 1 mg/kg/day.

Table 3 General Guidelines for Long-Term Prednisone Dosage and Regimens for Tapering Recipients Off Prednisone

Time posttransplant	Dosage (mg)
Tacrolimus-based immunosuppression	
0–2 weeks	20
2–6 weeks	15
6–12 weeks	10
3–6 months	7.5
6–9 months	5
9–12 months	2.5
>12 months	Discontinue[a]
Tacrolimus in patients with chronic hepatitis B and C	
0–2 weeks	20
2–4 weeks	15
4–8 weeks	10
8–12 weeks	7.5
3–6 months	5
6–9 months	2.5
>9 months	Discontinue[b]
Cyclosporine-based immunosuppression	
0–2 weeks	20
2–12 weeks	15
3–6 months	12.5
6–9 months	10
9–12 months	7.5
>12 months	5.0[c]

[a]Patients may experience rejection following discontinuation of prednisone; therefore, liver chemistries must be obtained twice weekly for 1 month to monitor for rejection.
[b]In patients with chronic hepatitis C, acute rejection may mimic recurrence of hepatitis; thus, careful monitoring of liver chemistries following withdrawal of prednisone is important.
[c]Most patients on cyclosporine will require small doses of prednisone indefinitely. Exceptions might include patients with recurrent hepatitis B or C, for whom specific recommendations will be made by transplant center physicians.

ified as culture results become available. Referral physicians should have a low threshold for contacting a physician at the transplant center for advice. When antibiotics are utilized, the potential of drug interactions—e.g., erythromycin and cyclosporine—should always be kept in mind.

Dental Problems

Liver transplant recipients should undergo routine dental examinations with prompt management of even minor gingival problems. Although there are no supporting data, most transplant centers recommend antibiotic prophylaxis on an empirical basis for dental procedures.

Prophylaxis of Infection

Patients are maintained on several different drugs for prophylaxis of frequently encountered infections after liver transplantation. Either nystatin swish and swallow or clotrimazole troches are prescribed for the prevention of oral candidiasis for the first 6–8 weeks. Acyclovir, at variable doses, is administered for the first 3–4 months for prophylaxis of cytomegalovirus infection. For 6–12 months or, as recommended by some liver transplant programs, on a lifelong basis, patients are given single-strength trimethoprim/sulfamethoxazole daily or three times weekly or, if sulfa allergy is present, aerosolized pentamidine monthly to prevent *Pneumocystis carinii* pneumonia. Patients undergoing cholangiography should receive broad-spectrum antibiotic therapy, typically a second- or third-generation cephalosporin. Some but not all studies suggest that patients with a Roux-en-Y biliary anastomosis who undergo a liver biopsy are at increased risk of bacterial sepsis, and broad-spectrum antibiotics may also be appropriate for these patients.

Immunizations

When appropriate according to age, routine immunizations should be given to patients prior to transplantation. Immunosuppressed patients are not given live attenuated immunizations for fear of causing disease. Even though hepatitis B vaccination has been associated with a poor protective antibody response in patients with advanced chronic liver disease, it is often given prior to liver transplantation. If patients lack immunity to hepatitis A, they should be given hepatitis A vaccine as well. Studies are under way to evaluate the efficacy of double-dose hepatitis B vaccination in end-stage liver disease similar to the regimen used for renal transplant recipients and chronic dialysis patients.

Elective Surgery

Transplant recipients may undergo anesthesia and elective surgery as needed. Some transplant centers will recommend that these procedures be performed at the transplant center so that transplant physicians can manage immunosuppressive drugs postoperatively, particularly the transitions between oral and intravenous dosing; but generally elective surgery can be performed at any facility after advice regarding postoperative management of immunosuppressive drugs is obtained.

Sexual Function, Birth Control, and Pregnancy

Chronic liver disease is associated with sexual dysfunction, and liver transplantation usually corrects these abnormalities with return of normal sexual functioning 6–9 months posttransplant. In two recent studies of menstrual function and pregnancy in women after liver transplantation, 28 of 34 patients resumed menstruation within 10 months of transplantation, while 5 patients appeared to be postmenopausal because of age and elevation of follicle stimulating hormone and luteinizing hormone. Transplant recipients should be advised regarding birth control. It is generally recommended that patients avoid pregnancy, at least during the first year. The safety and risks of oral contraceptives following liver transplantation are unknown, but concern regarding hepatotoxicity from thrombotic complications, interactions with other medications, and exacerbation of hypertension are reasons that these medications are generally avoided. Intrauterine devices are not recommended because of increased risk of infection. Barrier methods or elective sterilization for the spouse or recipient, if there is no desire to have children, is the usual recommendation.

The published experience regarding pregnancy after solid organ transplantation is expanding, and information is now available at the National Transplantation Pregnancy Registry at Thomas Jefferson University on approximately 1500 pregnancies in over 1000 transplant recipients. From this large data base, information is available on 57 female liver recipients who have had 86 pregnancies. It appears that maternal and newborn outcomes are favorable even though most pregnancies result in premature deliveries. Graft function appears to be maintained throughout pregnancy without an increased incidence of acute or chronic allograft rejection. An increased incidence of malformations has not been noted in the newborns. It is generally recommended that female liver transplant recipients not consider pregnancy until they have passed 1 year after transplantation with stable graft function.

ELEVATION OF LIVER CHEMISTRIES

There is a broad differential diagnosis when previously stable liver enzyme levels suddenly increase in the liver transplant recipient. The primary concerns after the patient has returned home 4–8 weeks after liver transplantation are acute cellular rejection, biliary obstruction, or hepatitis secondary to cytomegalovirus or recurrent or de novo hepatitis B or C. A logical approach to elevation of liver function tests is outlined in Table 4. Most transplant physicians will request that liver biopsies obtained locally by standard percutaneous techniques be sent by overnight mail to the transplant center for comparison with previous biopsies and review by the transplant staff.

Table 4 Approach to Elevation of Liver Function Tests

Mild → repeat in 3–7 days	
Moderate or severe → initial workup	
Early (<1 month) posttransplant → Doppler ultrasound	
Dilated bile ducts = obstruction → ERCP or PTC (in consultation with transplant center)	
No hepatic artery or portal vein visualized → notify transplant center (?angiography; exploration; retransplantation)	
Normal → liver biopsy[a]	
Later (>1 month) posttransplant → liver biopsy[a]	
Normal or nonspecific:	Rule out extrahepatic sepsis, hemolysis, drug-induced hepatotoxicity, or alcohol abuse
Acute rejection:	Notify transplant center immediately
Hepatitis	Check viral markers (HBV, HCV, CMV, and EBV); treatment per guidelines of transplant center
Obstruction	ERCP or PTC (in consultation with transplant center)

[a]Liver biopsies should be sent to transplant center to be reviewed by the transplant team and compared with previous liver biopsies; serial biopsies may be necessary to establish certain diagnoses posttransplant.

CONSEQUENCES OF IMMUNOSUPPRESSION

Common side effects of immunosuppressive drugs are noted in Table 5, and tacrolimus and cyclosporine drug interactions are listed in Tables 6 and 7.

Hypertension

Hypertension remains a major medical problem in liver transplant recipients and appears to be related primarily to cyclosporine therapy. Though the pathogenesis of cyclosporine-associated hypertension remains unclear, therapeutic efforts to decrease arterial pressure have focused on the renal and systemic hemodynamic effects of the drug, which increase vascular resistance. Probably two-thirds of patients taking cyclosporine will develop hypertension, which most often can be controlled relatively easily with medical therapy. The goal of antihypertensive therapy following liver transplantation in adults is to reduce blood pressure to < 140/90 mmHg with minimization of metabolic and electrolyte disturbances (hyperlipidemia, glucose intolerance, hypomagnesemia, and potassium shifts). As in all patients with hypertension, weight reduction and sodium restriction should be advocated.

Calcium-channel blockers probably represent the best first line of therapy in transplant recipients receiving cyclosporine therapy. This class of drugs improves renal hemodynamics and blocks vasoconstriction. If further control of blood pressure is required, introduction of beta blockade to potentiate antihypertensive effects and relieve the tachycardia sometimes provoked by calcium-channel blockers is a reasonable next step. Although diuretics may have some benefit, some physicians feel that hypovolemia may exacerbate cyclosporine-induced nephrotoxicity. Sympatholytics such as clonidine have proven useful in some patients with hypertension. Finally, one must remember that calcium-channel blockers such as verapamil and diltiazem may increase cyclosporine blood levels with an increase in the therapeutic or toxic activity of this drug.

Obesity, Diabetes Mellitus, Hyperlipidemia

Weight control is an important management problem once the patients return to a favorable sense of well-being. One recent study documented that excessive weight gain after liver

Table 5 Common Side Effects of Immunosuppressive Drugs

Corticosteroids	Azathioprine	Cyclosporine	Tacrolimus
Infection	Leukopenia	Nephrotoxicity	Nephrotoxicity
Poor wound healing	Thrombocytopenia	Hyperkalemia	Hyperglycemia
Osteonecrosis	Hepatotoxicity	Hypomagnesemia	Headache
Cataracts	Hair loss	Hypertension	GI toxicity
Diabetes		Hirsuitism	Peripheral neuropathy
Cushingoid habitus		Tremor	Skin rash
Peptic ulcer		Gingival hyperplasia	
Hypertension		Neurotoxicity	
Obesity		Hepatotoxicity	
CNS symptoms		Sinus congestion	

Table 6 Documented Drug Interactions with Cyclosporine (Sandimmune, Neoral)

Inhibitors of cyclosporine metabolism resulting in increased cyclosporine levels:	
Bromocriptine	Ketoconazole
Danazol	Methylprednisolone
Diltiazem	Metoclopramide
Erythromycin	Nicardipine
Fluconazole	Verapamil
Itraconazole	
Inducers of cyclosporine metabolism resulting in decreased cyclosporine levels:	
Carbamazepine	Rifampin
Phenobarbital	TMX-sulfa
Phenytoin	
Additive/synergistic in causing nephrotoxicity:	
Aminoglycosides	Ketoconazole
Amphotericin B	Melphalan
Cimetidine	Ranitidine
Cotrimoxazole	TMX-sulfa
Diclofenac	Vancomycin
Erythromycin	

transplantation is common and occurs between 2–16 months following transplantation. In the same study, obesity prior to transplantation predicted excessive weight gain after transplantation, although all patients were at risk.

Prednisone and tacrolimus are diabetogenic and may precipitate the new onset of diabetes or the need for insulin in preexisting diabetes. The prevalence of glucose intolerance is highest during the first year after transplantation, with as many as a third of patients exhibiting transient elevations of glucose. Only about 5% of patients without pretransplant diabetes will develop de novo diabetes mellitus. In general, the presence of diabetes does not affect survival or the incidence of complications after transplantation.

Lipid disorders are common in patients who have undergone liver transplantation and may be particularly severe in patients who have preexisting genetic hyperlipidemias. Prednisone is known to increase hepatic lipoprotein production and most frequently results in an increase in plasma triglycerides and very low density lipoprotein cholesterol. Azathioprine has no known effect on blood lipids. Cyclosporine enhances cholesterol biosynthesis and raises the levels of low density lipoprotein (LDL) cholesterol. The excessive weight gain following transplantation may lead to coexistent hyperglycemia and hyperinsulinism. Experience with lipid-lowering agents is limited in the setting of liver transplantation and should be considered only in patients with preexisting genetic lipid disorders and LDL cholesterol concentrations $>$ 160–190 mg/dL or triglycerides in excess of 1000 mg/dL.

Table 7 Potential Drug Interactions with Tacrolimus (Prograf)

Potential inhibitors of tacrolimus metabolism resulting in increased tacrolimus levels:	
Cimetidine	Itraconazole
Cyclosporine	Ketoconazole
Danazol	Nicardipine
Doxycycline	Troleandomycin
Erythromycin	Verapamil
Fluconazole	
Potential inducers of tacrolimus metabolism resulting in decreased tacrolimus levels:	
Carbamazepine	Phenobarbital
Corticosteroids	Phenytoin
Isoniazid	Rifampin
Potential additive/synergistic in causing nephrotoxicity:	
Aminoglycosides	Amphotericin B
Gentamicin	Cisplatin
Tobramycin	Cyclosporine
Streptomycin	Vancomycin
Amikacin	
Netilmicin	
Potential precipitants of hyperkalemia:	
Potassium supplements	Spironolactone
Triamterene	Amiloride
Possible additive/synergistic in causing neurotoxicity:	
Acyclovir	Imipenem
Ciprofloxacin	Norfloxacin
Ganciclovir	

[a]These interactions are theoretical and have not been documented in controlled studies.

De Novo Neoplasia

The overall incidence of de novo tumors after liver transplantation is approximately 6%. Specific cancers include carcinomas of the skin, lip, uterine cervix, vulva, and perineum Kaposi's sarcoma, and non-Hodgkin's lymphoma. Most of the lymphomas are extranodal are more aggressive than spontaneous lymphomas, and involve the central nervous system or gastrointestinal tract. These tumors are predominantly of B-cell origin and a majority have been shown to contain Epstein-Barr virus (EBV) genome, EBV nuclear antigens (EBNA), or both. The spectrum of EBV-related lesions ranges from benign polyclonal B-cell lymphoproliferative disease resembling infectious mononucleosis to malignant monoclonal B-cell lymphoma. The risk of developing a lymphoproliferative disorder, which is ~2% for liver transplant recipients, appears to be related in part to both cyclosporine and OKT_3 therapy. The median interval from liver transplantation to the development of this tumor was 6 months at the University of Pittsburgh. Liver biopsy may provide a clue to the diagnosis in the patient with lymphoproliferative disorder masquerading as rejection. In these patients, histology shows portal infiltrates with increasing predominance of plasma cells and immature lymphocytes. Although some patients respond to acyclovir therapy, discontinuance or reduction of immunosuppressive drugs is generally required.

BILIARY TRACT COMPLICATIONS

Biliary tract complications are relatively common following liver transplantation (10–30%) and some of these complications may present late, particularly anastomotic strictures, intrahepatic strictures, cholangitis, and bile peritonitis with T-tube removal. Other problems such as anastomotic leak, biliary fistulas, and dehiscence tend to occur early. The referral physician should be aware of the type of biliary construction performed when evaluating potential biliary tract complications. With a choledochocholedochostomy, biliary strictures can lead to near-complete biliary obstruction months to years following transplantation. The choice of percutaneous transhepatic, endoscopic retrograde, or surgical intervention depends upon the expertise and preference of the managing physicians. Broad-spectrum antibiotic therapy should be used before and immediately after invasive biliary procedures. Often immediate surgical intervention is utilized for high-grade, near-complete biliary obstruction. Complications following a Roux-en-Y choledochojejunostomy more typically occur early. Some patients may develop intrahepatic strictures that appear to result from hepatic arterial obstruction with ischemia to the biliary tree. These strictures are typically multiple and difficult to treat satisfactorily because of their intrahepatic location.

The T-tube placed across the choledochocholedochostomy is typically removed between the second and sixth month after liver transplantation. Approximately 10% of patients will experience bile leak with peritonitis, which may be treated with surgical intervention, endoscopic retrograde therapy with stenting, or nasobiliary cannula or symptomatic therapy with antibiotics and pain medication. There are no comparative studies to identify the best approach to this relatively common problem.

LATE INFECTIONS

Patients who experience late infections (6 or more months posttransplant) can generally be divided into three groups. Some patients will have ongoing problems with infections that recurred after liver transplantation, such as chronic hepatitis B or chronic hepatitis C. The majority of patients who have good allograft function and are receiving minimal doses of immunosuppressive drugs will be susceptible to the usual community-acquired infections, such as influenza, pneumococcal pneumonia, and urinary tract infections. A smaller group of patients with chronic allograft rejection or who have received larger doses of immunosuppressive drugs or repeated courses of corticosteroids or OKT_3 for acute rejection are susceptible to a broad range of opportunistic infections.

RECURRENCE OF DISEASE AFTER TRANSPLANTATION

Alcoholism

The rate of recidivism following liver transplantation in patients with alcoholism and end-stage liver disease averages approximately 15%. High-risk patients who have had short periods of sobriety (< 3–6 months) are most likely to return to drinking. It is likely that there is great motivation to remain abstinent during the early period after transplantation, but this motivation may fade with longer follow-up. Further studies are needed to document the long-term recidivism rate as patients are followed beyond 1–2 years after transplantation. It appears that the selection of patients with alcoholic liver disease for transplantation should be based not only on a fixed period of sobriety (> 6 months) but also on the presence of psychosocial parameters that predict sobriety. A multidisciplinary approach with assessment of medical, surgical, and psychiatric suitability is important. Factors such as admission of the disease of alcoholism by the patient and family members, participation in alcohol rehabilitation, and absence of psychiatric disease also predict long-term sobriety. Long-term monitoring for recidivism and referral for alcohol rehabilitation when needed are appropriate. All transplant recipients, irrespective of the cause of liver failure leading to transplantation, are counseled to refrain from drinking any alcohol.

Viral Hepatitis

In contrast to the overall 75–80% 3–5 year actuarial survival of patients undergoing liver transplantation in the late 1980s and early 1990s, patients with chronic hepatitis B had an approximate 25% reduction in survival with reported long-term survivals of only 45–50%. This reduced survival was related to reinfection of the graft, which was often associated with accelerated liver disease over several years or even rapid graft failure in a small subset of patients over several months. This latter syndrome is characterized clinically by progressive hyperbilirubinemia and only modest elevation of aminotransferases and has been termed fibrosing cholestatic hepatitis. The strongest predictor of recurrence of hepatitis B virus (HBV) infection posttransplant is the presence of active HBV replication pretransplant as defined by circulating HBeAg and/or HBV DNA. Patients with these markers appear to experience reinfection nearly universally, while patients who are negative for these markers are reinfected in approximately 70–80% of cases. HBV replication has been demonstrated in extrahepatic sites, such as bone marrow, spleen, and pancreas, and this factor likely accounts for allograft reinfection. On the other hand, coinfection with hepatitis delta virus inhibits HBV replication and may enhance clearance of HBsAg posttransplant.

Recent studies in European and U.S. centers demonstrate that hepatitis B immune globulin (HBIg) given intraoperatively and postoperatively long-term in doses (typically 10,000 IU or 45 mL) to maintain an anti-HBs level of > 100 mIU/mL reduces the HBV allograft reinfection rate to 10–30%. Lamivudine is undergoing study as an alternative or supplemental antiviral agent to prevent graft reinfection with HBV after liver transplantation. The use of the nucleoside analogue lamivudine and lower doses of immunosuppressive drugs, particularly prednisone, may reduce the pace of recurrent chronic hepatitis B when it occurs. Interferon therapy is unproven and potentially risky (it may precipitate rejection) posttransplant and is generally avoided.

Hepatitis C virus (HCV) is also recurrent in nearly 100% of patients following liver transplantation. Fortunately, in contrast to HBV infection, HCV infection is typically not associated with accelerated or progressive liver disease except in 10–15% of patients. HCV infection posttransplantation is the most common cause of hepatitis changes on liver biopsy, but allograft rejection may be difficult to distinguish from HCV infection on biopsy. Once rejection has been satisfactorily excluded and a hepatitis-like picture demonstrated on biopsy, most physicians are content to follow these patients who have stable but fluctuating abnormalities of aminotransferases. Lower doses of immunosuppressive drugs are often used, and interferon therapy remains unproven.

Cancer

Patients undergoing liver transplantation with cholangiocarcinoma have recurrent disease in more than 90% of cases. For this reason, these patients are typically excluded from liver transplantation if this tumor can be accurately documented pretransplant. Unfortunately, some patients with primary sclerosing cholangitis have tight benign strictures that cannot be reliably distinguished from cholangiocarcinoma prior to transplantation. The rapid onset of persistent jaundice, pruritus, and weight loss associated with a marked rise in bilirubin and alkaline phosphatase and cholangiography showing dilated intrahepatic bile ducts suggest cholangiocarcinoma. Patients undergoing transplantation for primary sclerosing cholangitis with unrecognized cholangiocarcinoma should be expected to develop recurrent disease on follow-up.

The use of liver transplantation for hepatocellular carcinoma is controversial because long-term survival with transplantation alone has been 30–40%. Fibrolamellar hepatocellular carcinoma is a clinicopathological variant that may have a more favorable outcome, although the data supporting this presumption are relatively scant. In general, patients with hepatocellular carcinoma are selected for liver transplantation if the malignancy is confined to the liver as documented preoperatively by abdominal, pelvic, and CT scans, as well as bone scan, and if the lesion is less than 5 cm in diameter. In addition, the tumor must not be resectable. Patients with hepatocellular carcinoma and poor hepatic function secondary to coexistent advanced cirrhosis are poor candidates for resection and are generally offered liver transplantation as the only reasonable alternative to resection. Many transplant centers will hospitalize a backup potential recipient, so that a donor graft will not be wasted should occult metastases be identified at the time of exploration. A number of adjuvant therapeutic modalities are available for hepatocellular carcinoma, particularly when tumors are small and single or few in number. These therapies—including intravenous doxorubicin given preoperatively, intraoperatively, and postoperatively or pretransplant chemoembolization—show promise in improving results of liver transplantation alone for hepatocellular carcinoma. Recently reported actuarial survival rates range from 60–75%. Patients should be monitored for recurrent hepatocellular carcinoma with alpha fetoprotein and imaging as appropriate. Recurrence in the allograft is not uncommon.

Autoimmune Diseases

Primary biliary cirrhosis may recur after liver transplantation, but generally it is manifest only on histological study of posttransplant liver biopsies and is not associated with elevated liver enzyme levels or clinical disease. Antimitochondrial antibody will disappear immediately after liver transplantation but typically recurs in reduced titer in the majority of patients. The difficulty in deciding whether or not primary biliary cirrhosis actually recurs lies in the similar histological features of primary biliary cirrhosis and chronic allograft rejection.

Although there have been a few case reports, it has been generally thought that autoimmune hepatitis does not usually recur after liver transplantation. The report of a few cases, however, raises concern that the total experience with liver transplantation for autoimmune hepatitis has not been large enough to definitively answer this question; there may not be any recurrence until many years after transplantation.

SUMMARY

The key elements of the routine outpatient management of liver transplant recipients include (1) gradually less frequent office visits for symptom survey, assessment of drug compliance, physical examination, and laboratory testing (CBC, chemistry panel, trough cyclosporine or tacrolimus levels); (2) monitoring and adjustment in immunosuppressive drugs in consultation with the transplant center; (3) symptomatic treatment of viral syndromes and prompt evaluation of temperature > 38.5 °C; (4) advice regarding exercise, diet, birth control, and pregnancy. Diagnosis of the cause of elevated liver tests may require imaging studies, liver biopsy, and/or cholangiography.

Management of the consequences of immunosuppression focuses on the following: (1) hypertension—calcium channel blockers, beta blockers, and diuretics; (2) obesity, diabetes mellitus, or hyperlipidemia—weight control, oral agents or insulin as needed for diabetes mellitus and lipid-lowering agents only for severe hyperlipidemia associated with genetic lipid disorders; (3) de novo neoplasia or EBV-related lymphoproliferative disease, which is treated with acyclovir, and major reduction in or discontinuation of immunosuppressive drugs.

Late biliary complications include anastomotic strictures, intrahepatic strictures, cholangitis, and bile peritonitis with T-tube removal. The choice of endoscopic, radiological, or operative therapy depends upon local expertise and preference.

Late infections after transplantation include ongoing viral infections associated with liver transplantation—such as chronic hepatitis B and C, community-acquired infections in patients receiving standard immunosuppressive drugs, and opportunistic infections in patients heavily immunosuppressed for recurrent acute or chronic allograft rejection.

A number of diseases may recur after liver transplantation. Patients with alcoholism have a short-term recidivism rate of approximately 15%, but long-term sobriety rates are unknown. Chronic HBV infection recurs in 10–30% of patients treated with HBIg, and the overall survival after liver transplantation for chronic hepatitis B without viral recurrence is 80–85%. The use of nucleoside analogues, such as lamivudine, and more rapid tapering of immunosuppression may reduce the pace of recurrent chronic hepatitis B when it recurs. Chronic HCV infection of the allograft occurs in more than 95% of patients, but clinical disease is typically mild. Chronic hepatitis C and rejection may be indistinguishable clinically and histologically. Liver transplantation for hepatocellular carcinoma has traditionally resulted in 30–40% long-term survival rates. Selection of patients with tumors less than 5 cm diameter and use of intravenous adjuvant chemotherapy with doxorubicin or chemoembolization may increase long-term survival rates to 60–75%.

BIBLIOGRAPHY

Armenti VT, Herrine SK, Moritz MJ. Reproductive function after liver transplantation. Clin Liver Dis 1997; 1:471–485.

Bzowej NH, Wright TL. Prophylaxis and treatment strategies for chronic viral hepatitis in liver transplant patients. Clin Liver Dis 1997; 1:323–339.

Farmer DG, Seu P, Swenson K, Economou J, Busuttil RW. Current and future treatment modalities for hepatocellular carcinoma. Clin Liver Dis 1997; 1:361–396.

Klion FM, Fabry TL. Late postoperative (outpatient) management. In Fabry TL, Klion FM, eds. Guide to Liver Transplantation. New York: Igaku-Shoin, 1992:197–214.

Maldonado JR, Keeffe EB. Liver transplantation for alcoholic liver disease: selection and outcome. Clin Liver Dis 1997; 1:305–321.

Palmer M, Schaffner F, Thung SN. Excessive weight gain after liver transplantation. Transplantation 1991; 51:797–800.

Shaw BW Jr, Stratta RJ, Donovan JP, Langnas AN, Wood RP, Markin RJ. Postoperative care after liver transplantation. Semin Liver Dis 1989; 9:202–230.

Tarterre Switala J, Arria A, Plail I, Van Thiel D. Quality of life before and after orthotopic hepatic transplantation. Arch Intern Med 1991; 151:1521–1526.

Testa G, Klintmalm GB. Cyclosporine and tacrolimus: the mainstay of immunosuppressive therapy for solid organ transplantation. Clin Liver Dis 1997; 1:417–437.

Index

About the Editor

EDWARD L. KRAWITT is Professor of Medicine at the University of Vermont, College of Medicine, Burlington, and Adjunct Professor of Medicine at Dartmouth College, Hanover, New Hampshire. A coeditor of *Autoimmune Liver Diseases*, his research focuses on the immunology, genetics, and treatment of autoimmune and chronic viral hepatitis. Dr. Krawitt received the B.A. degree (1955) in zoology from Cornell University, Ithaca, New York, and the M.D. degree (1959) from Cornell University Medical College, New York, New York.